Clinical Neurology: Role of Biomarkers

Clinical Neurology: Role of Biomarkers

Editor: Abbie Bardsley

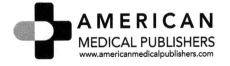

AMERICAN
MEDICAL PUBLISHERS
www.americanmedicalpublishers.com

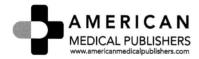

Cataloging-in-Publication Data

Clinical neurology : role of biomarkers / edited by Abbie Bardsley.
    p. cm.
Includes bibliographical references and index.
ISBN 978-1-63927-999-9
1. Neurology. 2. Nervous system--Diseases. 3. Biochemical markers.
4. Clinical medicine. I. Bardsley, Abbie.
RC346 .C553 2023
616.8--dc23

American Medical Publishers,
41 Flatbush Avenue,
1st Floor, New York,
NY 11217, USA

ISBN 978-1-63927-999-9 (Hardback)

Contents

Preface

The main aim of this book is to educate learners and enhance their research focus by presenting diverse topics covering this vast field. This is an advanced book which compiles significant studies by distinguished experts in the area of analysis. This book addresses successive solutions to the challenges arising in the area of application, along with it; the book provides scope for future developments.

The branch of medical science which focuses on the diagnosis and treatment of the ailments of the brain, the spinal cord and the peripheral nerves is known as clinical neurology. Biomarkers within this field are utilized for various purposes which include, determining the stage of a disease, guiding clinical diagnosis, monitoring progression or response to therapy, and assessing the risk associated with the disease. The biomarkers which are studied within the field of clinical neurology are found in the cerebral spinal fluid, and are not detectable in the blood. The blood brain barrier closely protects the brain and provides protection from various harmful substances present in the bloodstream. This barrier makes blood tests inconvenient and makes the brain's chemistry inaccessible. Latest advances used for detection through biomarkers are making the brain accessible while making the neurological disorders treatable. This book explores all the important aspects of clinical neurology in the modern day. The readers would gain knowledge that would broaden their perspective about the importance of biomarkers within this field.

It was a great honour to edit this book, though there were challenges, as it involved a lot of communication and networking between me and the editorial team. However, the end result was this all-inclusive book covering diverse themes in the field.

Finally, it is important to acknowledge the efforts of the contributors for their excellent chapters, through which a wide variety of issues have been addressed. I would also like to thank my colleagues for their valuable feedback during the making of this book.

Editor

No Effects of Anodal tDCS on Local GABA and Glx Levels in the Left Posterior Superior Temporal Gyrus

Gerard E. Dwyer[1,2]*, Alexander R. Craven[1,2], Marco Hirnstein[1,2], Kristiina Kompus[1,2], Jörg Assmus[3], Lars Ersland[1,2,4], Kenneth Hugdahl[1,2,5,6] and Renate Grüner[6,7]

[1] Department of Biological and Medical Psychology, University of Bergen, Bergen, Norway, [2] NORMENT Centre of Excellence, Haukeland University Hospital, Bergen, Norway, [3] Centre for Clinical Research, Haukeland University Hospital, Bergen, Norway, [4] Department of Clinical Engineering, Haukeland University Hospital, Bergen, Norway, [5] Division of Psychiatry, Department of Clinical Medicine, Haukeland University Hospital, Bergen, Norway, [6] Department of Radiology, Haukeland University Hospital, Bergen, Norway, [7] Department of Physics and Technology, University of Bergen, Bergen, Norway

*Correspondence:
Gerard E. Dwyer
gerard.dwyer@uib.no

A number of studies investigating the biological effects of transcranial direct current stimulation (tDCS) using magnetic resonance spectroscopy (MRS) have found that it may affect local levels of γ-aminobutyric acid (GABA), glutamate and glutamine (commonly measured together as "Glx" in spectroscopy), and N-acetyl aspartate (NAA), however, these effects depend largely on the stimulation parameters used and the cortical area targeted. Given that different cortical areas may respond to stimulation in different ways, the purpose of this experiment was to assess the as yet unexplored biological effects of tDCS in the posterior superior temporal gyrus (pSTG), an area that has attracted some attention as a potential target for the treatment of auditory verbal hallucinations in schizophrenia patients. Biochemical changes were monitored using continuous, online MRS at a field strength of 3 Tesla. Performing intrascanner stimulation, with continuous spectroscopy before, during and after stimulation, permitted the assessment of acute effects of tDCS that would otherwise be lost when simply comparing pre- and post-stimulation differences. Twenty healthy participants underwent a repeated-measures experiment in which they received both active anodal and sham intrascanner stimulation in a stratified, randomized, double-blind experiment. No significant changes in GABA, Glx, or NAA levels were observed as a result of anodal stimulation, or between active and sham stimulation, suggesting that a single session of anodal tDCS to the pSTG may be less effective than in other cortical areas that have been similarly investigated.

Keywords: tDCS, GABA, Glutamate, magnetic resonance spectroscopy, MRS

INTRODUCTION

Transcranial direct current stimulation (tDCS) is a non-invasive neurostimulation technique that uses constant, low level (0.5–2.0 mA) direct current to modulate cortical excitability in a polarity dependent manner (1). Nitsche and Paulus (2) used the magnitude of motor-evoked potentials (MEP) as generated by transcranial magnetic stimulation (TMS) as an indication of changes in excitability and found that tDCS was able to induce changes in excitability of up to 40%, with anodal stimulation having an excitatory effect, and cathodal stimulation having an inhibitory effect. Subsequent studies showed that effects may outlast the duration of stimulation, with short applications inducing excitability shifts during stimulation, and ~10 min or more of stimulation producing persistant effects lasting up to 90 min after current flow has ceased (3) suggesting that tDCS has the ability to induce long term potentiation (LTP)-like effects on synaptic plasticity (4).

Due to its purported effects on excitability and synaptic plasticity, tDCS has been investigated as a potential treatment for a range of neurological and psychiatric disorders such as Parkinson's disease (5), depression (6), and for the treatment of auditory verbal hallucinations in schziophrenia. A case reported by Homan et al. (7) found that cathodal tDCS halfway between T3 and P3 in the 10–20 electroencephelography (EEG) system was successful in alleviating both hallucinations (−60% Hallucination Change Scale (HCS) score) and global symptoms (−20% Postive and Negative Syndrome Scale (PANSS) score). A randomized control trial conducted by Brunelin et al. (8) using a similar stimulation paradigm at 2.0 mA also showed improvement in hallucinations (−31% Auditory Hallucination Rating Scale (AHRS) score) and global symptoms (−13% PANSS score). Subsequent studies, using similar stimulation parameters have found both reductions (9) and no significant differences (10, 11) in symptoms. While tDCS shows great promise as a potential treatment for schizophrenia, the lack of consistent findings between these studies highlight the need for a deeper understanding of the effects of tDCS.

Although generally accepted that anodal stimulation typically facilitates excitability and cathodal stimulation inhibits excitability (12), studies have shown that the effects of tDCS on excitability are not so simplistic, and depend on a number of factors such as electrode size and placement, stimulation intensity and duration, as well as the orientation of neurons relative to the stimulating electrodes (12–14). Furthermore, Batsikadze et al. (15) found that while 20 min of cathodal stimulation at 1.0 mA had an inhibitory effect, 20 min of cathodal stimulation at 2.0 mA had an excitatory effect, increasing the magnitude of measured MEPs. Esmaeilpour et al. (16) showed that the dose-response relationship in tDCS is not necessarily linear, and that although increasing current produces a corresponding increase in brain electric field, it may not necessarily enhance a neurophysiological, behavioral or clinical outcome. As Woods et al. (14) caution, it cannot be taken for granted that what is effective in a particular cortical area is transferable and applicable to others, rather recommending a "titration" of parameters.

Despite the observed effectiveness of tDCS, the exact mechanisms by which it works are not yet fully understood. Horvath et al. (17) show that changes in cognitive effects alone may be an unreliable measure of effectiveness. Computational forward models and simulations have been useful in imaging current flow, aiding in the design of stimulation paradigms (18) but do not provide information about neuronal responses to delivered current or whether the effect is excitatory or inhibitory in nature.

Krause et al. (19) suggest that tDCS may modulate the excitation/inhibition balance, that is, the relative contributions of excitatory and inhibitory inputs to a neural circuit corresponding to a neuronal event. Using in vivo magnetic resonance spectroscopy (MRS), the excitation-inhibition balance may be characterized in terms of the local concentrations of the excitatory neurotransmitter glutamate and inhibitory neurotransmitter gamma-aminobutyric acid (GABA). Studies that have used MRS to investigate the effect of tDCS have found anodal tDCS to reduce local cortical GABA concentration in the motor cortex (20, 21) and to increase local concentrations of glutamate and glutamine, measured together as "Glx," and N-acetyl aspartate (NAA) in the intraparietal and prefrontal cortices (22, 23), the observed reduction in inhibitory neurotransmitter levels and concurrent increases in excitatory neurotransmitter levels being consistent with the facilitatory nature of anodal stimulation. Thus, in vivo MRS provides a window into the biochemical events underlying tDCS that may also be used as a biomarker indicating the effectiveness and nature of a stimulation paradigm.

In this study, MRS was used to investigate the acute biochemical effects of tDCS in validating its potential for use as a treatment for auditory-verbal hallucinations in schizophrenia. However, rather than simply comparing pre- and post-stimulation spectral acquisitions, biochemical changes were measured continuously using online MRS in a manner similar to those used by Bachtiar et al. (24) and Hone-Blanchet et al. (23). By acquiring spectra continuously over the course of stimulation, spectral frames could be combined in such a way that metabolite levels could be measured and tracked before, during and post stimulation, allowing better insight into the acute effects of stimulation as opposed to the lasting effects. Findings in other cortical areas suggest that if anodal tDCS were to have a similar effect on the local excitation-inhibition balance, it may be measured as a statistically significant increase in Glx and NAA levels (22, 25) and decrease in GABA levels (20, 21, 24) and that these changes would be significantly different under active stimulation when compared to sham.

Abbreviations: BOLD, Blood Oxygen Level Dependent; EEG, Electroencephalography; ERETIC, Electronic reference to access in vivo concentrations; FWHM, Full width at half maximum; GABA, Gamma-aminobutyric acid; Glx, Glutamate and glutamine; GSH, Glutathione; LTP, Long-term potentiation; MEGA-PRESS, Mescher-Garwood point resolved spectroscopy; MEP, Motor evoked potential; MRS, Magnetic Resonance Spectroscopy; NAA, N-acetylaspartate; NAAG, N-acetylaspartylglutamate; pSTG, Posterior superior temporal gyrus; tDCS, Transcranial direct current stimulation; TE, Echo time; TMS, Transcranial Magnetic Stimulation; TR, Repetition time

MATERIALS AND METHODS

This study was carried out in accordance with the recommendations and ethical approval of the regional committee for medical and health research ethics (REK-Vest) REK case number 2013/2342. All subjects gave written informed consent in accordance with the Declaration of Helsinki and the guidelines drawn up by The Norwegian National Research Ethics Committee for medical and health research (NEM).

Participants

Twenty healthy participants (mean age: 25 years, range: 19–32; 10 male) participated in the study. All participants were required to complete a Norwegian language version of the Edinburgh handedness inventory (26) to determine right-handedness in an attempt to control for issues related to lateralization of cortical areas, such that stimulation in the left hemisphere affects approximately the same functional area in each participant. The test assessed dominance of right and left hand in performing 10 everyday activities to produce a score ranging between −100 (exclusively left handed) and +100 (exclusively right handed), participants with a score greater than +40 were considered to be right handed and were permitted into the study (mean score: +80, SD: 24). Based on self-report, participants were free from psychiatric and neurologic conditions and had not used any psychoactive/psychotropic substances, including no smoking or other tobacco based or nicotine containing products, for 6 months prior to participating in the experiment. Participants were also instructed not to consume alcohol for at least 24 h prior to participation.

Data from one female participant was omitted from final analyses due to abnormally high measurements of Glx more than three standard deviations above the group mean (Glx levels almost 5 times higher than average values), suggesting an error in spectral acquisition.

tDCS Stimulation

Stimulation was performed using an MR-compatible DC-Stimulator MR (neuroConn GmbH, Ilmenau, Germany) fitted with two 5×7 cm (35 cm^2) MR compatible rubber electrodes. Given that the motivation for this study was the potential for tDCS to be used as a treatment for schizophrenia, stimulation parameters were chosen to emulate those used in previous studies. Intensity was set at 2.0 mA (27) and although the majority of studies using tDCS as a treatment for auditory-verbal hallucinations have stimulated for 20 min, the prohibitively long scan time this would necessitate in order to have three equally long spectroscopy windows meant that stimulation had to be limited to 10 min. The anodal electrode was placed with the center of the pad on an area over the pSTG, such that the lower corners of the 7 cm edge of the electrode touch points T3 and T5 in the EEG 10-20 system. The cathodal electrode was placed over the contralateral orbitofrontal cortex, a site commonly used in tDCS montages for placement of the reference electrode (2, 12) such that the center of the electrode covered point AF8 in the EEG 10–20 system. Each electrode was coated with a layer of Ten20 conductive paste (Weaver and Company, Aurora, United States of America) at the interface between electrode and skin to improve both adhesion and conductivity. Once the electrodes were in place, participants were placed in the scanner with electrodes attached but not connected to the stimulation box. Electrodes were only connected prior to spectroscopy sequences.

This study followed a stratified, randomized, double-blind design, with both participants and experimenters blind to the stimulation condition. Each subject participated in two MR-scanning sessions with tDCS: one with active and one with sham stimulation, separated by a wash-out period of 1 h outside of the scanner (12, 28) counterbalanced for order. Double-blinding was performed by having the stimulation condition determined by a code, independently predetermined by a researcher not present at the stimulation, such that each participant underwent both active and sham stimulation conditions and that equal numbers experienced active and sham stimulation as the first condition.

MR-Imaging and Spectroscopy

All imaging and spectroscopy was performed on a 3 T GE 750 Discovery Scanner from GE Healthcare (General Electric, Milwaukee, United States of America) using a standard 8-channel head coil from Invivo (Invivo corp., Gainsville, Florida, United States of America).

Following a 3-plane localizer sequence (2D Spin Echo, TE $= 80$ ms, FOV $= 240$ mm, slice thickness $= 8$ mm, slice spacing $= 15$ mm) structural anatomical imaging was performed using a 3D T1 weighted fast spoiled gradient sequence (FSPGR) (number of slices $= 192$, slice thickness $= 1.0$ mm, repetition time (TR) $= 7.8$ ms, echo time (TE) $= 2.95$ ms, field of view $= 260 \times 260$ mm^2, flip angle $= 14$ degrees, matrix $= 256 \times 256$). These structural images were used to position a $24 \times 24 \times 24$ mm^3 voxel for the spectroscopy component of this experiment in the left pSTG, centered around the primary auditory cortex, aligned orthogonally in the axial scan plane with no angulation (**Figure 1**).

Since the aim of this study was to characterize acute biochemical changes in terms of the excitation-inhibition balance, a GABA specific MEGA-PRESS sequence (29) was used as it provides accurate and stable measurements of GABA, as well as a measurement of glutamate and glutamine combined as "Glx" (30). Spectroscopy was performed using a MEGA-PRESS sequence (TE $= 68$ ms, TR $= 1,500$ ms, 8-way phase cycling, editing at 1.9 and 7.5 ppm in alternating frames) of 628 paired repetitions, followed by 16 unsuppressed reference acquisitions for a total scan time of 31 min and 48 s. Once 10 min of spectroscopy had elapsed, stimulation was initiated at the control box located outside the scanner at the control room. Active stimulation was delivered for 10 min with 24 s of ramping time both before and after the stimulation/sham period at a constant intensity of 2.0 mA. For the sham stimulation condition, intensity was ramped up to 2.0 mA over 24 s, then delivered for another 40 s, before being ramped down to zero, giving participants a similar sensation to that they would experience during active stimulation. Spectroscopy acquisition continued for 10 min in order to assess post-stimulation effects (**Figure 2**).

Spectral Analysis

While no spectral artifacts were observed during steady-state tDCS stimulation, mild artifacts were seen in spectral frames acquired during the ramping periods for both active and sham stimulation. Frames from these periods were omitted from all subsequent analyses.

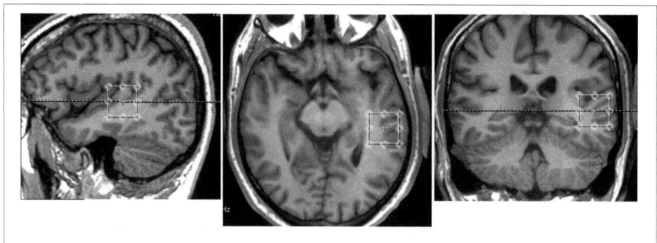

FIGURE 1 | Voxel placement in the pSTG in one participant: Sagittal (left), axial (middle), and coronal (right) views overlayed on an anatomical scan.

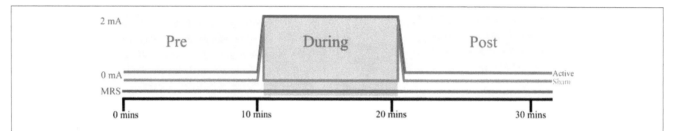

FIGURE 2 | tDCS and MRS: Each participant received both active and sham stimulation, separated by a washout period of 1 h, counterbalanced for order. 24 s of ramping up and down were incorporated into both active and sham stimulation. MRS was acquired constantly throughout each session. The pre-, during, and post-stimulation spectroscopy windows did not include frames acquired during ramping.

Following phase adjustment, coil combination, and realignment, each continuous acquisition was first subdivided into three smaller blocks of ~10 min, with exact length depending on how many frames were excluded due to ramping artifacts, comprising a pre-, during-, and post stimulation block for each session, hereafter referred to as a three point analysis. Frames within each block were then averaged together and within each block, ON, and OFF spectrum pairs were subtracted to produce a difference spectrum then subjected to quantitative analysis with LCModel (version 6.3-1J) (31, 32) using a simulated basis set (33) with Kaiser coupling constants (34) to provide an estimate of average levels of GABA, glutamate and glutamine measured together as Glx, glutathione (GSH), NAA, and N-acetyl aspartate glutamate (NAAG). Metabolite levels were scaled relative to the unsuppressed water signal acquired at the end of each spectroscopy sequence.

One issue that affects MEGA-edited GABA spectroscopy is co-editing of macromolecule (MM) resonances at 1.7 ppm contaminating the GABA signal in the difference spectrum. GABA, in this report, refers to both GABA and the co-edited macromolecule, typically denoted GABA+ (35).

To further investigate acute effects of tDCS, and eliminate the possibility short-lived metabolic fluctuations being obscured through averaging, a second analysis was performed in which the during- and post-stimulation blocks were further subdivided into two smaller windows in an attempt to uncover any changes in metabolite concentration during this period, thus providing five time points over the acquisition, hereafter referred to as the five point analysis: one 10 min pre-stimulation window, two 5 min during-, and two 5 min post-stimulation windows.

MRS signals have been demonstrated to be susceptible to line-broadening artifacts associated with local blood-oxygen-level dependent (BOLD) effects (36). As an indication of potential BOLD interference, the full width at half maximum (FWHM) values as determined by LCModel were used as a measure of quality control, to ensure the MRS signal had not been significantly affected between time points.

Statistical Analysis

Statistical analyses were performed using R (37) and the nlme package (38) to perform a linear mixed effects model analysis of the effect of tDCS on the concentrations of three metabolites of interest, namely NAA, Glx, and GABA, over time. This model specified two groups of participants (active-first and sham-first) and time period as fixed effects as well as an interaction effect between the two, with the subject as a random effect. This model was also used to investigate crossover effects between the active and sham stimulation conditions due to the within-subject design of the study, to determine whether order of stimulation, active first or sham first, may have had

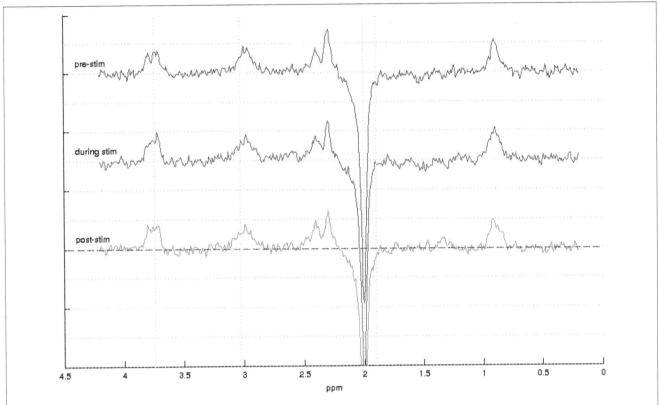

FIGURE 3 | MEGA-PRESS spectra from one participant showing spectra acquired during the pre-stimulation window (top, blue) during stimulation (middle, red) and post-stimulation (bottom, green).

any significant effect on results and whether the stimulation condition in the first session had any lasting effect on the second. The same model was used for both the 3-point and 5-point analyses.

RESULTS

Sample spectra from the three-point analysis of an individual participant are shown in **Figure 3** along with spectral quality metrics for all participants in **Table 1**. A linear mixed effects model of the average metabolite concentration across three time windows (pre-, during-, and post-stimulation) revealed no significant fluctuations in any of the metabolites of interest between any time points (**Figure 4** and **Appendix A**). Similarly, no significant fluctuations in any of the metabolites of interest were found between any time points in the five-time point analysis (**Figure 4** and **Appendix B**).

No significant crossover effects were found (**Figure 4**, **Appendices A, B**) indicating both that the order in which participants received the two different stimulation conditions had no significant effect on results and that there were no crossover effects from the first session significantly affecting the second. There was no significant difference in the change between groups over time, indicating no difference in fluctuations for any of the metabolite levels between active and sham conditions.

The FWHM as reported by LCModel was used as an indication of potential BOLD interference (**Tables 2, 3**), but saw very little fluctuation between time points, making BOLD interference an unlikely source of error.

DISCUSSION

The montage and stimulation parameters used in this experiment did not induce a statistically significant effect on Glx, GABA, or NAA levels as measured with the MRS sequence used, and there was no significant difference in response observed between the active and sham stimulation conditions.

The active hypothesis for this experiment was informed by previous studies in which active anodal stimulation was found to be associated with increases in Glx and NAA levels (22, 23) and decreases in GABA levels (20, 21, 24) as measured by MRS. In comparing these studies with the findings presented here, there are three key elements to be considered, namely the stimulation parameters, the MRS acquisition parameters and the site of stimulation and spectroscopy.

As stated in section tDCS Stimulation, due to limitations of the experimental design, stimulation could only be delivered for 10 min as opposed to the 20 min previously used in the treatment of schizophrenia symptoms. Although as little as 7 min of stimulation has been shown to induce lasting effects after stimulation has ceased (39), it cannot be taken for granted that the 10 min delivered in this session was sufficient to induce a change. While the stimulation window was shorter than the 30 min used by both Clark et al.

(22) and Hone-Blanchet et al. (23) and the 20 min and 15 min used by Bachtiar et al. (24) and Kim et al. (20), respectively, Stagg et al. (21) were able to detect significant changes in GABA and Glx levels in the left sensorimotor cortex using a similar

TABLE 1 | Spectral Quality: FWHM, SNR, and mean %CRLB for GABA and Glx for each stimulation window.

Window	FWHM (Hz)	SNR	Mean GABA %CRLB	Mean Glx %CRLB
Pre Stim	8.22 ± 2.34	20.47 ± 4.71	5.12	4.54
During Stim	8.39 ± 2.41	20.83 ± 4.20	5.16	4.41
Post Stim	8.03 ± 2.18	21.67 ± 4.04	4.91	4.24

TABLE 2 | Average FWHM and standard deviation (sd) as estimated by LCModel for the 3-point analysis.

	Mean FWHM–3-point analysis (Hz)					
	Pre	sd	During	sd	Post	sd
Active	7.95	1.86	7.98	1.79	7.59	1.38
Sham	8.46	2.24	8.64	2.24	8.32	2.30

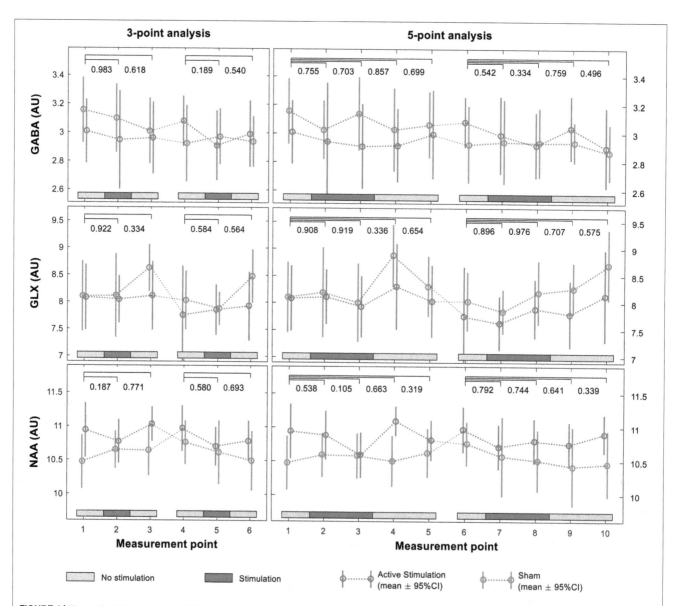

FIGURE 4 | Linear mixed effects model of GABA (upper row), Glx (middle row) and NAA (lower row) levels in the pSTG for both the first and second sessions using both 3-point (left) and 5-point (right) analyses. p-values shown above each plot indicate significance of interaction effects at each time point relative to baseline.

TABLE 3 | Average FWHM and standard deviation (sd) as estimated by LCModel for the 5-point analysis.

	Mean FWHM–5-point analysis (Hz)									
	Pre	sd	During1	sd	During2	sd	Post1	Sd	Post2	sd
Active	7.95	1.86	8.00	1.77	7.94	1.69	7.74	1.73	7.77	1.55
Sham	8.46	2.24	8.50	0.02	8.46	2.06	8.28	2.42	8.46	1.96

MEGA-PRESS sequence at 3 T given only 10 min of anodal stimulation at 1.0 mA. The findings of Batsikadze et al. (15) and Esmaeilpour et al. (16) suggest it is possible that stimulating at 2.0 mA had a different effect to the one predicted. However, studies conducted by Brunelin et al. (8) and Mondino et al. (9) both found significant reductions in symptoms of auditory-verbal hallucinations using stimulation in this area following cathodal stimulation at 2.0 mA, suggesting an issue more likely related to electrode polarity than stimulation intensity. While no significant changes, nor non-significant tendencies toward changes in any of the metabolites under investigation were seen during stimulation, even in the five-point analysis, it is unlikely that allowing a full 20 min of stimulation would induce a measureable effect, though it cannot be ruled out conclusively.

One of the unique features of this study was the use of continuous, online MRS as opposed to separate acquisitions. While Hone-Blanchet et al. (23) also acquired spectra during stimulation, also using a MEGA-PRESS sequence with an echo time of 68 ms and 11 min acquisition blocks, their study does not include a pre-stimulation window. Similarly, Clark et al. (22) acquired multiple spectra during the pre- and post-stimulation windows, also using a MEGA-PRESS sequence with an echo time of 68 ms, but with spectra acquired sequentially rather than continuously in blocks of 4 min and 48 s. While there is little difference in terms of the resultant spectra whether acquired continuously or sequentially, acquiring separate scans may introduce more variability as each pre-scan affects parameters such as shim, gain adjustment and center-frequency tuning between each segment. It may be considered more robust to acquire all spectra with the same parameters, as was done in this study with single continuous acquisitions. Compared with previous studies using similar sequences, comparable or shorter acquisition times, and smaller voxel sizes, i.e., 20 × 20 × 20 mm³ (21, 22, 24), there is little evidence to suggest an error in the MRS acquisition. Intuitively, a larger voxel size provides a higher signal-to-noise ratio, but may come at the expense of some focality in terms of covering the site of stimulation. It is possible that the larger voxel size used in this study may have incorporated spectra from cells not affected by stimulation. However, the voxel dimensions are still small compared to the surface area of the stimulating electrode, and tDCS is not a particularly focused stimulation technique.

The most significant difference between this study and other studies that have measured biochemical changes associated with tDCS with MRS is the cortical region being investigated, both as a stimulation site and volume of interest in spectroscopy. As Woods et al. (14) illustrated, it cannot be taken for granted

that all cortical areas will respond to stimulation in the same manner, and compared to areas such as the sensorimotor cortex and frontal areas such as the dorsolateral prefrontal cortex, the temporoparietal and temporal regions have not been quite as thoroughly investigated. One study investigating the use of anodal tDCS in an adjacent cortical area, namely the left mid-posterior temporal gyrus, on improving performance in a range or reading and naming tasks (40) did not find any significant improvement in performance. Although different stimulation parameters were used, the agreement between the null-findings of this and the present study suggest it is possible that the pSTG and adjacent areas in the region, are not as responsive to anodal stimulation as other areas that have been investigated, but that the effectiveness of tDCS as a treatment for hallucinations is based on its ability to modulate over-active areas in the brain with cathodal stimulation. That is to say, anodal stimulation may not affect excitability in the pSTG, but cathodal stimulation may be effective in modulating activity in over-active or pathologically active networks such as those that might be associated with hallucinations. Computer modeling may be able to determine whether the responsiveness of this cortical area may be due to anatomical features such as skull thickness or cerebrospinal fluid density. It may be of interest to repeat a similar experiment looking at the effects of cathodal stimulation in this area in conjunction with computer models that may be able to determine whether the absence of an observed affect may be attributed to issues of anatomy and current flow.

In an investigation into the effect of active, intrascanner tDCS on the BOLD response as measured with functional MRI, Antal et al. (41) found that the presence of an electric current in the magnetic field inside an MRI scanner produces artifacts that may result in confounding false-positive activity patterns. While mild artifacts were observed during the ramping periods before and after stimulation, and these spectral frames were removed from subsequent analyses, there were no artifacts observed during active or sham stimulation periods. Furthermore, there were no statistically significant differences observed between the pre- and post-stimulation windows, where no ongoing active or sham stimulation was present. This, coupled with the findings of previous studies using online MRS acquired during stimulation (23, 24) suggest that interference caused by ongoing intrascanner tDCS during spectral acquisition is not a likely source of error.

Another potential explanation for the null findings of this experiment is insufficient power as a result of too few participants. An analysis conducted in G*Power (42) determined there were enough participants to detect at least a medium sized effect (i.e., effect size > 0.6, 1-β = 0.8, α = 0.05). Many of the studies that have previously investigated biochemical effects of tDCS have noted significant findings with smaller sample sizes than the 19 used in this study, including $N = 12$ (22), $N = 17$ (23), and $N = 11$ (21). To this end it is believed that the study was sufficiently powered, in terms of the participant sample size, to detect a comparable effect. One of the problems with statistical power as outlined by Button et al. (43) is that while problems of low statistical power are typically associated with reduced chances of detecting a true effect, they may also reduce the likelihood of a statistically significant result being indicative of a true effect. That is, finding false positive effects due to inflated effect sizes. As Westwood et al. (40) illustrate, while it may be of value to include more participants in future studies, it calls the effectiveness of a single session of tDCS into question if the effects are so small. Referring to a meta-analysis in preparation, Westwood et al. (40) discuss an analysis of pooled studies looking at anodal stimulation in the frontal and temporal lobes which produced a sample size of almost 200 participants in which there was still no evidence of an effect of a single session of tDCS. In light of this, it is not believed that an increased sample size would have improved the outcome of this experiment.

One problem affecting the spectroscopy aspect of this study is that of how to quantify metabolite levels. Typical methods make use of water as an endogenous reference, or report the concentration as a ratio relative to an internal reference such as creatine or NAA. While creatine is typically favored as an internal reference (44) its use is complicated when using the MEGA-PRESS sequence as creatine signals are eliminated during subtraction and are not present in the difference edited spectrum, though they may be recovered from the spectra acquired without an editing pulse (commonly referred to as the "OFF" spectrum in the spectral pairs used to create the difference spectrum). NAA was not used as an internal reference as it has been demonstrated to be affected by anodal tDCS (22, 23), although no changes in NAA levels were measured over the course of the acquisition. The use of water as an endogenous reference can be problematic for studies such as this that attempt to measure metabolic changes in a dynamic manner, i.e., in relation to activity over time, as MRS signals have been shown to be susceptible to line-broadening artifacts associated with local BOLD effects (36). Using a fixed water reference taken at the end of the acquisition, as was done in this study, the reference signal was not subject to fluctuations as the result of a BOLD effect throughout the scan as the metabolites of interest were, i.e., comparing an unchanging reference to a signal subject to interference may increase the likelihood of a false change being detected. As a single, fixed water reference was used, it is difficult to decisively rule out any incidental BOLD-related fluctuations. However, such fluctuations would likely be manifest across all metabolites in the FWHM estimate given by LCModel, which is not seen in our data (**Tables 2, 3**), making it unlikely to be a significant source of error. Ideally, an experiment such as this would benefit from the use of external referencing, such as the Electronic Reference To access *in vivo* Concentrations (ERETIC) method (45, 46).

In interpreting these findings, it is important to consider that tDCS is regarded as a neuromodulatory technique, it does not induce activity or action potentials, but rather facilitates increases or decreases in neuronal excitability. Bikson and Rahman (47) discuss the idea of activity-selectivity and task-specific modulation, that is, that tDCS will preferentially modulate a neuronal network that is already active, while not modulating a separate network that is inactive. One of the problems with the region of interest in this study is that it contains the primary auditory cortex and adjacent areas responsible for the sensation of sound and processing of speech (48). While other paradigms have investigated cortical areas that may be associated with a task, e.g., the primary motor cortex and force adaptation task (20), that may distinguish between blocks of activity and rest, the auditory cortex will experience ongoing sensory input during scanning. It is possible that no biochemical changes were observed between blocks as the local cortical circuit was already in an active state during the pre-stimulation window and that tDCS was not able to drive a higher level of activity.

In conclusion, using continuous online MRS, no significant change in the levels of Glx, GABA, or NAA in the left pSTG was observed that could be attributed to an effect of active, anodal tDCS. Despite this, the method provides a useful insight into the acute effects of stimulation paradigms and their effect on local neuronal circuitry. Further research investigating an effect of tDCS in this area suggests performing a similar experiment using cathodal tDCS, redesigning the experiment to allow 20 min of stimulation, perhaps combining this experiment with computer models and also using an external referencing method to avoid possible confounding variables associated with how metabolite levels are measured.

AUTHOR CONTRIBUTIONS

GD, AC, MH, KK, KH, and RG were involved in the conception and design of the study. GD, AC, MH, and KK contributed to planning and performing of the experiments. AC performed the spectral analysis component of this study. JA performed statistical analyses. LE contributed to acquisition of MR-Spectra. GD wrote the manuscript with the assistance and critical feedback of all contributing authors.

FUNDING

The current research was partly funded by grants from the Research Council of Norway (#221550), European Research Council, ERC (#693124), and the Health Authority of Western Norway (#911783) to KH; the Bergen Research Foundation (grant BFS2016REK03) to MH; and Norway Grants (EMP180) to KK.

REFERENCES

1. Zaghi S, Acar M, Hultgren B, Boggio PS, Fregni F. Noninvasive brain stimulation with low-intensity electrical currents: putative mechanisms of action for direct and alternating current stimulation. *Neuroscientist* (2010) 16:285–307. doi: 10.1177/1073858409336227
2. Nitsche MA, Paulus W. Excitability changes induced in the human motor cortex by weak transcranial direct current stimulation. *J Physiol.* (2000) 527:633–9. doi: 10.1111/j.1469-7793.2000.t01-1-00633.x
3. Nitsche MA, Paulus W. Sustained excitability elevations induced by transcranial DC motor cortex stimulation in humans. *Neurology* (2001) 57:1899. doi: 10.1212/WNL.57.10.1899
4. Stagg CJ, Nitsche MA. Physiological basis of transcranial direct current stimulation. *Neuroscientist* (2011) 17:37–53. doi: 10.1177/1073858410386614
5. Benninger DH, Hallett M. Non-invasive brain stimulation for Parkinson's disease: current concepts and outlook 2015. *NeuroRehabilitation* (2015) 37:11–24. doi: 10.3233/NRE-151237
6. Brunoni AR, Moffa AH, Fregni F, Palm U, Padberg F, Blumberger DM, et al. Transcranial direct current stimulation for acute major depressive episodes: meta-analysis of individual patient data. *Br J Psychiatry* (2016) 208:522–31. doi: 10.1192/bjp.bp.115.164715
7. Homan P, Kindler J, Federspiel A, Flury R, Hubl D, Hauf M, et al. Muting the voice: a case of arterial spin labeling-monitored transcranial direct current stimulation treatment of auditory verbal hallucinations. *Am J Psychiatry* (2011) 168:853–4. doi: 10.1176/appi.ajp.2011.11030496
8. Brunelin J, Mondino M, Gassab L, Haesebaert F, Gaha L, Suaud-Chagny M-F, et al. Examining transcranial Direct-Current Stimulation (tDCS) as a treatment for hallucinations in schizophrenia. *Am J Psychiatry* (2012) 169:719–24. doi: 10.1176/appi.ajp.2012.11071091
9. Mondino M, Jardri R, Suaud-Chagny M-F, Saoud M, Poulet E, Brunelin J. Effects of fronto-temporal transcranial direct current stimulation on auditory verbal hallucinations and resting-state functional connectivity of the left temporo-parietal junction in patients with schizophrenia. *Schizophr Bull.* (2016) 42:318–26. doi: 10.1093/schbul/sbv114
10. Fitzgerald PB, McQueen S, Daskalakis ZJ, Hoy KE. A negative pilot study of daily bimodal transcranial direct current stimulation in schizophrenia. *Brain Stimul.* (2014) 7:813–6. doi: 10.1016/j.brs.2014.08.002
11. Fröhlich F, Burrello TN, Mellin JM, Cordle AL, Lustenberger CM, Gilmore JH, et al. Exploratory study of once-daily transcranial direct current stimulation (tDCS) as a treatment for auditory hallucinations in schizophrenia. *Eur Psychiatry* (2016) 33:54–60. doi: 10.1016/j.eurpsy.2015.11.005
12. Nitsche MA, Cohen LG, Wassermann EM, Priori A, Lang N, Antal A, et al. Transcranial direct current stimulation: state of the art 2008. *Brain Stimul.* (2008) 1:206–23. doi: 10.1016/j.brs.2008.06.004
13. Radman T, Ramos RL, Brumberg JC, Bikson M. Role of cortical cell type and morphology in subthreshold and suprathreshold uniform electric field stimulation in vitro. *Brain Stimul.* (2009) 2:215–28.e3. doi: 10.1016/j.brs.2009.03.007
14. Woods AJ, Antal A, Bikson M, Boggio PS, Brunoni AR, Celnik P, et al. A technical guide to tDCS, and related non-invasive brain stimulation tools. *Clin Neurophysiol.* (2016) 127:1031–48. doi: 10.1016/j.clinph.2015.11.012
15. Batsikadze G, Moliadze V, Paulus W, Kuo MF, Nitsche MA. Partially non-linear stimulation intensity-dependent effects of direct current stimulation on motor cortex excitability in humans. *J Physiol.* (2013) 591:1987–2000. doi: 10.1113/jphysiol.2012.249730
16. Esmaeilpour Z, Marangolo P, Hampstead BM, Bestmann S, Galletta E, Knotkova H, et al. Incomplete evidence that increasing current intensity of tDCS boosts outcomes. *Brain Stimul.* (2018) 11:310–21. doi: 10.1016/j.brs.2017.12.002
17. Horvath JC, Forte JD, Carter O. Quantitative review finds no evidence of cognitive effects in healthy populations from single-session transcranial Direct Current Stimulation (tDCS). *Brain Stimul.* (2015) 8:535–50. doi: 10.1016/j.brs.2015.01.400
18. Bikson M, Rahman A, Datta A. Computational models of transcranial direct current stimulation. *Clin EEG Neurosci.* (2012) 43:176–83. doi: 10.1177/1550059412445138
19. Krause B, Márquez-Ruiz J, Cohen Kadosh R. The effect of transcranial direct current stimulation: a role for cortical excitation/inhibition balance? *Front Hum Neurosci.* (2013) 7:602. doi: 10.3389/fnhum.2013.00602
20. Kim S, Stephenson MC, Morris PG, Jackson SR. tDCS-induced alterations in GABA concentration within primary motor cortex predict motor learning and motor memory: a 7T magnetic resonance spectroscopy study. *Neuroimage* (2014) 99:237–43. doi: 10.1016/j.neuroimage.2014.05.070
21. Stagg CJ, Best JG, Stephenson MC, Shea J, Wylezinska M, Kincses ZT, et al. Polarity-sensitive modulation of cortical neurotransmitters by transcranial stimulation. *J Neurosci.* (2009) 29:5202–6. doi: 10.1523/JNEUROSCI.4432-08.2009
22. Clark VP, Coffman BA, Trumbo MC, Gasparovic C. Transcranial direct current stimulation (tDCS) produces localized and specific alterations in neurochemistry: a 1H magnetic resonance spectroscopy study. *Neurosci Lett.* (2011) 500:67–71. doi: 10.1016/j.neulet.2011.05.244
23. Hone-Blanchet A, Edden RA, Fecteau S. Online effects of transcranial direct current stimulation in real time on human prefrontal and striatal metabolites. *Biol Psychiatry* (2016) 80:432–8. doi: 10.1016/j.biopsych.2015.11.008
24. Bachtiar V, Near J, Johansen-Berg H, Stagg CJ. Modulation of GABA and resting state functional connectivity by transcranial direct current stimulation. *Elife* (2015) 4:e08789. doi: 10.7554/eLife.08789
25. Hone-Blanchet A, Fecteau, S. Chapter 15 - The use of non-invasive brain stimulation in drug addictions. In: Kadosh RC, editor. *The Stimulated Brain.* San Diego, CA: Academic Press. (2014). p. 425–452. doi: 10.1016/B978-0-12-404704-4.00015-6
26. Oldfield RC. The assessment and analysis of handedness: the Edinburgh inventory. *Neuropsychologia* (1971) 9:97–113. doi: 10.1016/0028-3932(71)90067-4
27. Mondino M, Bennabi D, Poulet E, Galvao F, Brunelin J, Haffen E. Can transcranial direct current stimulation (tDCS) alleviate symptoms and improve cognition in psychiatric disorders? *World J Biol Psychiatry* (2014) 15:261–75. doi: 10.3109/15622975.2013.876514
28. Nitsche MA, Seeber A, Frommann K, Klein CC, Rochford C, Nitsche MS, et al. Modulating parameters of excitability during and after transcranial direct current stimulation of the human motor cortex. *J Physiol.* (2005) 568:291–303. doi: 10.1113/jphysiol.2005.092429
29. Mescher M, Merkle H, Kirsch J, Garwood M, Gruetter R. Simultaneous in vivo spectral editing and water suppression. *NMR Biomed.* (1998) 11:266–72. doi: 10.1002/(SICI)1099-1492(199810)11:6<266::AID-NBM530>3.0.CO;2-J
30. Henry ME, Lauriat TL, Shanahan M, Renshaw PF, Jensen JE. Accuracy and stability of measuring GABA, glutamate, and glutamine by proton magnetic resonance spectroscopy: a phantom study at 4Tesla. *J Magn Reson.* (2011) 208:210–8. doi: 10.1016/j.jmr.2010.11.003
31. Provencher SW. Estimation of metabolite concentrations from localized in vivo proton NMR spectra. *Magn Reson Med.* (1993) 30:672–9. doi: 10.1002/mrm.1910300604
32. Provencher SW. Automatic quantitation of localized in vivo 1H spectra with LCModel. *NMR Biomed.* (2001) 14:260–4. doi: 10.1002/nbm.698
33. Dydak U, Jiang Y-M, Long L-L, Zhu H, Chen J, Li W-M, et al. In vivo measurement of brain GABA concentrations by magnetic resonance spectroscopy in smelters occupationally exposed to manganese. *Environ Health Perspect.* (2011) 119:219–24. doi: 10.1289/ehp.1002192
34. Kaiser LG, Young K, Meyerhoff DJ, Mueller SG, Matson GB. A detailed analysis of localized J-difference GABA editing: theoretical and experimental study at 4 T. *NMR Biomed.* (2008) 21:22–32. doi: 10.1002/nbm.1150
35. Edden RAE, Puts NAJ, Barker PB. Macromolecule-suppressed GABA-edited magnetic resonance spectroscopy at 3T. *Magn Reson Med.* (2012) 68:657–61. doi: 10.1002/mrm.24391
36. Zhu X-H, Chen W. Observed BOLD effects on cerebral metabolite resonances in human visual cortex during visual stimulation: a functional 1H MRS study at 4 T. *Magn Reson Med.* (2001) 46:841–7. doi: 10.1002/mrm.1267
37. R Development Core Team. *R: A Language and Environment for Statistical Computing.* Vienna: R Foundation for Statistical Computing. (2016). Available online at: https://www.R-project.org/
38. Pinheiro J, Bates D, DebRoy S, Sarkar D, Team RC. *nlme: Linear and Nonlinear Mixed Effects Models: R Package Version 3.1-128.* (2016). Available online at: http://CRAN.R-project.org/package=nlme

39. Horvath JC, Forte JD, Carter O. Evidence that transcranial direct current stimulation (tDCS) generates little-to-no reliable neurophysiologic effect beyond MEP amplitude modulation in healthy human subjects: a systematic review. *Neuropsychologia* (2015) 66:213–36. doi: 10.1016/j.neuropsychologia.2014.11.021

40. Westwood SJ, Olson A, Miall RC, Nappo R, Romani C. Limits to tDCS effects in language: failures to modulate word production in healthy participants with frontal or temporal tDCS. *Cortex* (2017) 86:64–82. doi: 10.1016/j.cortex.2016.10.016

41. Antal A, Bikson M, Datta A, Lafon B, Dechent P, Parra LC, et al. Imaging artifacts induced by electrical stimulation during conventional fMRI of the brain. *Neuroimage* (2014) 85:1040–7. doi: 10.1016/j.neuroimage.2012.10.026

42. Faul F, Erdfelder E, Lang A-G, Buchner A. G*Power 3: a flexible statistical power analysis program for the social, behavioral, and biomedical sciences. *Behav Res Methods* (2007) 39:175–91. doi: 10.3758/BF03193146

43. Button KS, Ioannidis JPA, Mokrysz C, Nosek BA, Flint J, Robinson ESJ, et al. Power failure: why small sample size undermines the reliability of neuroscience. *Nat Rev Neurosci.* (2013) 14:365–76. doi: 10.1038/nrn3475

44. Bottomley PA, Griffiths JR. *Handbook of Magnetic Resonance Spectroscopy in vivo: MRS Theory, Practice and Applications.* Chichester: John Wiley & Sons Ltd. (2016).

45. Barantin L, Pape AL, Akoka S. A new method for absolute quantitation MRS metabolites. *Magn Reson Med.* (1997) 38:179–82. doi: 10.1002/mrm.1910380203

46. Heinzer-Schweizer S, De Zanche N, Pavan M, Mens G, Sturzenegger U, Henning A, et al. *In-vivo* assessment of tissue metabolite levels using 1H MRS and the Electric REference to access *in vivo* concentrations (ERETIC) method. *NMR Biomed.* (2010) 23:406–13. doi: 10.1002/nbm.1476

47. Bikson M, Rahman A. Origins of specificity during tDCS: anatomical, activity-selective, and input-bias mechanisms. *Front Hum Neurosci.* (2013) 7:688. doi: 10.3389/fnhum.2013.00688

48. Winer JA, Schreiner CE. *The Auditory Cortex.* New York, NY: Springer US. (2010).

2

Real-World Lab Data in Natalizumab Treated Multiple Sclerosis Patients Up to 6 Years Long-Term Follow Up

Maxi Kaufmann, Rocco Haase, Undine Proschmann, Tjalf Ziemssen *† and Katja Akgün †

MS Center Dresden, Center of Clinical Neuroscience, Carl Gustav Carus University Hospital, University of Technology Dresden, Dresden, Germany

*Correspondence:
Tjalf Ziemssen
tjalf.ziemssen@uniklinikum-dresden.de

† These authors have contributed to this work as senior authors

Natalizumab inhibits the transmigration of immune cells across the blood-brain barrier thus inhibiting inflammation in the central nervous system. Generally, this blockade at the blood-brain barrier has significant influence on the circulating lymphocytes. Up to date, only short-term data on peripheral blood parameters are available which are mostly from controlled clinical trials and not from real-world experience. Real-world lab data of 120 patients diagnosed with highly active disease course of relapsing-remitting multiple sclerosis (RRMS) were analyzed during natalizumab treatment. Patient sampling was performed by consecutive recruitment in the Multiple Sclerosis Center Dresden. Lab testing was performed before and at every third infusion up to 72 months follow-up. After first natalizumab infusion, absolute numbers of all major lymphocyte populations including CD4+ T-cells, CD8+ T-cells, CD19+ B-cells, and NK-cells significantly increased and remained stable during the whole observation period of 72 months. Upon lymphocyte subsets, CD19+ B-cells presented a disproportionate increase up to levels higher than normal level in most of the treated patients. Neutralizing antibodies to natalizumab abrogated the described changes. Intra-individual variation of lymphocytes and its subsets remained in a narrow range for the whole treatment period. CD4/CD8 ratio did not change compared to baseline measurement up to 6 years of natalizumab treatment. Monocytes, eosinophils, and basophils, but not neutrophils persistently increased during natalizumab treatment. Hematological parameters including erythrocyte, platelet count, hemoglobin, and hematocrit remained unchanged compared to baseline. Interestingly, immature precursor cells including erythroblasts were detectable in 36,8% of the treated patients during natalizumab therapy, but not in the pretreatment period. Asymptomatic elevations of liver enzymes were rare, mostly only transient and lower than 3x upper normal limit. Kidney function parameters remained stable within physiological ranges in most patients. CRP levels >20 mg/dl were recognized only in 10 patients during natalizumab therapy and were mostly linked to respiratory tract infections. In our present analysis, we report persistent, but stable increases of peripheral immune cell subtypes in natalizumab treated patients. Additional serological analyses confirm excellent tolerability and safety even 6 years after natalizumab initiation in post-marketing experience.

Keywords: natalizumab, multiple sclerosis, real-world lab data, peripheral immune cell subtypes, clinical practice

INTRODUCTION

Natalizumab (NAT) is a humanized monoclonal antibody selectively directed against the α4-subunit of the very late antigen-4 (VLA-4) integrin, a specific adhesion molecule on the surface of leukocytes except neutrophils. The α4-integrin interacts with the vascular cell adhesion molecule-1 (VCAM-1) expressed on endothelial cells of blood vessels to mediate extravasation and transmigration of immune cells across the blood-brain barrier into the central nervous system (CNS) (1–3). By its unique mechanism of action, NAT blocks the VLA-4/VCAM-1 mediated leukocyte-endothelial interaction (2, 4). Though, lymphocyte migration into brain tissue is prevented and the CNS inflammation is inhibited (5). NAT is highly effective in relapsing-remitting (RR) multiple sclerosis (MS) proven by marked decrease in relapse rate, MRI activity and disease progression (6, 7). There is a growing experience in selection of appropriated patients and use of NAT in everyday clinical practice since approval. Among disease-modifying treatments (DMT) in MS therapy, NAT is associated with an increased risk of progressive multifocal leukoencephalopathy (PML) especially in John Cunningham virus (JCV) positive and long-term treated patients (8). Since re-approval in 2006, a detailed and standardized management program was established which is now used in everyday clinical practice (8–10). As part of this risk management plan, standardized lab testing is recommended including complete blood count, peripheral immune cell status, and serological parameters to be aware of clinical relevant changes. Especially lymphocytosis has been already described in NAT-treated patients due to impaired lymphocyte extravasation into tissues as well as mobilization of hematopoetic precursor cells from bone marrow (11–16). As part of our NAT management, data from clinical practice are collected providing longitudinal information on different outcomes inclusive adverse affects (17). Such real-world evidence (RWE) and observational studies are becoming increasingly popular because they reflect the usefulness of drugs in real life and have the ability to discover uncommon or rare adverse drug reactions inclusive lab abnormalities (18). Therefore, RWE can assist to evaluate the drug profile in clinical practice and to link it with other clinical outcomes. The MSDS3D software which has been adapted to the NAT management in particular combines documentation of patient data with management of patients with MS implementing treatment-specific modules, to collect data of safety management inclusive lab data with regard to the characteristics of different treatments and populations (19).

Today, NAT has been successfully used in MS patients for more than 11 years. The increase in lymphocyte count was already discussed during the initial clinical trials (6, 20). Further

single evaluations followed after approval and in post-marketing experience (21–24). Nevertheless, a systematic and long-term evaluation of real-world routine lab testing data including peripheral cell subtypes and serological parameters is not yet available.

In this study, we present real world laboratory data of a cohort of NAT treated patients up to 72 months follow up. We aim to describe the biological impact of NAT on peripheral blood cell subset distribution during long period treatment observation in the real world. Additional serological analyses allow evaluation of tolerability and safety after NAT initiation in real world experience.

METHODS

Patients

We included 120 patients (91 females and 29 males) diagnosed with RRMS according the McDonald criteria and highly active disease course (25). After critical review of clinical and MRI data as well as available treatment options, NAT treatment was initiated. Patient sampling was performed by consecutive recruitment (**Figure 1**) in the MS center, University Hospital Dresden. Expanded Disability Status Scale (EDSS) was performed by an experienced, Neurostatus-certified neurologist (26). Patient baseline characteristics are reported in **Table 1**. Patients starting with NAT presented at an mean age about 33.7 ± 9.6 years, an median EDSS score about 3.5 and median duration since diagnosis of RRMS about 4.0. About 69.2% of patients received at least one DMT before NAT initiation, 30.8% patients were initiated to NAT without previous DMT. During a standardized treatment switch procedure, injectables were stopped 2 weeks before natalizumab start, fingolimod was stopped 8 weeks before natalizumab and other DMTs at least 6 months before natalizumab initiation. The proportion of patients without disease activity and NEDA-3 status defined by no relapses, no confirmed EDSS progression (≥ 1.0 point increase if EDSS baseline score was <4.0; ≥ 0.5 point increase if EDSS baseline score was ≥ 4.0), and no MRI progression (one or more new T2 or gadolinium enhancing lesions) during the 72 months observation period are presented in **Figure 2**. Data have been collected from the MSDS3D database. The study was approved by the institutional review board of the University Hospital of Dresden. Patients gave their written informed consent.

NAT Infusion Protocol and Blood Sampling

NAT infusion protocol used in our MS center was adapted to the standardized infusion protocol described in guidelines of diagnosis and treatment of MS patients of the German association of MS (27). NAT (300 mg) was given every 4 weeks intravenously (i.v.) over the course of 1 h. According to our standard operation procedure, routine blood analysis and EDSS evaluations were realized before NAT start and every 3 months. In this analysis, we evaluated these parameters up to 72 months follow up.

Abbreviations: ALAT, alanine aminotransferase; ASAT, aspartate aminotransferase; CNS, central nervous system; CRP, C-reactive protein; DMT, disease modifying drug; gamma-GT, gamma-glutamyltransferase; EDSS, Expanded Disability Status Scale; i.v., intravenously; JCV, John Cunningham virus; MRI, magnet resonance imaging; MS, multiples sclerosis; NAT, natalizumab; NEDA, no evidence of disease activity; NK cells, natural killer cells; PML, progressive multifocal leukoencephalopathy; RR, relapsing remitting; VCAM-1, vascular cell adhesion molecule-1; VLA-4, very late antigen 4.

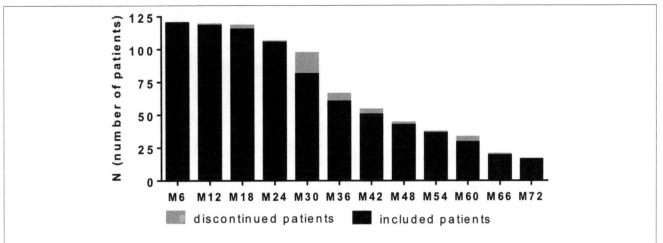

FIGURE 1 | Patient recruitment per 6 months period. One hundred and twenty patients with highly active MS were recruited and evaluated at data analysis. Based on consecutive sampling some of patients already reached 72 month follow up, whereas others did not yet at time point of data analysis. Number of patients included at defined time point are depicted (black bar). Additionally number of patients that discontinued NAT treatment at defined time point are presented (gray bar). Clinical and lab data were evaluated every 3 months.

TABLE 1 | Baseline characteristics.

Age (yr ± SD)	33.7 (9.6)
Male-[no. (%)]	29 (24.2)
Female-[no. (%)]	91 (75.8)
Previous use DMT-[no. (%)]	83 (69.2)
Interferon-beta	51 (42.5)
Glatiramer acetate	21 (17.5)
Fingolimod	4 (3.3)
Other approved medications	7 (5.8)
none-[no. (%)]	37 (30.8)
Duration since MS diagnosis (mean yr ± SD)	5.6 (5.8)
Mean score on EDSS	3.8 (1.8)

Baseline characteristics of evaluated patients. Other approved medications include, Triamcinolon (1), Azathioprin (1), Mitoxantron (4), Laquinimod (1). DMT, disease modifying therapy; yr, years; SD, standard deviation; no, number.

Routine Blood Analysis

Standardized blood testing was performed for routine blood parameters at the Institute of Clinical Chemistry and Laboratory Medicine, University Hospital in Dresden, Germany. The institute complies with standards required by DIN-EN-ISO-15189:2014 for medical laboratories. Routine blood testing included complete blood cell count, liver enzymes, creatinine, sodium, potassium, and C-reactive protein (CRP). Serological testing for JCV antibodies was performed before natalizumab start and every 6 months follow up and was measured at Unilabs, Denmark (Stratify JCV^TM Test).

Immune Cell Phenotyping by Fluorescence-Activated Cell Sorting (FACS)

After blood collection, subpopulations of T-cells, B-cells, and natural killer (NK) cells were characterized by surface staining with fluorescence labeled anti-CD3, anti-CD4, anti-CD8, anti-CD16, anti-CD14, anti-CD19, anti-CD56 (BD Biosciences, Heidelberg, Germany) according to the manufacturer's instructions. Negative controls included directly labeled or unlabeled isotype-matched irrelevant antibodies (BD Biosciences). Cells were evaluated on FACSCanto II flow cytometer.

Statistical Analysis

Data were analyzed applying Generalized Linear Mixed Models with Gamma distribution and log link function due to the right-skewed distribution pattern of the data. Bonferroni correction for pairwise tests was used. Correlations were calculated using Spearman's correlation model. At the time, there were no clear variables at hand that should have been treated as confounders. Since we had no determining groups to test for differences, confounders over time were left to be considered. In the graphs (**Figures 3–5, 7**), data are given as mean ± standard deviation (SD). In **Table 2**, data are additionally presented as mean ±95% confidence interval (CI) providing information about the precision of estimates over the course of the study. Values of $^{*}p < 0.05$, $^{**}p < 0.01$, and $^{***}p < 0.001$ were considered significant.

RESULTS

Complete Blood Cell Count and Its Variation During Long-Term NAT Therapy

In our analysis 120 patients were included starting on NAT therapy. Before NAT initiation, a wide range of leukocyte resp. lymphocyte counts (3.3–13.9 GPT/L, respectively, 0.4–3.7 GPT/L) was seen (**Figures 3A,B, Table 2**). Levels of baseline leukocyte resp. lymphocyte count did not significantly differ between patients without or with different previous DMT use in

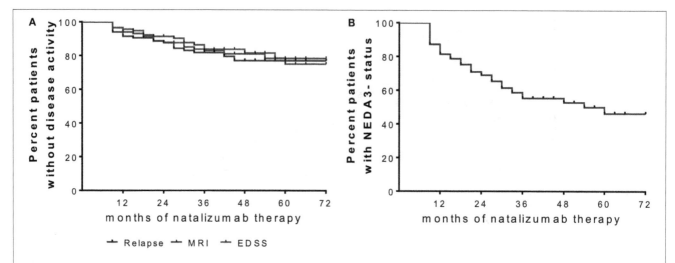

FIGURE 2 | Proportion of patients without disease activity and NEDA-3 status after NAT start. **(A)** Clinical parameters are depicted in a Kaplan–Meier survival curve analysis for relapses, confirmed EDSS progression (≥1.0 point increase if EDSS baseline score was <4.0; ≥0.5 point increase if EDSS baseline score was ≥4.0) and MRI progression (one or more new T2 or gadolinium enhancing lesions) after month 6 and during 72 months follow up. **(B)** No evidence of disease activity (NEDA)-3 status was confirmed when criteria of no relapses, no EDSS progression and no MRI progression were met.

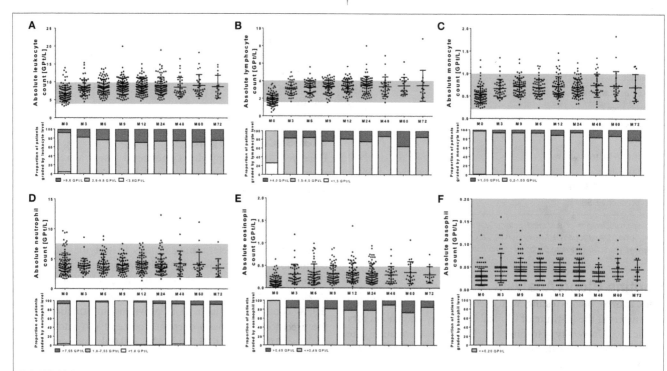

FIGURE 3 | Complete blood analysis during NAT treatment. Blood samples were taken before NAT started (M0) and every 3 months. Blood samples were analyzed in a certified medical laboratory. Analysis of complete blood count as leukocytes **(A)**, lymphocytes **(B)**, monocytes **(C)**, neutrophils **(D)**, eosinophils **(E)**, and basophils **(F)** were included. Data are shown for baseline analysis (M0), month 3 (M3), month 6 (M6), month 12 (M12), and every 12 months follow up (M24, M48, M60, M72). Results are depicted as mean ± standard deviation. Green background indicates reference range of depicted parameters. Additionally, proportion of patients graded by white blood cell levels are shown: lower than reference range (yellow), reference range (green), and higher than the reference range (blue). Levels of significance are presented in **Table 2**.

our cohort. At NAT start, 24 patients presented with lymphocyte counts <1.5 GPT/L without a specific pretreatment pattern.

After NAT initiation, leukocyte and lymphocyte counts increased significantly (global time effect $p < 0.001$,

Figures 3A,B, Table 2). On average, leukocyte count increased up to about 2.05 GPT/L absolutely and 37.33% relatively, lymphocytes up to about 1.63 GPT/L in absolute and 99.95% in relatively. The highest increase in leukocyte and lymphocyte

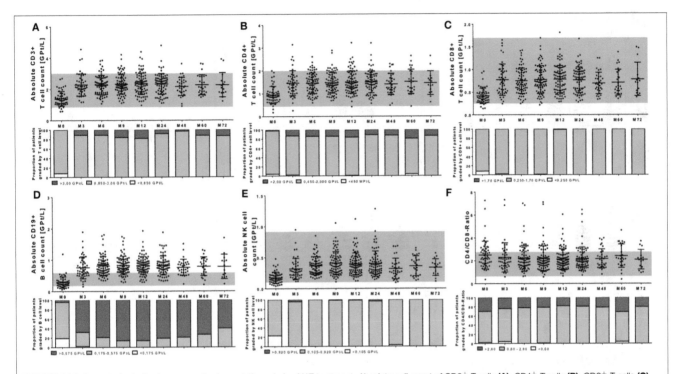

FIGURE 4 | Cell count of selective immune cell subpopulations during NAT treatment. Absolute cell count of CD3+ T cells **(A)**, CD4+ T cells **(B)**, CD8+ T cells **(C)**, CD19+ B cells **(D)**, NK cells **(E)**, and the CD4+/CD8+-Ratio **(F)** are depicted. Data are shown for baseline analysis (M0), month 3 (M3), month 6 (M6), month 12 (M12), and every 12 months follow up (M24, M48, M60, M72). Mean ± standard deviation are presented. Green background indicates reference range of depicted parameters. Additionally, proportion of patients graded by lymphocyte subtype level are shown: lower than reference range (yellow), reference range (green) and higher than the reference range (blue). Level of significance are presented in **Table 2**.

count was seen in patients pretreated with fingolimod (only 4 patients in our cohort included) before NAT start. Furthermore, there were no significant differences in leukocyte, respectively, lymphocyte increase or distribution during NAT treatment depending on pretreatment use. NAT treatment led to counts even higher than predefined upper normal limit for leukocytes in 28.8% of the treated patients and for lymphocytes in 21.4% of treated patients. Persistent lymphopenia <1.5 GPT/L was not seen during NAT treatment in our cohort.

Other leukocyte subtypes including monocytes, eosinophils, and basophils were significantly elevated and again increased even higher than upper normal level (global time effect $p < 0.001$, **Figures 3C,E,F, Table 2**). These effects were persistent without significant fluctuations during the entire observation period in all treated patients. Interestingly, no changes were seen regarding absolute number and distribution of neutrophils during the whole observation period (global time effect $p = 0.863$, **Figure 3D, Table 2**). Additional evaluation of blood parameters including hemoglobin, hematocrit, erythrocyte count, and platelets demonstrated stable parameters in normal range during the 72 months evaluation period. Immature precursor cells including erythroblasts were detectable in 36.8% of the treated patients during NAT therapy, whereas none of these patients presented erythroblasts in the pretreatment period.

Effects on Distinct Lymphocyte Subsets and Its Intra-Individual Variation

In addition to complete blood count analysis, distinct lymphocyte subsets were evaluated. Absolute count of T cell subtypes presented in the physiological reference range in most of the patients before NAT start (**Figures 4A–C**). Only in single patients, T cells below lower normal limit could be identified (two patients without pretreatment, one patient with previous fingolimod treatment, one patient with previous interferon-beta treatment). Interestingly, evaluating predefined reference ranges for B cells and NK cells, most of the patients with lower lymphocyte count at baseline were associated with lower B cell and NK cell count at baseline as well (**Figures 4D,F**). All investigated cell subtypes including CD3+ T cells, CD4+ T cells, CD8+ T cells, CD19+ B cells, and NK cells, significantly increased after NAT initiation (global time effect $p < 0.001$, **Figures 4A–E, Table 2**). A higher portion of patients with a more intense increase of CD8+ T cells was seen compared to CD4+ T cells (**Figures 4A–C**). For CD4+ T cells, an increase >10% was seen in 94.2% of treated patients, an increase >20% was seen in 88.5% of treated patients, an increase >50% was seen in 61.5% of treated patients, and an increase >100% was seen in 23.1% of treated patients. In contrast for CD8+ T cells, an increase >10% was found in 96.2%, an increase >20% was found on 92.3% of patients, an increase >50% was seen in 80.8% of patients, and an increase >100% was found in

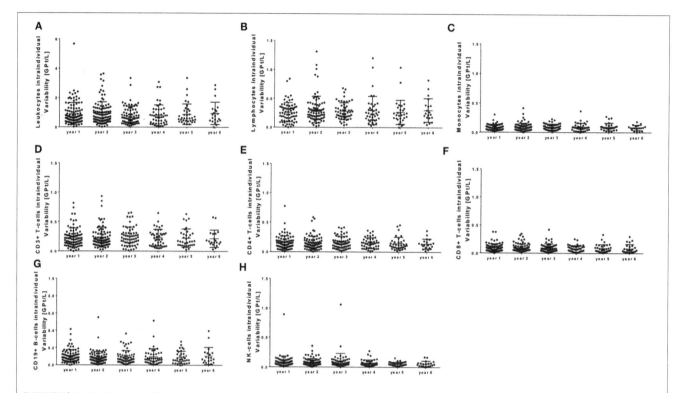

FIGURE 5 | Intra-individual variability of peripheral immune cell subsets during NAT treatment. Intra-individual variation of leukocytes **(A)**, lymphocytes **(B)**, monocytes **(C)**, CD3+ T cells **(D)**, CD4+ T cells **(E)**, CD8+ T cells **(F)**, CD19+ B cells **(G)**, and NK cells **(H)** are depicted for each year. Intra-individual variability was defined as the standard deviation of absolute cell counts every 3 months in every year after NAT start (starting at month 3). Mean ± standard deviation.

38.5% of NAT treated patients. Nevertheless, CD4/CD8 ratio was not significantly changed in our cohort during long-term NAT treatment (**Figure 4F**). Patients with increased CD4/CD8 ratio at baseline presented increased CD4/CD8 ratio during follow up as well. CD19+ B cells presented the most pronounced increase in their frequency distribution in almost all treated patients (**Figure 4D, Table 2**). Regarding CD19+ B cells, all patients increased more than 20%. An increase >50% was seen in 94.2% of treated patients and an increase >100% was seen in 86.5 % of treated patients. Additionally, NK cells markedly increased, remained in the reference range with stable levels during the whole period of investigation (**Figure 4E, Table 2**). An increase >20% was seen in 98.1% of treated patients, an increase >50% was seen in 90.4% of treated patients and an increase >100% was seen in 63.5% of treated patients.

There was a strong correlation between baseline count and relative increase for lymphocytes and its subtypes [r – (0.792 – 0.625); $p < 0.0001$], but no significant correlation between baseline count and absolute increase. Age [r – (0.221 – 0.109); $p > 0.05$] and different pretreatment conditions [r –(0.039 – 0.052); $p > 0.05$] could not predict changes and pattern of immune cell subtypes during NAT therapy. In addition, intra-individual variability of different immune cell subtypes was evaluated during NAT treatment (**Figure 5**). Intra-individual variability was defined as the standard deviation of absolute cell count every 3 months in every year after NAT start. Most pronounced variability was seen for the leukocyte count, whereas

lymphocytes and its subtypes varied only in a narrow range (**Figure 5**).

Reference to Clinical Parameters

The proportion of patients with or without disease activity and NEDA-3 status are presented in **Figure 2**. Evaluation of immune cell profiles in NEDA-3 positive patients vs. active patients could not confirm significant differences in the immune cell profile of leukocytes, lymphocytes, monocytes, T cell subsets, B cells, or NK cells during NAT treatment.

At NAT start, JCV antibody status was negative in 75 patients, positive in 19 patients, and unknown in 26 patients. During NAT treatment, 25.4% of JCV antibody negative patients switched to JCV antibody positive status. There were no cases of PML in our cohort. During the observation period, 39 patients stopped NAT treatment: 35 patients stopped because of positive JCV antibody status, three patients because of efficacy reasons and one patient because of the individual patient wish. Immune cell profile in patients that terminated NAT treatment was not statistically different to patients continuing NAT therapy.

Lymphocytes in a NAT Treated Patient With Neutralizing Antibodies Against NAT (nAbs)

This female patient was diagnosed RRMS in 02/2014 at an age of 25 years. In 05/2014 she started on dimethylfumarate treatment (**Figure 6A**). Due to side effects, treatment was changed to glatiramer acetate in 10/2015. In 03/2017 she suffered from a

TABLE 2 | Levels of statistical significance.

Time point	Leukocyte	Lymphocyte	Monocyte	Neutrophile granulocyte	Eosinophile granulocyte	Basophile granulocyte	CD3+ Tcell	CD4+ Tcell	CD8+ Tcell	CD19+ Bcell	NK cell
M0	6.73 (6.30; 7.18)	1.91 (1.78; 2.05)	0.53 (0.49; 0.57)	4.13 (3.77; 4.52)	0.13 (0.11; 0.16)	0.03 (0.02; 0.03)	1.41 (1.29; 1.54)	0.95 (0.85; 1.06)	0.42 (0.38; 0.47)	0.29 (0.25; 0.34)	0.18 (0.15; 0.20)
M3	8.37 (7.83; 8.95), $p < 0.001$	3.09 (2.87; 3.33), $P < 0.001$	0.67 (0.61; 0.73), $p = 0.005$	3.85 (3.51; 4.22), $P = 1.000$	0.34 (0.26; 0.45), $p = 0.001$	0.05 (0.04; 0.06), $P = 0.007$	2.29 (2.10; 2.50), $p < 0.001$	1.46 (1.32; 1.63), $p < 0.001$	0.77 (0.68; 0.88), $P < 0.001$	0.76 (0.66; 0.86), $p < 0.001$	0.36 (0.27; 0.47), $P = 0.011$
M6	8.56 (8.18; 9.03), $p < 0.001$	3.26 (3.07; 3.47), $P < 0.001$	0.69 (0.64; 0.74), $p < 0.001$	4.19 (3.81; 4.60), $P = 1.000$	0.34 (0.26; 0.44), $p = 0.001$	0.04 (0.04; 0.05), $p < 0.001$	2.29 (2.15; 2.43), $p < 0.001$	1.46 (1.36; 1.57), $p < 0.001$	0.75 (0.69; 0.82), $p < 0.001$	0.81 (0.74; 0.88), $p < 0.001$	0.37 (0.33; 0.40), $P < 0.001$
M9	8.74 (8.33; 9.18), $p < 0.001$	3.35 (3.17; 3.54), $P < 0.001$	0.71 (0.67; 0.75), $p < 0.001$	3.95 (3.67; 4.26), $P = 1.000$	0.34 (0.27; 0.42), $p < 0.001$	0.04 (0.04; 0.05), $p < 0.001$	2.33 (2.19; 2.47), $p < 0.001$	1.47 (1.38; 1.57), $p < 0.001$	0.78 (0.71; 0.85), $P < 0.001$	0.83 (0.76; 0.89), $p < 0.001$	0.41 (0.37; 0.45), $p < 0.001$
M12	8.77 (8.37; 9.18), $p < 0.001$	3.43 (3.25; 3.62), $P < 0.001$	0.71 (0.66; 0.76), $p < 0.001$	4.12 (3.78; 4.48), $P = 1.000$	0.36 (0.30; 0.43), $p < 0.001$	0.04 (0.04; 0.04), $P < 0.001$	2.35 (2.21; 2.51), $p < 0.001$	1.50 (1.40; 1.61), $p < 0.001$	0.78 (0.72; 0.85), $P < 0.001$	0.84 (0.77; 0.92), $p < 0.001$	0.39 (0.36; 0.43), $P < 0.001$
M24	8.86 (8.35; 9.41), $p < 0.001$	3.54 (3.31; 3.77), $P < 0.001$	0.69 (0.65; 0.73), $p < 0.001$	4.08 (3.69; 4.50), $P = 1.000$	0.33 (0.28; 0.38), $p < 0.001$	0.04 (0.04; 0.05), $p < 0.001$	2.33 (2.19; 2.49), $p < 0.001$	1.51 (1.40; 1.62), $p < 0.001$	0.77 (0.71; 0.84), $P < 0.001$	0.82 (0.76; 0.90), $p < 0.001$	0.40 (0.36; 0.45), $P < 0.001$
M48	8.57 (7.72; 9.51), $p = 0.010$	3.35 (2.98; 3.77), $P < 0.001$	0.74 (0.65; 0.84), $p < 0.001$	4.19 (3.49; 5.02), $P = 1.000$	0.29 (0.23; 0.37), $p = 0.001$	0.04 (0.03; 0.04), $p = 0.512$	2.16 (1.97; 2.37), $p < 0.001$	1.41 (1.26; 1.58), $p < 0.001$	0.70 (0.62; 0.78), $P < 0.001$	0.83 (0.68; 1.02), $p < 0.001$	0.32 (0.27; 0.38), $P = 0.001$
M60	9.04 (7.98; 10.24), $p = 0.006$	3.45 (3.07; 3.88), $P < 0.001$	0.73 (0.60; 0.88), $p = 0.193$	4.09 (3.31; 5.04), $P = 1.000$	0.35 (0.26; 0.47), $p = 0.002$	0.05 (0.04; 0.06), $P = 0.009$	2.27 (2.04; 2.53), $p < 0.001$	1.52 (1.33; 1.74), $p < 0.001$	0.71 (0.61; 0.83), $P < 0.001$	0.92 (0.68; 1.25), $p < 0.001$	0.36 (0.30; 0.43), $P < 0.001$
M72	8.73 (7.30; 10.43), $p = 0.448$	3.48 (2.64; 4.58), $p = 0.047$	0.69 (0.55; 0.88), $p = 1.000$	3.50 (2.76; 4.45), $P = 1.000$	0.30 (0.21; 0.42), $p = 0,051$	0.04 (0.03; 0.06), $P = 0.239$	2.26 (1.90; 2.69), $p = 0.002$	1.46 (1.22; 1.75), $p = 0.011$	0.78 (0.62; 0.99), $P = 0.006$	1.04 (0.62; 1.77), $p = 0.226$	0.34 (0.28; 0.412), $P = 0.001$

Mean and 95% confidence interval of each time-point of selected immune cell subsets. Level of significance with respective p-value (change compared to M0).

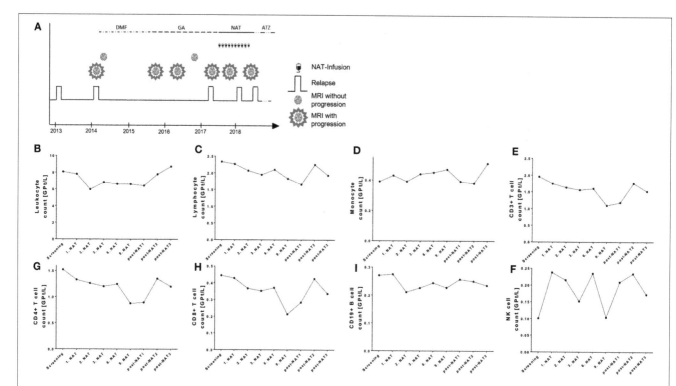

FIGURE 6 | Case presentation and course of peripheral immune cell subset in a NAT treated patient with positive nAbs. (A) Clinical data including relapse activity, MRI progression, and treatment conditions are presented. DMF, dimethylfumarate; GA, glatiramer acetate; NAT, natalizumab; ATZ, alemtuzumab. (B–I) Absolute cell count of leukocytes (B), lymphocytes (C), monocytes (D), CD3+ T cells (E), CD4+ T cells (F), CD8+ T cells (G), CD19+ B cells (H), and NK cells (I) are depicted. Data are shown for screening, NAT treatment period (1. NAT, 1st NAT infusion etc), and period after NAT cessation (post-NAT1, post-NAT2, post-NAT3; 1, 2, or 3 months after NAT stop).

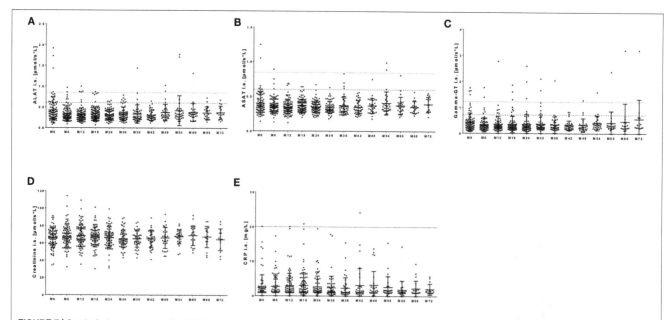

FIGURE 7 | Serological parameters during NAT treatment. Before each infusion started, blood samples were taken and analyzed in a certified medical laboratory. Analysis of serological parameters including ALAT (A), ASAT (B), gamma-GT (C), creatinine (D), and CRP (E) were included. Data are shown for baseline analysis (M0) and sixth months follow up (M6, M12, […], M72). Data are presented as mean ± standard deviation. Dotted line indicates the reverence range for men for ALAT and ASAT at a value of 0.85 μmol/s*L and for gamma-GT at 1.2 μmol/s*L. Broken line indicates reverence range for women for ALAT and ASAT at a value of 0.6 μmol/s*L and for gamma-GT at 0.7 μmol/s*L. There were no statistical significant changes.

severe relapse and cerebral MRI scan demonstrated new T2 lesions. JCV index was negative and first NAT infusion was performed in 06/2017. After 4 months, cerebral MRI scan presented two new T2 lesions. NAT infusions were continued. In 01/2018 after the 8. NAT infusion, the patient suffered again of an acute relapse that was treated with corticosteroids. Testing and re-testing of antibodies against NAT (nAbs) was done and high titers of nAbs were confirmed in 02/2018 and 03/2018 (testing was performed at the Department of Neurology, University Hospital Bochum, Prof. Dr. R. Gold). Evaluation of JCV index in 11/2017 and 04/2018 presented again negative results. MRI scan presented progress of >10 new T2 lesions in 05/2018. NAT treatment was stopped and treatment with alemtuzumab was started in 06/2018 (**Figure 6**).

Evaluation of blood cell count demonstrated that in contrast to our cohort presented above leukocytes and lymphocytes were not relevantly changed after starting NAT treatment in this patient (**Figures 6B,C**). Lymphocytes and its subsets were not increased during the NAT treatment and did not change in the post-treatment period as well (**Figures 6E,F**). We assume that nAbs developed quite early after NAT start. This case report demonstrates that real world lab data can potentially identify patients with nAbs development to NAT.

Standard Serological Parameters During NAT Treatment

Standard serological parameters were measured every 3 months as well (**Figure 7**). In most of the patients, liver enzymes including alanine aminotransferase (ALAT), aspartate aminotransferase (ASAT), and gamma-Glutamyltransferase (gamma-GT) demonstrated levels in the reference range over the whole observation period (**Figures 7A–C**). Nevertheless, out of our 120 patients few patients presented with transient and asymptomatic increase of ALAT, ASAT or gamma-GT (**Figures 7A–C**). After NAT initiation, ALAT levels were increased once during the whole observation period but reached reference range at re-test in 16 patients. Seven patients presented with repeated increase of ALAT level. In nine patients increased ASAT levels were seen once during NAT treatment with normalized values at re-testing. One patient presented repeated increase of ASAT levels threw observation. None of these patients reached levels >3x upper normal limit for ASAT, and only one patient reached levels >3x upper normal limit for ALAT, but presented with normalized values after re-test. (**Figures 7A,B**). Gamma-GT was elevated in 21 patients during NAT therapy. Elevation of gamma-GT was transient and appeared only once in eight of the investigated patients. In 13 patients, repeated elevations of gamma-GT levels were seen. Only three patients presented with gamma-GT levels >3x upper normal limit. This increase was asymptomatic and without any clinical significance.

Kidney function parameters including creatinine (**Figure 7D**) as well as sodium and potassium levels (data not shown) remained stable within physiological ranges in most of the patients. Only few patients appeared with transient elevation in creatinine levels at least once during NAT therapy in our cohort (**Figure 7D**). Creatinine levels lower than physiological reference ranged appeared primarily in immobilized patients and did not reflect any clinical relevance (**Figure 7D**). CRP levels ≥20

mg/dL were defined as clinical significant. In our observation, almost all patients presented with normal CRP levels during the whole observation period (**Figure 7E**). Nevertheless, 10 patients presented with an increase in CRP up to 144 mg/dL during NAT therapy. Six of these 10 patients showed clinical symptoms of an infection. At onset of CRP increase, six of these 10 patients suffered from respiratory tract infection that resolved during follow up. In four of these patients, CRP increase was paralleled by clinical significant increase of leukocyte but not lymphocyte count.

DISCUSSION

In our longitudinal observational study, we systematically collected real world lab data including specific immune cell subsets and routine laboratory parameters in NAT treated patients during long-term NAT treatment. Upon NAT treated patients, there are a huge amount of reports available discussing long period outcome and clinical parameters including relapse rate, MRI-activity, and disease progression presenting long-term efficacy (28–30), whereas analyses of immune cell subsets and standard lab analyses are restricted only up to 24–48 months follow up (15, 23, 24). Compared to previous studies, we analyzed a representative large number of patients for a treatment period up to 6 years. Our cohort demonstrated the excellent clinical effectiveness of NAT in the real world scenario as well. NAT selectively directs the α4 subunit of VLA-4 on the surface of leukocytes (2). The interplay of VLA-4 on white blood cells and VCAM-1 expressed on endothelial cells enables peripheral immune cells to cross the blood-brain barrier and boosting CNS inflammation as known in MS pathology (1, 31). While NAT treatment, leukocyte extravasation especially into the CNS is inhibited and immune cells are sequestered in peripheral blood (13, 21). In line with previous data, our results confirm early increase of peripheral lymphocyte subsets in NAT treated patients (21, 22, 24, 32, 33). Additionally we demonstrate an early and persistent biological response of NAT treatment in different leukocyte subsets over the entire period of 6 years evaluation. Interestingly, pretreatment conditions could not predict the course of leukocytes and lymphocytes after NAT start in our cohort, baseline leukocyte and lymphocyte count was correlated with relative but not absolute increase. Regarding lymphocyte subsets, increase of CD8+ and CD19+ lymphocytes was most pronounced and especially CD19+ B cells were higher than normal level in most of the treated patients. These data were also reported by others (24, 33). Previous observations confirmed the relevance of VLA-4 also on B cells for the CNS recruitment and inflammation in MS pathogenesis (34). Though selective inhibition of VLA-4 dependent B cells may contributes to the efficacy during NAT therapy (34). The risk of nAbs development during NAT therapy is a well-known phenomenon and may interfere with NAT efficacy (35). Here we demonstrate that the typical immunological effects in the periphery are missing in a patient with nAbs to NAT. Though, even standard blood count can probably assist to identify insufficient impact of NAT treatment and to consider further testing. Of course, this has to be systematically proven in a larger cohort.

Previous studies presented various expression levels of VLA-4 on different lymphocyte subtypes with higher levels on B lymphocytes than on T lymphocytes and also more pronounced on CD8+ T cells than on CD4+ T cells (21, 32, 36). Though, the VLA-4/VCAM-1 mediated transmigration of immune cells is differently affected among different peripheral immune cells in NAT treated patients that lead to different sequestration in peripheral blood. Additional to peripheral lymphocyte sequestration due to impaired transmigration mechanisms, effects on the lymphocyte release from bone marrow are discussed (11, 12, 14, 16). Different studies presented mobilization of hematopoietic lymphoid precursor cells from the bone marrow by NAT mediated blocking of retention signals (11, 12, 14). In the line with this, an increase in erythroblasts was seen as well in our cohort. This mobilization additionally contributes to increase of circulating B cells especially with naïve and memory phenotype in NAT treated patients (16). Furthermore, NAT-associated but not clinically relevant morphologic changes in lymphocytes have been described defined by enhanced fraction of atypical lymphocytes (37, 38).

During our observation, CD4/CD8 ratio did not change during the entire period of therapy compared to baseline. These findings are comparable with other results of shorter evaluation periods (24), whereas some early reports presented a decrease in CD4/CD8 ratio suggesting increased risk of opportunistic infections including PML in such patients (23, 39). These studies were usually characterized by smaller samples size and shorter period of evaluation compared to our analysis. In our cohort, NAT lead to increase and re-distribution of peripheral immune cell subsets, which happened early and remained constant without relevant variation during the whole period of 6 years evaluation. Although some immune cell subsets increased out of reference range, no serious adverse events including severe infections or opportunistic infections appeared, no malignancies, or hematological abnormalities were detectable.

Additionally to T and B cell subsets, NK cells increased early directly after NAT initiation. In comparison with other lymphocyte subtypes, NK cells presented one of the most pronounced increases in periphery. These data are in line with other observations that additionally discussed a link between increase of NK cells and response during NAT treatment (21, 24, 40, 41). Here we show, that NAT induced changes in NK cell count persist even years after treatment initiation possible additionally contributing to efficacy in long-term treatment.

Monocytes, eosinophils, and basophils showed a lower but significant increase. In contrast to another study in which monocytes steadily increased over the whole observational period (15), in our analysis monocyte cell count increased to a constant level already after 1 month of treatment start and kept stable. Blocking VLA-4 by NAT leads to sequestration of monocytes and granulocyte subsets in peripheral blood, but does not affect migration of myeloid progenitor cells as seen for the lymphoid progenitors described above (42). These aspects may explain the moderate increase in monocytes and granulocyte subsets compared to lymphocytes. No significant changes were seen in cell count and distribution of neutrophils. Neutrophils do not express VLA-4, therefore,

NAT does not affect its distribution (15, 43). Furthermore, we confirmed stable hematological parameters including erythrocyte count, hemoglobin, hematocrit, and platelet count during longterm evaluation of NAT treatment (15). In our evaluation, no association between the distribution of peripheral immune cell subsets and clinical disease activity parameters during NAT treatment could be found. The immune cell phenotyping presented in our study is part of the routine lab testing in our treated MS patients and is characterized by limitations in comparison to more detailed immune cell profiling as presented in other immune profiling studies using e.g., high-dimensional cytometry (44). These studies are more complex in immune cell profiling techniques but may elucidate more details in immune cell patterns and clinical response.

Although controlled data regarding peripheral immune cell subsets within first years of NAT treatment are available, reports on standard testing of serological parameters especially in long-term evaluation are missing. Based on the known excellent safety profile of NAT, hepatic, or kidney dysfunction is not common. Nevertheless, frequent testing of routine lab parameters is recommended and part of the monitoring program applied in NAT treated patients (45). During our observation period of 6 years, there were no relevant or long lasting abnormalities in serological testing of liver enzymes or kidney function. In general, patients presented these parameters in physiological ranges with rare, only transient and not clinical significant increases during the whole period of NAT treatment. Evaluation of CRP levels is a helpful tool to define infectious conditions. NAT therapy does not impair variation of CRP levels as seen by other MS treatments e.g., after alemtuzumab initiation (46, 47). In our cohort, only few patients with transient increase of CRP levels were found. In six out of ten patients with increased CRP levels, a clinical relevant infection was apparent. These data are important to demonstrate that evaluation of CRP levels maybe a helpful tool to identify acute infections even in NAT treated patients when changes in peripheral blood cells are a common phenomenon.

Here, we presented real world lab data on NAT demonstrating the consistent and safe impact of NAT on peripheral immune cell subsets and routine lab parameters within real world conditions and everyday clinical practice. We have already shown the value of real world lab data for fingolimod recently (48). Patients included in our investigation have a different clinical profile compared to those included in randomized clinical trials with limiting inclusion criteria allowing the assessment of real world lab data. The broad and unselected patient population is a great advantage of our study, which does represent the common patient in daily clinical practice. Because of the differences in disease duration, previous medication use and various pre-existing conditions, they describe the real world patient population best. Nevertheless, differences in monitoring procedures and data collection in different centers impact the quality and comparability of such real world data (17). Standardized treatment protocols and monitoring tools (e.g., the MSDS3D software approach) can assist to achieve comparable requirements for patient care as well as data collection even at multiple centers and in every-day clinical practice (18). So NAT real world data on pregnancy are available (49). This standardized collection of real world data and observational studies providing longitudinal information on drug profile and different outcomes in real life are essential to improve decision-making and optimize treatment management.

AUTHOR CONTRIBUTIONS

KA and TZ study concept and design. MK acquisition of data. MK, KA, and RH analysis and interpretation of data. MK, KA,

and TZ drafting of the manuscript. UP and RH critical revision of the manuscript for important intellectual content. RH and MK statistical analysis.

ACKNOWLEDGMENTS

We are grateful to Prof. Dr. T. Chavakis from the Institute of Clinical Chemistry and Laboratory Medicine, University Clinic Dresden for performing the analysis and providing the data. We acknowledge support by the Open Access Publication Funds of the SLUB/TU Dresden.

REFERENCES

1. Elices MJ, Osborn L, Takada Y, Crouse C, Luhowskyj S, Hemler ME, et al. VCAM-1 on activated endothelium interacts with the leukocyte integrin VLA-4 at a site distinct from the VLA-4/fibronectin binding site. *Cell* (1990) 60:577–84. doi: 10.1016/0092-8674(90)90661-W
2. Yednock TA, Cannon C, Fritz LC, Sanchez-Madrid F, Steinman L, Karin N. Prevention of experimental autoimmune encephalomyelitis by antibodies against alpha 4 beta 1 integrin. *Nature* (1992) 356:63–6. doi: 10.1038/356063a0
3. Lobb RR, Hemler ME. The pathophysiologic role of alpha 4 integrins *in vivo*. *J Clin Invest.* (1994) 94:1722–8. doi: 10.1172/JCI117519
4. Sehr T, Proschmann U, Thomas K, Marggraf M, Straube E, Reichmann H, et al. New insights into the pharmacokinetics and pharmacodynamics of natalizumab treatment for patients with multiple sclerosis, obtained from clinical and *in vitro* studies. *J Neuroinflammation* (2016) 13:164. doi: 10.1186/s12974-016-0635-2
5. Skarica M, Eckstein C, Whartenby KA, Calabresi PA. Novel mechanisms of immune modulation of natalizumab in multiple sclerosis patients. *J Neuroimmunol.* (2011) 235:70–6. doi: 10.1016/j.jneuroim.2011.02.010
6. Polman CH, O'connor PW, Havrdova E, Hutchinson M, Kappos L, Miller DH, et al. A randomized, placebo-controlled trial of natalizumab for relapsing multiple sclerosis. *N Engl J Med.* (2006) 354:899–910. doi: 10.1056/NEJMoa044397
7. Rudick RA, Stuart WH, Calabresi PA, Confavreux C, Galetta SL, Radue EW, et al. Natalizumab plus interferon beta-1a for relapsing multiple sclerosis. *N Engl J Med* (2006) 354:911–23. doi: 10.1056/NEJMoa044396
8. Bloomgren G, Richman S, Hotermans C, Subramanyam M, Goelz S, Natarajan A, et al. Risk of natalizumab-associated progressive multifocal leukoencephalopathy. *N Engl J Med.* (2012) 366:1870–80. doi: 10.1056/NEJMoa1107829
9. Gorelik L, Lerner M, Bixler S, Crossman M, Schlain B, Simon K, et al. Anti-JC virus antibodies: implications for PML risk stratification. *Ann Neurol.* (2010) 68:295–303. doi: 10.1002/ana.22128
10. Ziemssen T, Gass A, Wuerfel J, Bayas A, Tackenberg B, Limmroth V, et al. Design of TRUST, a non-interventional, multicenter, 3-year prospective study investigating an integrated patient management approach in patients with relapsing-remitting multiple sclerosis treated with natalizumab. *BMC Neurol.* (2016) 16:98. doi: 10.1186/s12883-016-0625-0
11. Bonig H, Wundes A, Chang KH, Lucas S, Papayannopoulou T. Increased numbers of circulating hematopoietic stem/progenitor cells are chronically maintained in patients treated with the CD49d blocking antibody natalizumab. *Blood* (2008) 111:3439–41. doi: 10.1182/blood-2007-09-112052
12. Zohren F, Toutzaris D, Klarner V, Hartung HP, Kieseier B, Haas R. The monoclonal anti-VLA-4 antibody natalizumab mobilizes CD34+ hematopoietic progenitor cells in humans. *Blood* (2008) 111:3893–5. doi: 10.1182/blood-2007-10-120329

13. Kivisakk P, Healy BC, Viglietta V, Quintana FJ, Hootstein MA, Weiner HL, et al. Natalizumab treatment is associated with peripheral sequestration of proinflammatory T cells. *Neurology* (2009) 72:1922–30. doi: 10.1212/WNL.0b013e3181a8266f
14. Jing D, Oelschlaegel U, Ordemann R, Holig K, Ehninger G, Reichmann H, et al. CD49d blockade by natalizumab in patients with multiple sclerosis affects steady-state hematopoiesis and mobilizes progenitors with a distinct phenotype and function. *Bone Marrow Transplant.* (2010) 45:1489–96. doi: 10.1038/bmt.2009.381
15. Bridel C, Beauverd Y, Samii K, Lalive PH. Hematologic modifications in natalizumab-treated multiple sclerosis patients: an 18-month longitudinal study. *Neurol Neuroimmunol Neuroinflamm.* (2015) 2:e123. doi: 10.1212/NXI.0000000000000123
16. Mattoscio M, Nicholas R, Sormani MP, Malik O, Lee JS, Waldman AD, et al. Hematopoietic mobilization: potential biomarker of response to natalizumab in multiple sclerosis. *Neurology* (2015) 84:1473–82. doi: 10.1212/WNL.0000000000001454
17. Ziemssen T, Hillert J, Butzkueven H. The importance of collecting structured clinical information on multiple sclerosis. *BMC Med.* (2016) 14:81. doi: 10.1186/s12916-016-0627-1
18. Haase R, Wunderlich M, Dillenseger A, Kern R, Akgun K, Ziemssen T. Improving multiple sclerosis management and collecting safety information in the real world: the MSDS3D software approach. *Expert Opin Drug Saf.* (2018) 17:369–78. doi: 10.1080/14740338.2018.1437144
19. Ziemssen T, Kempcke R, Eulitz M, Grossmann L, Suhrbier A, Thomas K, et al. Multiple sclerosis documentation system (MSDS): moving from documentation to management of MS patients. *J Neural Transm.* (2013) 120:S61–6. doi: 10.1007/s00702-013-1041-x
20. Miller DH, Khan OA, Sheremata WA, Blumhardt LD, Rice GP, Libonati MA, et al. A controlled trial of natalizumab for relapsing multiple sclerosis. *N Engl J Med.* (2003) 348:15–23. doi: 10.1056/NEJMoa020696
21. Putzki N, Baranwal MK, Tettenborn B, Limmroth V, Kreuzfelder E. Effects of natalizumab on circulating B cells, T regulatory cells and natural killer cells. *Eur Neurol.* (2010) 63:311–7. doi: 10.1159/000302687
22. Zanotti C, Chiarini M, Serana F, Sottini A, Garrafa E, Torri F, et al. Peripheral accumulation of newly produced T and B lymphocytes in natalizumab-treated multiple sclerosis patients. *Clin Immunol.* (2012) 145:19–26. doi: 10.1016/j.clim.2012.07.007
23. Marousi S, Karkanis I, Kalamatas T, Travasarou M, Paterakis G, Karageorgiou CE. Immune cells after prolonged Natalizumab therapy: implications for effectiveness and safety. *Acta Neurol Scand.* (2013) 128:e1–5. doi: 10.1111/ane.12080
24. Koudriavtseva T, Sbardella E, Trento E, Bordignon V, D'agosto G, Cordiali-Fei P. Long-term follow-up of peripheral lymphocyte subsets in a cohort

of multiple sclerosis patients treated with natalizumab. *Clin Exp Immunol.* (2014) 176:320–6. doi: 10.1111/cei.12261

25. Polman CH, Reingold SC, Banwell B, Clanet M, Cohen JA, Filippi M, et al. Diagnostic criteria for multiple sclerosis: 2010 revisions to the McDonald criteria. *Ann Neurol.* (2011) 69:292–302. doi: 10.1002/ana.22366

26. Kurtzke JF. Rating neurologic impairment in multiple sclerosis: an expanded disability status scale (EDSS). *Neurology* (1983) 33:1444–52. doi: 10.1212/WNL.33.11.1444

27. Kknms A. (ed.). *Qualitätshandbuch MS/NMOSD Empfehlungen zur Therapie der Multiple Sklerose Neuro- myelitis-optica-Spektrum- Erkrankungen für Ärzte* (2017).

28. Hoepner R, Faissner S, Salmen A, Gold R, Chan A. Efficacy and side effects of natalizumab therapy in patients with multiple sclerosis. *J Cent Nerv Syst Dis.* (2014) 6:41–9. doi: 10.4137/JCNSD.S14049

29. Van Pesch V, Sindic CJ, Fernandez O. Effectiveness and safety of natalizumab in real-world clinical practice: review of observational studies. *Clin Neurol Neurosurg.* (2016) 149:55–63. doi: 10.1016/j.clineuro.2016.07.001

30. Shirani A, Stuve O. Natalizumab for multiple sclerosis: a case in point for the impact of translational neuroimmunology. *J Immunol.* (2017) 198:1381–6. doi: 10.4049/jimmunol.1601358

31. Hickey WF. Migration of hematogenous cells through the blood-brain barrier and the initiation of CNS inflammation. *Brain Pathol.* (1991) 1:97–105. doi: 10.1111/j.1750-3639.1991.tb00646.x

32. Niino M, Bodner C, Simard ML, Alatab S, Gano D, Kim HJ, et al. Natalizumab effects on immune cell responses in multiple sclerosis. *Ann Neurol.* (2006) 59:748–54. doi: 10.1002/ana.20859

33. Krumbholz M, Meinl I, Kumpfel T, Hohlfeld R, Meinl E. Natalizumab disproportionately increases circulating pre-B and B cells in multiple sclerosis. *Neurology* (2008) 71:1350–4. doi: 10.1212/01.wnl.0000327671.91357.96

34. Lehmann-Horn K, Sagan SA, Bernard CC, Sobel RA, Zamvil SS. B-cell very late antigen-4 deficiency reduces leukocyte recruitment and susceptibility to central nervous system autoimmunity. *Ann Neurol.* (2015) 77:902–8. doi: 10.1002/ana.24387

35. Vennegoor A, Rispens T, Strijbis EM, Seewann A, Uitdehaag BM, Balk LJ, et al. Clinical relevance of serum natalizumab concentration and anti-natalizumab antibodies in multiple sclerosis. *Mult Scler.* (2013) 19:593–600. doi: 10.1177/1352458512460604

36. Ryan DH, Nuccie BL, Abboud CN, Winslow JM. Vascular cell adhesion molecule-1 and the integrin VLA-4 mediate adhesion of human B cell precursors to cultured bone marrow adherent cells. *J Clin Invest.* (1991) 88:995–1004. doi: 10.1172/JCI115403

37. Leclerc M, Lesesve JF, Gaillard B, Troussard X, Tourbah A, Debouverie M, et al. Binucleated lymphocytes in patients with multiple sclerosis treated with natalizumab. *Leuk Lymphoma* (2011) 52:910–2. doi: 10.3109/10428194.2010.551156

38. Robier C, Amouzadeh-Ghadikolai O, Bregant C, Diez J, Melinz K, Quehenberger F, et al. The frequency of occurrence of atypical lymphocytes in peripheral blood smears of natalizumab-treated patients with multiple sclerosis. *Int J Lab Hematol.* (2017) 39:469–74. doi: 10.1111/ijlh.12662

39. Stuve O, Marra CM, Bar-Or A, Niino M, Cravens PD, Cepok S, et al. Altered CD4+/CD8+ T-cell ratios in cerebrospinal fluid of natalizumab-treated patients with multiple sclerosis. *Arch Neurol.* (2006) 63:1383–7. doi: 10.1001/archneur.63.10.1383

40. Mellergard J, Edstrom M, Jenmalm MC, Dahle C, Vrethem M, Ernerudh J. Increased B cell and cytotoxic NK cell proportions and increased T cell responsiveness in blood of natalizumab-treated multiple sclerosis patients. *PLoS ONE* (2013) 8:e81685. doi: 10.1371/journal.pone.0081685

41. Caruana P, Lemmert K, Ribbons K, Lea R, Lechner-Scott J. Natural killer cell subpopulations are associated with MRI activity in a relapsing-remitting multiple sclerosis patient cohort from Australia. *Mult Scler.* (2016) 23:1479–1487. doi: 10.1177/1352458516679267

42. Planas R, Jelcic I, Schippling S, Martin R, Sospedra M. Natalizumab treatment perturbs memory- and marginal zone-like B-cell homing in secondary lymphoid organs in multiple sclerosis. *Eur J Immunol.* (2012) 42:790–8. doi: 10.1002/eji.201142108

43. Bochner BS, Luscinskas FW, Gimbrone MA Jr, Newman W, Sterbinsky SA, Derse-Anthony CP, et al. Adhesion of human basophils, eosinophils, and neutrophils to interleukin 1-activated human vascular endothelial cells: contributions of endothelial cell adhesion molecules. *J Exp Med.* (1991) 173:1553–7. doi: 10.1084/jem.173.6.1553

44. Lohmann L, Janoschka C, Schulte-Mecklenbeck A, Klinsing S, Kirstein L, Hanning U, et al. Immune cell profiling during switching from natalizumab to fingolimod reveals differential effects on systemic immune-regulatory networks and on trafficking of non-t cell populations into the cerebrospinal fluid-results from the tofingo successor study. *Front Immunol.* (2018). 9:1560. doi: 10.3389/fimmu.2018.01560

45. Klotz L, Berthele A, Bruck W, Chan A, Flachenecker P, Gold R, et al. Monitoring of blood parameters under course-modified MS therapy. Substance-specific relevance and current recommendations for action. *Nervenarzt* (2016) 87:645–59. doi: 10.1007/s00115-016-0077-1

46. Targan SR, Feagan BG, Fedorak RN, Lashner BA, Panaccione R, Present DH, et al. Natalizumab for the treatment of active Crohn's disease: results of the ENCORE Trial. *Gastroenterology* (2007) 132:1672–83. doi: 10.1053/j.gastro.2007.03.024

47. Thomas K, Eisele J, Rodriguez-Leal FA, Hainke U, Ziemssen T. Acute effects of alemtuzumab infusion in patients with active relapsing-remitting MS. *Neurol Neuroimmunol Neuroinflamm.* (2016) 3:e228. doi: 10.1212/NXI.0000000000000228

48. Kaufmann M, Haase R, Proschmann U, Ziemssen T, Akgün K. Real world lab data: Patterns of lymphocyte counts in fingolimod treated patients. *Frontiers in Immunology* (2018) 9: 460–11. doi: 10.3389/fimmu.2018.02669

49. Proschmann U, Thomas K, Thiel S, Hellwig K, Ziemssen T. Natalizumab during pregnancy and lactation. *Multiple Sclerosis* (2018) 24:1627–34. doi: 10.1177/1352458517728813

3

Quantitative EEG and Verbal Fluency in DBS Patients: Comparison of Stimulator-On and -Off Conditions

Florian Hatz[1], Antonia Meyer[1], Anne Roesch[1], Ethan Taub[2], Ute Gschwandtner[1] and Peter Fuhr[1]*

[1] Department of Neurology, Hospitals of University of Basel, Basel, Switzerland, [2] Department of Neurosurgery, Hospitals of University of Basel, Basel, Switzerland

*Correspondence:
Peter Fuhr
peter.fuhr@usb.ch

Introduction: Deep brain stimulation of the subthalamic nucleus (STN-DBS) ameliorates motor function in patients with Parkinson's disease and allows reducing dopaminergic therapy. Beside effects on motor function STN-DBS influences many non-motor symptoms, among which decline of verbal fluency test performance is most consistently reported. The surgical procedure itself is the likely cause of this decline, while the influence of the electrical stimulation is still controversial. STN-DBS also produces widespread changes of cortical activity as visualized by quantitative EEG. The present study aims to link an alteration in verbal fluency performance by electrical stimulation of the STN to alterations in quantitative EEG.

Methods: Sixteen patients with STN-DBS were included. All patients had a high density EEG recording (256 channels) while testing verbal fluency in the stimulator on/off situation. The phonemic, semantic, alternating phonemic and semantic fluency was tested (Regensburger Wortflüssigkeits-Test).

Results: On the group level, stimulation of STN did not alter verbal fluency performance. EEG frequency analysis showed an increase of relative alpha2 (10–13 Hz) and beta (13–30 Hz) power in the parieto-occipital region ($p \leq 0.01$). On the individual level, changes of verbal fluency induced by stimulation of the STN were disparate and correlated inversely with delta power in the left temporal lobe ($p < 0.05$).

Conclusion: STN stimulation does not alter verbal fluency performance in a systematic way at group level. However, when in individual patients an alteration of verbal fluency performance is produced by electrical stimulation of the STN, it correlates inversely with left temporal delta power.

Keywords: Parkinson, DBS, quantitative EEG, automated artifact removal, verbal fluency

INTRODUCTION

Deep brain stimulation of the subthalamic nucleus (STN-DBS) is widely used in advanced Parkinson's disease (PD) to treat motor complications. The subthalamic nucleus is the preferred target for DBS in most cases (1). STN-DBS improves motor manifestations in the limbs, while axial motor manifestations and language are improved variably, to a lesser extent, or not at all (2).

As for neuropsychological performance, verbal fluency (VF) performance is reportedly impaired by STN-DBS (3–7), while there is less evidence for GPi-DBS causing a decline in VF (8). The pathophysiological reason for this decline is still in debate (8). Chouiter et al. found that lesions by stroke or tumor of the left basal ganglia impair semantic and phonemic VF performance (9). However, to our current knowledge there is no study showing a direct long-term effect of precise microsurgical placement of electrodes on neuropsychological capacity. Interestingly, in a study by Isler et al. (10) reduction in cognitive flexibility after microsurgical penetration of the caudate nucleus recovered after 12 months. Anatomical studies in non-human primates have yielded evidence of a subdivision of the STN into a motor portion, an associative portion, and a smaller limbic portion (11, 12), while the associative portion is highly connected to the dorsolateral prefrontal and lateral orbitofrontal cortex. STN stimulation lessens the amount of language-related basal ganglia output via the thalamus and thus reduces thalamo-cortical drive (13). As striatal dysfunction is thought to induce set-shifting deficits by way of secondary dysfunction of the prefrontal cortex (4), this may partly account for decrease of VF after DBS. While it has been shown that the decline of VF after STN-DBS is an effect of the surgical procedure/perioperative activities (14), the influence of the electrical stimulation on VF performance is still controversial.

Both, the temporal and frontal lobes are involved in semantic and phonemic fluency tests. The left hemisphere is generally more important for VF than the right, and frontal lobes are more relevant for phonemic than for semantic fluency (15, 16).

Reduction of VF performance correlates with a reduction of median frequency or an increase of relative power in lower frequency bands in EEG (17).

In this study we aim to characterize the STN-stimulation-related changes in semantic, phonemic, and alternating fluency tasks and quantitative EEG (QEEG) measures (band powers, median frequency) in a group of PD patients. As VF is reduced by DBS, potentially by the stimulation itself, and as changes in VF performance are linked to frontal and temporal lobes, we expect a reduction of VF performance in the DBS-on compared to the DBS-off condition along with an increase of lower band power in frontal and temporal lobes.

METHODS

Patients

Eighteen patients with STN-DBS were included. Sixteen completed the study protocol and were included in the analysis. Fifteen patients were right-handed and one was ambidextrous. Subjects characteristics are shown in **Table 1**. All of them underwent high-density resting-state EEG recordings (256 channels) and testing of VF in the DBS-on and DBS-off conditions. The phonemic, semantic, alternating phonemic, and alternating semantic fluency was evaluated RWT, Regensburger Wortflüssigkeits-Test, 2 min testing per task, no counting of errors, (18). Median age was 68.0 (IQR 60–71), 9 males and 7 females. Median duration of education was 14 years (IQR 12–16.5). Median years after first symptoms of PD were 12.5 (IQR 10.75–19). Patients were included 32 months (IQR 26–58) after

TABLE 1 | Subjects characteristics.

Age (years)	68.0 (59.2–71.8)
Education (years)	14 (12–16.5)
Years since diagnosis of PD (years)	12.5 (10.75–19)
Levodopa-equivalence-dose (mg)	562 (219–798)
Duration since DBS implantation (months)	32 (25.75–58.25)

Median values and lower/upper quartiles are shown.

STN-DBS operation and had a median levodopa equivalents dose of 562 (IQR 219–798).

EEG Recording

After initial testing of VF performance, QEEGs from all patients were initially recorded with the DBS-on. For EEG recordings a 256-channel Geodesic DC-EEG System 300 was used. Sampling rate was set to 1,000 Hz, first high pass filter to 0.01 Hz. Impedances of EEG electrodes were kept below 40 kΩ. Subjects were seated comfortably in a reclining chair in a dimly lit, sound attenuated and electromagnetically shielded room. They were instructed to relax, but to stay awake and to minimize eye and body movements. After 12 min recording DBS was turned off and QEEG was recorded for additional 12 min, followed by VF testing. As for all subjects in the study STN-DBS consisted in a monopolar stimulation.

EEG Post-processing

DBS-stimulation generates an artifact of considerably larger amplitude than the intrinsic brain signal recorded by EEG (19); the latter can only be analyzed once the former has been removed. Different methods of artifact removal have been proposed. The method described by Sun et al. for subtracting a reconstructed artifact is difficult to apply to real-life data (20). Lio et al. applied a combination of low-pass filter and a frequency-domain filter tracking outliers (21). Santillan-Guzman et al. proposed a temporal-frequency-domain filter (22). This method takes advantage of the known frequency characteristics of the artifact but does not exploit the similarity of signal shape at all of the recording electrodes due to the effect of volume conduction. We therefore used principal-component analysis to delete the first component, followed by an independent component analysis. These components were averaged using the DBS artifact as a trigger, and components with remaining signals after averaging were eliminated. Finally a 70 Hz low-pass filter (high-order, least-square filter) was applied (**Figure 1**). All steps for DBS-artifact elimination were integrated and performed in the toolbox "TAPEEG" (23), allowing fully automated artifact removal. Visually, frequency spectra for every patient in the ON- and OFF-condition were compared, showing a convincing reduction/elimination of the DBS artifact (**Supplemental Figure 1**).

Inverse Solution (Frequency Domain)

Using a previously published method (24), resulting EEG data was re-referenced to average reference and bad channels were interpolated with spherical spline method. Power spectra were calculated from epochs of 4 s duration (spectral resolution 0.25 Hz) using Welch's method (20, 25). Source-space data was

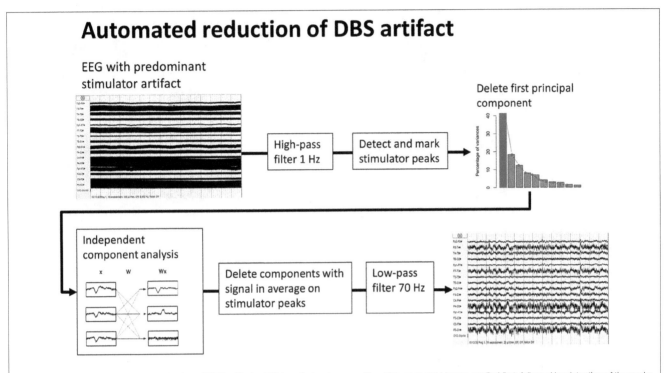

FIGURE 1 | Workflow of automated reduction of DBS artifacts. A high-order least-square filter, high-pass at 1 Hz was applied first, followed by detection of the peaks of the stimulator artifacts. Second, a principal-component analysis was performed. A large part of the stimulator artifact is accounted for by the first principal component. This component was then deleted and the EEG reconstructed. Third, after an independent component analysis, all resulting components were averaged on the previously detected peaks for identification of the components, including DBS artifacts. These components were deleted and, again, the EEG was reconstructed. Finally, a high order least-square filter, low-pass at 70 Hz, was applied.

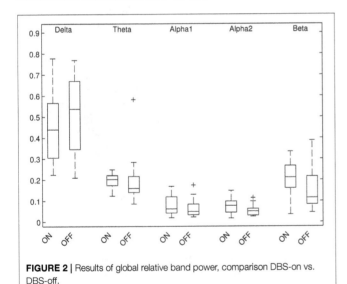

FIGURE 2 | Results of global relative band power, comparison DBS-on vs. DBS-off.

calculated by LORETA inverse solution for spectral data as described by Frei et al. (26), using a vector transposition matrix calculated with the software-package Cartool (27), based on the MNI brain atlas (28) and without using a normalization. The calculation was achieved using 5,011 solution points with subsequent reduction to 78 regions of interest (ROIs) based on the AAL atlas (29). According to previous studies by our group, median frequency and relative power in the delta- (1–4 Hz),

theta- (4–8 Hz), alpha1- (8–10 Hz), alpha2- (10–13 Hz) and beta- (13–30 Hz) bands were calculated.

Statistics

The relative band powers, median frequencies, and results of VF testing in the DBS-on and DBS-off conditions were compared with paired t-tests. The changes in relative power and VF tests were calculated ("value DBS-on" minus "value DBS-off") and Spearman rank correlations calculated. Due to large intersubject power differences, relative power is the preferred measure for group data, while due to intrasubject stability of the EEG, absolute power is the preferred measure for longitudinal data within subjects. Permutation was used to correct for multiple testing and non-normal distributions of the resulting values.

The study was carried out in accordance with the recommendations of the Ethikkommission beider Basel (EKBB). The protocol was approved by the EKBB. All subjects gave written informed consent in accordance with the Declaration of Helsinki.

RESULTS

Results of relative band power are shown in **Figure 2**. In the DBS-on condition, the relative alpha2 power was higher in parieto-occipital regions bilaterally (**Figure 3**, $p \leq 0.01$) and the relative beta power was higher in the left parieto-occipital region (**Figure 3**, $p \leq 0.05$).

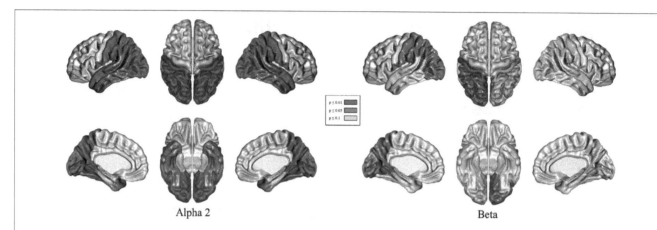

FIGURE 3 | Topographical differences in relative alpha2 and beta power: DBS-on vs. DBS-off. Results of *t*-tests with permutation (red = regions with *p* < 0.01/light red = regions with *p* < 0.05/rose = regions with *p* < 0.1).

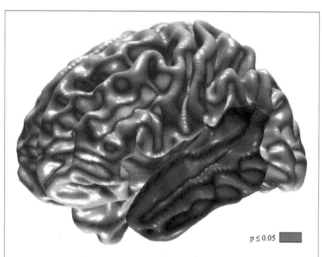

FIGURE 4 | Inverse correlation of changes in phonemic verbal fluency and relative delta power. For calculation the difference of VF (VF with DBS-on minus VF with DBS-off) and relative delta power (delta with DBS-on minus delta with DBS-off). Results of *t*-tests with permutation (red = regions with *p* < 0.05).

Changes of relative delta power in the left temporal lobe and the phonemic VF were inversely correlated (**Figure 4**, *p* < 0.05).

Alternating semantic fluency performance slightly decreased after switching off stimulation, but this result is below statistical significance. For all other VF tests, no difference between the two conditions was found (**Figure 5**).

DISCUSSION

Switching off the STN-DBS did not improve VF performance in the present study in PD patients at least 6 months after operation. This finding accords with that of previous studies (14, 30) and supports the hypothesis that impairment in VF tests after operation is due to STN-DBS procedure rather than to the electrical stimulation. In addition to the surgical microtrauma,

STN-DBS procedure includes anesthesia, changes in medication and sometimes post-operative delirium. Especially, the reduction of dopaminergic pharmacotherapy after the STN-DBS procedure may be an important factor, as VF performance is known to be ameliorated by dopaminergic drugs (31).

According to the present results, bilateral STN-DBS stimulation increases alpha2 and beta power in posterior regions in the resting-state EEG compared to the stimulator off condition. High alpha2 power is linked to increased capacity to initiate new tasks (32, 33) and probably facilitates switching between different tasks as tested in alternating VF. Alpha activity requires an intact thalamo-cortical loop (34), and its increase may reflect a partial functional normalization of this loop in the DBS-on condition, contributing to improved motor function and VF. This concept is compatible with the observation of a trend toward ameliorated alternating semantic fluency in the DBS-on state and is further supported by a previous study including 14 patients with PD, showing a slight positive effect of stimulation in the STN on phonemic fluency (30). However, this effect may be not strong enough to compensate for the decline of VF after STN-DBS procedure including a reduction of dopaminergic drugs.

The present result of increased beta power in the DBS-on state seems to contradict previous studies, which showed an improvement of motor function associated with a decrease of beta power over the sensorimotor, premotor and prefrontal cortex during STN stimulation and movement (35). However, in the present study the increase of beta power in the DBS-on situation occurs in resting state EEG and, therefore, the results are not directly comparable to studies analyzing event-related EEG alterations. Two MEG studies recorded also in resting state showed in contrast to the present results a decrease of beta band activity by STN-DBS (36, 37). While recordings in the study by Abbasi et al. took place 1 day after implantation and, therefore, were obtained in a different situation, the study by Luoma et al. with a latency of at least 3 months after implantation is better

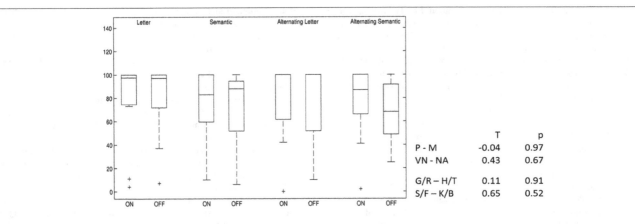

FIGURE 5 | Differences in verbal fluency: DBS-on vs. DBS-off. Percent ranks of test results, boxplots showing median, upper and lower quartiles. P–M, comparison of phonemic fluency with "P" and "M" letters; VN–NA, comparison of semantic fluency with "Names" and "Food"; G/R–H/T, comparison of phonemic fluency with alternating "G" and "R" and alternating "H" and "T" letters; S/F–K/B, comparison of semantic fluency with alternating "Sport" and "Fruits" and alternating "Clothes" and "Flowers".

comparable to our results obtained at a latency of at least 6 months.

However, the present result is in line with the observation of a correlation between beta power in the paracentral region and motor function as well as sensorimotor integration after L-dopa intake (38) and with the results of a study by Cao et al. (39). The reason for these contradictory results is currently unclear; medication may play a role.

Changes of absolute delta power in the left temporal lobe and the phonemic fluency on the individual level correlate inversely. The fact that neither delta power nor phonemic fluency changes significantly between DBS-on and DBS-off conditions on the group level does not contradict such a correlation on the individual level as observed here. However, according to a post-stroke study using voxel-based volumetry phonemic fluency is a dysfunction of the left frontal rather than the left temporal lobe (15).

One limitation of this study is its small sample size. Speculations can be made about the underlying mechanisms of DBS-induced changes in brain rhythms, but no inferences can be drawn about therapeutic language effects in individual patients. For practical and ethical reasons, the time spent in the DBS-off condition was limited, and this necessitated the retesting of VF after only 12 min in off-time. Although this was longer than the 3 min off-time in the study by Yilmaz et al. (14), it may still not have been long enough for the effects of DBS on VF to disappear entirely.

AUTHOR CONTRIBUTIONS

FH conceived and conducted the study, processed the EEG data, and drafted the manuscript. AM and AR conducted neuropsychological and linguistical testing of all patients. PF and UG initiated and designed the study, cared for the patients and critically reviewed the manuscript. ET had operated all patients and critically reviewed the manuscript. All authors read and approved the final manuscript.

ACKNOWLEDGMENTS

We thank the participating subjects and caregivers. The financial support of the Freiwillige Akademische Gesellschaft Basel, the Gottfried und Julia Bangerter-Rhyner-Stiftung, the Hedwig Widmer Stiftung, the Swiss National Science Foundation (grants: 33CM30-140338, 33CM30-124115, 326030-128775/1) and the Novartis Research Foundation is gratefully acknowledged.

REFERENCES

1. Volkmann J. Deep brain stimulation for the treatment of Parkinson's disease. *J Clin Neurophysiol Off Publ Am Electroencephalogr Soc.* (2004) 21:6–17.
2. Fasano A, Aquino CC, Krauss JK, Honey CR, Bloem BR. Axial disability and deep brain stimulation in patients with Parkinson disease. *Nat Rev Neurol.* (2015) 11:98–110. doi: 10.1038/nrneurol.2014.252
3. Combs HL, Folley BS, Berry DTR, Segerstrom SC, Han DY, Anderson-Mooney AJ, et al. Cognition and depression following deep brain stimulation of the subthalamic nucleus and globus pallidus pars internus in Parkinson's disease: a meta-analysis. *Neuropsychol Rev.* (2015) 25:439–54. doi: 10.1007/s11065-015-9302-0

4. Marshall DF, Strutt AM, Williams AE, Simpson RK, Jankovic J, York MK. Alternating verbal fluency performance following bilateral subthalamic nucleus deep brain stimulation for Parkinson's disease. *Eur J Neurol.* (2012) 19:1525–31. doi: 10.1111/j.1468-1331.2012.03759.x

5. Parsons TD, Rogers SA, Braaten AJ, Woods SP, Tröster AI. Cognitive sequelae of subthalamic nucleus deep brain stimulation in Parkinson's disease: a meta-analysis. *Lancet Neurol.* (2006) 5:578–88. doi: 10.1016/S1474-4422(06)70475-6

6. Daniels C, Krack P, Volkmann J, Pinsker MO, Krause M, Tronnier V, et al. Risk factors for executive dysfunction after subthalamic nucleus stimulation in Parkinson's disease. *Mov Disord.* (2010) 25:1583–9. doi: 10.1002/mds.23078

7. Witt K, Granert O, Daniels C, Volkmann J, Falk D, Eimeren T. van, et al. Relation of lead trajectory and electrode position to neuropsychological outcomes of subthalamic neurostimulation in Parkinson's disease: results from a randomized trial. *Brain* (2013) 136:2109–19. doi: 10.1093/brain/awt151

8. Højlund A, Petersen MV, Sridharan KS, Østergaard K. Worsening of verbal fluency after deep brain stimulation in Parkinson's disease: a focused review. *Comput Struct Biotechnol J.* (2016) 15:68–74. doi: 10.1016/j.csbj.2016.11.003

9. Chouiter L, Holmberg J, Manuel AL, Colombo F, Clarke S, Annoni J-M, et al. Partly segregated cortico-subcortical pathways support phonologic and semantic verbal fluency: a lesion study. *Neuroscience* (2016) 329:275–83. doi: 10.1016/j.neuroscience.2016.05.029

10. Isler C, Albi A, Schaper FL, Temel Y, Duits A. Neuropsychological outcome in subthalamic nucleus stimulation surgeries with electrodes passing through the caudate nucleus. *Stereotact Funct Neurosurg.* (2016) 94:413–20. doi: 10.1159/000453278

11. Haynes WIA, Haber SN. The organization of prefrontal-subthalamic inputs in primates provides an anatomical substrate for both functional specificity and integration: implications for basal ganglia models and deep brain stimulation. *J Neurosci Off J Soc Neurosci.* (2013) 33:4804–14. doi: 10.1523/JNEUROSCI.4674-12.2013

12. Wise SP, Murray EA, Gerfen CR. The frontal cortex-basal ganglia system in primates. *Crit Rev Neurobiol.* (1996) 10:317–56.

13. Barbas H, García-Cabezas MÁ, Zikopoulos B. Frontal-thalamic circuits associated with language. *Brain Lang.* (2013) 126:49–61. doi: 10.1016/j.bandl.2012.10.001

14. Yilmaz R, Akbostanci MC, Mercan FN, Sorgun MH, Savas A. No effect of different stimulation conditions on verbal fluency and visuospatial orientation in patients with subthalamic nucleus deep brain stimulation. *Stereotact Funct Neurosurg.* (2015) 93:326–32. doi: 10.1159/000438996

15. Baldo JV, Schwartz S, Wilkins D, Dronkers NF. Role of frontal versus temporal cortex in verbal fluency as revealed by voxel-based lesion symptom mapping. *J Int Neuropsychol Soc.* (2006) 12:896–900. doi: 10.1017/S1355617706061078

16. Metternich B, Buschmann F, Wagner K, Schulze-Bonhage A, Kriston L. Verbal fluency in focal epilepsy: a systematic review and meta-analysis. *Neuropsychol Rev.* (2014) 24:200–18. doi: 10.1007/s11065-014-9255-8

17. Zimmermann R, Gschwandtner U, Hatz F, Schindler C, Bousleiman H, Ahmed S, et al. Correlation of EEG slowing with cognitive domains in nondemented patients with Parkinson's disease. *Dement Geriatr Cogn Disord.* (2015) 39:207–14. doi: 10.1159/000370110

18. Aschenbrenner S. *Regensburger Wortflüssigkeits-Test: RWT* (2000). Hogrefe: Verlag für Psychologie.

19. Frysinger RC, Quigg M, Elias WJ. Bipolar deep brain stimulation permits routine EKG, EEG, and polysomnography. *Neurology* (2006) 66:268–70. doi: 10.1212/01.wnl.0000194272.79084.7e

20. Sun Y, Farzan F, Garcia Dominguez L, Barr MS, Giacobbe P, Lozano AM, et al. A novel method for removal of deep brain stimulation artifact from electroencephalography. *J Neurosci Methods* (2014) 237:33–40. doi: 10.1016/j.jneumeth.2014.09.002

21. Lio G, Thobois S, Ballanger B, Lau B, Boulinguez P. Removing deep brain stimulation artifacts from the electroencephalogram: issues, recommendations and an open-source toolbox. *Clin Neurophysiol.* (2018) 129:2170–85. doi: 10.1016/j.clinph.2018.07.023

22. Santillan-Guzman A, Heute U, Muthuraman M, Stephani U, Galka A. DBS artifact suppression using a time-frequency domain filter. In: *2013 35th Annual International Conference of the IEEE Engineering in Medicine and Biology Society (EMBC)*. Osaka (2013). p. 4815–8. doi: 10.1109/EMBC.2013.6610625

23. Hatz F, Hardmeier M, Bousleiman H, Rüegg S, Schindler C, Fuhr P. Reliability of fully automated versus visually controlled pre- and post-processing of resting-state EEG. *Clin Neurophysiol Off J Int Fed Clin Neurophysiol.* (2015) 126:268–74. doi: 10.1016/j.clinph.2014.05.014

24. Hatz F, Benz N, Hardmeier M, Zimmermann R, Rueegg S, Schindler C, et al. Quantitative EEG and apolipoprotein E-genotype improve classification of patients with suspected Alzheimer's disease. *Clin Neurophysiol Off J Int Fed Clin Neurophysiol.* (2013) 124:2146–52. doi: 10.1016/j.clinph.2013.04.339

25. Welch P. The use of fast Fourier transform for the estimation of power spectra: a method based on time averaging over short, modified periodograms. *IEEE Trans Audio Electroacoust.* (1967) 15:70–3.

26. Frei E, Gamma A, Pascual-Marqui R, Lehmann D, Hell D, Vollenweider FX. Localization of MDMA-induced brain activity in healthy volunteers using low resolution brain electromagnetic tomography (LORETA). *Hum Brain Mapp.* (2001) 14:152–65. doi: 10.1002/hbm.1049

27. Brunet D, Murray MM, Michel CM. Spatiotemporal analysis of multichannel EEG: CARTOOL. *Comput Intell Neurosci.* (2011) 2011:813870. doi: 10.1155/2011/813870

28. Aubert-Broche B, Evans AC, Collins L. A new improved version of the realistic digital brain phantom. *Neuroimage* (2006) 32:138–45. doi: 10.1016/j.neuroimage.2006.03.052

29. Tzourio-Mazoyer N, Landeau B, Papathanassiou D, Crivello F, Etard O, Delcroix N, et al. Automated anatomical labeling of activations in SPM using a macroscopic anatomical parcellation of the MNI MRI single-subject brain. *Neuroimage* (2002) 15:273–89. doi: 10.1006/nimg.2001.0978

30. Ehlen F, Vonberg I, Kühn AA, Klostermann F. Effects of thalamic deep brain stimulation on spontaneous language production. *Neuropsychologia* (2016) 89:74–82. doi: 10.1016/j.neuropsychologia.2016.05.028

31. Herrera E, Cuetos F, Ribacoba R. Verbal fluency in Parkinson's disease patients on/off dopamine medication. *Neuropsychologia* (2012) 50:3636–40. doi: 10.1016/j.neuropsychologia.2012.09.016

32. Klimesch W. EEG alpha and theta oscillations reflect cognitive and memory performance: a review and analysis. *Brain Res Rev.* (1999) 29:169–95. doi: 10.1016/S0165-0173(98)00056-3

33. Sadaghiani S, Scheeringa R, Lehongre K, Morillon B, Giraud A-L, Kleinschmidt A. Intrinsic connectivity networks, alpha oscillations, and tonic alertness: a simultaneous electroencephalography/functional magnetic resonance imaging study. *J Neurosci.* (2010) 30:10243–50. doi: 10.1523/JNEUROSCI.1004-10.2010

34. Schreckenberger M, Lange-Asschenfeld C, Lochmann M, Mann K, Siessmeier T, Buchholz H-G, et al. The thalamus as the generator and modulator of EEG alpha rhythm: a combined PET/EEG study with lorazepam challenge in humans. *Neuroimage* (2004) 22:637–44. doi: 10.1016/j.neuroimage.2004.01.047

35. Brown P, Marsden CD. Bradykinesia and impairment of EEG desynchronization in Parkinson's disease. *Mov Disord.* (1999) 14:423–9. doi: 10.1002/1531-8257(199905)14:3<423::AID-MDS1006>3.0.CO;2-V

36. Abbasi O, Hirschmann J, Storzer L, Özkurt TE, Elben S, Vesper J, et al. Unilateral deep brain stimulation suppresses alpha and beta oscillations in sensorimotor cortices. *Neuroimage* (2018) 174:201–7. doi: 10.1016/j.neuroimage.2018.03.026

37. Luoma J, Pekkonen E, Airaksinen K, Helle L, Nurminen J, Taulu S, et al. Spontaneous sensorimotor cortical activity is suppressed by deep brain stimulation in patients with advanced Parkinson's disease. *Neurosci Lett.* (2018) 683:48–53. doi: 10.1016/j.neulet.2018.06.041

38. Melgari J-M. Alpha and beta EEG power reflects L-dopa acute administration in parkinsonian patients. *Front Aging Neurosci.* (2014) 6:302. doi: 10.3389/fnagi.2014.00302

39. Cao C, Li D, Jiang T, Ince NF, Zhan S, Zhang J, et al. Resting state cortical oscillations of patients with Parkinson disease and with and without subthalamic deep brain stimulation: a magnetoencephalography study. *J Clin Neurophysiol.* (2015) 32:109–18. doi: 10.1097/WNP.0000000000000137

4

Vacuolated PAS-Positive Lymphocytes on Blood Smear: An Easy Screening Tool and a Possible Biomarker for Monitoring Therapeutic Responses in Late Onset Pompe Disease (LOPD)

Daniela Parisi[1†], Olimpia Musumeci[1†], Stefania Mondello[2], Teresa Brizzi[1,3], Rosaria Oteri[1], Alba Migliorato[2], Annamaria Ciranni[1], Tiziana E. Mongini[4], Carmelo Rodolico[1], Giuseppe Vita[1] and Antonio Toscano[1]*

[1] Department of Clinical and Experimental Medicine, University of Messina, Messina, Italy, [2] Department of Biomedical and Dental Sciences and Morphofunctional Imaging, University of Messina, Messina, Italy, [3] DIBIMIS University of Palermo, Palermo, Italy, [4] Department of Neurosciences Rita Levi Montalcini, University of Turin, Turin, Italy

*Correspondence:
Antonio Toscano
atoscano@unime.it

[†] These authors have contributed equally to this work

Background: Primary aim was to investigate the diagnostic value of PAS-positive vacuolated lymphocytes on blood smear in Late Onset Pompe Disease (LOPD) patients and, secondly, to evaluate its potential utility in monitoring treatment effects.

Methods: We examined blood smear of 26 LOPD patients. We evaluated 10 treated and 16 untreated LOPD patients. Among the latter group, 7 patients later initiated ERT and were tested again 6 months after start. Blood smear was also sampled from 82 controls and 19 patients with other muscle glycogenoses (MGSDs). PAS staining was used to evaluate: (1) presence of lymphocytes with glycogen-filled vacuoles, (2) quantification of vacuolated lymphocytes.

Results: We found that PAS-positive lymphocytes were significantly higher in LOPD patients than in controls or other MGSDs ($p < 0.05$ and $p < 0.001$, respectively). ROC curve for discriminating between untreated LOPD patients and controls yielded an AUC of 1.00 (95%CI 1.00–1.00; $p < 0.0001$). PAS-positive lymphocyte cutoff level of >10 yielded sensitivity of 100% (95%CI 78–100%), specificity of 100% (95%CI 96–100%), and positive predictive value of 100%. Patients studied before and after ERT showed a dramatic decrease of PAS-positive vacuolated lymphocytes number ($p = 0.016$). In other MGSDs, PAS-positive lymphocytes were significantly lower that untreated LOPD patients but higher than controls.

Conclusions: Our data suggest that the Blood Smear Examination (BSE) for PAS-positive lymphocytes quantification could be used as a simple and sensitive test for a quick screening of suspected Pompe disease. The quantification of vacuolated lymphocytes appears to be also a valuable tool for monitoring the efficacy of treatment in LOPD patients.

Keywords: PAS-positive lymphocytes, blood smear, LOPD screening test, therapeutic monitoring, Pompe disease

INTRODUCTION

Pompe disease (glycogen storage disease type II, OMIM#232300) is a rare autosomal recessive lysosomal storage disorder caused by deficiency of acid alpha-glucosidase (GAA), a lysosomal enzyme that is responsible for the cleavage of the α-1,4- and α-1,6-glycosidic bonds of glycogen to glucose (1, 2).

GAA deficiency leads to the accumulation of glycogen in the lysosomes of several tissues, demonstrating a multisystemic disorder although cardiac and skeletal muscles involvement remains more prominent (3, 4).

Two different clinical forms are conventionally described: a severe infantile form (IOPD) characterized by muscular hypotonia, hypertrophic cardiomyopathy and respiratory failure, and a more heterogeneous late onset form (LOPD) with a predominant progressive proximal, axial and respiratory muscle weakness (5–7).

In LOPD, initial clinical manifestations as muscle weakness, exercise intolerance, myalgia, or even isolated hyperCKemia appear often unspecific and may mimic a large variety of other muscle disorders as limb-girdle muscular dystrophies (LGMD), congenital, metabolic or inflammatory myopathies (8–11).

[1]According to the recent European Pompe Consortium (EPOC) recommendations for a correct Pompe disease diagnosis, a rapid and appropriate Dried Blood Spot (DBS) test may detect reduced GAA activity (12–14). This method may allow a fast screening of LOPD high-risk populations, so providing an addressing role in the diagnostic algorithm (14–16). In case of positive result it is necessary to perform a second biochemical confirmatory test on a different tissue (leucocytes, fibroblasts, or skeletal muscle) and/or the molecular genetic analysis (12).

However, muscle biopsy remains an important tool in the evaluation of muscle disorders; in most of Pompe disease cases, the morphological study shows a pattern of vacuolar myopathy with glycogen storage but sometimes it can result unspecific (17).

Since 2006, Enzyme Replacement Therapy (ERT) with recombinant human α-glucosidase (rGAA) became available. Early initiation of ERT in symptomatic patients seems to be essential to limit the progressive muscle damage, emphasizing the need for an early diagnosis (12, 18–20).

Abnormal cytoplasmic vacuolation of lymphocytes, identifiable on blood smear examination (BSE), has been proposed as a possible screening tool in Pompe patients (21–23).

The aim of the present study was to primarily investigate the diagnostic value of BSE of vacuolated lymphocytes in a cohort of LOPD patients compared to sex- and age-matched healthy individuals and to other patients with different muscle glycogenoses (MGSDs). Further, we evaluated the possibility of using BSE of vacuolated lymphocytes as a biomarker for monitoring and assessing treatment effects in LOPD.

---

[1]Abbreviations: LOPD - Late onset Pompe disease; GSD glycogenoses - MGSD - muscle glycogenoses; LGMW - limb girdle muscle weakness; MGG - MayGrünwald/Giemsa; PAS - Periodic Acid-Schiff; GAA - acid alpha-glucosidase; DBS - dried bloodspot; BSE - Blood Smear Examination; GAA - acid alpha-glucosidase; IOPD – infantile onset Pompe disease; EPOC - European Pompe Consortium; ERT – Enzyme Replacement Therapy; ROC - Receiver operating characteristic; IQR - interquartile range; AUC - area under the curve.

METHODS

Study Population

The study was approved by the local ethics committee (University Policlinic of Messina). The research was conducted according to the revised Declaration of Helsinki (1998) and all participants provided written informed consent prior to participation in the study.

Between April 2015 and March 2017, we examined blood smears of 26 patients defined diagnosis of LOPD, followed at our Neuromuscular Unit. Subjects were 15 males and 11 females, aged from 3 to 78 years. In all patients, the diagnosis of Pompe disease was confirmed by GAA activity assay on skeletal muscle and genetic analysis as recently suggested by EPOC recommendations (12).

When the study began, a blood sample was obtained from 10 treated and 16 untreated LOPD patients. During the study course, 7 out of the 16 untreated patients initiated ERT and, to monitor the effects of therapy on lymphocytes vacuolations, patients were tested again 6 months after ERT start.

Control values were obtained from 82 age-matched healthy individuals —40 M and 42 F—aged from 12 to 90 years.

We also collected blood smears from 19 patients affected by other muscle glycogenoses: 9 with glycogenosis type V (GSD V), 2 with GSD VII, 5 with GSD III, 1 with GSD X, 1 with GSD XIII and another one with GSD 0.

Assessment of Vacuolated Peripheral Blood Lymphocytes

A blood sample was taken and two blood films were prepared for each subject. Using routine staining procedures for light microscopy, blood smears were stained by Periodic Acid-Schiff (PAS) stain to evaluate the lymphocytes with glycogen-filled vacuoles (23, 24). Laboratory staff performing sample analysis was blinded to clinical information.

The number of vacuolated PAS positive lymphocytes per 100 lymphocytes (percentage of PAS-positive lymphocytes) was counted.

Figure 1 shows PAS-stained blood smear of a healthy individual (A), of an untreated LOPD (B) and of the same LOPD patient after ERT (C).

Statistical Analyses

Data were assessed for equality of variance and distribution. Descriptive statistics with means and median, as appropriate, and proportions were used to describe continuous and categorical variables. The association between categorical variables and population group was evaluated using the chi-square test. Because of the skewed distribution, Mann–Whitney U test was used for 2 continuous group comparisons and or the Kruskal–Wallis test for 3 or more continuous group comparisons. To compare pre and post-ERT PAS-positive lymphocytes values, we used the Wilcoxon paired rank test. Receiver operating characteristic (ROC) curves were created to explore the ability of PAS-positive lymphocytes to distinguish between LOPD patients and controls. Estimates of the area under the curves were obtained (area under the curve = 0.5

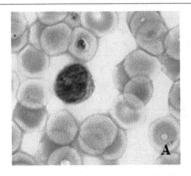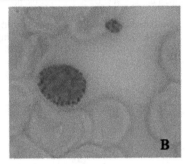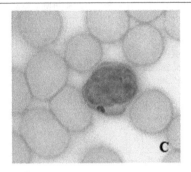

FIGURE 1 | Periodic acid-Schiff (PAS)-stained blood smear at 40 X magnification. **(A)** Healthy control, **(B)** Untreated LOPD patient showing a lymphocyte with a larger number of PAS-positive inclusions, **(C)** Same LOPD patient after 6 months of ERT.

indicates no discrimination and an area under the curve = 1.0 indicates a perfect diagnostic test). PAS-positive lymphocyte cut point was selected to maximize the sensitivity and specificity. Classification performance was assessed by sensitivity, specificity, and positive predictive values with 95% CIs. All statistical tests were two-sided and a p-value < 0.05 was considered statistically significant. Statistical analysis was carried out using SAS software package version 9.4 (SAS Institute Inc., Cary, NC) and R software (www.r-project.org; version 3.3.3).

RESULTS

We studied a total of 26 LOPD patients, 82 healthy individuals and 19 patients with other MGSD, enrolled from April 2015 until March 2017. The demographic and clinical characteristics of patients and controls are shown in **Table 1**.

In this LOPD cohort, 7 patients only showed presymptomatic hyperCKemia whereas 19 manifested with axial and limb girdle muscle weakness. Muscle biopsy, performed in 24 out of 26 LOPD patients, showed a variable amount of fibers with glycogen-filled vacuoles in 92% of patients.

The 19 patients with other MGSDs (10 M and 9 F) aged from 6 to 58 years. 9 GSD V and 2 GSD VII patients presented hyperCKemia, exercise intolerance and myoglobinuria without muscle weakness. GSD X and XIII patients complained of exercise intolerance, myalgia and contractures and rhabdomyolysis episodes. GSD III patients presented axial and limb-girdle muscle weakness. GSD 0 patient presented dysmorphic features with short stature, long face and low ears, exercise intolerance, and respiratory failure.

In all Pompe patients, we found, on a blood smear, a high percentage of vacuolated PAS-positive lymphocytes ranging from 10 to 57% in untreated and from 2 to 28% in treated patients that resulted significantly different than controls ($p < 0.01$ and $p < 0.001$, respectively) (**Table 2**).

GAA activity showed a strong negative correlation with PAS-positive lymphocytes in both treated and untreated LOPD patients ($r = -0.75$, $p = 0.01$, and $r = -0.60$, $p = 0.02$, respectively). On the other hand, PAS-positive lymphocytes

TABLE 1 | Summary of demographic and clinical data of LOPD cases as well as healthy individuals included in this study.

	Healthy individuals (n = 82)	Patients with LOPD (n = 26)	p-Value[a]
Age, years, median (IQR) Range	53 (34–71) (12–90)	50 (37–55) (3–78)	0.09
Male, n (%)	40 (49%)	15 (57.69%)	0.63
Age at Onset years, median (IQR)	NA	32.5 (20–40)	
Age at Diagnosis, years, median (IQR)	NA	43 (34–51)	
CLINICAL PRESENTATION, n (%)			
– Isolated hyperCKemia	NA	7 (26.92%)	
– LGMW	NA	19 (73.08%)	
ERT, n (%)			
– Yes	NA	10 (38.46%)	
– No	NA	16 (61.54.08%)	

[a]Mann–Whitney U test for continuous variables, cross-tabulations and 2-test for categorical variables.
NA, not applicable.

weakly correlated with age in controls ($r = -0.27$, $p = 0.015$) and approached the significance in treated LOPD patients ($r = -0.58$, $p = 0.07$). Conversely, PAS-positive lymphocytes were not associated to clinical phenotype ($p = 0.53$) or any other correlation. No correlation with genotype was found.

PAS-positive lymphocytes in patients with MGSD, although they were significantly higher than in controls ($p < 0.05$), appeared to be statistically lower than untreated LOPD patients ($p < 0.01$), and tended to be lower compared to treated patients (**Figure 2**). Intriguingly, in GSD III cases, the presence of vacuolated lymphocytes was higher than in the other MGSD making the MGSD mean values in the lower level of the untreated LOPD patients.

ROC curve for discriminating between untreated LOPD patients and controls yielded an area under the curve (AUC) of 1.00 (95% CI 1.00–1.00; $p < 0.0001$) (**Figure 3**).

Classification performance at a PAS-positive lymphocyte cutoff level of >10 yielded a sensitivity of 100% (95% CI 78 to

TABLE 2 | Number of vacuolated-PAS positive lymphocytes in the study cohort of LOPD patients, in other MGSDs and in healthy individuals.

	Healthy individuals (n = 82)	Untreated LOPD patients (n = 16)	Treated LOPD patients (n = 10)	Other MGSDs (n = 19)	P-Value[a]
Number of vacuolated PAS positive lymphocytes (IQR)	1 (0–3)	37 (18–45)	9 (2–17)	3(1–9)	<0.0001
Range	(0–9)	(10–57)	(2–28)	(0–17)	

[a]Kruskal-Wallis test for continuous variables, IQR, interquartile range.

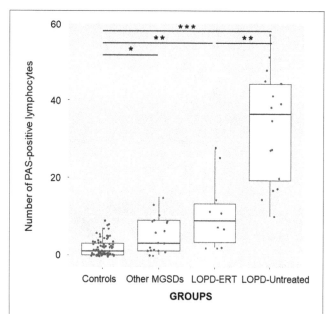

FIGURE 2 | A comparison of the number of vacuolated lymphocytes in patients with LOPD dichotomized into untreated and ERT-treated vs. controls and other MGSD. The black horizontal line in each box represents the median, with the boxes representing the interquartile range. Significant differences are indicated with *p < 0.05, **p < 0.01, or ***p < 0.001.

100%), a specificity of 100% (95% CI 96 to 100%), and a positive predictive value of 100%.

We compared PAS- positive lymphocytes in blood samples, obtained from 7 patients before starting ERT and after 6 month of treatment. Patients showed a dramatic decrease in the number of PAS-positive lymphocytes after 6 months on ERT compared to baseline values (P = 0.016) (**Figure 4**).

DISCUSSION

Since the availability of ERT, as first line treatment for patients with Pompe disease, it became evident that an early diagnosis is crucial to achieve efficient therapeutic responses. The use of the DBS as a key screening method to identify patients with GAA deficiency has been proposed in several studies (14–16).

In Pompe disease, glycogen storage is present in different tissues including lymphocytes in the peripheral blood. It has been reported that on BSE, patients with Pompe disease may show vacuolated lymphocytes (21–23).

In 1977, von Bassewitz et al observed vacuoles in peripheral lymphocytes by light microscopy and, using electron microscopy, detected glycogen-filled lysosomes in 5 IOPD cases (21). In the following years, vacuolated lymphocytes have been described on blood smear also in other storage and metabolic disorders as Batten's disease (neuronal ceroid lipofuscinosis), Salla disease, β galactosidase deficiency, mucopolysaccharidoses, Niemann-Pick disease, fucosidosis, mannosidosis, and Wolman's disease. In 2005, a retrospective review of 2.550 blood films of patients with a clinical history suggestive of metabolic diseases, identified vacuolated lymphocytes in 156 cases, 23% were recognized as Pompe disease (15 IOPD and 8% LOPD) PAS staining was performed to better characterize glycogen storage in the lymphocytes vacuoles (22). In 2010, Hagemans et al collected peripheral blood films from patients with Pompe disease and controls showing that PAS-positive lymphocytes were more common in Pompe disease compared to controls and suggesting their possible role as diagnostic screening procedure (23). More recently Pascarella et al. suggested that quantification of PAS-positive lymphocytes in blood films is useful to identify autophagic vacuolar myopathies and should be routinely used for Pompe disease diagnosis (25).

In this study, we investigated the presence of glycogen-filled vacuoles in peripheral blood lymphocytes of LOPD patients to evaluate its use as screening test as well as surrogate biomarker to monitor therapeutic efficacy. Our data confirmed that PAS staining is a reliable marker of glycogen accumulation in LOPD patients lymphocytes. Comparing the number of PAS-positive lymphocytes of all 26 LOPD patients vs. controls or others MSGDs patients, we found that they were significantly higher in LOPD (**Figure 2**), proving that this method is quite specific to detect Pompe disease patients. A strong correlation was found between presence of vacuolated lymphocytes and GAA residual activity but not with other clinical parameters as age, disease duration or phenotype.

On the other hand, considering treated and untreated LOPD patients, we found that PAS-positive lymphocytes were significantly higher in untreated than in treated patients (p < 0.01). Diagnostic accuracy of the PAS-positive lymphocytes in blood was quite impressive showing an AUC of 100%. With a cutoff value of 10 as a percentage of PAS positive lymphocytes, a sensitivity of 100% and a specificity of 100% were reached (**Figure 3**). Thus, these results indicate that this test may play a role as valid and reliable indicator of LOPD.

It is worthwhile to outline that, in 7 LOPD patients, the percentage of PAS-positive lymphocytes, counted in blood smears before ERT and 6 months after, was significantly lower

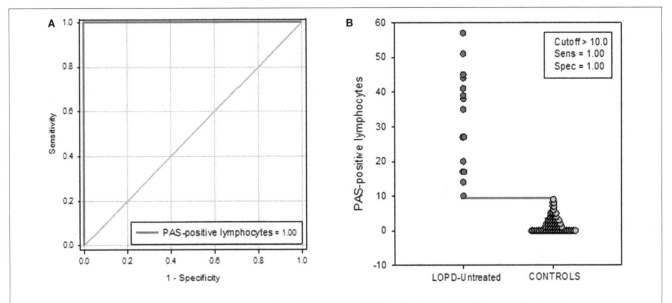

FIGURE 3 | (A) Receiver operating characteristic (ROC) curve for distinguishing untreated LOPD patients vs. controls. The area under the receiver operating characteristic curve (AUC) demonstrates that the levels of PAS-positive lymphocytes assessed in serum are able to discriminate between untreated LOPD patients and controls, with an AUC of 1.00 (95% CI 1.00 to 1.00). (B) Levels of PAS-positive lymphocytes in untreated LOPD patients and in controls. The red horizontal line represents the optimal cutoff value for distinguishing between untreated LOPD patients and controls.

after treatment (**Figure 4**). Although number of samples is quite limited, the latter finding could suggest that the percentage of the PAS-positive lymphocytes could be utilized as a surrogate biomarker to check therapeutic efficacy, even in future trials. Similarly in Fabry disease, another lysosomal disorder which share several commonalities with Pompe disease, GB3 and Lyso-GB3 in plasma and urine are considered as reliable biomarkers for staging the disease and monitor ERT response (26).

PAS-positive lymphocytes values of patients with other MGSDs were significantly reduced than in untreated LOPD patients. They also tended to be lower compared to treated LOPD patients (**Figure 2**), suggesting that BSE could be usefully applied as a screening tool in LOPD high-risk population, even in combination with DBS. Of course, it is worthwhile to outline that in the LOPD diagnostic algorithm, BSE as well as DBS results need to be confirmed by biochemical and genetic testing.

Being based on a simple histochemical test, BSE could be even easier to be applied in patients screening rather than DBS methods that require a fluorimetric or a tandem mass spectrometry, equipment that could be not universally available in the setting of diagnostic laboratories.

However, GSD III patients seem to have higher PAS-positive lymphocytes than other MGSDs; they appeared quite similar to the lowest Pompe disease untreated values in this cohort although GSD III clinical features are usually distinctive from Pompe disease (27). A possible explanation of a similar morphological appearance of vacuolated lymphocytes in GSD II and III, should take into account the fact that even debrancher enzyme is located in lymphocytes and its deficiency may lead to glycogen accumulation (28).

Our results have shown that residual GAA activity strongly correlated with PAS-positive lymphocytes in both treated and

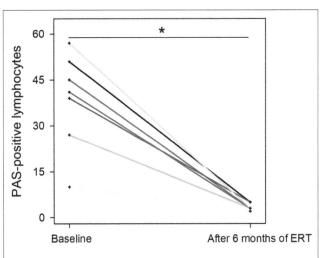

FIGURE 4 | Trends over time in the number of vacuolated lymphocytes *P = 0.016. Individual patient values are showed.

untreated LOPD patients. One limit of the study could be considered the relatively small sample size that precluded meaningful multivariate analyses.

CONCLUSIONS

Our data suggest that quantification of PAS-positive lymphocytes in peripheral blood films could be used either as a simple screening method to support a diagnosis in patients with a suspected Pompe disease or also as surrogate biomarker for therapeutic management purposes.

AUTHOR CONTRIBUTIONS

OM had full access to all the data in the study and takes responsibility for the integrity of the data and accuracy of data analysis. DP, OM, AT, TM, CR, GV contributed to study design. DP, OM, TB, RO, AC, AM, AT contributed to data collection. DP, OM, AT drafted the manuscript. OM, TB, CR, TM provided clinical information. SM performed statistical analysis. All authors read and approved the final manuscript.

ACKNOWLEDGMENTS

The authors thank Prof. A. van der Ploeg and RL Stigter for their helpful suggestions to optimize the technical performance of BS staining. The authors wish to thank Telethon Foundation for the Grant GUP13013 (AT). Some of these data were presented by AT at the 20th International World Muscle Society Congress.

REFERENCES

1. Hirschhorn R, Reuser AJJ. Glycogen storage disease type II: acid alpha-glucosidase (acid maltase) deficiency. In: Valle D, Beaudet AL, Vogelstein B, Kinzler KW, Antonarakis SE, Ballabio A, editors. *The Metabolic and Molecular Bases of Inherited Disease.* New York, NY: McGraw-Hill (2001). p. 3389–420.

2. van der Ploeg AT, Reuser AJ. Pompe's disease. *Lancet* (2008) 372:1342–53. doi: 10.1016/S0140-6736(08)61555-X

3. Toscano A, Musumeci O. Pathophysiological mechanisms in Glycogenosis type II. In: Filosto M, Toscano A, Padovani A, editors. *Advances in Diagnosis and Management of Glycogenosis II.* New York, NY: Nova Science Publisher Inc. (2012). p. 17–21.

4. Angelini C, Semplicini C, Ravaglia S, Bembi B, Servidei S, Pegoraro E, et al. Italian GSDII Group Observational clinical study in juvenile-adult glycogenosis type 2 patients undergoing enzyme replacement therapy for up to 4 years. *J Neurol.* (2012) 259:952–8 doi: 10.1007/s00415-011-6293-5

5. van Capelle CI, van der Meijden JC, van den Hout JM, Jaeken J, Baethmann M, Voit T, et al. Childhood Pompe disease: clinical spectrum and genotype in 31 patients. *Orphanet J Rare Dis.* (2016) 11:65. doi: 10.1186/s13023-016-0442-y

6. Montagnese F, Barca E, Musumeci O, Mondello S, Migliorato A, Ciranni A, et al. Clinical and molecular aspects of 30 patients with late-onset Pompe disease (LOPD): unusual features and response to treatment. *J Neurol.* (2015) 262:968–78. doi: 10.1007/s00415-015-7664-0

7. Wokke JH, Escolar DM, Pestronk A, Jaffe KM, Carter GT, van den Berg LH, et al. Clinical features of late-onset Pompe disease: a prospective cohort study. *Muscle Nerve* (2008) 38:1236–45. doi: 10.1002/mus.21025

8. Preisler N, Lukacs Z, Vinge L, Madsen KL, Husu E, Hansen RS, et al. Late-onset Pompe disease is prevalent in unclassified limb-girdle muscular dystrophies. *Mol Genet Metab.* (2013) 110:287–9. doi: 10.1016/j.ymgme.2013.08.005

9. Savarese M, Di Fruscio G, Torella A, Fiorillo C, Magri F, Fanin M, et al. The genetic basis of undiagnosed muscular dystrophies and myopathies: results from 504 patients. *Neurology* (2016) 87:71–6. doi: 10.1212/WNL.0000000000002800

10. Chan J, Desai AK, Kazi ZB, Corey K, Austin S, Hobson-Webb LD, et al. The emerging phenotype of late-onset Pompe disease: a systematic literature review. *Mol Genet Metab.* (2017) 120:163–17. doi: 10.1016/j.ymgme.2016.12.0042

11. Roberts M, Kishnani PS, van der Ploeg AT, Müller-Felber W, Merlini L, Prasad S, et al. The prevalence and impact of scoliosis in Pompe disease: lessons learned from the Pompe Registry. *Mol Genet Metab.* (2011) 104:574–82. doi: 10.1016/j.ymgme.2011.08.011

12. van der Ploeg AT, Kruijshaar ME, Toscano A, Laforêt P, Angelini C, Lachmann RH, et al. European Pompe consortium european consensus for starting and stopping enzyme replacement therapy in adult patients with Pompe disease: a 10-year experience. *Eur J Neurol.* (2017) 24:768–e31. doi: 10.1111/ene.13285

13. Wagner M, Chaouch A, Müller JS, Polvikoski T, Willis TA, Sarkozy A, et al. Presymptomatic late-onset Pompe disease identified by the dried blood spot test. *Neuromuscul Disord.* (2013) 23:89–92 doi: 10.1016/j.nmd.2012.09.004

14. Musumeci O, la Marca G, Spada M, Mondello S, Danesino C, Comi GP, et al. Italian GSD II group LOPED study: looking for an early diagnosis in a late-onset Pompe disease high-risk population. *J Neurol Neurosurg Psychiatry* (2016) 87:5–11. doi: 10.1136/jnnp-2014-310164

15. Spada M, Porta F, Vercelli L, Pagliardini V, Chiadò-Piat L, Boffi P, et al. Screening for later-onset Pompe's disease in patients with paucisymptomatic hyperCKemia. *Mol Genet Metab.* (2013) 109:171–3. doi: 10.1016/j.ymgme.2013.03.002

16. Lukacs Z, Nieves Cobos P, Wenninger S, Willis TA, Guglieri M, Roberts M, et al. Prevalence of Pompe disease in 3,076 patients with hyperCKemia and limb-girdle muscular weakness. *Neurology* (2016) 87:295–8. doi: 10.1212/WNL.0000000000002758

17. Vissing J, Lukacs Z, Straub V. Diagnosis of Pompe disease: muscle biopsy vs blood-based assays. *JAMA Neurol.* (2013) 70:923–7. doi: 10.1001/2013.jamaneurol.486

18. Toscano A, Schoser B. Enzyme replacement therapy in late-onset Pompe disease: a systematic literature review. *J Neurol.* (2013) 260:951–9. doi: 10.1007/s00415-012-6636-x

19. Schoser B, Stewart A, Kanters S, Hamed A, Jansen J, Chan K, et al. Survival and long-term outcomes in late-onset Pompe disease following alglucosidase alfa treatment: a systematic review and meta-analysis. *J Neurol.* (2017) 264:621–30. doi: 10.1007/s00415-016-8219-8

20. Chien YH, Hwu WL, Lee NC. Pompe disease: early diagnosis and early treatment make a difference. *Pediatr Neonatol.* (2013) 54:219–27. doi: 10.1016/j.pedneo.2013.03.009

21. von Bassewitz DB, Bremer HJ, Bourgeois M, Gröbe H, Stoermer J. Vacuolated lymphocytes in type II glycogenosis–a diagnostic approach? *Eur J Pediatr.* (1977) 127:1–7.

22. Anderson G, Smith VV, Malone M, Sebire NJ. Blood film examination for vacuolated lymphocytes in the diagnosis of metabolic disorders; retrospective experience of more than 2500 cases from a single centre. *J Clin Pathol.* (2005) 58:1305–10. doi: 10.1136/jcp.2005.027045

23. Hagemans MLC, Stigter RL, van Capelle CI, van der Beek NAM, Winkel LPF, van Vliet L, et al. PAS-positive lymphocyte vacuoles can be used as diagnostic screening test for Pompe disease. *J Inherit Metab Dis.* (2010) 33:133–9. doi: 10.1007/s10545-009-9027-4

24. de Barsy T, Hers HG. Biochemical and ultrastructural study of leucocytes in type II glycogenosis. *Arch Int Physiol Biochim.* (1975) 83:954–5.

25. Pascarella A, Terracciano C, Farina O, Lombardi L, Esposito T, Napolitano F, et al. Vacuolated PAS-positive lymphocytes as an hallmark of Pompe disease and other myopathies related to impaired autophagy. *J Cell Physiol.* (2018) 233:5829–37. doi: 10.1002/jcp. 26365

26. Krämer J, Weidemann F. Biomarkers for diagnosing and staging of Fabry disease. *Curr Med Chem.* (2018) 25:1530–7. doi: 10.2174/0929867324666170616102112

27. Lucchiari S, Pagliarani S, Salani S, Filocamo M, Di Rocco M, Melis D, et al. Hepatic and neuromuscular forms of glycogenosis type III: nine mutations in AGL. *Hum Mutat.* (2006) 27:600–1. doi: 10.1002/humu.9426

28. Hoffmann GF. Metabolic myopathies. In: Hoffmann GF, Zschocke J, Nyhan WL, editors. *Inherited Metabolic Diseases.* Philadelphia, PA: Lippincott William and Wilkins (2002) p. 261.

5

IL-6 Plasma Levels Correlate with Cerebral Perfusion Deficits and Infarct Sizes in Stroke Patients without Associated Infections

Benjamin Hotter[1,2]*, Sarah Hoffmann[1,2], Lena Ulm[3], Christian Meisel[4], Jochen B. Fiebach[1,2] and Andreas Meisel[1,2]

[1] Charité – Universitätsmedizin Berlin, Corporate Member of Freie Universität Berlin, Berlin Institute of Health, Humboldt-Universität zu Berlin, Berlin, Germany, [2] Center for Stroke Research Berlin, NeuroCure Clinical Research Center and Department of Neurology, Charité University Hospital Berlin, Berlin, Germany, [3] Centre for Clinical Research, University of Queensland, Herston, QLD, Australia, [4] Department of Medical Immunology, Charité University Medicine & Labor Berlin - Charité Vivantes, Berlin, Germany

*Correspondence:
Benjamin Hotter
benjamin.hotter@charite.de

Introduction: We aimed to investigate several blood-based biomarkers related to inflammation, immunity, and stress response in a cohort of patients without stroke-associated infections regarding their predictive abilities for functional outcome and explore whether they correlate with MRI markers, such as infarct size or location.

Methods: We combined the clinical and radiological data of patients participating in two observational acute stroke cohorts: the PREDICT and 1000Plus studies. The following blood-based biomarkers were measured in these patients: monocytic HLA-DR, IL-6, IL-8, IL-10, LBP, MRproANP, MRproADM, CTproET, Copeptin, and PCT. Multiparametric stroke MRI was performed including T2*, DWI, FLAIR, TOF-MRA, and perfusion imaging. Standard descriptive sum statistics were used to describe the sample. Associations were analyzed using Fischer's exact test, independent samples t-test and Spearmans correlation, where appropriate.

Results: Demographics and stroke characteristics were as follows: 94 patients without infections, mean age 68 years (SD 10.5), 32.2% of subjects were female, median NIHSS score at admission 3 (IQR 2–5), median mRS 3 months after stroke 1 (IQR 0–2), mean volume of DWI lesion at admission 5.7 ml (SD 12.8), mean FLAIR final infarct volume 10 ml (SD 14.9), cortical affection in 61% of infarctions. Acute DWI lesion volume on admission MRI was moderately correlated to admission/maximum IL-6 as well as maximum LBP. Extent of perfusion deficit and mismatch were moderately correlated to admission/maximum IL-6 levels. Final lesion volume on FLAIR was moderately correlated to admission IL-6 levels.

Conclusion: We found IL-6 to be associated with several parameters from acute stroke MRI (acute DWI lesion, perfusion deficit, final infarct size, and affection of cortex) in a cohort of patients not influenced by infections.

Clinical Trial Registration: www.ClinicalTrials.gov, identifiers NCT01079728 and NCT00715533

Keywords: stroke, biomarker, MRI, IL-6, neuroinflammation

INTRODUCTION

Stroke is globally recognized as a leading cause for mortality and adult disability. While the advent of intravenous thrombolysis and recanalization has significantly improved the outcome of stroke, a significant proportion of patients persist to suffer from deficits and disabilities. This is partly explained by the course of stroke itself, but also depending on neurological and medical complications (1–3). Prognosis and precise prediction of outcome remains challenging, especially during the hyperacute phase of the disease. While demographic and clinical characteristics, such as i.e., age and severity of acute clinical syndrome, allow for an educated guess (4), the accuracy of prediction is limited (5). For the post-acute phase of the disease, recent progress has been made in prediction of motor and cognitive recovery (6, 7).

Development of more accurate scores to predict outcome in the acute setting may benefit from the inclusion of biomarkers. While individual association of sanguine parameters with stroke characteristics and functional outcome has been reported, no single biomarker stands out in the field. Immune parameters including cytokines and other acute phase proteins are indicative

to the risk of post-stroke infections but have also been associated to functional outcome after stroke (8).

We aimed to investigate a range of inflammation-, immunity-, and stress-related biomarkers in a cohort of patients without stroke-associated infections regarding their predictive abilities for functional outcome and explore whether they correlate with MRI markers, such as infarct size or location.

METHODS

We combined the clinical and radiological data of patients participating in two observational acute stroke cohorts: the PREDICT and 1000Plus studies (clinicaltrials.gov NCT01079728 and NCT00715533). Both studies received full approval by the institutional ethics' committee, including the pooling of data for combined analysis. All patients (or if necessary, their legal representatives) gave informed consent to participation. Protocol details of both studies have been previously published (9, 10). Briefly, both studies recruited acute ischemic stroke patients to investigate either the prediction of stroke-associated pneumonia (PREDICT) or the natural course of multimodal MRI parameters (1000Plus), especially the evolution of DWI-perfusion imaging-

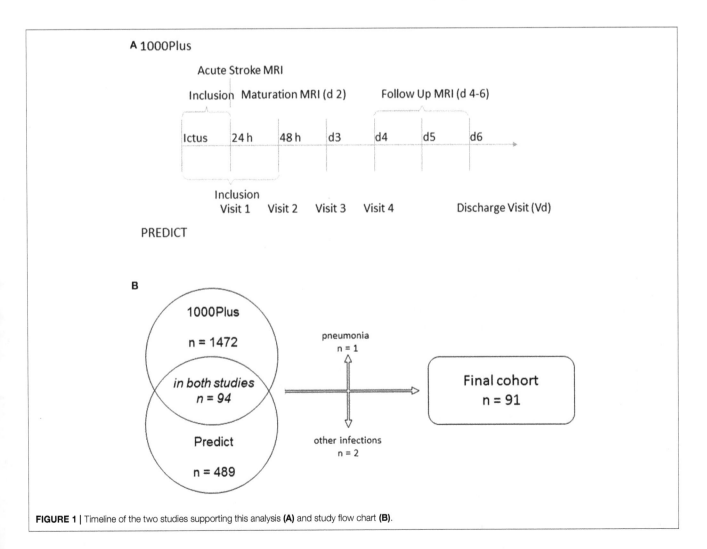

FIGURE 1 | Timeline of the two studies supporting this analysis **(A)** and study flow chart **(B)**.

mismatch. There was significant overlap of visit time points throughout the course of the study (see **Figure 1**). PREDICT was a multicentric study, with one of the participating centers (Charité Campus Benjamin Franklin) being the only study site in the 1000Plus study. PREDICT recruited 189 patients on that common site, 94 of which also participating in the 1000Plus study. We excluded patients suffering from an infection during their time of hospital admission for this analysis.

Blood samples parameters were obtained within the first 4 days of hospital admission. Samples were immediately post-processed and then frozen at −80°C in order to allow for batch analyses at the end of the study. Serum levels of mid-regional pro atrial natriuretic peptide (MRproANP), mid-regional pro adrenomedullin (MRproADM), C-terminal pro endothelin (CTproET), ultrasensitive copeptin (CPus), and ultrasensitive procalcitonin (PCTus) were measured using fluorescent immunoassays on the automated BRAHMS KRYPTOR compact PLUS™ analyzer (BRAHMS GmbH/Thermo Fisher Scientific, Henningsdorf, Germany) according to the manufacturer's protocol. The lower limits of quantitation were 4.5 pmol/l for MRproANP, 0.05 nmol/l for MRproADM, 3 pmol/l for CTproET, 1.9 pmol/l for CPus, and 0,02 µg/l for PCTus. Plasma concentrations of IL-6, IL-8, IL-10, and LBP were determined with the IMMULITE™ semi-automatic chemiluminescent immunoassay (Siemens Medical Solutions, Bad Nauheim, Germany). The detection limit for IL-6 and IL-8 is 2, 1 pg/ml for IL-10 and 0.8 µg/ml for LBP. Expression of human leukocyte antigen-DR (HLA-DR) on monocytes was determined in EDTA whole blood samples by flow cytometry using a highly standardized quantitative assay, as described earlier (9).

Multiparametric stroke MRI was performed on a 3T scanner (Tim Trio; Siemens AG, Erlangen, Germany) at admission (always within 24 h of the event), the following day and lastly 4–6 days after the event. Applied sequences contained T2*, DWI, FLAIR, TOF-MRA, and for the first two imaging time points also perfusion imaging. For further detail please refer to the published protocol (10). Admission MRI was performed as initial imaging upon presentation, or if outside of regular hours as the first examination the next morning. Follow-up MRIs were performed in the morning of the respective days. Blood samples were collected for the first day as soon as the patients and/or their legal representatives consented. The following samples were drawn with the routine laboratory rounds in the morning. Hence, delay between imaging and blood sampling was kept as short as logistically possible.

Standard descriptive sum statistics were used to describe demographics and stroke characteristics as well as biomarker and imaging results. Associations were analyzed by use of Fischer's exact test, independent samples t-test and Spearmans correlation, depending on character of variables. Alpha-error level was set at 2-tailed $p = 0.05$. All statistics were performed using SPSS (version 24.0, IBM, Armonk, NY, USA). In view of the small sample size and the explorative nature of the study, we decided against statistical correction such as Bonferroni.

RESULTS

We identified 94 patients participating in both Predict and 1000Plus. Three of them suffered from an infection during the course of their hospital stay and were excluded from this analysis (see **Figure 1B** for further detail). Mean age was 68 years (SD 10.5) and 32.2% of subjects were female. Median NIHSS score at admission was 3 (IQR 2–5). At 3 months, median mRS was 1 (IQR 0–2). Thrombolysis was applied in 23% of patients. For further details on clinical syndrome on admission, risk factors and stroke etiology refer to **Table 1**.

Initial MRI was performed at a median of 549.5 min (IQR 130.25–860) after event. Mean volume of DWI lesion at admission was 5.7 ml (SD 12.8), mean final infarct volume as measured on FLAIR was 10 ml (SD 14.9). The right hemisphere was more frequently affected than the left hemisphere (52 vs. 37%) and cortex was involved in 61% of infarctions. Blood samples were collected during the first 4 days of hospitalization after stroke, and values for day of admission as well as maximum/minimum values are outlined in **Table 2**.

Age of patients was associated with IL-6, MRproANP, MRproADM, and CTproET. Stroke severity at admission as measured by National Institute of Health Stroke Scale

TABLE 1 | Demographics and clinical stroke characteristics.

n	91
Sex, n (%) female	29 (32.2)
Age, years, mean (SD)	68.0 (10.5)
Admission NIHSS, median (IQR)	3 (2-5)
Admission mRS, median (IQR)	2 (1-3)
ADMISSION SYMPTOMS	
Aphasia [7]	10 (11.9)
Motor deficit	67 (77.9)
Dysarthria [7]	46 (54.8)
Dysphagia [11]	5 (6.3)
RISK FACTORS	
Diabetes mellitus	25 (28.7)
Atrial fibrillation	14 (16.1)
Previous stroke	16 (18.4)
Arterial hypertension	74 (85.1)
Hyperlipidemia	55 (63.2)
Smoking [61]	5 (16.1)
Thrombolysis	20 (23.0)
TOAST	
Large artery occlusion	56 (64.4)
Cardioembolism	18 (20.7)
Small artery disease	6 (6.9)
Other etiology	3 (3.4)
Unknown etiology	3 (3.4)
Concurring etiology	1 (1.1)
mRS 90 days after event, median (IQR) [17]	1 (0–2)

Values given are n (%) if not explicitly stated otherwise, missing cases reported if >5 as [n]. NIHSS, National Institute of Health Stroke Scale; mRS, modified Rankin Scale; TOAST, Trial of Org10172 in Acute Stroke Treatment.

TABLE 2 | Imaging and blood-based biomarker results.

Hemisphere of DWI lesion	
Right	46 (51.7)
Left	32 (36.0)
Bilateral	11 (12.4)
DWI lesion volume on acute MRI, ml	5.7 (12.8)
PI deficit volume on acute MRI, ml	45.1 (78.0)
DWI-PI mismatch on acute MRI, ml	26.4 (58.5)
TYPE OF INFARCTION	
Territorial	76 (85.4)
Lacunar infarction	12 (13.5)
Borderzone infarction	1 (1.1)
REGIONS AFFECTED	
Any Cortex	54 (60.7)
Caudate	3 (3.3)
Lenticulate	4 (4.4)
Capsula interna	8 (8.8)
Insula	11 (12.1)
ASPECT M1	6 (6.6)
ASPECT M2	17 (18.7)
ASPECT M3	14 (15.4)
ASPECT M4	15 (16.5)
ASPECT M5	34 (37.4)
ASPECT M6	21 (23.1)
FLAIR lesion volume on Follow Up, ml [33]	10.0 (14.9)
HLA-DR, EPITOPES/CELL, MEDIAN (IQR)	
At inclusion [3]	18,387 (14,434–25,788)
Lowest [1]	16,505 (11,386–21,285)
IL-6, PG/ML, MEDIAN (IQR)	
At inclusion [3]	2.8 (2.0–5.2)
Highest [1]	5.2 (2.7–11.0)
IL-8, PG/ML, MEDIAN (IQR)	
At inclusion [3]	5.0 (5.0–5.0)
Highest [1]	5.0 (5.0–5.2)
IL-10, PG/ML, MEDIAN (IQR)	
At inclusion [3]	5.0 (5.0–5.0)
Highest [1]	5.0 (5.0–5.0)
LBP, µG/ML, MEDIAN (IQR)	
At inclusion [3]	7.23 (5.48–9.34)
Highest [1]	8.90 (6.68–11.65)
MPproANP, PG/ML, MEDIAN (IQR)	
At inclusion [29]	111.4 (65.5–180.9)
Highest [23]	122.5 (79.1–195.8)
MPproADM, PG/ML, MEDIAN (IQR)	
At inclusion [29]	0.703 (0.593–0.868)
Highest [22]	0.751 (0.613–0.917)
CTproET, PG/ML, MEDIAN (IQR)	
At inclusion [30]	61.4 (50.7–75.9)
Highest [22]	64.4 (54.6–83.1)
CPus, PG/ML, MEDIAN (IQR)	
At inclusion [29]	8.84 (5.27–14.22)
Highest [22]	10.19 (5.60–17.40)
PCT us, PG/ML, MEDIAN (IQR)	
At inclusion [30]	0.031 (0.024–0.041)
Highest [23]	0.039 (0.028–0.050)

Values given are n (%) if not explicitly stated otherwise, missing cases reported if >5 as [n]. HLA-DR, Human leukocyte antigen expression on monocytes; IL-6, IL-8, IL-10, three interleukins; LBP, lipopolysaccharide-binding protein; MRproANP, mid-regional pro atrial natriuretic peptide; MRproADM, mid-regional pro adrenomedullin; CTproET, C-terminal pro endothelin; CPus, ultrasensitive copeptin; PCTus, ultrasensitive procalcitonin.

(NIHSS) score was associated with IL-6. Functional outcome as measured by modified Rankin Scale (mRS) at day 90 was associated with admission levels of ultrasensitive Copeptin, maximum MRproADM, IL-6, and minimum HLA-DR levels (**Table 3**).

Acute volume of DWI restriction on admission MRI scans was moderately correlated to admission (Spearman's ρ 0.336) and maximum (Spearman's ρ 0.276) IL-6 as well as maximum LBP (Spearman's ρ 0.222) levels. Extent of perfusion imaging (PI) deficit and DWI-PI-Mismatch were moderately correlated to admission (Spearman's ρ 0.306 and 0.231, respectively) and maximum (Spearman's ρ 0.277 and 0.215, respectively) IL-6 levels. Final lesion volume on FLAIR was moderately correlated to admission IL-6 levels (Spearman's ρ 0.364) (**Table 4**). Cortical infarcts were associated with higher IL-6 levels at admission. By use of the ASPECT scoring system we only found inconsistent associations of biomarker levels with infarct location (**Supplementary Table 1**).

DISCUSSION

We examined the relationship of inflammatory, immune, and stress biomarkers with MRI parameters in 91 stroke patients not suffering from stroke-associated infections during the course of the study. Interleukin-6 was associated with infarct size and tissue at risk, as well as final infarct volume. The other studied biomarkers did not show any associations with imaging markers in the absence of infection. Overall, the studied cohort was rather mildly affected by stroke (median admission NIHSS 3 IQR 2–5 and 3 months mRS 1 IQR 0–2).

The biological role of IL-6 in ischemic stroke remains uncertain. Astrocytes and microglia express IL-6, but whether it primarily exerts neurotoxic or—protective effects is a matter of scientific discourse (11, 12). Our study found a significant association of IL-6 levels with NIHSS scores at admission, although Spearman's ρ only showed moderate correlation. Furthermore, we found a significant correlation of IL-6 levels with lesion volume, whether on DWI scans at admission, PI deficit, DWI-PI mismatch or on follow-up FLAIR images, which is in line with the association of IL-6 levels and NIHSS scores at admission. Infarct size has previously been reported to correlate at least with intrathecal levels, but not consistently with serum levels, of IL-6 (13–15). IL-6 was repeatedly associated with poor functional outcome, but whether this is an independent effect or a signal due to infection remains unclear (8). Our data shows a significant association of IL-6 with functional outcome as measured by mRS in a cohort of patients not suffering from infection, further corroborating an association independent of infections. IL-6 has been previously linked to small vessel disease and silent cerebral infarctions (16–18). IL-6 and also IL-10 were associated with the presence of diffusion-perfusion- or clinical-diffusion-mismatch on acute stroke MRI (19–21). Furthermore, cortical infarcts were associated with IL-6. The associations of several other biomarkers with localization of lesions have to be interpreted with caution considering the sample size and plausibility.

TABLE 3 | Association of biomarkers at inclusion and lowest/highest measurement with clinical parameters.

		Aphasia	Motor deficit	Dysarthria	Dysphagia	Sex	NIHSS	mRS d90	Age
HLA-DR	Inclusion	0.405	0.979	0.548	0.757	0.606	0.409	0.052	0.249
	Lowest	0.987	0.436	0.959	0.173	0.340	0.099	**0.030**	0.069
IL-6	Inclusion	0.410	0.478	0.912	0.739	0.824	**0.005**	0.252	**0.001**
	Highest	0.369	0.281	0.983	0.438	0.884	**0.005**	**0.015**	**0.030**
IL-8	Inclusion	0.443	**0.050**	0.640	0.552	0.803	0.073	0.226	0.339
	Highest	0.633	0.393	0.386	0.467	0.597	0.331	0.683	0.566
IL-10	Inclusion	0.416	0.468	0.136	0.611	0.564	0.916	0.248	0.460
	Highest	0.247	0.360	0.257	0.727	0.989	0.683	0.587	0.236
LBP	Inclusion	0.086	0.364	0.958	0.660	0.227	0.291	0.952	0.148
	Highest	0.857	0.861	0.442	0.353	0.621	0.062	0.637	0.152
MPproANP	Inclusion	0.486	0.640	**0.012**	**0.029**	0.914	0.163	0.654	**0.005**
	Highest	0.521	0.287	**0.047**	**0.005**	0.926	0.068	0.911	**0.005**
MPproADM	Inclusion	**0.001**	0.320	0.310	0.915	0.296	0.241	0.264	**<0.001**
	Highest	0.351	0.209	0.618	0.979	0.547	0.158	**0.043**	**0.001**
CTproET	Inclusion	0.398	0.323	0.613	0.994	0.962	0.160	0.344	**0.018**
	Highest	**0.015**	0.330	0.893	0.888	0.933	0.092	0.169	**0.039**
Copeptin us	Inclusion	0.720	0.455	0.548	0.436	0.357	0.768	**0.006**	0.540
	Highest	0.335	0.910	0.354	0.441	0.115	0.918	0.144	0.298
PCT us	Inclusion	0.643	0.381	**0.007**	0.736	0.286	0.254	0.962	0.975
	Highest	0.855	0.560	0.056	0.908	0.362	0.634	0.230	0.711

Values given are two-sided p-values obtained by a students' t-test; Bold text denotes significant associations; HLA-DR, Human leukocyte antigen expression on monocytes; IL-6, IL-8, IL-10, three interleukins; LBP, lipopolysaccharide-binding protein; MRproANP, mid-regional pro atrial natriuretic peptide; MRproADM, mid-regional pro adrenomedullin; CTproET, C-terminal pro endothelin; CPus, ultrasensitive copeptin; PCTus, ultrasensitive procalcitonin.

Interestingly, in our cohort of patients not suffering from infections, plasma levels of IL-8 and IL-10 were mostly not detectable and below the upper limit of normal (5.0 pg/ml). This is in line with previous findings by us and Chamorro et al. showing increased IL-10 levels in patients with stroke-associated infections (22, 23). These cytokines may therefore be mainly triggered by systemic inflammation in the course of infectious complications after stroke, whereas neuroinflammation within the CNS does not seem to trigger their expression.

As previously described, we found functional outcome after 3 months to be inversely correlated to HLA-DR (24), and furthermore correlated to MRproADM and ultrasensitive Copeptin. Expression of monocytic HLA-DR is a marker of monocyte activation and has been shown to be a key marker for stroke-induced immune depression (9, 25). Lower HLA-DR expression is a strong predictor of stroke-associated pneumonia and is associated with worse functional outcome (9, 24). The latter association is further corroborated in our data independent of infection.

Several biomarkers showed an association with age, and while this has previously been reported for CTproET (26) and appears plausible for a vascular stress marker as MRproANP, the relationship for MRproADM and IL-6 is less seemingly obvious. LBP is a marker of bacterial translocation and higher levels are found in patients with post-stroke infection (27). It is also associated with a worse short-term stroke outcome (28). We could not reproduce this finding in stroke patients not suffering from infection or show any association with

imaging characteristics. MRproANP is used as a biomarker for hemodynamic stress and was previously shown to indicate higher risk for ischemic stroke (29). There were no significant associations with imaging characteristics or functional outcome in our cohort. MRproADM exerts vasodilating, vasoprotective, and angiogenic effects and is associated with post-stroke infections (30) and functional outcome after stroke (31). MRproADM has been associated with progression of small vessel disease accompanying cognitive decline (32). We could not reproduce the association with poor outcome or find an association with imaging characteristics. The vasopressin surrogate CP has been associated with higher risk of all-cause mortality, poor functional outcome and infections after ischemic stroke (33–36). Furthermore, it has been proposed to improve prediction of recurring cerebrovascular events (37). CTproET is influenced by age, renal function, and hemodynamic parameters of healthy subjects, and is a strong vasoconstrictor (26). While it has not been studied as biomarker in ischemic stroke before, its derivative endothelin has been associated with carotid atherosclerosis and silent cerebral infarctions (38). Both biomarkers were not associated with outcome in our cohort, and did not show any significant correlations with imaging findings. PCT is a blood-based marker for infection in general and was shown to be associated with post-stroke infections and functional outcome (36, 39, 40). Furthermore, higher levels of PCT are associated with extent of small vessel disease and silent infarctions on MRI (41). Our data did not show an association with functional outcome or imaging characteristics.

IL-6 Plasma Levels Correlate with Cerebral Perfusion Deficits and Infarct Sizes in Stroke Patients...

41

TABLE 4 | Association of biomarkers at inclusion and lowest/highest measurement with imaging parameters.

		Initial DWI volume	Initial PI deficit	Initial mismatch	Final FLAIR volume
HLA-DR	At Inclusion	0.933	0.936	0.716	0.397
	Lowest	0.678	0.234	0.443	0.300
IL-6	At Inclusion	**0.002**	**0.016**	**0.030**	**0.006**
	Highest	**0.009**	**0.029**	**0.042**	0.383
IL-8	At Inclusion	0.955	0.667	0.928	0.068
	Highest	0.787	0.798	0.099	0.347
IL-10	At Inclusion	0.290	0.555	0.701	0.822
	Highest	0.081	0.101	0.595	0.435
LBP	At Inclusion	0.084	0.877	0.625	0.546
	Highest	**0.037**	0.349	0.431	0.688
MPproANP	At Inclusion	0.949	0.945	0.566	0.830
	Highest	0.853	0.795	0.486	0.941
MPproADM	At Inclusion	0.882	0.901	0.123	0.130
	Highest	0.682	0.801	0.267	0.340
CTproET	At Inclusion	0.923	0.887	0.665	0.827
	Highest	0.834	0.906	0.541	0.849
Copeptin us	At Inclusion	0.144	0.801	0.457	0.701
	Highest	0.487	0.673	0.648	0.815
PCT us	At Inclusion	0.804	0.214	0.224	0.637
	Highest	0.418	0.151	0.381	0.513

Values given are two-sided p-values obtained by a Spearman's correlation; Bold text denotes significant associations; HLA-DR, Human leukocyte antigen expression on monocytes; IL-6, IL-8, IL-10, three interleukins; LBP, lipopolysaccharide-binding protein; MRproANP, mid-regional pro atrial natriuretic peptide; MRproADM, mid-regional pro adrenomedullin; CTproET, C-terminal pro endothelin; CPus, ultrasensitive copeptin; PCTus, ultrasensitive procalcitonin.

Our study suffers from several limitations: the sample size, while average for a study in this field, is limited, especially considering the amount of analyses performed. While multiple testing was a concern for us, the purpose of this study was purely exploratory. Our findings need to be corroborated by further confirmatory studies. Furthermore, our study cohort was overall rather mildly affected by stroke, not necessarily reflecting a cohort of severely impaired patients. Strengths of this report are the prospective collection of data with an in-depth clinical and neuroradiological assessment during the acute course of the disease avoiding recall H bias.

Our data supports the conclusion that IL-6 is an inflammatory marker of cerebral parenchymal damage independent of systemic infections.

AUTHOR CONTRIBUTIONS

BH wrote the manuscript and conducted all statistical analyses. SH and LU co-designed the PREDICT study and revised the manuscript. JF designed the 1000Plus study and was a major contributor in writing the manuscript. CM was a major contributor in writing the manuscript. AM designed the trial and was a major contributor in writing and revising the manuscript. All authors read and approved the final manuscript.

FUNDING

This analysis was based on the PREDICT study funded by German Research Foundation (Exc257), German Federal Ministry of Education and Research (01EO0801), European Community FP7 (201024), and Siemens Healthcare Diagnostics, and the 1000Plus study funded by the Federal Ministry of Education and Research (01 EO 0801). Additional funding was received from Thermo Fisher Scientific BRAHMS GmbH, Germany. Design of the study, as well as collection, analysis, and interpretation of data, as well as writing of the manuscript were independent of all funding sources.

REFERENCES

1. Kumar S, Selim MH, Caplan LR. Medical complications after stroke. *Lancet Neurol.* (2010) 9:105–18. doi: 10.1016/S1474-4422(09)70266-2

2. Weimar C, Roth MP, Zillessen G, Glahn J, Wimmer MLJ, Busse O, et al. Complications following acute ischemic stroke. *Eur Neurol.* (2002) 48:133–40. doi: 10.1159/000065512

3. Heuschmann PU, Wiedmann S, Wellwood I, Rudd A, Di Carlo A, Bejot Y, et al. Three-month stroke outcome: the European Registers of Stroke (EROS) investigators. *Neurology* (2011) 76:159–65. doi: 10.1212/WNL.0b013e318206ca1e

4. Ntaios G, Faouzi M, Ferrari J, Lang W, Vemmos K, Michel P. An integer-based score to predict functional outcome in acute ischemic stroke: the ASTRAL score. *Neurology* (2012) 78:1916–22. doi: 10.1212/WNL.0b013e3182 59e221

5. Byblow WD, Stinear CM. It is difficult to make predictions, especially about the future. *Stroke* (2017) 48:3187–8. doi: 10.1161/STROKEAHA.117. 019071

6. Scrutinio D, Lanzillo B, Guida P, Mastropasqua F, Monitillo V, Pusineri M, et al. Development and validation of a predictive model for functional outcome after stroke rehabilitation: the maugeri model. *Stroke* (2017) 48:3308–15. doi: 10.1161/STROKEAHA.117.018058

7. Stinear CM. Prediction of motor recovery after stroke: advances in biomarkers. *Lancet Neurol.* (2017) 16:826–36. doi: 10.1016/S1474-4422(17)30283-1

8. Bustamante A, Sobrino T, Giralt D, García-Berrocoso T, Llombart V, Ugarriza I, et al. Prognostic value of blood interleukin-6 in the prediction of functional outcome after stroke: a systematic review and meta-analysis. *J Neuroimmunol.* (2014) 274:215–24. doi: 10.1016/j.jneuroim.2014.07.01

9. Hoffmann S, Harms H, Ulm L, Nabavi DG, Mackert B-M, Schmehl I, et al. Stroke-induced immunodepression and dysphagia independently predict stroke-associated pneumonia - The PREDICT study. *J Cereb Blood Flow Metab.* (2016) 37:3671–82. doi: 10.1177/0271678X16671964

10. Hotter B, Pittl S, Ebinger M, Oepen G, Jegzentis K, Kudo K, et al. Prospective study on the mismatch concept in acute stroke patients within the first 24 h after symptom onset - 1000Plus study. *BMC Neurol.* (2009) 9:60. doi: 10.1186/1471-2377-9-60

11. Van Wagoner NJ, Benveniste EN. Interleukin-6 expression and regulation in astrocytes. *J Neuroimmunol.* (1999) 100:124–39. doi: 10.1016/S0165-5728(99)00187-3

12. Müller B. Cytokine imbalance in non-immunological chronic disease. *Cytokine* (2002) 18:334–9. doi: 10.1006/cyto.2002.0882

13. Tarkowski E, Rosengren L, Blomstrand C, Wikkelso C, Jensen C, Ekholm S, et al. Early intrathecal production of interleukin-6 predicts the size of brain lesion in stroke. *Stroke* (1995) 26:1393–8. doi: 10.1161/01.STR. 26.8.1393

14. Ormstad H, Aass HCD, Lund-Sørensen N, Amthor K-F, Sandvik L. Serum levels of cytokines and C-reactive protein in acute ischemic stroke patients, and their relationship to stroke lateralization, type, and infarct volume. *J Neurol.* (2011) 258:677–85. doi: 10.1007/s00415-011-6006-0

15. Waje-Andreassen U, Krakenes J, Ulvestad E, Thomassen L, Myhr KM, Aarseth J, et al. IL-6: an early marker for outcome in acute ischemic stroke. *Acta Neurol Scand.* (2005) 111:360–5. doi: 10.1111/j.1600-0404.2005.00416.x

16. Satizabal CL, Zhu YC, Mazoyer B, Dufouil C, Tzourio C. Circulating IL-6 and CRP are associated with MRI findings in the elderly: the 3C-Dijon Study. *Neurology* (2012) 78:720–7. doi: 10.1212/WNL.0b013e3182 48e50f

17. Miwa K, Tanaka M, Okazaki S, Furukado S, Sakaguchi M, Kitagawa K. Relations of blood inflammatory marker levels with cerebral microbleeds. *Stroke* (2011) 42:3202–6. doi: 10.1161/STROKEAHA.111.621193

18. Hoshi T, Kitagawa K, Yamagami H, Furukado S, Hougaku H, Hori M. Relations of serum high-sensitivity C-reactive protein and interleukin-6 levels with silent brain infarction. *Stroke* (2005) 36:768–72. doi: 10.1161/01.STR.0000158915.28329.51

19. Montaner J, Rovira A, Molina CA, Arenillas JF, Ribó M, Chacón P, et al. Plasmatic level of neuroinflammatory markers predict the extent of diffusion-weighted image lesions in hyperacute stroke. *J Cereb Blood Flow Metab.* (2003) 23:1403–7. doi: 10.1097/01.WCB.0000100044.07481.97

20. Rodríguez-Yánez M, Sobrino T, Arias S, Vázquez-Herrero F, Brea D, Blanco M, et al. Early biomarkers of clinical-diffusion mismatch in acute ischemic stroke. *Stroke* (2011) 42:2813–8. doi: 10.1161/STROKEAHA.111.614503

21. Rodríguez-Yánez M, Castellanos M, Sobrino T, Brea D, Ramos-Cabrer P, Pedraza S, et al. Interleukin-10 facilitates the selection of patients for systemic thrombolysis. *BMC Neurol.* (2013) 13:62. doi: 10.1186/1471-2377-13-62

22. Chamorro A, Amaro S, Vargas M, Obach V, Cervera A, Torres F, et al. Interleukin 10, monocytes and increased risk of early infection in ischaemic stroke. *J Neurol Neurosurg Psychiatr.* (2006) 77:1279–81. doi: 10.1136/jnnp.2006.100800

23. Klehmet J, Harms H, Richter M, Prass K, Volk HD, Dirnagl U, et al. Stroke-induced immunodepression and post-stroke infections: lessons from the preventive antibacterial therapy in stroke trial. *Neuroscience* (2009) 158:1184–93. doi: 10.1016/j.neuroscience.2008.07.044

24. Urra X, Cervera Á, Obach V, Climent N, Planas AM, Chamorro A. Monocytes are major players in the prognosis and risk of infection after acute stroke. *Stroke* (2009) 40:1262–8. doi: 10.1161/STROKEAHA.108. 532085

25. Hug A, Dalpke A, Wieczorek N, Giese T, Lorenz A, Auffarth G, et al. Infarct volume is a major determiner of post-stroke immune cell function and susceptibility to infection. *Stroke* (2009) 40:3226–32. doi: 10.1161/STROKEAHA.109.557967

26. Bhandari SS, Davies JE, Struck J, Ng LL. Plasma C-terminal proEndothelin-1 (CTproET-1) is affected by age, renal function, left atrial size and diastolic blood pressure in healthy subjects. *Peptides* (2014) 52:53–7. doi: 10.1016/j.peptides.2013.12.001

27. Worthmann H, Tryc AB, Dirks M, Schuppner R, Brand K, Klawonn F, et al. Lipopolysaccharide binding protein, interleukin-10, interleukin-6 and C-reactive protein blood levels in acute ischemic stroke patients with post-stroke infection. *J Neuroinflammation* (2015) 12:13. doi: 10.1186/s12974-014-0231-2

28. Klimiec E, Pera J, Chrzanowska-Wasko J, Golenia A, Slowik A, Dziedzic T. Plasma endotoxin activity rises during ischemic stroke and is associated with worse short-term outcome. *J Neuroimmunol.* (2016) 297:76–80. doi: 10.1016/j.jneuroim.2016.05.006

29. Katan M, Moon YP, Paik MC, Mueller B, Huber A, Sacco RL, et al. Procalcitonin and midregional proatrial natriuretic peptide as markers of ischemic stroke: the Northern Manhattan study. *Stroke* (2016) 47:1714–9. doi: 10.1161/STROKEAHA.115.011392

30. Bustamante A, García-Berrocoso T, Penalba A, Giralt D, Simats A, Muchada M, et al. Sepsis biomarkers reprofiling to predict stroke-associated infections. *J Neuroimmunol.* (2017) 312:19–23. doi: 10.1016/j.jneuroim.2017. 08.012

31. Seifert-Held T, Pekar T, Gattringer T, Simmet NE, Scharnagl H, Bocksrucker C, et al. Plasma midregional pro-adrenomedullin improves prediction of functional outcome in ischemic stroke. *PLoS ONE* (2013) 8:e68768. doi: 10.1371/journal.pone.0068768

32. Kuriyama N, Ihara M, Mizuno T, Ozaki E, Matsui D, Watanabe I, et al. Association between mid-regional proadrenomedullin levels and progression of deep white matter lesions in the brain accompanying cognitive decline. *J Alzheimers Dis.* (2017) 56:1253–62. doi: 10.3233/JAD-160901

33. Xu Q, Tian Y, Peng H, Li H. Copeptin as a biomarker for prediction of prognosis of acute ischemic stroke and transient ischemic attack: a meta-analysis. *Hypertens Res.* (2017) 40:465–71. doi: 10.1038/hr. 2016.165

34. Tu W-J, Ma G-Z, Ni Y, Hu X-S, Luo D-Z, Zeng X-W, et al. Copeptin and NT-proBNP for prediction of all-cause and cardiovascular death in ischemic stroke. *Neurology* (2017) 88:1899–905. doi: 10.1212/WNL.00000000 00003937

35. Katan M, Fluri F, Morgenthaler NG, Schuetz P, Zweifel C, Bingisser R, et al. Copeptin: a novel, independent prognostic marker in patients with ischemic stroke. *Ann Neurol.* (2009) 66:799–808. doi: 10.1002/ana.21783

36. Fluri F, Morgenthaler NG, Mueller B, Christ-Crain M, Katan M. Copeptin, procalcitonin and routine inflammatory markers-predictors of infection after stroke. *PLoS ONE* (2012) 7:e48309. doi: 10.1371/journal.pone. 0048309

37. De Marchis GM, Weck A, Audebert H, Benik S, Foerch C, Buhl D, et al. Copeptin for the prediction of recurrent cerebrovascular events after transient

ischemic attack: results from the CoRisk study. *Stroke* (2014) 45:2918–23. doi: 10.1161/STROKEAHA.114.005584

38. Minami S, Yamano S, Yamamoto Y, Sasaki R, Nakashima T, Takaoka M, et al. Associations of plasma endothelin concentration with carotid atherosclerosis and asymptomatic cerebrovascular lesions in patients with essential hypertension. *Hypertens Res.* (2001) 24:663–70. doi: 10.1291/hypres.24.663

39. Ulm L, Hoffmann S, Nabavi DG, Hermans M, Mackert B-M, Hamilton F, et al. The Randomized Controlled STRAWINSKI Trial: procalcitonin-guided antibiotic therapy after stroke. *Front Neurol.* (2017) 8:153. doi: 10.3389/fneur.2017.00153

40. Wang C, Gao L, Zhang Z-G, Li Y-Q, Yang Y-L, Chang T, et al. Procalcitonin is a stronger predictor of long-term functional outcome and mortality than high-sensitivity C-reactive protein in patients with ischemic stroke. *Mol Neurobiol.* (2016) 53:1509–17. doi: 10.1007/s12035-015-9112-7

41. Li G, Zhu C, Li J, Wang X, Zhang Q, Zheng H, et al. Increased level of procalcitonin is associated with total MRI burden of cerebral small vessel disease in patients with ischemic stroke. *Neurosci Lett.* (2018) 662:242–6. doi: 10.1016/j.neulet.2017.10.040

6

CSF-Progranulin and Neurofilament Light Chain Levels in Patients with Radiologically Isolated Syndrome—Sign of Inflammation

Marc Pawlitzki[1,2]*, Catherine M. Sweeney-Reed[1], Daniel Bittner[1], Anke Lux[3], Stefan Vielhaber[1], Stefanie Schreiber[1], Friedemann Paul[4,5,6] and Jens Neumann[1]

[1] Department of Neurology, Otto-von-Guericke University, Magdeburg, Germany, [2] Department of Neurology with Institute of Translational Neurology, University Hospital of Muenster, Münster, Germany, [3] Department for Biometrics and Medical Informatics, Otto-von-Guericke-University, Magdeburg, Germany, [4] Charité – Universitätsmedizin Berlin, Corporate Member of Freie Universität Berlin, Humboldt-Universität zu Berlin, and Berlin Institute of Health, NeuroCure Clinical Research Center, Berlin, Germany, [5] Charité – Universitätsmedizin Berlin, Corporate Member of Freie Universität Berlin, Humboldt-Universität zu Berlin, and Berlin Institute of Health, Department of Neurology, Berlin, Germany, [6] Experimental and Clinical Research Center, Max Delbrueck Center for Molecular Medicine and Charité – Universitätsmedizin Berlin, Corporate Member of Freie Universität Berlin, Humboldt-Universität zu Berlin, and Berlin Institute of Health, Berlin, Germany

*Correspondence:
Marc Pawlitzki
marc.pawlitzki@ukmuenster.de

Background: Cerebrospinal fluid (CSF) markers of disease in patients with radiologically isolated syndrome (RIS) are the subject of intense investigation, because they have the potential to enhance our understanding of the natural disease course and provide insights into similarities and differences between RIS and other multiple sclerosis (MS) disease identities.

Methods: Here we compared neurofilament light chain (NFL) and progranulin (PGRN) levels in the CSF in RIS patients with levels in patients with different subtypes of MS and healthy controls (HC) using Kruskal–Wallis one-way analysis of variance.

Results: Median CSF NFL concentrations in RIS patients did not differ to those in HC and clinically isolated syndrome (CIS) patients, but were significantly lower than in relapsing remitting (RRMS) and primary progressive (PPMS) MS patients. In contrast, RIS patients exhibited higher median CSF PGRN levels than HC and showed no significant differences compared with CIS, RRMS, and PPMS cases.

Conclusion: We postulate that elevated PGRN values in the CSF of RIS patients might indicate inflammatory and repair activity prior to axonal disintegration.

Keywords: multiple sclerosis, radiologically isolated syndrome, cerebrospinal fluid, neurofilament light chain, progranulin

INTRODUCTION

Widespread routine clinical implementation of magnetic resonance imaging (MRI) leads to incidental detection of MRI abnormalities suggestive of multiple sclerosis (MS) in patients undergoing cerebral MRI due to non-specific neurological symptoms (e.g., headache, dizziness) (1). Among these patients, a considerable number, mainly young men, develop radiological and clinical progression to relapsing (RRMS) or primary progressive (PPMS) forms of MS within 5

CSF-Progranulin and Neurofilament Light Chain Levels in Patients with Radiologically Isolated...

45

years (2, 3). This observation led to the establishment of the definition of the radiologically isolated syndrome (RIS) (4) as a probable preclinical variant of MS (5, 6). Additionally, a fraction of these patients exhibit oligoclonal bands (OCBs) in the cerebrospinal fluid (CSF), similar to those found in patients with a clinically isolated syndrome (CIS) (7).

Because early disease-modifying treatment (DMT) could delay the conversion from CIS to clinical MS (8), and repeated MRI examinations have led to early identification of progression to MS from CIS, with the offer of more powerful therapies, the question arises as to whether RIS patients could profit from these procedures as well. To address this question, the understanding of pro- and anti-inflammatory activity, repair mechanisms, and axonal loss, in the absence of noticeable clinical events, needs to be expanded to estimate the clinical relevance of incidentally diagnosed MRI lesions.

We consider CSF progranulin (PGRN) and neurofilament light chain (NFL) to serve as *in vivo* measures of inflammatory activity, tissue repair and neuroaxonal damage. In short, in the central nervous system, PGRN is mainly expressed in neurons and microglia (9). Considering anti-inflammatory and repair activity, progranulin (PRGN) has been identified as a molecule, which could regulate inflammation after axonal injury in the context of MS-associated relapses and continuous inflammation in progressive forms of MS by overexpression in activated microglia (10).

Neurofilaments are structural constituents of the neuroaxonal cytoskeleton and integral components of synapses; they are essential for axonal growth, transport, and signaling pathways (11, 12). White matter and cortical injury is related to elevated CSF NFL that represents a downstream effect of neuroaxonal loss (13), and CSF NFL increase has been found in early MS disease stages with axonal injury as well (14).

In the current study, we assessed the concentrations of CSF PGRN and NFL in RIS patients as potential markers of early repair mechanisms/inflammation and axonal loss, to compare them with the CSF PGRN and NFL concentrations in controls and patients at different MS disease stages and with different MS subtypes.

METHODS

Patients, Controls, and Clinical Assessment

Our cross-sectional study included $n = 23$ RIS patients, diagnosed according to the criteria proposed by Okuda et al. (4) and MAGNIMS (15), and $n = 15$ CIS, $n = 15$ RRMS and $n = 26$ PPMS patients, diagnosed according to the McDonald criteria (2010) (16). All patients were recruited retrospectively at the Department of Neurology, Otto-von-Guericke University Magdeburg, Germany, between 2012 and 2017. Due to the retrospective character of the study, written informant consent was not obtained, but all analyses were taken from diagnostic procedures in clinical routine.

All patients underwent a lumbar puncture (LP) and their clinical disability was assessed applying the Expanded Disability

TABLE 1 | Summary of the clinical and radiologic data of all investigated groups.

	HC (N = 30)	RIS (N = 23)	CIS (N = 15)	RRMS (N = 15)	PPMS (N = 26)
Age at lumbar puncture (years)	35 (18–49)	37 (18–72)	44 (21–61)	33 (17–55)	52 (25–71)
Male SEX, N (%)	12 (33)	8 (35)	3 (16)	6 (30)	15 (60)
Disease duration (months)	–	6 (0–89)	4 (1–78)	19 (2–174)	61 (12–255)
EDSS	–	0 (0–1.5)	1 (0–3.5)	1.5 (0–6)	4.5 (2–7.5)
Presence of Gd+ lesions, n (%)	–	0 (0)	0 (0)	4 (29)	3 (11.5)
Presence of periventricular lesions, n (%)	–	22 (96)	13 (87)	13 (87)	25 (96)
Presence of infratentorial lesions, n (%)	–	9 (39)	3 (20)	7 (46)	16 (62)
Presence of juxtacortical lesions, n (%)	–	14 (61)	8 (53)	10 (67)	20 (77)
Presence of spinal cord lesions lesions, n (%)	–	4 (17)	5 (33)	8 (53)	20 (77)

N, number of participants; unless otherwise reported median (range) is given. CSF, cerebrospinal fluid; CIS, Clinically isolated syndrome; EDSS, Expanded Disability Status Scale; Gd+, Gadolinium enhancing; HC, healthy controls; PPMS, primary progressive multiple sclerosis; RRMS, relapsing remitting multiple sclerosis; RIS, radiologically isolated syndrome. Disease duration was defined as the timespan between symptom onset and the date of lumbar puncture.

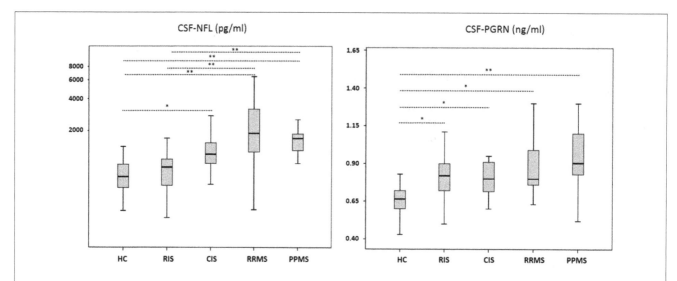

FIGURE 1 | Neurofilament light (NFL) and Progranulin (PGRN) in cerebrospinal fluid (CSF). CIS, clinically isolated syndrome; HC, healthy controls; PPMS, primary progressive multiple sclerosis; RIS, radiologically isolated syndrome; RRMS, relapsing remitting multiple sclerosis. Boxes indicate the interquartile range, bars indicates median CSF-NFL/PGRN values, and Whiskers present the 95% CI. Group comparisons were conducted using a Kruskal–Wallis one way analysis of variance with *post-hoc* Dunn–Bonferroni-testing. $P < 0.05$ were deemed to be statistically significant. RIS, CIS, RRMS, and PPMS showed higher CSF PGRN values than HC, while PPMS and RRMS also differed in contrast to RIS cases. RJS, CIS, RRMS, and PPMS showed higher CSF PGRN values than HC. $^{*}P < 0.005$; $^{**}P < 0.001$.

Status Scale (EDSS) (17). Reasons for performing a MRI examination in RIS patients were non-specific complaints including headache ($n = 7$ [30%]), non-specific dizziness ($n = 5$ [22%]), tinnitus ($n = 3$ [13%]), transitory ischemic attack (5 [22%]), back pain ($n = 2$ [9%]) and idiopathic peripheral facial palsy ($n = 1$ [4%]). In MS patients, disease duration was defined as time in months from symptom onset to the LP, while in RIS cases it was defined as time from the patients' first complaints to the LP. CIS, RRMS and PPMS patients neither presented with a relapse within the last 4 weeks, nor did they received any disease-modifying treatment.

CSF was additionally acquired from a hospital-based cohort of $n = 30$ healthy controls (HC). The CSF from the HC group was obtained from individuals in whom the presence of a neurological disorder had been suspected, but these individuals were deemed to be healthy in retrospect and in particular have normal cerebral MRI scans. In addition to the clinical classification, patients included in the control group also fulfilled the following Reiber laboratory criteria defining a non-inflammatory CSF [<5 cells/µl, >500 mg protein/ml, <2 mmol/l lactate, no disruption of the blood/CSF barrier, no oligoclonal bands (OCB) in the CSF, and no intrathecal immunoglobulin (Ig) G, IgA, or IgM synthesis] (18).

The study was approved by the local ethics committee (No. 07/17).

Neuro-Imaging Investigations

Brain and spinal cord MRI scans from patients originated from non-standardized protocols from differing MRI units and magnetic field strengths (1.5 or 3.0 Tesla) were performed within 6 months or after CSF measurement. All examinations included T1- and T2-weighted spin-echo sequences with the

administration of gadolinium (Gd). Abnormalities including T1-hypointesities, T2-hyperintesities, and Gd-enhanced T1-lesions were initially identified by a neuroradiologist and they were subsequently verified by a MS specialist (M.P.). Brain and spinal cord scans of all RIS cases were reviewed to confirm the fulfillment of dissemination in space (DIS) criteria (4).

CSF Measures

Immediately after LP, CSF cells were counted, and total protein, albumin quotient (Q_{alb}), and OCBs were measured. The remaining CSF material was centrifuged at 4°C, aliquoted, and stored at −80°C until PGRN and NFL analysis was performed. PGRN and NFL levels were measured using commercially available ELISA kits (PGRN: Human Progranulin ELISA kit, Mediagnost, Reutlingen, Germany; NFL: UmanDiagnostics NF-light®, Umeå, Sweden) following the instructions provided by the manufacturer. All samples were processed in duplicate, in serial procedures, and the mean was taken for statistical analysis.

Statistical Analysis

Statistical analysis was conducted using SPSS 21 (IBM, Armonk, New York, USA). Comparisons of categorical variables (e.g., sex or OCBs) were performed using a α^2-test. Moreover, a univariate analysis of variance, including the estimated marginal means was performed to evaluate between-subject-effects and the effect of age, sex on PGRN and NFL. For further group comparisons of continuous variables (e.g., age, CSF NFL, CSF PGRN, disease duration, EDSS), a Kruskal–Wallis one-way analysis of variance was conducted with group (HC vs. RIS vs. CIS vs. RRMS vs. PPMS patients) as the independent variable, applying pairwise *post-hoc* testing (Dunn-Bonferroni-test).

TABLE 2 | Summary of the cerebrospinal fluid results of all investigated groups.

	HC (N = 30)	RIS (N = 23)	CIS (N = 15)	RRMS (N = 15)	PPMS (N = 26)	p-values									
						HC vs. RIS	HC vs. CIS	HC vs. RRMS	HC vs. PPMS	RIS vs. CIS	RIS vs. RRMS	RIS vs. PPMS	CIS vs. RRMS	CIS vs. PPMS	RRMS vs. PPMS
CSF Cell count /µl	1 (0–4)	1 (0–14)	3 (0–19)	3 (1–25)	4 (1–16)	**0.001**	0.08	**0.01**	1.0	1.0	1.0	0.09	1.0	1.0	**0.04**
CSF protein (mg/dl)	311 (178–460)	371 (238–909)	321 (226–491)	421 (255–650)	410 (248–1047)	0.2	1.0	**0.04**	**0.001**	1.0	1.0	1.0	1.0	1.0	1.0
Positive OCB, N (%)	0 (0)	19 (83)	15 (100)	15 (100)	25 (96)	–	–	–	–	–	–	–	–	–	–
Qalb	4.3 (2.3–6.4)	4.7 (2.8–11.8)	4.03 (3.0–7.2)	5.5 (2.5–8.9)	5.0 (2.0–18.8)	0.05	0.05	0.05	0.05	0.05	0.05	0.05	0.05	0.05	0.05
CSF NFL (pg/ml)	742 (357–1424)	914 (306–2552)	1206 (628–2762)	1699 (990–4275)	1893 (364–6458)	1.0	**0.03**	**<0.001**	**<0.001**	0.3	**<0.001**	**<0.001**	0.8	0.5	1.0
CSF PGRN (pg/ml)	0.67 (0.43–1.12)	0.82 (0.50–1.20)	0.80 (0.60–1.20)	0.80 (0.63–1.30)	0.91 (0.52–1.59)	**0.004**	**0.04**	**0.004**	**<0.001**	1.0	1.0	0.7	1.0	0.6	1.0

N, number of participants; unless otherwise reported median (range) is given. CIS, clinically isolated syndrome; CSF, cerebrospinal fluid; HC, healthy controls; NFL, neurofilament light chain; PGRN, progranulin; PPMS, primary progressive multiple sclerosis; Qalb, albumin quotient; RIS, radiologically isolated syndrome; RRMS, relapsing remitting multiple sclerosis. Disease duration was defined as the timespan between symptom onset and time of lumbar puncture. For group comparisons a Kruskal-Wallis one-way analysis of variance with post-hoc Dunn-Bonferroni-testing were conducted. Bold value indicates P-values < 0.05 were deemed to be statistically significant.

RESULTS

Cohort Characterization and MRI Examination

The demographics, the clinical and MRI data of the cohorts are provided in **Table 1**. Median age and sex [$\chi^2(4) = 0.07$] did not differ between SC, RIS, CIS, and RRMS patients, whereas PPMS patients were significantly older than SC, RIS ($p < 0.001$, respectively) and RRMS patients ($p = 0.002$). Median disease duration was longer in PPMS compared to RIS and CIS ($p < 0.001$, respectively). Median EDSS at the time of LP differed between RIS compared to RRMS and PPMS ($p = 0.007$; $p < 0.001$), as well as between CIS and PPMS ($p < 0.001$) and RRMS vs. PPMS ($p = 0.02$).

CSF Examination

CSF cell count was significantly higher in RRMS compared with PPMS patients and HC as well as between RIS and HC patients. OCBs were present exclusively in the CSF of 19 (83%) RIS, 25 (96%) PPMS, and all (100%) CIS and RRMS patients (Table 2). Univariate analysis underlined the group difference in particular, and the absence of an effect of age and sex on PGRN and NFL levels.

The concentration of CSF NFL was significantly higher in CIS, RRMS, and PPMS compared to RIS and HC, while there were no significant differences between RIS and HC (**Figure 1** and **Table 2**). The comparison of CSF PRGN between groups revealed significantly higher levels in CIS, RIS, RRMS, and PPMS than detected in HC (**Figure 1** and **Table 2**).

DISCUSSION

Detection and characterization of early biomarkers in RIS patients, in order to investigate whether they could reflect MS disease courses, is an ongoing challenge. We compared the concentrations of CSF PGRN and NFL in RIS patients with the concentrations in healthy controls and in patients at different disease stages and with different subtypes of treatment-naive MS in the absence of an acute clinical relapse. Our analysis revealed similar PGRN concentrations in RIS patients to those found in several MS subtypes. PGRN levels were significantly higher, on the other hand, in RIS patients than in HC, while NFL concentrations did not differ between the RIS and HC cohorts.

To the best of our knowledge, the current study provides the largest comparison of CSF PGRN levels in different subtypes of MS, including RIS patients, to date. Surprisingly, while NFL values in the CSF of RIS patients were comparable with the HC cohort and significant lower compared with those in patients at different MS disease stages, the RIS cohort exhibited significantly higher concentrations of PRGN in comparison with the HC cohort and showed similar concentrations to those found in patients with the different MS subtypes.

Former studies have reported elevated (19) or unchanged CSF PGRN values in MS but included patients who had experienced an acute relapse (20). The absence of differences of CSF PGRN thus seems to be unusual, because acute inflammation is considered to provoke PGRN expression (19). Furthermore, it has been shown that disease-modifying treatment could decrease PGRN levels (19). In order to exclude heterogeneity, we divided the cohorts into distinct subtypes (RIS, CIS, RRMS, PPMS), comprising only patients without an acute clinical relapse and also without disease-modifying treatments.

The role of PGRN is currently under intense investigation, and microglia cells have been identified as expressing and secreting PGRN after axonal injury (21). CSF PGRN level seems to be largely unaffected by blood PGRN concentration and in turn potential blood-CSF barrier disruption which underline the specificity of intrathecal produced PRGN (22). In addition, PGRN levels correlate with the concentration of the proinflammatory cytokine interleukin 6, which is elevated after acute (19) and chronic axonal injury (10). However, NFL levels were not increased in our RIS cohort, indicating that PGRN could be secreted even before axonal injury is detectable in the CSF via elevated NFL concentrations. This finding leads us to speculate tentatively that PGRN may be upregulated early, at the beginning of disease activity, and that RIS might in turn be a prodromal stage of MS. PGRN may thus shed new light on, clinically silent, disease-related alterations at the earliest MS stages. In line with histological findings that inflammation is the primary hallmark of MS and induces neuronal injury (23, 24), we suggest that PGRN might be more sensitive to detecting early disease-related abnormalities, also in RIS cases, in the face of (still) normal axonal integration, as measured by NFL levels (25).

The finding of missing NFL elevation in RIS patients is surprising, given the early, MRI-detectable neurodegeneration already found in the RIS cohorts (26) and the recognized association between raised CSF NFL and GD-enhancing white matter lesions in RIS patients (27). However, no GD-enhancing white matter lesions were present in our RIS group, suggesting that our cohort is more homogeneous or less severely affected, and acute axonal loss might thus play an insignificant role and be therefore not detectable via the elevated NFL concentrations that are seen in relapsing and progressive MS patients (14, 28, 29).

In addition to the MRI findings resulting in a diagnosis of RIS, we identified CSF abnormalities, e.g., OCBs in the CSF, in almost all of our RIS patients, which is in line with previous studies, in which OCBs were identified as independent predictors for early conversion to MS (27, 30). Our RIS-cohort may thus be characterized as high-risk patients (27) for conversion. However, the prevalence of OCBs is not specific for MS (31), nor does it mirror acute or continuous inflammatory activity (32).

Here we demonstrated significantly elevated CSF PGRN levels in RIS and MS patients during the clinically silent or non-relapsing phase, presumably suggesting ongoing inflammation, while only the later disease stages revealed an increased CSF NFL, thus mirroring axonal injury in addition. We here report the results from a pilot study. The limitations are the relatively small sample size and the higher mean age of PPMS patients. Standardized MRI, in addition, might assist to improve the evaluation of the relationship between white matter lesion volume and CSF-PGRN in MS patients. Hence, longitudinal studies with a larger sample size are needed to overcome these limitations and to determine the prognostic role of PGRN in MS and in particular in RIS patients.

AUTHOR CONTRIBUTIONS

All authors listed have made a substantial, direct and intellectual contribution to the work, and approved it for publication.

ACKNOWLEDGMENTS

We thank Kerstin Kaiser and Jeanette Witzke, Department of Neurology, Otto-von-Guericke University, Magdeburg, Germany, for excellent technical assistance.

REFERENCES

1. Granberg T, Martola J, Kristoffersen-Wiberg M, Aspelin P, Fredrikson S. Radiologically isolated syndrome–incidental magnetic resonance imaging findings suggestive of multiple sclerosis, a systematic review. *Mult Scler.* (2013) 19:271–80. doi: 10.1177/135245851245 1943

2. Okuda DT, Siva A, Kantarci O, Inglese M, Katz I, Tutuncu M, et al. Radiologically isolated syndrome: 5-year risk for an initial clinical event. *PLoS ONE* (2014) 9:e90509. doi: 10.1371/journal.pone.0090509

3. Lebrun C, Bensa C, Debouverie M, De Seze J, Wiertlievski S, Brochet B, et al. Unexpected multiple sclerosis: follow-up of 30 patients with magnetic resonance imaging and clinical conversion profile. *J Neurol Neurosurg Psychiatr.* (2008) 79:195–8. doi: 10.1136/jnnp.2006.108274

4. Okuda DT, Mowry EM, Beheshtian A, Waubant E, Baranzini SE, Goodin DS, et al. Incidental MRI anomalies suggestive of multiple sclerosis: the radiologically isolated syndrome. *Neurology* (2009) 72:800–5. doi: 10.1212/01.wnl.0000335764.14513.1a

5. Makhani N, Lebrun C, Siva A, Brassat D, Carra Dallière C, Seze J, et al. Radiologically isolated syndrome in children: clinical and

radiologic outcomes. *Neurol Neuroimmunol Neuroinflamm.* (2017) 4:e395. doi: 10.1212/NXI.0000000000000395

6. Alcaide-Leon P, Cybulsky K, Sankar S, Casserly C, Leung G, Hohol M, et al. Quantitative spinal cord MRI in radiologically isolated syndrome. *Neurol Neuroimmunol Neuroinflamm.* (2018) 5:e436. doi: 10.1212/NXI.0000000000000436

7. Gabelić T, Radmilović M, Posavec V, Skvorc A, Bošković M, Adamec I, et al. Differences in oligoclonal bands and visual evoked potentials in patients with radiologically and clinically isolated syndrome. *Acta Neurol Belg.* (2013) 113:13–7. doi: 10.1007/s13760-012-0106-1

8. Leist TP, Comi G, Cree BA, Coyle PK, Freedman MS, Hartung HP, et al. Effect of oral cladribine on time to conversion to clinically definite multiple sclerosis in patients with a first demyelinating event (ORACLE MS): A phase 3 randomised trial. *Lancet Neurol.* (2014) 13:257–67. doi: 10.1016/S1474-4422(14)70005-5

9. Eriksen JL, Mackenzie IRA. Progranulin: normal function and role in neurodegeneration. *J Neurochem.* (2008) 104:287–97. doi: 10.1111/j.1471-4159.2007.04968.x

10. Vercellino M, Grifoni S, Romagnolo A, Masera S, Mattioda A, Trebini C, et al. Progranulin expression in brain tissue and cerebrospinal

fluid levels in multiple sclerosis. *Mult Scler.* (2011) 17:1194–201. doi: 10.1177/1352458511406164

11. Oberstadt M, Claßen J, Arendt T, Holzer M. TDP-43 and Cytoskeletal Proteins in ALS. *Mol Neurobiol.* (2018) 55:3143–51. doi: 10.1007/s12035-017-0543-1

12. Petzold A, Gveric D, Groves M, Schmierer K, Grant D, Chapman M, et al. Phosphorylation and compactness of neurofilaments in multiple sclerosis: indicators of axonal pathology. *Exp Neurol.* (2008) 213:326–35. doi: 10.1016/j.expneurol.2008.06.008

13. Bergman J, Dring A, Zetterberg H, Blennow K, Norgren N, Gilthorpe J, et al. Neurofilament light in CSF and serum is a sensitive marker for axonal white matter injury in MS. *Neurol Neuroimmunol Neuroinflamm.* (2016) 3:e271. doi: 10.1212/NXI.0000000000000271

14. Kuhle J, Plattner K, Bestwick JP, Lindberg RL, Ramagopalan SV, Norgren N, et al. A comparative study of CSF neurofilament light and heavy chain protein in MS. *Mult Scler.* (2013) 19:1597–603. doi: 10.1177/1352458513482374

15. De Stefano N, Giorgio A, Tintoré M, Pia Amato M, Kappos L, Palace J, et al. Radiologically isolated syndrome or subclinical multiple sclerosis: MAGNIMS consensus recommendations. *Mult Scler.* (2018) 24:214–21. doi: 10.1177/1352458517717808

16. Polman CH, Reingold SC, Banwell B, Clanet M, Cohen JA, Filippi M, et al. Diagnostic criteria for multiple sclerosis: 2010 revisions to the McDonald criteria. *Ann Neurol.* (2011) 69:292–302. doi: 10.1002/ana.22366

17. Kurtzke JF. Rating neurologic impairment in multiple sclerosis: an expanded disability status scale (EDSS). *Neurology* (1983) 33:1444–52. doi: 10.1212/WNL.33.11.1444

18. Reiber H, Lange P. Quantification of virus-specific antibodies in cerebrospinal fluid and serum: sensitive and specific detection of antibody synthesis in brain. *Clin Chem.* (1991) 37:1153–60.

19. Kimura A, Takemura M, Saito K, Serrero G, Yoshikura N, Hayashi Y, et al. Increased cerebrospinal fluid progranulin correlates with interleukin-6 in the acute phase of neuromyelitis optica spectrum disorder. *J Neuroimmunol.* (2017) 305:175–81. doi: 10.1016/j.jneuroim.2017.01.006

20. Riz M, de Galimberti D, Fenoglio C, Piccio LM, Scalabrini D, Venturelli E, et al. Cerebrospinal fluid progranulin levels in patients with different multiple sclerosis subtypes. *Neurosci Lett.* (2010) 469:234–6. doi: 10.1016/j.neulet.2009.12.002

21. Naphade SB, Kigerl KA, Jakeman LB, Kostyk SK, Popovich PG, Kuret J. Progranulin expression is upregulated after spinal contusion in mice. *Acta Neuropathol.* (2010) 119:123–33. doi: 10.1007/s00401-009-0616-y

22. Feneberg E, Steinacker P, Volk AE, Weishaupt JH, Wollmer MA, Boxer A, et al. Progranulin as a candidate biomarker for therapeutic trial in patients with ALS and FTLD. *J Neural Transm.* (2016) 123:289–96. doi: 10.1007/s00702-015-1486-1

23. Bitsch A, Schuchardt J, Bunkowski S, Kuhlmann T, Brück W. Acute axonal injury in multiple sclerosis. Correlation with demyelination and inflammation. *Brain* (2000) 123:1174–83. doi: 10.1093/brain/123.6.1174

24. Brück W. The pathology of multiple sclerosis is the result of focal inflammatory demyelination with axonal damage. *J Neurol.* (2005) 252(Suppl. 5):v3–9. doi: 10.1007/s00415-005-5002-7

25. Giorgio A, Stromillo ML, De Leucio A, Rossi F, Brandes I, Hakiki B, et al. Appraisal of brain connectivity in radiologically isolated syndrome by modeling imaging measures. *J Neurosci.* (2015) 35:550–8. doi: 10.1523/JNEUROSCI.2557-14.2015

26. Azevedo CJ, Overton E, Khadka S, Buckley J, Liu S, Sampat M, et al. Early CNS neurodegeneration in radiologically isolated syndrome. *Neurol Neuroimmunol Neuroinflamm.* (2015) 2:e102. doi: 10.1212/NXI.0000000000000102

27. Matute-Blanch C, Villar LM, Álvarez-Cermeño JC, Rejdak K, Evdoshenko E, Makshakov G, et al. Neurofilament light chain and oligoclonal bands are prognostic biomarkers in radiologically isolated syndrome. *Brain* (2018) 141:1085–93. doi: 10.1093/brain/awy021

28. Lycke JN, Karlsson JE, Andersen O, Rosengren LE. Neurofilament protein in cerebrospinal fluid: a potential marker of activity in multiple sclerosis. *J Neurol Neurosurg Psychiatr.* (1998) 64:402–4. doi: 10.1136/jnnp.64.3.402

29. Semra YK, Seidi OA, Sharief MK. Heightened intrathecal release of axonal cytoskeletal proteins in multiple sclerosis is associated with progressive disease and clinical disability. *J Neuroimmunol.* (2002) 122:132–9. doi: 10.1016/S0165-5728(01)00455-6

30. Thouvenot E, Hinsinger G, Demattei C, Uygunoglu U, Castelnovo G, Pitton-Vouyovitch S, et al. Cerebrospinal fluid chitinase-3-like protein 1 level is not an independent predictive factor for the risk of clinical conversion in radiologically isolated syndrome. *Mult Scler.* (2018). doi: 10.1177/1352458518767043. [Epub ahead of print].

31. Jarius S, Eichhorn P, Franciotta D, Petereit HF, Akman-Demir G, Wick M, et al. The MRZ reaction as a highly specific marker of multiple sclerosis: re-evaluation and structured review of the literature. *J Neurol.* (2017) 264:453–66. doi: 10.1007/s00415-016-8360-4

32. Haertle M, Kallweit U, Weller M, Linnebank M. The presence of oligoclonal IgG bands in human CSF during the course of neurological diseases. *J Neurol.* (2014) 261:554–60. doi: 10.1007/s00415-013-7234-2

7

Driving Ability in Alzheimer Disease Spectrum: Neural Basis, Assessment and Potential Use of Optic Flow Event-Related Potentials

Takao Yamasaki[1,2]* and Shozo Tobimatsu[1]

[1] Department of Clinical Neurophysiology, Neurological Institute, Graduate School of Medical Sciences, Kyushu University, Fukuoka, Japan, [2] Department of Neurology, Minkodo Minohara Hospital, Fukuoka, Japan

*Correspondence:
Takao Yamasaki
yamasa@neurophy.med.kyushu-u.ac.jp

Driving requires multiple cognitive functions including visuospatial perception and recruits widespread brain networks. Recently, traffic accidents in dementia, particularly in Alzheimer disease spectrum (ADS), have increased and become an urgent social problem. Therefore, it is necessary to develop the objective and reliable biomarkers for driving ability in patients with ADS. Interestingly, even in the early stage of the disease, patients with ADS are characterized by the impairment of visuospatial function such as radial optic flow (OF) perception related to self-motion perception. For the last decade, we have studied the feasibility of event-related potentials (ERPs) in response to radial OF in ADS and proposed that OF-ERPs provided an additional information on the alteration of visuospatial perception in ADS (1, 2). Hence, we hypothesized that OF-ERPs can be a possible predictive biomarker of driving ability in ADS. In this review, the recent concept of neural substrates of driving in healthy humans are firstly outlined. Second, we mention the alterations of driving performance and its brain network in ADS. Third, the current status of assessment tools for driving ability is stated. Fourth, we describe ERP studies related to driving ability in ADS. Further, the neural basis of OF processing and OF-ERPs in healthy humans are mentioned. Finally, the application of OF-ERPs to ADS is described. The aim of this review was to introduce the potential use of OF-ERPs for assessment of driving ability in ADS.

Keywords: Alzheimer disease spectrum, radial optic flow perception, event-related potentials, driving ability, Alzheimer's disease, mild cognitive impairment

INTRODUCTION

Driving is a complicated skill that needs to integrate multiple cognitive, perceptual and motor abilities (3), and is supported by widely distributed brain network responsible for these complex processes (4–8). The driving ability can be disturbed by a decline in these brain networks due to normal aging and cognitive impairment such as dementia (3, 9–11). In recent years, the number of individuals with dementia is steadily increasing due to aging of the population (12). Under such circumstances, traffic accidents in individuals with dementia have increased and become an urgent social problem (11).

Among dementia, Alzheimer's disease (AD) is the most common (12). AD progresses on a spectrum with three stages, so-called, "AD spectrum (ADS)" (13); (1) preclinical AD (14), (2) mild cognitive impairment (MCI) due to AD (15), and (3) AD dementia (16). AD dementia is characterized by the impairment of short-term episodic memory, orientation, visuospatial function, language and executive function (12). The major neuropathological hallmarks of AD are deposition of β amyloid (senile plaques) and accumulation of neurofibrillary tangles, which cause a series of toxic events that result in synaptic dysfunction, neuronal loss and brain atrophy (12). Overall, multiple cognitive function associated with distributed brain network are impaired due to the AD pathology, resulting in the decline of driving ability in patients with AD.

There are various methods to assess driving ability, which include on-road test, driving simulation, and neuropsychological tests. However, recent systematic review and meta-analysis on these methods have demonstrated a lack of consistency of the findings among the studies though the several cognitive tests are considered to be the predictors of driving performance in AD patients (3, 17). So far, there have been no tests sufficient to determine driving safety, so it is necessary to establish a reliable method that can accurately evaluate driving ability in ADS. Interestingly, visuospatial dysfunction is often an early symptom even in the early stage of ADS (18, 19). Specifically, psychophysical studies demonstrated that AD patients exhibited selective elevation of motion coherence thresholds for radial optic flow (OF) motion which was related to self-motion perception (20), compared with those of coherent horizontal (HO) motion and static forms (19). In addition, the impaired OF perception was correlated with poor performance of the spatial navigation test (19). These findings suggest that the deficits of OF perception is responsible for the impairment of spatial navigation including the driving performance in AD patients. Some patients with MCI also exhibited selective impairment of coherent OF motion perception (18).

Event-related potentials (ERPs) are a pertinent tool to assess the visual function as well as dysfunction in humans because ERPs are non-invasive, objective, rapid, repeatable with the low cost. ERPs are also characterized by excellent temporal resolution (< 1 ms) and can measure neural activity directly compared with functional magnetic resonance imaging (fMRI) (21, 22). Therefore, radial OF-ERPs may be a neural biomarker for decline of driving performance in ADS.

In this review, we first outline the neural basis of driving ability in healthy humans. Second, we describe the alterations of performance and associated brain function for driving in ADS. Third, we refer to current status of the assessment tests for driving and its problems. Fourth, ERP studies related to driving ability in ADS are stated. Further, we mention the neural basis of OF perception and findings of OF-related ERPs in healthy humans. Finally, we introduce the potential use of OF-ERPs for assessing driving ability of ADS. The aim of this review was to stress the feasibility of neurophysiological evaluation of OF perception that can be a neural biomarker for altered driving ability in ADS.

NEURAL BASIS OF DRIVING ABILITY IN HEALTHY INDIVIDUALS

Driving requires the coordination of multiple cognitive functions and recruitment of associated multiple brain regions. Several fMRI studies on various driving tasks have demonstrated the activation of widespread brain network including occipital, parietal, frontal, motor and cerebellar regions and others to maintain safe driving (4–8). **Figure 1** shows an example of activated brain regions while driving in a recent fMRI study (4). In their study, during driving only condition, the occipital activations were observed in the inferior, superior and middle occipital gyri and lingual gyrus. The activated areas of parietal lobe were superior and inferior parietal lobe, postcentral gyrus, and precuneus. The activations of frontal regions consisted of the inferior, middle and superior frontal gyri and precentral gyrus. The superior and middle temporal gyri were the activated areas of temporal regions. The activations of the cerebellum included the uvular, declive, and cerebellar tonsil. In addition, the limbic region such as cingulate gyrus, sub-lobar region including insula and lentiform nucleus were activated (4).

During driving, occipital and parietal regions plays a crucial role in visuospatial perception and attention to visual motion and fixed landmarks during vehicle movement. The frontal region is important for the executive function, working memory, processing thoughts, and decision-making. The motor and cerebellar regions engage in fine-control and action planning during movement execution (4–8). Furthermore, the recruitment of these brain regions is changeable but not uniform while driving. For instance, during distracted driving, brain activations shift the posterior regions to the frontal regions, particularly in the prefrontal areas (6). Taken together, because brain networks related to driving are broadly distributed, they may be susceptible to brain disorder such as ADS which shows extensive brain damage.

ALTERED DRIVING PERFORMANCE IN ADS

Older drivers are at higher risk for traffic accidents such as crashes, injuries and deaths than other age groups (11). Further, individuals with AD dementia have an increased risk of traffic accidents compared to healthy older drivers (11). Severity of decline in driving performance was correlated with a degree of cognitive impairment in AD dementia (23). Individuals with MCI also had significantly more errors (collisions, center line crossings, road edge excursions, stop sign missed, speed limit exceedance) compared with healthy control drivers (10). MCI is classified into two types: amnestic MCI (aMCI) (with memory impairment) and non-aMCI (without memory impairment) (24). MCI is further classified into single-domain MCI (with impairment in single cognitive domain) and multiple-domain MCI (with impairment in multiple cognitive domain) (24). Patients with multiple-domain aMCI have the two or more impairments of memory, attention, viusospatial function, and executive function. Comparing multiple-domain aMCI with single-domain aMCI, the former demonstrates greater driving difficulty compared with the latter and healthy controls (10). Since all these cognitive functions are important for driving performance, multiple-domain aMCI may exhibit a greater driving difficulty than single-domain aMCI.

A single-photon emission computed tomography (SPECT) study has demonstrated that severity of impaired driving

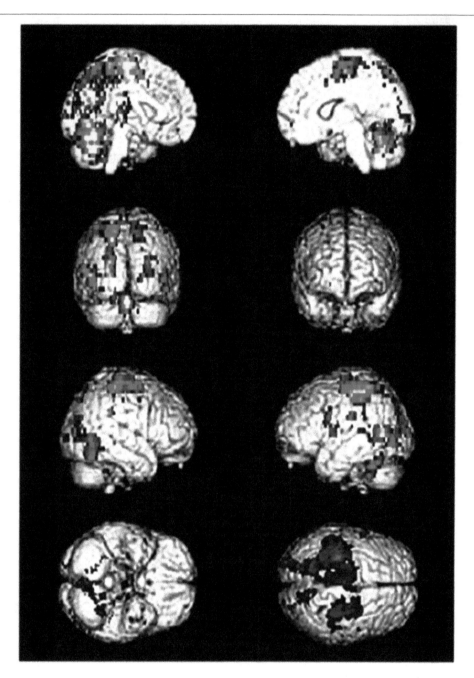

FIGURE 1 | Activated brain regions during driving in fMRI. Distributed brain networks including occipital, parietal, frontal, motor, and cerebellar regions are mainly activated while driving only task. fMRI, functional magnetic resonance imaging. [Modified from (4), licensed under Creative Commons].

performance is significantly correlated with the changes of cerebral blood flow in the temporo-parietal regions in early stage of AD (25). A positron emission tomography (PET) study showed that the executive functioning was correlated with metabolism in the temporo-parietal regions, which was impaired in early stage of AD (26). Neuropsychological studies also reported a significant relationship between driving performance and visuospatial perceptual ability in AD (17). These findings

indicate that the hypoperfusion or hypometabolism of temporo-parietal regions reflects the impairments of visuospatial perception and executive function, which result in impaired driving performance in early stage of AD. Moreover, with increased severity of driving impairment, the perfusion of frontal region was also reduced in addition to temporo-parietal regions in SPECT (25). The AD pathology is observed in the temporo-parietal regions in the early stage of the disease while that pathology spread into the frontal regions in the later stage (27). Therefore, the impairment of executive function involving the frontal regions can be more correlated with the driving impairment for the late stage of AD. Interestingly, a recent PET study have revealed that driving risk is strongly correlated with accumulation of amyloid even in the preclinical stage of AD (28). In another study using tau and amyloid PET, participants at Stage 2 [amyloid (+) and tau (+)] of preclinical AD (14) were more likely to receive a marginal/fail rating compared to participants at Stage 0 [amyloid (-) and tau (-)] or 1 [amyloid (+) and tau (-)] (11, 14). This finding suggests that individuals with preclinical AD (Stage 2) may already decline in driving skills.

Overall, the driving performance is gradually worsening along with the course of ADS from preclinical AD to AD dementia. These alterations of driving performance seem to be induced by the progression of AD pathology. In particular, the early pathological change in the posterior temporo-parietal regions associated with visuospatial function (OF perception) may be responsible for the impaired driving in the early stage of ADS.

ASSESSMENT TOOLS FOR DRIVING ABILITY IN ADS

Various methods including on-road test, driving simulation and neuropsychological tests have been used for evaluating driving ability (3, 17, 29). The on-road test is the gold standard for assessing fitness to drive, but it requires much time for patients. There is also a need for someone who is proficient in the judgment. The driving simulation is similar to the on-road test, but it is expensive. Therefore, these two

tests cannot be routinely performed at the medical clinics. For this reason, neuropsychological tests are commonly used. Neuropsychological tests can evaluate various aspects of brain function including attention, executive function and visuospatial abilities known to be impaired in patients with ADS. For example, the following tests are frequently used; the Mini-Mental State Examination (MMSE) for memory, attention and language skill, the Trail Making Test Part A and B (TMT-A and -B) for cognitive flexibility, Drawing test for visuo-constructive ability, and Maze test for visual orientation (29). However, these neuropsychological examinations, especially when doing multiple tests, require a long time to perform, so that patients often get tired. Characteristics with some pros and cons of these assessment tools are briefly summarized in **Table 1**.

There have been many studies that investigate the usefulness of above mentioned tests as predictors of driving ability (3, 17, 29). However, a recent systematic review (17) demonstrated a lack of consistency in the findings, with some studies showing a relationship between cognitive test and driving performance for individuals with AD, whereas others did not. Further, this review suggested that deficits in a single cognitive ability were not a reliable predictor of driving performance. In contrast, a composite battery that assessed the multiple cognitive domains required to be an efficient driver was the best predictor of driving performance in individuals with AD (17). Another study compared the predictive value of the three types of assessment such as clinical interview, neuropsychological test battery (including multiple tests) and driving simulation (29). They found that neuropsychological assessment provided the best prediction of fitness to drive. Clinical interviews were less objective and less standardized than neuropsychological

TABLE 1 | Assessment tools for driving ability in ADS.

Assessment tools	Characteristics	Pros	Cons
On-road test	- Gold standard - Evaluate driving abilities using actual vehicle by a trained expert	- Close to driving in the natural environment	- Expensive - Limited availability - Need a trained expert - Long time to perform - Cannot examine the driving ability under hazardous conditions
Driving simulators	- Mimic real-world driving using a front monitor, a handle, an accelerator, a brake pedal, etc. which resemble an actual vehicle	- Wide range of test conditions (e.g., night and day, different weather conditions, or road environments) - Especially, we can safely examine the driving performance under hazardous conditions	- Expensive - Limited availability
Neuropsychological tests	- Assess various cognitive functions indispensable for driving (e.g., attention, executive function and visuospatial abilities, etc)	- Widely available - Multiple options for standardized measures	- Long time to perform - Need a trained expert
ERPs	- Directly measure neural activity from scalp electrodes while watching OF stimuli in the case of OF-ERPs	- Widely available - Non-invasive - Inexpensive - Short time to perform - Easy to use	- Currently not standardization for driving assessment

ERPs, event-related potentials; OF, optic flow.

tests and driving simulation. Driving simulation is also not sufficiently predictive if used alone. However, combining all three types of assessments yielded the best prediction for fitness to drive in patients with AD (29). Other systematic review and meta-analysis have demonstrated that executive function, attention, visuospatial function and global cognition revealed by neuropsychological tests may be predictive of driving performance in patients with MCI and AD. Specifically, TMT-A and -B and Maze test emerged as the best single predictors of driving performance though there were variability and inconsistencies. On-road and simulator assessments have yielded inconsistent results in terms of the safety to drive in patients with MCI and AD (3).

From the results of these studies, there has been no single test sufficient to determine driving safety in patients with MCI and AD though the combined use of these tests is somewhat useful. Accordingly, it is necessary to establish an objective method that can be performed easily, in a short time, at a low cost, but has high reliability. Note that ERPs have all such features, therefore, ERPs are suitable for evaluating driving ability in ADS. In the following section, we describe ERP researches on driving evaluation in ADS.

ASSESSMENT OF DRIVING ABILITY IN ADS USING ERPS

ERPs are electrical potential generated by the brain time-locked to a sensory, cognitive, or motor event and provide a powerful, non-invasive technique with superb temporal resolution, for studying the brain's synaptic function (30–32). In general, early ERP components (< 200 ms) reflect sensory processes as they depend mainly on the physical parameters of the stimulus, so-called exogenous component. Conversely, later ERP components (> 200 ms) are relatively more dependent on the mental operations performed on the stimuli as well as on non-sensory factors such as predictability, higher perceptual and semantic features, so-called endogenous component.

ERPs have been extensively used for functional evaluation of brain in ADS (30–32). The P300 component (around at 300–500 ms) elicited by an oddball paradigm has been most studied in ADS as the convenient measure of the cognitive dysfunction. In general, early sensory components at around 50–100 ms are relatively spared whereas potentials starting around 200 ms and beyond are more consistently abnormal even in the early stage of AD and MCI. Thus, ERPs may reveal neurophysiological changes related to the expansion of the neocortical association areas of AD pathology (32).

For the ERP research on driving, the P300 cognitive component is often used as an index of driving performance in healthy individuals (33–36). However, there have been no P300-ERP studies on driving ability in ADS. To our knowledge, only two ERP studies used N200 component for the driving ability of AD (37, 38) (**Table 2**). In a study of (37), ERPs were recorded in young and older normal controls, and early AD patients while participants viewed real-world videos and dot motion stimuli (OF) simulating self-movement scenes.

In both stimulus conditions, N200 latencies were delayed by aging whereas AD patients exhibited the diminished N200 amplitude. In addition, AD patients were uniquely unresponsive to increments in motion speed. Since OF is crucial for speed judgments and braking during vehicular navigation, the authors proposed that the AD unresponsiveness to accelerations might reveal some of the mechanism involved in their driving impairment and potentially help identify high-risk individuals at earlier stage. In another study (abstract form) (38), early AD patients and older normal control took a virtual reality driving evaluation that incorporates multiple cognitive, visual and motor tests. OF-ERPs were also recorded. Compared to older normal control, AD patients had significantly lower driving scores and smaller N200 amplitudes. Furthermore, there was a highly significant correlation between driving scores and N200 amplitudes. The authors concluded that significant correlations between vehicular driving scores and N200 amplitudes supported the role of extrastriate cortical dysfunction in impaired driving capacity and that the potential use of ERPs as screening tools for selective functional impairments and as biomarkers of AD.

These two studies (37, 38) suggest that OF-ERPs (sensory N200 component) may be useful for evaluation of driving ability in AD. However, it remains unknown whether the N200 component is the best predictor of driving ability in AD, and whether or not OF-ERPs can be an index of driving ability even in aMCI. For the last decade, we have been studying the feasibility of sensory ERPs in response to radial OF in aMCI and AD and proposed that OF-ERPs provided an additional information on the alteration of visuospatial perception in ADS (1, 2). The visuospatial deficits (impaired OF perception) related to the posterior temporo-parietal dysfunction play a key role in the navigational or driving impairment in ADS (18, 19, 25). Hence, we hypothesized that sensory ERPs elicited by OF but not P300 cognitive ERPs could be a neural biomarker in driving impairment even in the early stage of ADS. In the following section, we describe neural basis of OF processing in healthy humans and the potential use of OF-ERPs as a driving evaluation method.

NEURAL BASIS OF OF PERCEPTION IN HEALTHY HUMANS

When we move through our environment with walking or cars, the radial pattern of OF is produced at the retina (**Figure 2A**). The ability of visual motion system that analyzes OF is biologically important because it provides visual cues that can be used to perceive the direction of self-motion, to guide locomotion and to avoid obstacles (20, 39). Thus, the drivers must analyze radial OF information continuously to control his/her vehicle during driving, so that the OF processing is indispensable for safe driving.

In humans, there are two functionally and anatomically segregated visual pathways: the ventral and dorsal pathways (**Figure 3**) (21, 22, 42). Both pathways begin in the retina and project to the primary visual cortex (V1). After V1, the ventral

TABLE 2 | ERP studies on driving ability in ADS.

References	Participants	Study design and protocol	Outcome measure	Summary of main findings
Fernandez and Duffy (2012) (37)	- [OF (dot motion)] - Early AD (n = 15; age, 78.6 ± 8.0) - Older normal control (n = 16; age, 76.2 ± 10.0) - Young normal control (n = 12; age, unknown) [Real-world video motion stimuli] - Early AD (n = 6; age, 73.2 ± 6.3) - Older normal control (n = 5; age, 70.6 ± 6.4) - Young normal control (n = 9; age, 29.33 ± 8.5)	- Cross-sectional study - ERPs evoked by OF (dot motion) (Changes of coherence and speed) - ERPs evoked by real-world video motion stimuli (Changes of coherence and speed)	- N200 amplitude and latency	- Diminished N200 amplitude in early AD - Increasing speed elicits smaller N200 amplitudes in early AD
Fernandez-Romero and Cox (2016) (38) (abstract form)	- Early AD (n = unknown; age, unknown) - Older normal control (n = unknown; age, unknown)	- Cross-sectional study - ERPs evoked by OF - Virtual reality driving evaluation	- N200 amplitude and latency - Multiple cognitive, visual and motor tests	- Smaller N200 amplitude in early AD - Lower driving score in early AD - Significant correlations between vehicular driving scores and N200 amplitudes
Yamasaki et al (1)	- aMCI (n = 18; age, 72.4 ± 6.9) - Early AD (n = 18; age, 75.5 ± 5.7) - Older normal control (n = 18; age, 71.8 ± 4.1) - Young normal control (n = 18; age, 28.2 ± 5.1)	- Cross-sectional study - ERPs evoked by OF and HO (dot motion)	- N170 and P200 amplitudes and latencies	- Prolonged latency of OF-specific P200 in aMCI - Prolonged latencies of N170 and P200 in early AD - Significant correlation between OF-specific P200 latency and MMSE score
Yamasaki et al (2)	- aMCI (n = 15; age, 74.4 ± 4.4) - Older normal control (n = 15; age, 73.5 ± 4.5) - Young normal control (n = 15; age, 27.9 ± 5.0)	- Cross-sectional study - ERPs evoked by OF (dot motion), faces, words, chromatic and achromatic gratings	- N170 and P200 amplitudes and latencies for OF - N170 amplitudes and latencies for faces and words - N120 amplitude and latency for chromatic gratings - Steady-state response for achromatic gratings	- Prolonged N170 and P200 latencies for OF in aMCI - Prolonged N170 latencies for faces and words in aMCI - Normal N120 for chromatic gratings in aMCI - Normal steady-state response for achromatic gratings in aMCI - Significant correlations between N170 latency for OF and LM WMS-R scores, and between P200 amplitude for OF and LM WMS-R scores - High AUC in N170 and P200 latencies for OF in ROC analysis

aMCI, amnestic mild cognitive impairment; AD, Alzheimer's disease; ERPs, event-related potentials; OF, optic flow; MMSE, Mini-Mental State Examination; LM WMS-R, logical memory in Wechsler Memory Scale-Revised; ROC, receiver operating characteristic; AUC, area under the curve.

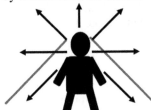 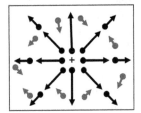

A Radial OF pattern produced by forward self-movement

B Coherent radial OF motion stimuli

FIGURE 2 | Radial OF motion. **(A)** When we move through our environment, radial OF pattern is produced by forward self-movement. **(B)** Coherent radial OF motion stimuli used in our study. We can create radial OF motion stimuli easily using random dots. Dots radiate from the focus of expansion, which corresponds to the observer's direction of heading. OF, optic flow.

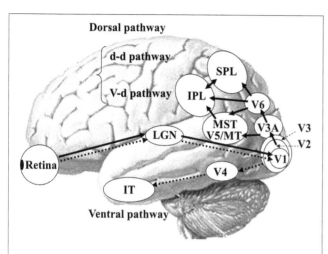

FIGURE 3 | Parallel visual pathways in humans. There are two major parallel streams: ventral and dorsal pathways in humans. Detailed functions of the two streams are provided in the text (see section Neural Basis of OF Perception in Healthy Humans). A recent study has revealed the importance of interconnection between IPL and SPL for OF processing (40) so that we modified this figure considering this point. d-d pathway, dorso-dorsal pathway; v-d pathway, ventro-dorsal pathway; LGN, lateral geniculate nucleus; MT, middle temporal area; MST, medial superior temporal area; IPL, inferior parietal lobule, SPL, superior parietal lobule; IT, inferior temporal cortex. [Modified from (41), Copyright (2012) with permission from IOS press].

stream is important for form and color perception, projecting to V4 and the inferior temporal (IT) cortex. In contrast, the dorsal stream is responsible for motion perception, connecting to V5/middle temporal (MT)+ (V5/MT and medial superior temporal area [MST]), V6 and the posterior parietal cortex (21). The dorsal stream also comprises two distinct functional flows; the dorso-dorsal (d-d) and ventro-dorsal (v-d) streams (43). The d-d stream consists of V6 and the superior parietal lobule (SPL) while the v-d stream involves V5/MT and the inferior parietal lobule (IPL). From the concept of such visual processing mechanism, the OF perception is mainly processed by the dorsal stream.

Primate studies have reported a number of cortical areas that selectively respond to OF, including the dorsal part of the MST (44), the ventral intraparietal area (VIP) (45), area 7a (46) as well as area PEc (47). Conversely, V5/MT neurons do not show such specific selectivity (48). In humans, several OF selective areas have been identified by neuroimaging studies within the dorsal streams (49–57). These OF selective areas contain visual areas such as MST and V6, multisensory areas such as the VIP, the precuneus motion area (PcM) and cingulate sulcus visual area, and vestibular areas such as the putative area 2v (p2v) and parieto-insular vestibular cortex (PIVC). A recent fMRI study have demonstrated that the posterior-insular cortex (PIC) area plays an important role in the integration of visual and vestibular stimuli for the perception of self-motion while the PIVC is selectively responsive to vestibular stimulation (58, 59). Overall, the VIP, PcM and p2V are located within the d-d stream (SPL) while the v-d stream (IPL) consists of PIC (40).

OF-ERPS IN HEALTHY HUMANS

In order to compare OF processing with HO processing in healthy humans, we recorded ERPs for coherent OF and HO motion stimuli in healthy young subjects by using a high-density EEG system (60) (**Figures 2B, 4**). We used coherent motion stimuli as the visual stimuli, which consisted of 400 white square dots randomly distributed on a black background. The white dots moved at a velocity of 5.0°/s. Two types of motion stimuli (OF and HO) were used. OF stimuli contained dots that moved in a radial outward pattern while HO contained dots that moved leftward or rightward. The coherent level was 90% in both stimuli. Both stimuli had the same dot density, luminance, contrast and average dot speed. Random motion (RM) was used as a baseline condition. The OF and HO stimuli were presented for 750 ms, with the presentation of RM for 1,500–3,000 ms alternately. The N170 [analogous to N200 in previous ERP studies (37, 38), about 170 ms] and P200 (about 200 ms) were recorded as major components. We analyzed the peak latencies, amplitudes, scalp distribution and the sources in both components.

The N170 was distributed over occipito-temporal regions in response to both OF and HO stimuli. The distribution of the OF-N170 extended further into the parietal region compared with those of HO-N170 (**Figure 4B**). The OF-N170 amplitude was significantly larger and its latency was significantly shorter than those of HO-N170 (**Figure 4A**). Exact low resolution brain electromagnetic tomography (eLORETA) analysis of the N170 revealed that the current density was significantly elevated over the occipito-temporal areas including V5/MT+ in response to both stimuli compared with RM baseline (**Figure 5A**). These findings were consistent with those of minimum-norm estimate (MNE) of visual evoked magnetic fields (VEFs) (61). A direct comparison between OF and HO stimuli revealed no significant difference in the current density of the N170. Current density estimation with eLORETA in ERPs and MNE in VEFs provided strong evidence that the generator source of the N170 was located in V5/MT+ for both stimuli. Therefore, the N170 constitutes a non-specific motion component derived from an area close to V5/MT+. However, OF stimuli elicited an N170 with a higher amplitude and shorter latency, compared with HO (**Figure 4A**), which may reflect a higher activity of V5/MT+ during OF processing. Alternatively, V5/MT+ can be subdivided into V5/MT and MST (50, 62). V5/MT neurons respond to both OF and HO stimuli (48), whereas MST selectively responds to OF (44, 46). Thus, the selective activation of MST neurons may contribute to the higher amplitude and shorter latency of the OF-N170 response.

The P200 component exhibited distinct characteristics between OF and HO. The OF-P200 was distributed over the parieto-central region (**Figure 4**). HO stimulus also evoked an observable P200, but its topography was limited to the central region (**Figure 4**). The P200 amplitude was significantly larger for OF compared with HO stimuli. Similarly, the latency of OF-P200 was significantly faster compared with that of HO-P200 (**Figure 4A**). Regarding the parietal OF-P200, the current density was significantly elevated in the IPL (**Figure 5B**, top

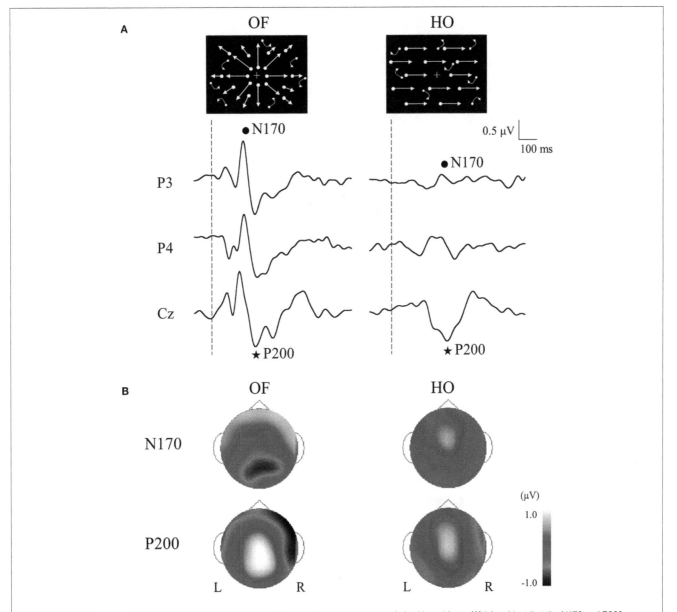

FIGURE 4 | ERPs in response to coherent OF and HO motion stimuli and their scalp topography in healthy subjects. **(A)** It is evident that the N170 and P200 are distinct motion-related components. The N170 component was distributed over occipito-temporal areas regardless of the stimulus type, extending further to the parietal region in the OF condition only. **(B)** The P200 component in response to OF stimuli was distributed over the parieto-central region while that of HO was distributed over the central region. The color bar represents the amplitude value (red = positive, blue = negative). Please note that this figure was presented at 2009 International Symposium on Early Detection and Rehabilitation Technology of Dementia. December 11–12, 2009, Okayama, Japan. ERPs, event-related potentials; HO, horizontal motion.

row). In contrast, for the central HO-P200, the current density was distributed over the SPL (**Figure 5B**, middle row). A direct comparison revealed that the current density of the IPL in response to OF stimuli compared with HO stimuli was significantly elevated (red color). Conversely, the current density of SPL was significantly elevated in HO compared with OF (blue color) (**Figure 5B**, bottom row). Overall, these findings suggest that the parietal OF-P200 is functionally coupled with the IPL (the v-d stream) and that it is the OF-specific component.

Conversely, the central HO-P200 is related to the SPL (the d-d stream) (60). These functional dissociations between IPL (OF perception) and SPL (HO perception) were consistent with our fMRI study (41). Therefore, we propose that different spatio-temporal processing is driven by these motion stimuli within the two distinct dorsal streams in humans. From these findings, it is likely that ERPs with coherent OF and HO motion are useful for functional evaluation of the dorsal stream. More specifically, OF-related ERPs (OF-N170 and OF-P200 components) are

...

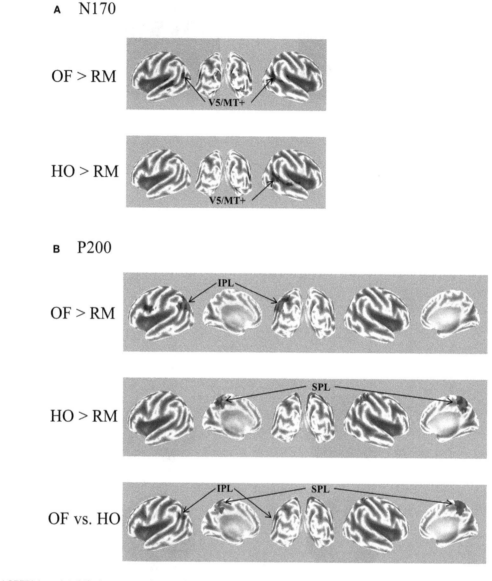

FIGURE 5 | eLORETA-based statistical nonparametric maps for a comparison between OF and HO in GFP peaks of N170 and P200. **(A)** The current density of N170 was significantly elevated over the occipito-temporal areas including V5/MT+ in both stimulus conditions. **(B)** The current density of the parietal P200 for OF was significantly elevated in the left IPL (BA 39/40). Conversely, there was a significant elevation of the current density of the central P200 for HO in the bilateral SPL (BA 7). In the figure at the bottom, red and blue mean OF and HO, respectively. Please note that this figure was presented at 2009 International Symposium on Early Detection and Rehabilitation Technology of Dementia. December 11–12, 2009, Okayama, Japan. eLORETA, exact low resolution brain electromagnetic tomography; GFP, global field power; RM, random motion.

considered to be able to identify subtle changes of visuospatial function (OF perception) associated with driving ability in individuals.

OF-ERPS IN ADS

To examine whether we can detect the impairment of OF perception in aMCI and AD, ERPs for OF and HO were recorded in patients with aMCI and AD, and in healthy old and young adults (1) (**Table 2**). aMCI was defined according to the criteria of Petersen (24). The patients with AD met the criteria for probable

AD according to NINCDS-ADRDA (63). Neuropsychological tests including MMSE and the Clinical Dementia Rating (CDR) were performed. Regarding ERPs, visual stimuli and analysis were same as the former study in healthy young subjects (60). There was no significant difference in both OF-N170 and HO-N170 responses between aMCI patients and healthy old adults (**Figure 6**). In contrast, the latency of OF-P200 was significantly prolonged in aMCI patients compared with healthy old adults (**Figure 6**). Therefore, within the dorsal stream, the v-d stream (IPL) related to OF perception, but not the d-d stream (SPL) associated with HO perception, is selectively impaired in aMCI

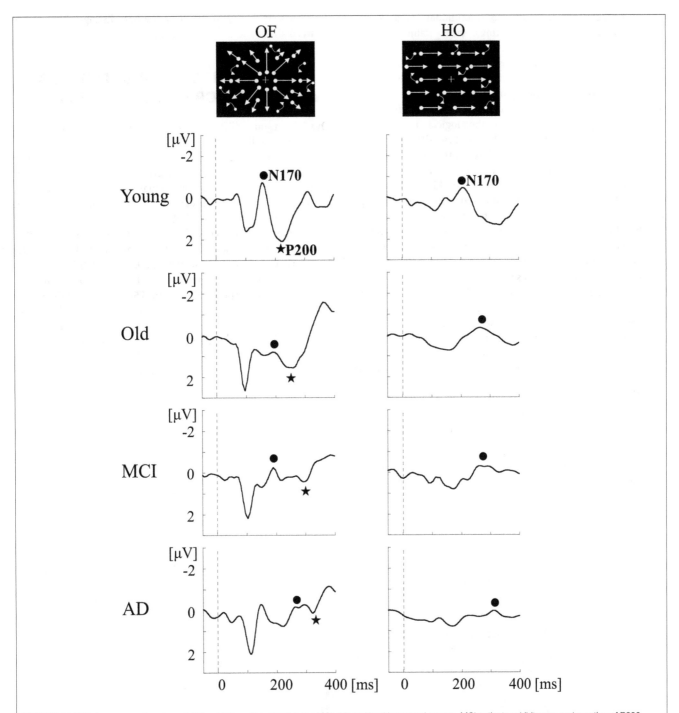

FIGURE 6 | ERPs in response to coherent OF and HO motion stimuli in the MCI, AD and healthy control groups. MCI patients exhibit more prolongation of P200 latency for OF than healthy elderly adults, but no prolongation of N170 latency for both stimuli. AD patients show a prolongation of both N170 and P200 latencies compared with other groups. MCI, mild cognitive impairment. [Modified from (64), Copyright (2012) with permission from IEEE].

patients. On the other hand, AD patients showed a prolongation of N170 and P200 latencies for both OF and HO stimuli compared with healthy old adults and aMCI patients (**Figure 6**). Our results indicate that aMCI patients exhibit a selective impairment of OF perception related to the higher-level of dorsal stream (v-d stream including IPL). Conversely, AD patients show the impairments of both OF and HO perception associated with the distributed higher-level dorsal stream (both v-d and d-d streams including IPL, SPL and V5/MT+). These findings were consistent with the spread of AD pathology following disease progression (1, 64). Thus, we can detect the impairment of OF perception even in patients with aMCI by using OF-ERPs.

We further recorded ERPs to multimodal visual stimuli (chromatic and achromatic gratings, faces, kanji and kana words and OF motion) in aMCI patients, healthy old and young adults (2) (**Table 2**). Inclusion criteria for aMCI patients and healthy old adults followed the criteria of the Japanese Alzheimer's Disease Neuroimaging Initiative (65). These criteria were based on several neuropsychological tests: MMSE, CDR, Geriatric Depression Scale and the logical memory test (delayed recall) of the Wechsler Memory Scale-Revised (WMS-R). Multimodal visual stimuli were optimized to activate elements of each visual stream separately. The OF stimulus was same as the former studies (1, 60). ERP responses to lower (V1) level stimuli (chromatic and achromatic gratings) were not significantly differed between aMCI patients and healthy old adults. Conversely, ERP latencies for higher-ventral (faces and kanji words) and higher-dorsal (kana words and OF motion) were significantly prolonged in aMCI patients. Interestingly, OF-related ERPs were significantly correlated with the logical memory test (delayed recall) of the WMS-R (OF-N170 latency, $r = -0.507$; OF-P200 amplitude, $r = 0.493$) (**Figure 7A**). Furthermore, the receiver operating characteristic (ROC) analysis exhibited that the highest area under the curve (AUC) was observed for OF-ERP latencies (OF-N170 latency, AUC = 0.856; OF-P200 latency, AUC = 0.831) (**Figure 7B**).

This suggests that OF-ERPs have the best distinguishing ability between aMCI and healthy old adults.

A POTENTIAL USE OF OPTIC FLOW-ERPS IN ASSESSING DRIVING ABILITY IN ADS

Overall, in our ERP studies (1, 2), OF-related visuospatial perception indispensable for driving was associated with cognitive function in ADS. As previously mentioned, severity of decline in driving ability was correlated with the degree of cognitive function (23) or visuospatial function (17). Therefore, we assume that OF-ERPs can detect early signs of decline in driving ability in patients with ADS.

In support of our view that altered OF-related visuospatial perception is associated with the driving disability in ADS, Vilhelmsen et al. (66) found that the latency of N2 (analogous to N170 in our study) increased as the speed of OF-motion increased (driving speeds 25, 50, and 75 km/h) in healthy young subjects. They supposed that the subjects perceived the OF stimulus with higher speeds as more complex than that of the lower speeds, which resulted in the increased N2 latency. Healthy individuals can handle our OF stimulus easily but the damaged ADS brain may need more effort because of an excessive

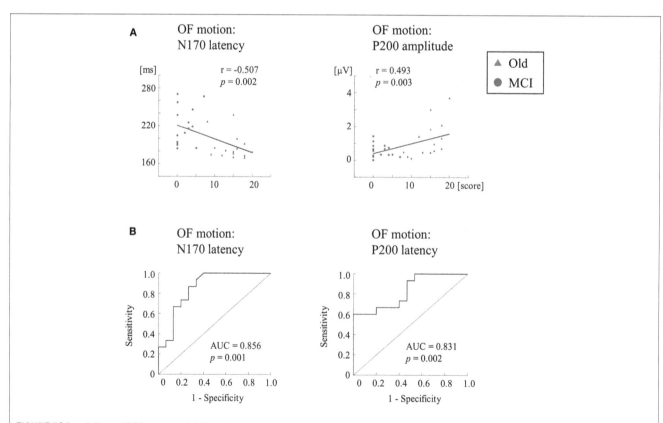

FIGURE 7 | Correlation and ROC analyses. **(A)** Correlation of ERPs with delayed LM WMS-R scores. ERPs for OF motion stimuli are significantly correlated with delayed LM WMS-R scores. **(B)** The results of ROC curve analysis for discriminability of ERP components. The N170 and P200 latencies for OF motion have AUCs ≥ the threshold of 0.7 for acceptable discrimination. Please note that AD group was not recruited in this study [Modified from (1), Copyright (2016) with permission from IOS press]. LM WMS-R, logical memory in Wechsler Memory Scale-Revised; ROC, receiver operating characteristic; AUC, area under the curve.

load for the visuospatial processing system. This interpretation may explain the delayed N170 and P200 latencies in our study (1, 2).

Based on ERP findings of our (1, 2) and other groups (37, 38), OF-ERPs (both N170 and P200 components) may be useful for evaluation of driving ability in aMCI and AD patients. However, it should be kept in mind that the relationship between OF-ERPs and the performance of on-road and driving simulator tests has not established. In addition, we have not yet determined the reference values of OF-ERPs (amplitude and latency) on driving ability. Thus, in the near future, we will perform a large-scale longitudinal ERP study for determining the relationship between driving ability and OF perception in a wide range of ADS. By doing so, we can assess driver's aptitude to prevent the traffic accidents in patients with ADS. Meanwhile, we are currently trying to develop the simple and reliable touch panel-type assessment system of driving ability using radial OF stimuli (measuring OF-detection threshold) (https://kaken.nii.ac.jp/en/grant/KAKENHI-PROJECT-17K09801/). This system may be useful for driving performance evaluation, which is much simpler than ERPs.

CONCLUSIONS

To maintain safe driving, widespread brain networks including occipital, parietal, frontal, motor and cerebellar regions are recruited. These brain networks are vulnerable in ADS pathology that shows extensive neocortical brain damage. In ADS, the driving ability continues to gradually decline accompanied by the course of AD pathology. Especially, the early pathological change in the posterior temporo-parietal regions related to OF

perception is responsible for the impaired driving in the early stage of ADS. Although various methods including on-road test, driving simulation and neuropsychological tests are used for evaluating driving ability, there is no single test sufficient to determine driving safety in ADS patients. Conversely, ERPs are non-invasive and objective method that can be performed easily, in a short time, at a low cost, but has high reliability. Based on previous and our ERP studies, OF-ERPs can be an indicative neural biomarker for assessing the decline of driving ability in ADS.

AUTHOR CONTRIBUTIONS

All authors listed have made a substantial, direct and intellectual contribution to the work, and approved it for publication.

FUNDING

This study was partly supported by the following grants: JSPS KAKENHI Grant Number JP17K09801 to TY, and Grant from the Research on Innovative Areas (No.15H05875) from the Ministry of Education, Culture, Sports, Science, and Technology to ST.

ACKNOWLEDGMENTS

We wish to thank Drs. Yasumasa Ohyagi (Department of Neurology and Geriatric Medicine, Ehime University), Jun-ichi Kira (Department of Neurology, Kyushu University) and Shigenobu Kanba (Department of Neuropsychiatry, Kyushu University) for their research assistance.

REFERENCES

1. Yamasaki T, Goto Y, Ohyagi Y, Monji A, Munetsuna S, Minohara M, et al. Selective impairment of optic flow perception in amnestic mild cognitive impairment: evidence from event-related potentials. *J Alzheimers Dis.* (2012) 28:695–708. doi: 10.3233/JAD-2011-110167

2. Yamasaki T, Horie S, Ohyagi Y, Tanaka E, Nakamura N, Goto Y, et al. A potential VEP biomarker for mild cognitive impairment: evidence from selective visual deficit of higher-level dorsal pathway. *J Alzheimers Dis.* (2016) 53:661–76. doi: 10.3233/JAD-150939

3. Hird MA, Egeto P, Fischer CE, Naglie G, Schweizer TA. A systematic review and meta-analysis of on-road simulator and cognitive driving assessment in Alzheimer's disease and mild cognitive impairment. *J Alzheimers Dis.* (2016) 53:713–29. doi: 10.3233/JAD-160276

4. Choi MH, Kim HS, Yoon HJ, Lee JC, Baek JH, Choi JS, et al. Increase in brain activation due to sub-tasks during driving: fMRI study using new MR-compatible driving simulator. *J Physiol Anthropol.* (2017) 36:11. doi: 10.1186/s40101-017-0128-8

5. Just MA, Keller TA, Cynkar J. A decrease in brain activation associated with driving when listening to someone speak. *Brain Res.* (2008) 1205:70–80. doi: 10.1016/j.brainres.2007.12.075

6. Schweizer TA, Kan K, Hung Y, Tam F, Naglie G, Graham SJ. Brain activity during driving with distraction: an immersive fMRI study. *Front Hum Neurosci.* (2013) 7:53. doi: 10.3389/fnhum.2013.00053

7. Spiers HJ, Maguire EA. Neural substrates of driving behaviour. *Neuroimage* (2007) 36:245–55. doi: 10.1016/j.neuroimage.2007.02.032

8. Uchiyama Y, Ebe K, Kozato A, Okada T, Sadato N. The neural substrates of driving at a safe distance: a functional MRI study. *Neurosci Lett.* (2003) 352:199–202. doi: 10.1016/j.neulet.2003.08.072

9. Allison S, Babulal GM, Stout SH, Barco PP, Carr DB, Fagan AM, et al. Alzheimer disease biomarkers and driving in clinically normal older adults: role of spatial navigation abilities. *Alzheimer Dis Assoc Disord.* (2018) 32:101–6. doi: 10.1097/WAD.0000000000000257

10. Hird MA, Vesely KA, Fischer CE, Graham SJ, Naglie G, Schweizer TA. Investigating simulated driving errors in amnestic single- and multiple-domain mild cognitive impairment. *J Alzheimers Dis.* (2017) 56:447–52. doi: 10.3233/JAD-160995

11. Roe CM, Babulal GM, Mishra S, Gordon BA, Stout SH, Ott BR, et al. Tau and amyloid positron emission tomography imaging predict driving performance among older adults with and without preclinical Alzheimer's disease. *J Alzheimers Dis.* (2018) 61:509–13. doi: 10.3233/JAD-170521

12. Alzheimer's Association. 2018 Alzheimer's disease facts and figures. *Alzheimers Dement.* (2018) 14:367–429. doi: 10.1016/j.jalz.2018.02.001

13. Petersen RC. New clinical criteria for the Alzheimer's disease spectrum. *Minn Med.* (2012) 95:42–5.

14. Sperling RA, Aisen PS, Beckett LA, Bennett DA, Craft S, Fagan AM, et al. Toward defining the preclinical stages of Alzheimer's disease: recommendations from the National Institute on Aging-Alzheimer's Association workgroups on diagnostic guidelines for Alzheimer's disease. *Alzheimers Dement.* (2011) 7:280–92. doi: 10.1016/j.jalz.2011.03.003

15. Albert MS, DeKosky ST, Dickson D, Dubois B, Feldman HH, Fox NC, et al. The diagnosis of mild cognitive impairment due to Alzheimer's disease: recommendations from the National Institute on Aging-Alzheimer's

Association workgroups on diagnostic guidelines for Alzheimer's disease. *Alzheimers Dement.* (2011) 7:270–9. doi: 10.1016/j.jalz.2011.03.008

16. McKhann GM, Knopman DS, Chertkow H, Hyman BT, Jack CRJr, Kawas CH, et al. The diagnosis of dementia due to Alzheimer's disease: recommendations from the national institute on aging-alzheimer's association workgroups on diagnostic guidelines for alzheimer's disease. *Alzheimers Dement.* (2011) 7:263–9. doi: 10.1016/j.jalz.2011.03.005

17. Bennett JM, Chekaluk HE, Batchelor J. Cognitive tests and determining fitness to drive in dementia: a systematic review. *J Am Geriatr Soc.* (2016) 64:1904–17. doi: 10.1111/jgs.14180

18. Mapstone M, Steffenella TM, Duffy CJ. A visuospatial variant of mild cognitive impairment: getting lost between aging and AD. *Neurology* (2003) 60:802–8. doi: 10.1212/01.WNL.0000049471.76799.DE

19. Tetewsky SJ, Duffy CJ. Visual loss and getting lost in Alzheimer's disease. *Neurology* (1999) 52:958–65.

20. Gibson JJ. *The Perception of the Visual World.* Boston, MA: Houghton Mifflin (1950).

21. Tobimatsu S, Celesia GG. Studies of human visual pathophysiology with visual evoked potentials. *Clin Neurophysiol.* (2006) 117:1414–33. doi: 10.1016/j.clinph.2006.01.004

22. Yamasaki T, Tobimatsu S. Electrophysiological assessment of the human visual system. In: Harris JM, Scott J, editors. *Neuroscience Research Progress, Visual Cortex: Anatomy, Functions and Injuries.* New York, NY: Nova Science Publishers (2012). p. 37–67.

23. Ott BR, Heindel WC, Papandonatos GD, Festa EK, Davis JD, Daiello LA, et al. A longitudinal study of drivers with Alzheimer disease. *Neurology* (2008) 70:1171–8. doi: 10.1212/01.wnl.0000294469.27156.30

24. Petersen RC. Mild cognitive impairment as a diagnostic entity. *J Intern Med.* (2004) 256:183–94. doi: 10.1111/j.1365-2796.2004.01388.x

25. Ott BR, Heindel WC, Whelihan WM, Caron MD, Piatt AL, Noto RB. A single-photon emission computed tomography imaging study of driving impairment in patients with Alzheimer's disease. *Dement Geriatr Cogn Disord.* (2000) 11:153–60. doi: 10.1159/000017229

26. Matías-Guiu JA, Cabrera-Martín MN, Valles-Salgado M, Pérez-Pérez A, Rognoni T, Matías-Guiu J, et al. Neural basis of cognitive assessment in Alzheimer disease, amnestic mild cognitive impairment, and subjective memory complaints. *Am J Geriatr Psychiatry* (2017) 25:730–40. doi: 10.1016/j.jagp.2017.02.002

27. Braak H, Braak E. Neuropathological stageing of Alzheimer-related changes. *Acta Neuropathol.* (1991) 82:239–59. doi: 10.1007/BF00308809

28. Ott BR, Jones RN, Noto RB, Yoo DC, Snyder PJ, Bernier JN, et al. Brain amyloid in preclinical Alzheimer's disease is associated with increased driving risk. *Alzheimers Dement.* (2017) 6:136–42. doi: 10.1016/j.dadm.2016.10.008

29. Piersma D, Fuermaier AB, de Waard D, Davidse RJ, de Groot J, Doumen MJ, et al. Prediction of fitness to drive in patients with Alzheimer's dementia. *PLoS ONE* (2016) 11:e0149566. doi: 10.1371/journal.pone.0149566

30. Horváth A, Szucs A, Csukly G, Sákovics A, Stefanics G, Kamondi A. EEG and ERP biomarkers of Alzheimer's disease: a critical review. *Front Biosci.* (2018) 23:183–220. doi: 10.2741/4587

31. Scally B, Calderon PL, Anghinah R, Parra MA. Event-related potentials in the continuum of Alzheimer's disease: would they suit recent guidelines for preclinical assessment? *J Clin Diagn Res.* (2016) 4:127. doi: 10.4172/2376-0311.1000127

32. Olichney JM, Yang JC, Taylor J, Kutas M. Cognitive event-related potentials: biomarkers of synaptic dysfunction across the stages of Alzheimer's disease. *J Alzheimers Dis.* (2011) 26:215–28. doi: 10.3233/JAD-2011-0047

33. Ou B, Wu C, Zhao G, Wu J. P300 amplitude reflects individual differences of navigation performance in a driving task. *Int J Ind Ergon.* (2012) 42:8–16. doi: 10.1016/j.ergon.2011.11.006

34. Ebe K, Itoh K, Kwee IL, Nakada T. Covert effects of "one drink" of alcohol on brain processes related to car driving: an event-related potential study. *Neurosci Lett.* (2015) 593:78–82. doi: 10.1016/j.neulet.2015.03.020

35. Chai J, Qu W, Sun X, Zhang K, Ge Y. Negativity bias in dangerous drivers. *PLoS ONE* (2016) 11:e0147083. doi: 10.1371/journal.pone.0147083

36. Solís-Marcos I, Galvao-Carmona A, Kircher K. Reduced attention allocation during short periods of partially automated driving: an

37. Fernandez R, Duffy CJ. Early Alzheimer's disease blocks responses to accelerating self-movement. *Neurobiol Aging* (2012) 33:2551–60. doi: 10.1016/j.neurobiolaging.2011.12.031

38. Fernandez-Romero R, Cox DJ. Impaired driving capacity in early stage Alzheimer's is associated with decreased cortical responsiveness to simulated self-movement. *Alzheimers Dement.* (2016) 12:882. doi: 10.1016/j.jalz.2016.06.1824

39. Warren WH, Hannon DJ. Direction of self-motion is perceived from optic flow. *Nature* (1988) 336:162–3. doi: 10.1038/336162a0

40. Uesaki M, Takemura H, Ashida H. Computational neuroanatomy of human stratum proprium of interparietal sulcus. *Brain Struct Funct.* (2018) 223:489–507. doi: 10.1007/s00429-017-1492-1

41. Yamasaki T, Horie S, Muranaka H, Kaseda Y, Mimori Y, Tobimatsu S. Relevance of in vivo neurophysiological biomarkers for mild cognitive impairment and Alzheimer's disease. *J Alzheimers Dis.* (2012) 31:S137–54. doi: 10.3233/JAD-2012-112093

42. Livingstone M, Hubel D. Segregation of form, color, movement, and depth: anatomy, physiology, and perception. *Science* (1988) 240:740–9. doi: 10.1126/science.3283936

43. Rizzolatti G, Matelli M. Two different streams form the dorsal visual system: anatomy and functions. *Exp Brain Res.* (2003) 153:146–57. doi: 10.1007/s00221-003-1588-0

44. Tanaka K, Saito H. Analysis of motion of the visual field by direction, expansion/contraction and rotation cells in the dorsal part of the medial superior temporal area of the macaque monkey. *J Neurophysiol.* (1989) 62:642–56. doi: 10.1152/jn.1989.62.3.642

45. Zhang T, Heuer HW, Britten KH. Parietal area VIP neuronal responses to heading stimuli are encoded in head-centered coordinates. *Neuron* (2004) 42:993–1001. doi: 10.1016/j.neuron.2004.06.008

46. Siegel RM, Reid HL. Analysis of optic flow in the monkey parietal 7a. *Cereb Cortex* (1997) 7:327–46. doi: 10.1093/cercor/7.4.327

47. Raffi M, Squatrito S, Maioli MG. Neuronal responses to optic flow in the monkey parietal area PEc. *Cereb Cortex* (2002) 12:639–46. doi: 10.1093/cercor/12.6.639

48. Lagae L, Maes H, Raiguel S, Xiao DK, Orban GA. Responses of macaque STS neurons to optic flow components: a comparison of MT and MST. *J Neurophysiol.* (1994) 71:1597–626. doi: 10.1152/jn.1994.71.5.1597

49. de Jong BM, Shipp S, Skidmore B, Frackowiak RS, Zeki S. The cerebral activity related to the visual perception of forward motion in depth. *Brain* (1994) 117:1039–54. doi: 10.1093/brain/117.5.1039

50. Morrone MC, Tosetti M, Montanaro D, Fiorentini A, Cioni G, Burr DC. A cortical area that responds specifically to optic flow, revealed by fMRI. *Nat Neurosci.* (2000) 3:1322–8. doi: 10.1038/81860

51. Peuskens H, Sunaert S, Dupont P, Van Hecke P, Orban GA. Human brain regions involved in heading estimation. *J Neurosci.* (2001) 21:2451–61. doi: 10.1523/JNEUROSCI.21-07-02451.2001

52. Ptito M, Kupers R, Faubert J, Gjedde A. Cortical representation of inward and outward radial motion in man. *Neuroimage* (2001) 14:1409–15. doi: 10.1006/nimg.2001.0947

53. Wunderlich G, Marshall JC, Amunts K, Weiss PH, Mohlberg H, Zafieris O, et al. The importance of seeing it coming: a functional magnetic resonance imaging study of motion-in-depth towards the human observer. *Neuroscience* (2002) 112:535–40. doi: 10.1016/S0306-4522(02)00110-0

54. Cardin V, Smith AT. Sensitivity of human visual and vestibular cortical regions to egomotion-compatible visual stimulation. *Cereb Cortex* (2010) 20:1964–73. doi: 10.1093/cercor/bhp268

55. Biagi L, Crespi SA, Tosetti M, Morrone MC. BOLD response selective to flow-motion in very young infants. *PLoS Biol.* (2015) 13:e1002260. doi: 10.1371/journal.pbio.1002260

56. Uesaki M, Ashida H. Optic-flow selective cortical sensory regions associated with self-reported states of vection. *Front Psychol.* (2015) 6:775. doi: 10.3389/fpsyg.2015.00775

57. Wada A, Sakano Y, Ando H. Differential responses to a visual self-motion signal in human medial cortical regions revealed by wide-view stimulation. *Front Psychol.* (2016) 7:309. doi: 10.3389/fpsyg.2016.00309

58. Frank SM, Baumann O, Mattingley JB, Greenlee MW. Vestibular and visual responses in human posterior insular cortex. *J Neurophysiol.* (2014) 112:2481–91. doi: 10.1152/jn.00078.2014

59. Frank SM, Wirth AM, Greenlee MW. Visual-vestibular processing in the human Sylvian fissure. *J Neurophysiol.* (2016) 116:263–71. doi: 10.1152/jn.00009.2016

60. Yamasaki T, Tobimatsu S. Motion perception in healthy humans and cognitive disorders. In: Wu J, editor. *Early Detection and Rehabilitation Technologies for Dementia: Neuroscience and Biomedical Applications.* Hershey, PA: IGI Global (2011). p. 156–61.

61. Yamasaki T, Inamizu S, Goto Y, Tobimatsu S. Visual system: clinical applications. In: Tobimatsu S, Kakigi R, editors. *Clinical Applications of Magnetoencephalography.* Tokyo: Springer Japan KK (2016). p. 145–59.

62. Huk AC, Dougherty RF, Heeger DJ. Retinotopy and functional subdivision of human area MT and MST. *J Neurosci.* (2002) 22:7195–205. doi: 10.1523/JNEUROSCI.22-16-07195.2002

63. McKhann G, Drachman D, Folstein M, Katzman R, Price D, Stadlan EM. Clinical diagnosis of alzheimer's disease: report of the NINCDS-ADRDA work group under the auspices of department of health and human services task force on Alzheimer's disease. *Neurology* (1984) 34:939–44.

64. Yamasaki T, Goto Y, Ohyagi Y, Monji A, Munetsuna S, Minohara M, et al. A deficit of dorsal stream function in patients with mild cognitive impairment and Alzheimer's disease. In: *2012 IEEE/ICME International Conference on Complex Medical Engineering* (Kobe) (2012). p. 28–31.

65. Ikari Y, Nishio T, Makishi Y, Miya Y, Ito K, Koeppe RA, et al. Head motion evaluation and correlation for PET scans with 18F-FDG in the Japanese Alzheimer's disease neuroimaging initiative (J-ADNI) multi-center study. *Ann Nucl Med.* (2012) 26:535–44. doi: 10.1007/s12149-012-0605-4

66. Vilhelmsen K, van der Weel FR, van der Meer ALH. A high-density EEG study of differences between three high speeds of simulated forward motion from optic flow in adult participants. *Front Syst Neurosci.* (2015) 9:146. doi: 10.3389/fnsys.2015.00146

8

A Smart Device System to Identify New Phenotypical Characteristics in Movement Disorders

Julian Varghese[1]*, Stephan Niewöhner[2], Iñaki Soto-Rey[1], Stephanie Schipmann-Miletić[3], Nils Warneke[3], Tobias Warnecke[4] and Martin Dugas[1]

[1] Institute of Medical Informatics, University of Münster, Münster, Germany, [2] Department of Information Systems, University of Münster, Münster, Germany, [3] Department of Neurosurgery, University Hospital Münster, Münster, Germany, [4] Department of Neurology, University Hospital Münster, Münster, Germany

Correspondence:
Julian Varghese
julian.varghese@uni-muenster.de

Parkinson's disease and Essential Tremor are two of the most common movement disorders and are still associated with high rates of misdiagnosis. Collected data by technology-based objective measures (TOMs) has the potential to provide new promising and highly accurate movement data for a better understanding of phenotypical characteristics and diagnostic support. A technology-based system called Smart Device System (SDS) is going to be implemented for multi-modal high-resolution acceleration measurement of patients with PD or ET within a clinical setting. The 2-year prospective observational study is conducted to identify new phenotypical biomarkers and train an Artificial Intelligence System. The SDS is going to be integrated and tested within a 20-min assessment including smartphone-based questionnaires, two smartwatches at both wrists and tablet-based Archimedean spirals drawing for deeper tremor-analyses. The electronic questionnaires will cover data on medication, family history and non-motor symptoms. In this paper, we describe the steps for this novel technology-utilizing examination, the principal steps for data analyses and the targeted performances of the system. Future work considers integration with Deep Brain Stimulation, dissemination into further sites and patient's home setting as well as integration with further data sources as neuroimaging and biobanks. Study Registration ID on ClinicalTrials.gov: NCT03638479.

Keywords: Parkinson's Disease, Essential Tremor, smart wearables, artificial intelligence, neural networks

INTRODUCTION

Tremor-related diseases as Parkinson's Disease (PD) and Essential Tremor (ET) are two of the most common movement disorders (1). Disease classification is primarily based on clinical criteria and remains challenging (2, 3). Smart wearables with multi-sensor technology provide a source of objective movement monitoring allowing for greater precision in recording subtle changes unlike current clinical rating scales in hospital routine (4, 5). A technology-based system—called Smart Device System (SDS)—was implemented to monitor and visualize multi-modal high-resolution data. The project is going to be conducted in close collaboration with the local departments of Neurology and Neurosurgery and the Task Force on Technology by the International Movement Disorder Society. Though there is an increasing number of existent mobile apps from application stores or mature medical devices as the Parkinson's KinetiGraph™ system, there is a low number of large-scale deployments to capture and analyze the monitored data (6). More importantly, two key barriers—mentioned in a review by the International Movement Disorder Society—hamper integration into routine healthcare and identification of new phenotypical characteristics (7):

- First, there is poor integration of clinically relevant motor and non-motor phenomena. Especially, changes in tremor characteristics in relation to provoking circumstances (e.g., specific motor or cognitive actions) are currently not integrated into electronic tremor analyses. The SDS system utilizes different monitoring settings in one easy-to-follow examination at a health care facility: (A) Movement monitoring using two smartwatches at both patient wrists in a pre-defined neurological examination that provokes different tremor types. (B) Electronic questionnaires regarding medication/drug consumption, family history and non-motor symptoms on a smartphone. (C) Archimedean Spirals drawn by the patient on a tablet. Each of these three settings viewed individually already show high potential to classify or stratify tremor-related diseases (7–9). However, synchronization of these multimodal data (A–C) and advanced pattern recognition analyses such as Deep Learning would unlock a new integrative approach to boost classification performance and to find new phenotypical characteristics. In particular, Deep Learning methods have recently shown high classification performance in pattern recognition in other medical domains if a large amount of expert-tagged training data is available (10, 11).
- Second, there is a lack of open data repositories and data standards to share best practices of existing smart wearable solutions. This project uses the Medical-Data-Models Portal (MDM Portal) that has evolved to the largest European information infrastructure for medical data models (12). This portal will be used to harmonize and enrich developed data models toward established data standards and foster interoperability with other health information systems. Moreover, active collaboration with the Neurology Department and Task Force on Technology will align clinical and technical key requirements with current ongoing developments.

A 2-year prospective exploratory study is going to be conducted in which the SDS system will be applied within a 20-min data capture session for each included participant. The objective is to train a Deep Neural Network that is capable of predicting the disease entity (PD, ET, none of them) and to identify new phenotypical characteristics based on the fully integrated and pseudonymized study data.

MATERIALS AND EQUIPMENT

The project is planned as a 2-year prospective exploratory study at the Movement Disorders outpatient clinic at the University Hospital Münster. Each patient diagnosed with PD (ICD 10-GM: G20.-) or ET (ICD-10-GM G25.0) and visiting the outpatient clinic is going to be a potential study participant. To be included, each patient must receive, fully understand and sign the informed consent form. All requirements of the updated EU data protection regulation from the start of May 2018 will be strictly adhered to. The study design is registered on Clinicaltrial.gov (Identifier: NCT03638479).

Figure 1 provides an overview of the SDS system and its intended processing steps. Three Apple-based mobile devices will be customized for different monitoring settings. Smartwatch-based examination takes 10-min including calibration and putting them on both wrists. The total assessment time including questionnaires (8 min), drawing one spiral (1–2 min) is 20 min.

The examiner smartphone (iPhone at least Series 7) constitutes the first step of examination and provides short questionnaires about non-motor symptoms, family history and medication. Two smartwatches (Series 4.0) constitute the second step and enables high-resolution tremor capture from both wrists in a neurological examination (see **Table 1**). The captured data will be sent via Bluetooth to the smartphone. Since only one smartwatch can be paired with one smartphone at the same time, another smartphone is necessary to forward data from the second smartwatch to the examiner iPhone. The iPad Pro constitutes the final step of the assessment and will enable drawing of Archimedean spirals after protocol-based neurological examination. Captured data will be sent to the examiner smartphone, from which all captured data will be pseudonymized and securely transmitted in JSON format into a European General Data Protection Regulation-compliant research database. This connection to the research database is implemented within a REST-based client-server architecture using HTTPS as encryption. Two exemplary JSON files are attached as **Supplementary Files** that show structure of the transmitted raw data for two subject cases (one healthy subject, one with Parkinson's disease). The raw data from each JSON file will then be imported into a PostgreSQL-based research database. The overview of all data items is listed in the **Table S1**. All data processing, transmission, and storage processes were approved by the local data protection officer.

The software development for smartwatch-based and smartphone-based data capture is already finished. Tablet-based data capture will be included as soon as development and tests are completed. The first 3 months of the study consist of a setting up and testing phase, regardless of the tablet-based component. Only then, patients will be recruited and data capture commences and endures for 21 months. Based on a database report of the local EMR system, we expect 120 patients with ET and 954 patients with PD at our local site. A fixed number of follow up visits is not planned during this study. However, patients that will re-appear at the local site according to the usual treatment plan will be identified as follow-up patients to enable data analysis on disease progression.

STEPWISE PROCEDURES

The following sections describe data capture settings in detail to provide a highly structured and reproducible data basis. Principal steps regarding data processing, analysis and model training are

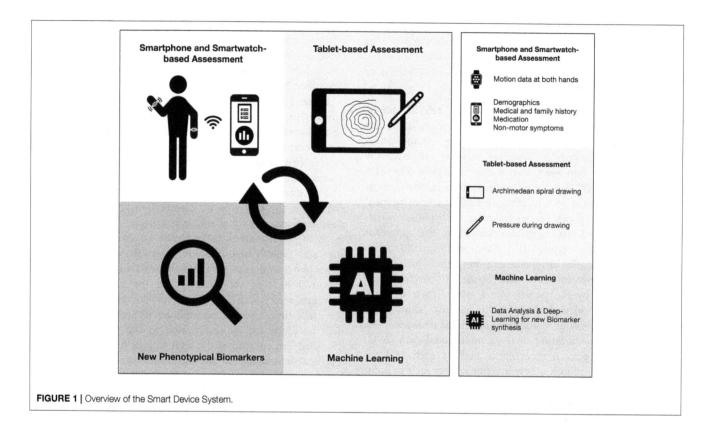

FIGURE 1 | Overview of the Smart Device System.

listed in the *Methods and Anticipated Results* section and will be subject to further refinements once the data is collected and evaluated.

Recruitment

Each patients and his/her accompanying person (e.g., life partner), who visit the movement disorders outpatient clinic at the University Hospital in Münster and fulfill the aforementioned criteria will be asked to participate in the study. In most cases, each patient will be accompanied by a familiar person. These companions represent age-matched healthy controls. Each participant will be informed about the SDS system, the data to be captured, pseudonymized, transferred and stored for data analysis. Study inclusion starts once informed consent form has been signed.

Data Capture and Neurological Examination

Preceded by a literature review of tremor-related medical history, clinical phenomenology and the new tremor classification (8, 13–18) a series of workshops were conducted with neurologists specialized in Movement Disorders. As a result, a set of questionnaire items and a short technology-based examination were designed to capture data features, which were regarded to have highest predictive power for differential diagnoses of ET and PD. The questionnaire items will be captured first and are listed in **Table S1**. Then, neurological examination will start with one smartwatch at each participant's wrist, see **Table 1**. All steps in this examination are illustrated in a video (19) and

the examiner initiates the next step or can repeat the current step. Thus, the acceleration data is always labeled with the corresponding examination step, which will provide essential context information for training the Deep-Learning model. The final assessment is to have the participant draw a spiral with a provided stylus and tablet (**Figure 2**), starting with the right hand and then with left hand. All components of the SDS-system (smartphone, smartwatches, and tablet) will only capture, pseudonymize, and submit data to a research database for Deep Learning. No components of the system will apply any analyses that intends to confirm or change any routine diagnostic or therapeutic procedures. Instead, all advanced data analyses will be conducted subsequently on the pseudonymized data at the research database server and none of analyses results will be sent back to the patient-level.

METHODS AND ANTICIPATED RESULTS

Acceleration data by the smartwatches will be analyzed with signal processing methods (including Fast Fourier Transform and band-pass filters) to infer average tremor amplitude and frequency in each examination section. **Figure 3** illustrates a number of readily implemented graphical user interfaces and functioning initial results analyses.

Data captured by spiral drawing will be processed for angular feature detection, direction inversion and pattern deviation from ideal spiral according to Zham et al. (8). The sum of all captured and processed data will train a neural network model to predict the diagnosis label (PD, ET,

TABLE 1 | Smartwatch-based steps of neurological examination.

Step	Duration (s)	Description
1a	20	Rest tremor. Participant is seated in resting position, standardized to Zhang et al. (9)
1b	20	Rest tremor and serial sevens. Participant starts from 100, subtracts 7, and stops after five answers.
2	10	Hold arms lifted.
3	10	Lift and extend arms according to Zhang et al. (9)
4	20	Hold 1 kg weight in every hand for 10 s. Start with the right hand. Then, have the participant's arm rested again as in 1a.
5	20	Finger pointing. Participant should point with his index fingers repetitively to examiner's lifted hand for 10 s. Start with participant's right index, then left.
6	20	Drink from glass. Have the participant grasp an empty glass with his right hand as if he/she would drink from it. Then repeat with his/her left hand.
7	10	Cross and extend both arms.
8	10	Bring both index fingers to each other, repeat until time expires.
9	20	Let participant's both index fingers tap his/her nose. Repetitively with the right (10 s), then with left index (10 s).
10	20	Entrainment. While holding the arms extended, have the participant stamp with his/her right foot according to the stamp frequency of the examiner. Then have him/her repeat with the left foot.

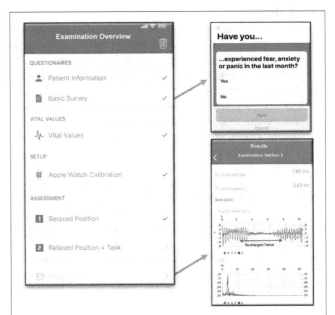

FIGURE 3 | Overview screen **(left)**: the full examination takes approximately 20-min and starts with questionnaires and heart frequency measurement by the smartwatch. Before hand-tremor assessment starts, smart-watch calibration is required. Questionnaire screen **(upper right)**: showing one item of the PD-NMS instrument. Initial signal processing on the smartphone **(bottom right)**: visualization of average amplitude and frequency, raw acceleration data during examination section 3 and frequency spectrum. The acceleration data illustrates a simulated case of re-emergent tremor on the time axis. FFT, Fast Fourier Transform. Data capture and analyses of tablet-based spiral drawing is not implemented yet.

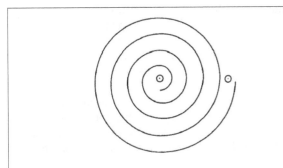

FIGURE 2 | Archimedean spiral to be drawn with a pressure-sensing stylus on a 10.5 inch screen on an Apple iPad Touch, starting from the point in the middle.

none of them) and identify data patterns that could represent new biomarkers. The model will be trained applying Google Tensor Flow-based Network architectures using Convolutional neural networks (CNN) as they have shown highly promising pattern recognition results in medical images (11). In addition, long short-term memories (LSTM) networks will enable time-series analysis to account for temporal dynamics within the protocol-based examination and tablet-based spiral drawing. Both core methods (CNN + LSTM) will continuously be evaluated separately and in combination (e.g., using LSTM on top of CNN-extracted features). Sensitivity, positive predictive value/precision and accuracy will be calculated based on existent diagnosis labels using nested cross-validation. Statistical

significance of classification results will be calculated by permutation tests. Univariate and Multivariate Analyses will be performed based on standard statistical regression analyses (e.g., logistic regression). This is necessary, first, to continuously and critically compare performance of Deep Learning black boxes with classical statistical approaches and second, to get a deeper understanding of the inter-related input features and their predictive power to classification results.

A concrete formulation of hypotheses is limited since we did not find any similar systems that were evaluated in studies from which we can derive a reliable patient sample size calculation based on statistical power analyses. Therefore, following key performance indicators (KPI) are aimed at the end of the study period based on classification performances in other disease domains (11, 20):

- **KPI 1:** >80% of all recruited participant cases will provide complete data as described in data capture **Table S1** in the pseudonymized research database.
- **KPI 2:** >90% accuracy, >90% sensitivity, >90% positive predictive value for classifying ET and PD by the tested model using nested cross validation.

All data items from smartwatch-based data and questionnaires that are relevant for data analysis are specified in the standardized Operational Data Model by the clinical data interchange standards consortium and will be available on the MDM-Portal.

Limitations

A proper sample size calculation was not performed, since it cannot be inferred how many samples the model will require to approach the targeted key performance indicators as—to our knowledge—there was no similar model trained and tested within this domain. However, there are basic assumptions of machine learning principles, stating that the size of training samples should be a multiple of the number input variables and output classes of the model to perform reasonably well (21). The smart-watch-based examination is the most data-consuming procedure capturing acceleration (A) and rotation (R) in 3 axes in 10 different examination sections at 2 different hands. This results in approximately 2 (A+R)* 3 * 10 * 2 = 120 input variables. Three output classes are modeled (PD, ET, control: none of them or healthy). Ideally, we require a multiple of 120 * 3 training samples. Based on the EMR report, we can expect at least 500 patients with PD or ET at our local site, if every second will provide consent. Additionally, most of the patients will attend the ambulance with their spouses or partners, who will also be asked to participate as controls. We are convinced that the required recruitment number is approachable within the study phase, since the data capture is non-obtrusive without any interventional character.

In the case of reaching the targeted key performance indicators, they should still be taken with caution. The predictive capability will never be 100% flawless. This is even more likely to be the case if the system is tested in different environments with different examiners. The study will acquire at least two different regular examiners to train robustness for inter-examiner differences. We believe that this work has established a straight forward and fully-documented examination framework, that can be reproduced in other environments. After study completion, the resulting model, implementation code and execution description will be published as open source and supplied with anonymized training data samples.

INTERPRETATION OF ANTICIPATED RESULTS

Results

Each of the three technology-driven data capture settings is expected to show high potential to classify tremor-related diseases. Synchronization of these multimodal data and integrative pattern recognition analyses are expected to provide deeper insights into tremor characteristics. All of the technical devices used within this study have recently evolved to affordable mass products. Coupled with highly customizable apps, some of these devices already received FDA approval as for instance the Kardiaband app by AliveCor, the first FDA-cleared smartwatch-based ECG reader (22). This demonstrates the qualified use of such smart wearables not only for fitness or wellness purposes but also for valid medical use. A further advantage of the SDS system—compared to commercial and proprietary systems as the KinetiGraph™ system—is that all of its devices can be programmed and adapted by any Apple-based App developer through well-established Software Development kits and therefore preventing vendor lock-in. Once our system has reached the required level of accuracy, sensitivity and precision, regulatory steps will be taken for medical device approval and rollout to further sites. As a consequence, the system will not replace but could decisively extend diagnostic processes, which are currently suffering from high misdiagnoses rates in this domain (2, 3).

Future Work

Deep brain stimulation (DBS) is an effective surgical treatment option and shows significant benefit for tremor and quality of life in patients with PD, ET, and other tremor etiologies (23–26). Intraoperative neurophysiological and clinical testing is important for optimal targeting of the DBS leads. Currently, evaluation of effects and symptoms is performed by an experienced neurologist and might be influenced by individual perception. Methods that enable an objective evaluation of the neurological status might help improving positioning of the DBS leads aiming at more accurate positioning and better results. A major challenge is to obtain medical clearance for the aforementioned devices or to establish sensors which comply with high regulatory requirements for intraoperative usage. In addition, the devices might help detecting minor changes in tremor pre- and post-operatively during the course of the disease and facilitate adjustment of DBS systems.

Extending the hospital-based setting, continuous and longitudinal measurement of movement and patient questionnaire-based input will be captured to provide patient home-based data for detailed monitoring of individual disease courses. This feature will be implemented after this study, because new phenotypical key characteristics from the IMF funded phase will first need to be identified and then captured with highest priority in the home-based setting. Moreover, the timely relations between medication intake and tremor effects will elucidate therapeutic effects in a long-term setting.

Further characteristics from Neuroimaging data are going to be identified and integrated to the research database. To elaborate on a larger patient sample size and ongoing genetic testing approaches of PD and ET, the need of a multi-center study and biobanks for genome-wide association analyses will be discussed.

AUTHOR CONTRIBUTIONS

JV has written the study design, acquired the funding, supervised the implementation of the system and written the manuscript. SN has implemented the system. IS-R has made significant contributions to the study design, acquisition of funding the project. SS-M and NW provided significant input to the study design and neurosurgical applications. TW has provided significant input to the study design, system requirements and the neurologic examination. MD has supervised and guided the project. All authors have received, critically revised and approved the manuscript.

ACKNOWLEDGMENTS

This is a short text to acknowledge the contributions of specific colleagues, institutions, or agencies that aided the efforts of the authors.

FUNDING

The study is funded by Innovative Medizinische Forschung of the University of Münster, Germany (Grant ID: VA111809).

REFERENCES

1. Louis ED, Ottman R, Hauser WA. How common is the most common adult movement disorder? Estimates of the prevalence of essential tremor throughout the world. *Mov Disord.* (1998) 13:5–10. doi: 10.1002/mds.870130105
2. Newman EJ, Breen K, Patterson J, Hadley DM, Grosset KA, Grosset DG. Accuracy of Parkinson's disease diagnosis in 610 general practice patients in the West of Scotland. *Mov Disord.* (2009) 24:2379–85. doi: 10.1002/mds.22829
3. Jain S, Lo SE, Louis ED. Common misdiagnosis of a common neurological disorder: how are we misdiagnosing essential tremor? *Arch Neurol.* (2006) 63:1100–4. doi: 10.1001/archneur.63.8.1100
4. Heldman DA, Espay AJ, LeWitt PA, Giuffrida JP. Clinician versus machine: reliability and responsiveness of motor endpoints in Parkinson's disease. *Parkinsonism Relat Disord.* (2014) 20:590–5. doi: 10.1016/j.parkreldis.2014.02.022
5. Papapetropoulos S, Mitsi G, Espay AJ. Digital health revolution: is it time for affordable remote monitoring for Parkinson's disease? *Front Neurol.* (2015) 6:34. doi: 10.3389/fneur.2015.00034
6. Silva de Lima AL, Hahn T, Evers LJW, Vries NM de, Cohen E, Afek M, et al. Feasibility of large-scale deployment of multiple wearable sensors in Parkinson's disease. *PLoS ONE* (2017) 12:e0189161. doi: 10.1371/journal.pone.0189161
7. Espay AJ, Bonato P, Nahab FB, Maetzler W, Dean JM, Klucken J, et al. Technology in Parkinson's disease: challenges and opportunities. *Mov Disord.* (2016) 31:1272–82. doi: 10.1002/mds.26642
8. Zham P, Arjunan S, Raghav S, Kumar DK. Efficacy of guided spiral drawing in the classification of Parkinson's disease. *IEEE J Biomed Health Inform.* (2017) 22:1648–52. doi: 10.1109/JBHI.2017.2762008
9. Zhang B, Huang F, Liu J, Zhang D. A novel posture for better differentiation between Parkinson's tremor and essential tremor. *Front Neurosci.* (2018) 12:317. doi: 10.3389/fnins.2018.00317
10. LeCun Y, Bengio Y, Hinton G. Deep learning. *Nature* (2015) 521:436–44. doi: 10.1038/nature14539
11. Esteva A, Kuprel B, Novoa RA, Ko J, Swetter SM, Blau HM, et al. Dermatologist-level classification of skin cancer with deep neural networks. *Nature* (2017) 542:115–8. doi: 10.1038/nature21056
12. Dugas M, Neuhaus P, Meidt A, Doods J, Storck M, Bruland P, et al. Portal of medical data models: Information infrastructure for medical research and healthcare. *Database (Oxford)* (2016) 2016:bav121. doi: 10.1093/database/bav121
13. Deuschl G, Bhatia KP, Elble R, Hallett M. Understanding the new tremor classification. *Mov Disord.* (2018) 33:1267–8. doi: 10.1002/mds.27368
14. Gövert F, Becktepe J, Deuschl G. Die neue Tremorklassifikation der International Parkinson and Movement Disorder Society. *Der Nervenarzt* (2018) 89:376–85. doi: 10.1007/s00115-018-0489-1
15. Hopfner F, Deuschl G. Is essential tremor a single entity? *Eur J Neurol.* (2018) 25:71–82. doi: 10.1111/ene.13454
16. Papengut F, Raethjen J, Binder A, Deuschl G. Rest tremor suppression may separate essential from parkinsonian rest tremor. *Parkinsonism Relat Disord.* (2013) 19:693–7. doi: 10.1016/j.parkreldis.2013.03.013
17. Alty JE, Kempster PA. A practical guide to the differential diagnosis of tremor. *Postgrad Med J.* (2011) 87:623–9. doi: 10.1136/pgmj.2009.089623
18. Bötzel K, Tronnier V, Gasser T. The differential diagnosis and treatment of tremor. *Dtsch Arztebl Int.* (2014) 111:225–35; quiz 236. doi: 10.3238/arztebl.2014.0225
19. Varghese J. *Examination Video and Supplement for Smartwatch-Based Data Capturing.* (2018). Available online at: https://uni-muenster.sciebo.de/s/gLxVcl7mF5mfb4W (Accessed October 5, 2018).
20. Bangor A, Kortum PT, Miller JT. An empirical evaluation of the system usability scale. *Int J Hum Comput Interact.* (2008) 24:574–94. doi: 10.1080/10447310802205776
21. Natarajan P, Frenzel JC, Smaltz DH. *Demystifying Big Data and Machine Learning for Healthcare.* Taylor & Francis (2017). Available online at: https://books.google.de/books?id=omxdDgAAQBAJ
22. Food and Drug Administration. *November 2017 510(k) Clearances, Including Kardia Band System.* (2017). Available online at: https://www.fda.gov/medicaldevices/productsandmedicalprocedures/deviceapprovalsandclearances/510kclearances/ucm587897.htm (Accessed August 29, 2018).
23. Paschen S, Deuschl G. Patient evaluation and selection for movement disorders surgery: the changing spectrum of indications. *Prog Neurol Surg.* (2018) 33:80–93. doi: 10.1159/000480910
24. Deuschl G, Paschen S, Witt K. Clinical outcome of deep brain stimulation for Parkinson's disease. *Handb Clin Neurol.* (2013) 116:107–28. doi: 10.1016/B978-0-444-53497-2.00010-3
25. Fasano A, Romito LM, Daniele A, Piano C, Zinno M, Bentivoglio AR, et al. Motor and cognitive outcome in patients with Parkinson's disease 8 years after subthalamic implants. *Brain* (2010) 133:2664–76. doi: 10.1093/brain/awq221
26. Deuschl G, Raethjen J, Hellriegel H, Elble R. Treatment of patients with essential tremor. *Lancet Neurol.* (2011) 10:148–61. doi: 10.1016/S1474-4422(10)70322-7

9

Identification of Blood Biomarkers for Alzheimer's Disease Through Computational Prediction and Experimental Validation

Fang Yao[1,2], Kaoyuan Zhang[1], Yan Zhang[1], Yi Guo[3], Aidong Li[4], Shifeng Xiao[1], Qiong Liu[1]*, Liming Shen[1]* and Jiazuan Ni[1]

[1] Shenzhen Key Laboratory of Marine Biotechnology and Ecology, College of Life Science and Oceanography, Shenzhen University, Shenzhen, China, [2] Key Laboratory of Optoelectronic Devices and Systems of Ministry of Education and Guangdong Province, College of Optoelectronic Engineering, Shenzhen University, Shenzhen, China, [3] Department of Neurology, Shenzhen People's Hospital, Shenzhen, China, [4] Department of Rehabilitation, The Eighth Affiliated Hospital of Sun Yat-sen University, Shenzhen, China

*Correspondence:
Qiong Liu
liuqiong@szu.edu.cn
Liming Shen
slm@szu.edu.cn

Background: Alzheimer's disease (AD) is the major cause of dementia in population aged over 65 years, accounting up to 70% dementia cases. However, validated peripheral biomarkers for AD diagnosis are not available up to present. In this study, we adopted a new strategy of combination of computational prediction and experimental validation to identify blood protein biomarkers for AD.

Methods: First, we collected tissue-based gene expression data of AD patients and healthy controls from GEO database. Second, we analyzed these data and identified differentially expressed genes for AD. Third, we applied a blood-secretory protein prediction program on these genes and predicted AD-related proteins in blood. Finally, we collected blood samples of AD patients and healthy controls to validate the potential AD biomarkers by using ELISA experiments and Western blot analyses.

Results: A total of 2754 genes were identified to express differentially in brain tissues of AD, among which 296 genes were predicted to encode AD-related blood-secretory proteins. After careful analysis and literature survey on these predicted blood-secretory proteins, ten proteins were considered as potential AD biomarkers, five of which were experimentally verified with significant change in blood samples of AD vs. controls by ELISA, including GSN, BDNF, TIMP1, VLDLR, and APLP2. ROC analyses showed that VLDLR and TIMP1 had excellent performance in distinguishing AD patients from controls (area under the curve, AUC = 0.932 and 0.903, respectively). Further validation of VLDLR and TIMP1 by Western blot analyses has confirmed the results obtained in ELISA experiments.

Conclusion: VLDLR and TIMP1 had better discriminative abilities between ADs and controls, and might serve as potential blood biomarkers for AD. To our knowledge, this is the first time to identify blood protein biomarkers for AD through combination of computational prediction and experimental validation. In addition, VLDLR was first reported here as potential blood protein biomarker for AD. Thus, our findings might provide important information for AD diagnosis and therapies.

Keywords: Alzheimer's disease, blood, protein, biomarker, computation

INTRODUCTION

Alzheimer's disease (AD) is the major cause of dementia in population aged over 65 years, accounting up to 70% dementia cases (1). This disease is pathologically characterized with extracellular senile plaques (amyloid-β, Aβ) and intraneuronal neurofibrillary tangles (NFTs), which are the prime suspects in damaging and killing nerve cells (2). AD has become a major health problem in the world due to the lack of effective treatment. It was reported that there were approximate 48 million people worldwide affected by AD in 2015, and the number was estimated to reach 86 million by the year 2050 (3). Clearly, the increasing AD cases would load great burden on families and society, urging the physicians and scientists to find precise and effective ways to diagnose and treat this disease.

Currently, the clinical diagnosis of AD requires a series of examinations including medical history, neuropsychological assessment, and various radiological investigations (4). However, those diagnosis processes could not be used as routine examinations for AD, because they are time-consuming and largely depend on physician's experience. In order to diagnose AD objectively and accurately, researchers have used biotechnologies and bioinformatics methods to search for disease biomarkers. As cerebrospinal fluid (CSF) is affinity with brain, it is considered to contain potential biomarkers of AD pathologies. Several studies have indicated that the decreased concentration of $A\beta_{42}$ peptide and increased concentration of tau proteins in CSF of AD patients compared to controls might work as diagnostic biomarkers for AD (5, 6). While CSF collection by lumbar puncture is invasive and may lead to some side effects such as headache (7), which limits the application of these biomarkers for large-scale AD screening. Blood contains large number of disease-associated proteins and its obtaining is non-invasive, thus it becomes a good source for discovery of AD biomarkers.

Extensive researches have been done to discover plasma or serum biomarkers for AD. For example, Ray and colleagues used antibody arrays to identify an 18-panel protein signature from 120 cell-signaling proteins, which could differentiate ADs from non-demented controls and could also distinguish mild cognition impairment (MCI) patients who later progressed to AD from those unchanged or converted to other dementia (8). Liao and colleagues recognized 6 possible plasma biomarkers for AD patients by combining 2D-PAGE and LC-MS/MS methods (9). Pratico' et al disclosed that the F2-IsoPs, resulting from peroxidation of poly-unsaturated fatty acid (10), have high levels in plasma of AD and MCI patients by using GC-MS technology (11, 12). However, the identified AD biomarkers are discrepant dramatically due to the variations in research methods. Generally, discovery of blood biomarkers for disease was conducted through

comparing the proteome of blood samples from disease and control. But this no-targeted method is very challenging because there are lots of proteins with relatively low abundance or with a wide range of orders of magnitude in blood, which could not all be covered by one mass spectrometer (13). As of today, there are no valid biomarkers for AD diagnosis in blood.

In this study, we conducted a combination of computational prediction and experimental validation to identify potential blood protein biomarkers for AD. We firstly analyzed previously published gene expression data of brain tissues from AD patients to identify differentially expressed genes for AD. Furthermore, we applied a blood-secretory protein prediction program on these genes to predict AD-related proteins in blood. Finally, several potential blood protein biomarkers for AD were selected and verified by enzyme-linked immunosorbent assay (ELISA) experiments and Western blot analyses on blood samples from AD patients and healthy controls. This work provides a more specific and effective way to investigate blood protein biomarkers for AD.

MATERIALS AND METHODS

The schematic diagram of the workflow in this study was given as **Figure S1**.

Gene Expression Data of Brain Tissues From AD Patients

Brain tissue-based gene expression data of AD patients were collected from GEO database (14). Two series of datasets, GSE48350 (15, 16) and GSE5281 (17), were selected for data analyses according to the criteria described as follows: first, the datasets we used for analysis are gene expression data of brain tissues from AD patients and healthy controls; second, each dataset must contain both samples of AD patients and healthy controls; third, the number of AD samples and healthy controls are no less than 10 respectively in each dataset. After analysis, we found that these two datasets meet our screening criteria, and have a relatively large number of samples for data analysis. The two datasets are all generated from the platform of Affymetrix Human Genome U133 Plus 2.0 Array, which includes 43285 probes corresponding to 21246 genes. There are 253 samples (80 ADs and 173 controls) in GSE48350, and 161 samples (87 ADs and 74 controls) in GSE5281. All CEL files of each dataset were downloaded from the database, and normalized by using Robust Multi-array Averaging (RMA) method (18) for further analysis. Detailed information about these samples can be accessed from GEO database.

Identification of Differentially Expressed Genes for AD

We first identified differentially expressed probes (DEPs), and then mapped these probes to their genes. The following procedure was used to identify DEPs for each dataset. Kolmogorov–Smirnov test (19) was used to examine whether the data come from a normal distribution. If they were from normal distribution, Student's t-test would be used to detect DEPs.

Abbreviations: AD, Alzheimer's disease; ROC, receiver operating characteristic; Aβ, amyloid-β; NFT, neurofibrillary tangles; CSF, cerebrospinal fluid; MCI, mild cognition impairment; ELISA, enzyme-linked immunosorbent assay; DEPs, differentially expressed probes; FDR, false discovery rate; FC, fold change; SVM, support vector machines; DSM-IV, Diagnostic and Statistical Manual of Mental Disorders-Fourth Edition; BBB, blood-brain barrier; AUC, area under the curve; ROS, reactive oxygen species; SEM, standard errors of the means.

However, our results showed that the values of many examined probes did not fit normal distribution, Wilcoxon rank sum test (20) was applied to identify DEPs for AD with p-value < 0.05 as cutoff for significance. Additionally, Benjamini and Hochberg (21) method was used to control the false discovery rate (FDR) of the selected DEPs with q-value < 0.05 as cutoff. In order to further determine which probes were up-regulated and down-regulated in ADs, fold change (FC) was computed across samples for each probe. As a whole, probes with q-value < 0.05 and FC > 1.2 were considered up-regulated, and those with q-value < 0.05 and FC < 0.833 were down-regulated. Finally, we chose the differentially expressed probes with consistent change trend in these two datasets to map to their corresponding genes, which were considered to be differentially expressed genes for AD.

Prediction of AD-Related Blood Proteins Based on Differentially Expressed Genes

All differentially expressed genes were analyzed for prediction whether their protein products could be secreted into blood through a program developed by Juan Cui et al (22). The basic idea of this program was summarized as follows. First, human proteins that are known to be secretory proteins and can be detected in plasma/serum due to various pathological conditions were collected to form positive dataset. Second, non-blood-secretory proteins, which include proteins unrelated to secretory pathway and secreted proteins not involved in the circulatory system, were selected as negative dataset. Third, these proteins' physical and chemical properties, amino acid sequence and structural features were collected to identify what these blood-secretory proteins have in common. Fourth, a list of protein features such as signal peptides, glycosylation sites, secondary structural content, hydrophobicity and polarity measures etc. was identified due to their great power in distinguishing blood-secretory proteins from those that were deemed not. Finally, a classifier based on support vector machines (SVM) (23) was constructed to predict the blood-secretory proteins by using the positive and negative datasets and the identified protein features.

Validation of Potential Blood Protein Biomarkers of AD by ELISA Experiments

In this work, ELISA experiments were carried out on blood samples from AD patients and healthy individuals to validate the predicted blood protein biomarkers for AD. The research protocol of this study was approved by the Human Research Ethics Committee of Shenzhen University and had been performed in accordance with the ethical standards. A total of 123 subjects were enrolled in experiment from Shenzhen People's Hospital and the Eighth Affiliated Hospital of Sun Yat-sen University, including 54 AD patients and 69 healthy subjects. Informed consents were obtained from all participants in accordance with the Declaration of Helsinki prior to their inclusion in this study. All the patients were diagnosed by neuropsychiatrists in the hospital according to the criteria of Diagnostic and Statistical Manual of Mental Disorders-Fourth Edition (DSM-IV). The average age of the patients and controls were 74.3 (ranged from 52 to 93) and 73.9 (ranged from 53

to 94), respectively. The ratio of male to female was about 2:3. In each ELISA experiment, blood samples were selected from AD patients and age- and gender-matched healthy controls. Blood samples (5 ml) were collected using glass tubes. Serums were separated by centrifugation at 3000 g for 10 min, and then subdivided into aliquots and stored at $-80°C$ for further use.

For ELISA experiments, commercial ELISA kits for proteins gelsolin (GSN), brain-derived neurotrophic factor (BDNF), metalloproteinase inhibitor 1 (TIMP1), pigment epithelium-derived factor (SERPINF1) and amyloid-like protein 2 (APLP2) were bought from Uscn Life Science Inc. (Wuhan, China). The catalog numbers of these ELISA kits were SEA372Hu, SEA011Hu, SEA552Hu, SEB972Hu, and SEG122Hu, respectively. Additionally, ELISA kits of inositol 1,4,5-trisphosphate receptor-interacting protein (ITPRIP), transmembrane emp24 domain-containing protein 10 (TMED10), very low-density lipoprotein receptor (VLDLR), mitogen-activated protein kinase 8 (MAPK8) and mitogen-activated protein kinase 1 (MAPK1) were bought from Sbj Biological technology Co., Ltd. (Nanjing, China) with catalog numbers of SBJ-H2157, SBJ-H2158, SBJ-H1100, SBJ-H2160, and SBJ-H2161, respectively. The concentrations of these proteins were measured under the manufacturer's instructions. The total protein concentrations of samples were determined using bicinchoninic acid (BCA) protein assay kit with product No. 23227 (Beyotime, Jiangsu, China).

Statistical Analyses for ELISA Experiments

Protein concentration of each sample detected by ELISA was normalized with its total protein concentration. For the normalized protein concentrations, G-test (24) was applied to detect the outliers for each group. Software GraphPad Prism 5 was used to visualize the normalized protein concentrations of AD samples and healthy controls. T-test was applied to make differential analysis on normalized protein concentrations of AD samples vs. controls, and then FDR (21) was employed to adjust the p-values obtained from T-test, using 0.05 as significant cutoff. Furthermore, receiver operating characteristic (ROC) curve analysis was carried out to evaluate the power of these proteins in distinguishing AD samples from healthy controls, which was generated by using package pROC on R (25, 26).

Further Validation of the Potential Protein Biomarkers of AD by Western Blot Analyses

To further validate the potential protein biomarkers of AD in blood, Western blot analyses were carried out on un-depleted serum samples of AD patients and healthy controls by specific antibodies. Total protein concentrations of these samples were measured by the BCA assay. Proteins (10 μg) were separated by SDS-PAGE on 12% polyacrylamide gels. After electrophoresis, the proteins were transferred onto 0.2 μm polyvinylidene fluoride (PVDF) membranes (Millipore, Massachusetts, USA), and the membranes were blocked with 5% nonfat-dried milk in Tris-buffered saline (TBS: 100 mM Tris, and 1.5 M NaCl, pH 7.6) for 1 h and then washed with TBS containing 0.4% (v/v) tween

20 (TBST), followed by incubation with primary antibodies (Bioss Biotechnology, Beijing, China) against VLDLR and TIMP1 overnight at 4°C and horseradish peroxidase (HRP)-conjugated secondary antibody (1:8000, Abmart Inc, Shanghai, China) for 2 h at room temperature. The membranes were washed three times each for 10 min in TBST and developed with enhanced chemiluminescence (ECL) kit (FDbio-Femto ECL kit, FDbio Science Biotech co., Ltd, Hangzhou, China). Immunoreactive signals were detected using a Kodak Image Station 4000M imaging system (Carestream Health Inc., Rochester, NY, USA). Quantitative analysis was performed on the protein bands by ImageJ analysis software (National Institutes of Health, USA). Equal amount of proteins were separated by SDS-PAGE and stained with Coomassie blue, which was used as the loading control.

Statistical Analysis for Western Blot

The data of Western blot were analyzed using the two-tailed Student's t-test to examine any significant differences between ADs and controls by GraphPad Prism 7 software (GraphPad Software, USA) and presented as the means ± the standard errors of the means (SEM). Differences were considered significant with p-value < 0.05.

RESULTS

Identification of Differentially Expressed Genes in the Brain Tissues of AD Patients

Two brain tissue-based gene expression datasets of AD patients were downloaded from GEO database. There were 5481 DEPs (2511 up-regulated and 2970 down-regulated) identified in GSE48350 and 12115 DEPs (4675 up-regulated and 7440 down-regulated) in GSE5281. Further comparing analysis was made on these two groups of DEPs, and 1545 probes (corresponding to 1186 genes) and 1981 probes (corresponding to 1568 genes) were found consistently up- and down-regulated in these two datasets, respectively (27). In addition, pathway enrichment analysis was conducted on these genes and showed that focal adhesion, TGF-β signaling pathway, and MAPK signaling pathway were significantly enriched by up-regulated genes, and synapse transmission, neuronal system, and calcium signaling pathway were significantly enriched by down-regulated genes [complete list shown in our previous study (27)]. These pathways are consistent with previous observations that AD is associated with neuronal damage and apoptosis, synaptic dysfunction, neuronal activity alteration, blood brain barrier dysfunction, neuro inflammation, oxidative stress, mitochondrial function and aberrant lipid metabolism (28). Therefore, these differentially expressed genes are speculated to be associated with AD pathogenesis.

Prediction of AD-Related Protein in Blood

It is well known that blood-brain barrier (BBB) controls substances exchange strictly between brain and blood. However, some evidence indicates that breakdown of BBB may account for AD occurrence or aggravation and could enhance the movement of proteins between brain and blood in either direction (29, 30). Thereby, there might be some protein biomarkers reflecting AD pathology in blood. Based on the information described above, we applied a program developed by Juan Cui et al (22) on the differentially expressed genes of AD to predict whether the corresponding proteins could be secreted into blood. Consequently, a total of 296 proteins encoded by 115 up-regulated and 181 down-regulated genes were predicted to be blood-secretory proteins, suggesting that they might be AD-related proteins in blood (**Table S1**). Some of these proteins have been previously reported as AD biomarkers, such as gelsolin (31), serotransferrin (32, 33), metalloproteinase inhibitor 1 (34), mitogen-activated protein kinase 1 (35), pigment epithelium-derived factor (36) and brain-derived neurotrophic factor (37, 38).

To gain a comprehensive understanding of these predicted AD-related blood-secretory proteins, we carried out GO enrichment analysis using DAVID (39). A variety of GO terms were enriched, including 66 biological processes, 30 cellular components and 30 molecular functions (**Table S2**). We found that the biological processes such as protein phosphorylation and microtubule-based process, cellular components like mitochondrion and neuronal cell body, and molecular functions like ATP binding and MAP kinase activity were enriched, which are all known to be involved in the development of AD. The top 10 GO terms of biological processes, cellular components and molecular functions are shown in **Figure 1**.

To further choose precise and important candidate biomarkers for AD, we manually checked the relationship between these proteins and AD through database and literature studies. First, we collected a total of 1493 AD-related genes from three databases, 1291 from GAD (40), 169 from KEGG (41), and 197 from MALACARDS (42). Generally, if genes were related with AD, their corresponding protein products were considered to be AD-related as well. Thus, 1493 proteins encoded by these AD-related genes were AD-related proteins. Second, we made literature searches and compiled 167 proteins that have been reported as potential blood biomarkers of AD. Third, we combined the AD-related proteins collected from database and literature, and obtained a total of 1590 AD-related proteins. Finally, we made a comparison analysis between these reported AD-related proteins with 296 predicted blood-secretory proteins, and found that 35 proteins were consistent in these two groups (**Table 1**).

In order to explore the relationship between these 35 proteins and AD pathology, we made a protein-protein interaction analysis through the online sever LENS (43). A network was generated, which contains the 35 AD-related proteins presented by red nodes, 4 key AD pathology related proteins (APP, APOE, PSEN1, and PSEN2) presented by blue nodes and other proteins presented by gray nodes, which connect the 35 proteins with the 4 key proteins (**Figure 2**). In the network, most proteins are connected to these 4 key proteins except PFKFB3, HMGCS1, ATAD1, and PADI2, suggesting that almost all these proteins were associated with AD pathogenesis.

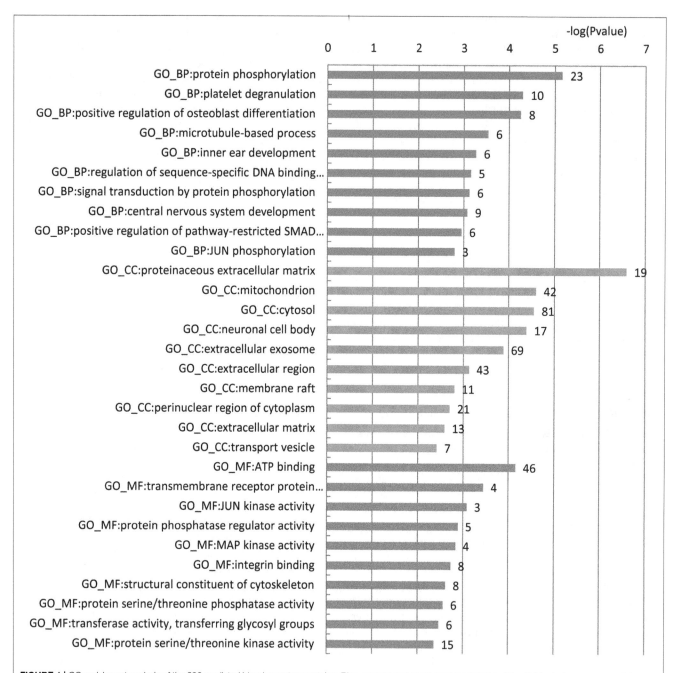

FIGURE 1 | GO enrichment analysis of the 296 predicted blood-secretory proteins. Blue, orange and green bars represent enriched biological processes, cellular components and molecular functions, respectively. The number of proteins enriched in each GO term is shown along with each bar.

Validation of Potential Protein Biomarkers of AD in Blood by ELISA Experiments

Based on the gene expression levels of these 35 proteins in AD samples and their functional annotations, 10 proteins were chosen for experimental verification. They are GSN, BDNF, TIMP1, SERPINF1, ITPRIP, TMED10, VLDLR, MAPK8, APLP2, and MAPK1.

ELISA experiments were performed to examine the protein levels in blood samples from AD patients and healthy controls.

Figure 3 shows that the expression levels of five proteins were significantly changed in AD samples vs. controls, among which GSN and TIMP1were increased in AD samples, while BDNF, VLDLR and APLP2 were decreased. Furthermore, comparison analyses were carried out on the results of computational prediction and experimental validation (**Table 2**). We found that these five proteins were consistent in their change trend among prediction and validation. In order to investigate whether age and gender would affect our validation results, further statistical

TABLE 1 | The list of 35 AD-related blood-secretory proteins.

Uniprot ID	Protein name	Gene name
P17655	Calpain-2 catalytic subunit	CAPN2
P19438	Tumor necrosis factor receptor superfamily member 1A	TNFRSF1A
P02654	Apolipoprotein C-I	APOC1
P01033	Metalloproteinase inhibitor 1	TIMP1
P02787	Serotransferrin	TF
Q15165	Serum paraoxonase/arylesterase 2	PON2
Q16875	6-phosphofructo-2-kinase/fructose-2,6-bisphosphatase 3	PFKFB3
Q8IWB1	inositol 1,4,5-trisphosphate receptor interacting protein	ITPRIP
Q9UQE7	Structural maintenance of chromosomes protein 3	SMC3
P25774	Cathepsin S	CTSS
P49716	CCAAT/enhancer-binding protein delta	CEBPD
Q9Y2G2	Caspase recruitment domain-containing protein 8	CARD8
P36894	Bone morphogenetic protein receptor type-1A	BMPR1A
P49755	Transmembrane emp24 domain-containing protein 10	TMED10
Q9Y2J8	Protein-arginine deiminase type-2	PADI2
P28482	Mitogen-activated protein kinase 1	MAPK1
P16298	Serine/threonine-protein phosphatase 2B catalytic subunit beta isoform	PPP3CB
P98155	Very low-density lipoprotein receptor	VLDLR
P23560	Brain-derived neurotrophic factor	BDNF
Q00005	Serine/threonine-protein phosphatase 2A 55 kDa regulatory subunit B beta isoform	PPP2R2B
P29120	Neuroendocrine convertase 1	PCSK1
O76003	Glutaredoxin-3	GLRX3
P05019	Insulin-like growth factor I	IGF1
Q01581	Hydroxymethylglutaryl-CoA synthase, cytoplasmic	HMGCS1
Q8NBU5	ATPase family AAA domain-containing protein 1	ATAD1
Q96FJ0	AMSH-like protease	STAMBPL1
O14975	Very long-chain acyl-CoA synthetase	SLC27A2
P02753	Retinol-binding protein 4	RBP4
P40938	Replication factor C subunit 3	RFC3
O00451	GDNF family receptor alpha-2	GFRA2
Q06481	Amyloid-like protein 2	APLP2
P45983	Mitogen-activated protein kinase 8	MAPK8
P53779	Mitogen-activated protein kinase 10	MAPK10
P06396	Gelsolin	GSN
P36955	Pigment epithelium-derived factor	SERPINF1

analyses were made on the concentrations of these five proteins according to the different age stages and genders of samples with AD and healthy controls (**Figures S2, S3**). We found that almost all these five proteins were significantly changed in samples of AD vs. control at different age stages and genders. Even though APLP2 is not changed with statistical significance in samples of AD vs. control at age stage 70–89, and BDNF and APLP2 are not significantly changed in male samples of AD vs. control, they still have downward trend in AD samples compared to controls, indicating that age and gender do not affect our experimental validation results.

ROC curve analyses were used to evaluate the performance of the five significantly changed proteins in distinguishing AD samples from controls (**Figure 4**). We found that VLDLR had the most discriminative ability with the area under the curve (AUC) of 0.932 (sensitivity 80.8%, specificity 96.7%), the AUC of TIMP1

was 0.903 (sensitivity 80.0%, specificity 100%) and the AUCs of GSN, BDNF and APLP2 were 0.826, 0.714, and 0.682 respectively. Since VLDLR and TIMP1 were with AUCs larger than 0.85, suggesting that they are more powerful in identifying ADs from controls, and might serve as potential protein biomarkers for AD in blood. Even though the AUCs of GSN, BDNF, and APLP2 were less than 0.85, they could also provide important information for AD diagnosis and therapies.

Further Validation of Potential Protein Biomarkers for AD by Western Blot Analyses

Based on the ELISA analyses, VLDLR and TIMP1 were chosen for further validation of their abilities in identifying the samples of AD patients by Western blot analyses. The serum samples

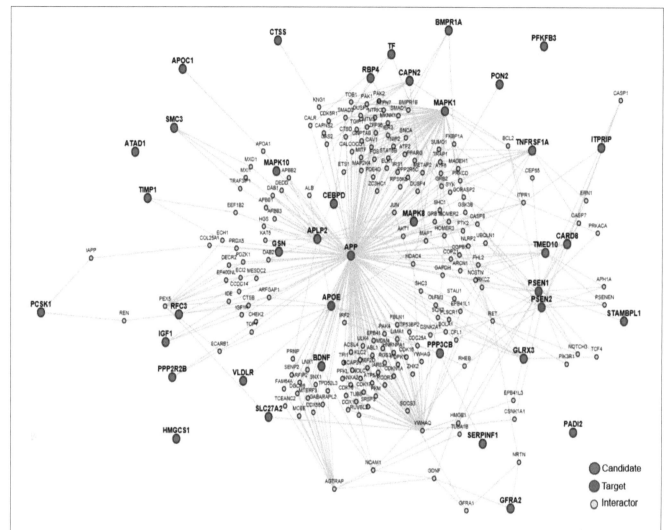

FIGURE 2 | The protein-protein interaction network of the 35 proteins. The red notes are 35 proteins worked as candidates, and the blue notes are AD pathology related proteins worked as targets.

of 5 AD patients and 5 age- and gender-matched healthy controls were used to detect the expression levels of these two proteins. After densitometry analysis on Western blots, VLDLR and TIMP1 were found down- and up-regulated in AD patients respectively as shown in **Figure 5**, which confirmed the results obtained in the ELISA experiments.

DISCUSSION

AD is the major cause of dementia. However, there are no valid biomarkers for AD diagnosis in blood so far. In this study, we searched for potential protein biomarkers of AD in blood through computational prediction combined with experimental verification. Based on this strategy, we predicted 296 AD-related blood-secretory proteins, which were predominant enriched in protein phosphorylation, microtubule-based process, mitochondria and MAP kinase activity. As widely known, AD is

characterized by neurodegenerative plaques and neurofibrillary tangles in brain (44). Tau protein is microtubule-associated phosphoprotein, whose homeostasis plays a critical role in maintaining the microtubule stability. Hyperphosphorylation of tau has been confirmed to cause dynamic instability and disintegration of microtubule, and then formation of neurofibrillary tangles, which would result in neurodegeneration in the end (45). In addition, reactive oxygen species (ROS) have been reported to involve in the AD pathology mechanisms (46). Mitochondria are the most important places to generate ROS in AD. Some evidence indicated that mitochondria dysfunction in the patients of AD enhanced the oxidative stress and the cellular apoptosis (44). Since these predicted proteins were mainly involved in the processes related to AD pathogenesis (47), we considered that these proteins might be associated with AD pathology.

After careful analyses on these 296 proteins, 10 proteins were chosen for experimental validation by ELISA. Five proteins

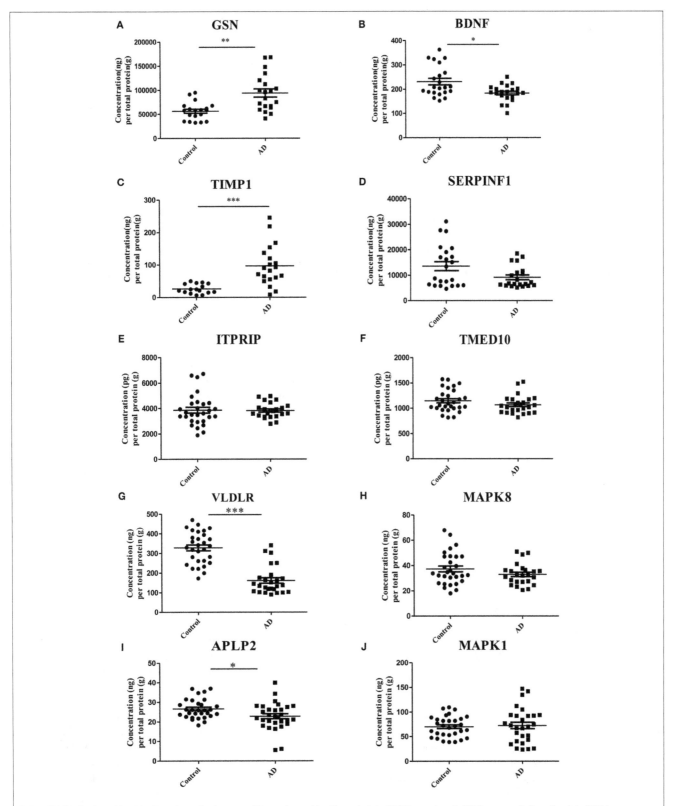

FIGURE 3 | Validation of the 10 selected proteins between AD samples and health controls by ELISA experiment. **(A)** The concentration of protein GSN in serum samples of AD and control. **(B)** The concentration of protein BDNF in serum samples of AD and control. **(C)** The concentration of protein TIMP1 in serum samples of AD and control. **(D)** The concentration of protein SERPINF1 in serum samples of AD and control. **(E)** The concentration of protein ITPRIP in serum samples of AD and control. **(F)** The concentration of protein TMED10 in serum samples of AD and control. **(G)** The concentration of protein VLDLR in serum samples of AD and control. **(H)** The concentration of protein MAPK8 in serum samples of AD and control. **(I)** The concentration of protein APLP2 in serum samples of AD and control. **(J)** The concentration of protein MAPK1 in serum samples of AD and control. *$p < 0.05$ vs. controls; **$p < 0.05$ vs. controls; ***$p < 0.0005$ vs. controls.

TABLE 2 | The results of 10 proteins in computational prediction and experimental validation.

Proteins	Computational result	Up/down	Means of protein concentrations		Means of relative protein concentrations		P-value	FDR
			Control	AD	Control	AD		
GSN	Up	Up	3512.06 (ng/ml)	5661.87 (ng/ml)	56470.35 (ng/g)	94026.19 (ng/g)	0.0004	0.0013
BDNF	Down	Down	15.55 (ng/ml)	12.04 (ng/ml)	231.09 (ng/g)	183.97 (ng/g)	0.0042	0.0105
TIMP1	Up	Up	1.65 (ng/ml)	5.18 (ng/ml)	26.49 (ng/g)	96.86 (ng/g)	0.0001	0.0005
SERPINF1	Down	Down	789.96 (ng/ml)	515.23 (ng/ml)	13508.58 (ng/g)	9117.03 (ng/g)	0.0345	0.0575
ITPRIP	Up	–	295.20 (pg/ml)	279.96 (pg/ml)	3855.06 (pg/g)	3825.37 (pg/g)	0.916	0.916
TMED10	Up	–	75.51 (pg/ml)	78.10 (pg/ml)	1145.62 (pg/g)	1066.62 (pg/g)	0.1542	0.1933
VLDLR	Down	Down	26.36 (ng/ml)	11.77 (ng/ml)	327.92 (ng/g)	161.63 (ng/g)	0.0001	0.0005
MAPK8	Down	–	2.48 (ng/ml)	2.41 (ng/ml)	37.33 (ng/g)	32.98 (ng/g)	0.1546	0.1933
APLP2	Down	Down	1.80 (ng/ml)	1.68 (ng/ml)	26.62 (ng/g)	22.83 (ng/g)	0.0184	0.0368
MAPK1	Down	–	5.45 (ng/ml)	5.30 (ng/ml)	70.31 (ng/g)	72.60 (ng/g)	0.7631	0.8479

In the table, up and down represent up-regulated and down-regulated proteins in the blood samples of AD patients when compared with those of controls.

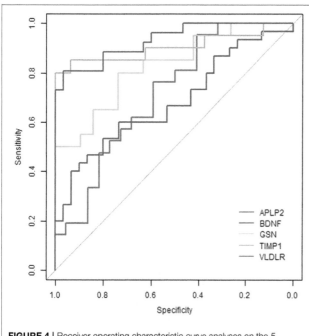

FIGURE 4 | Receiver operating characteristic curve analyses on the 5 proteins. The blue line represents protein APLP2, the red line is BDNF, the green line is GSN, the orange line is TIMP1 and the purple line is VLDLR.

(GSN, BDNF, TIMP1, VLDLR, and APLP2) were verified to be differentially expressed in AD patients vs. controls, suggesting that they might serve as potential biomarkers for AD in blood. Among them, GSN, BDNF, and TIMP1 have been reported to be potential blood protein biomarkers for AD in previous studies (34, 38, 48, 49), while VLDLR and APLP2 were first time reported here as potential protein biomarkers for AD in blood. To further understand the role of these proteins in the pathogenesis of AD, we present the relationship of these proteins with AD in details in the following parts.

GSN was reported to be implicated in AD due to its level changed with AD progression (50). GSN could bind amyloid

beta (Aβ) peptide, inhibit its fibrillization, solubilize reformed Aβ fibrils, and promote its clearance from brain (51). Some studies found that the expression level of GSN was increased in serums of AD compared to controls (49), but others found the decreased expression level of GSN in plasm of AD vs. controls (48). In this study, we predicted and verified that the level of GSN was significantly higher in serums of AD comparing with controls, which was inferred that high expression level of GSN might attribute to the neuroprotective response in AD subjects through immune compensatory system.

BDNF could support the survival of existing neurons and encourage the growth and differentiation of new neurons and synapses (52, 53). Previous studies suggested that BDNF had protective effects on neurons by reducing amyloid beta toxicity (54). BDNF depletion led to an increase in the numbers and size of the cortical amyloid plaque through analyzing on transgenic mouse model of AD (55). It has been reported that BDNF is lower in brain tissue of AD patients (54), which is consistent with our analysis. Kim BY and colleagues made a comprehensive systematic review and meta-analysis on articles and found that BDNF was increased in early AD serum samples and decreased in AD with low MMSE scores respectively comparing with healthy individuals (38). In this study, lower BDNF expression was predicted and experimentally confirmed in blood of AD patients.

TIMP1 is a tissue inhibitor of MMP9 and plays an important role in the development of AD for its function of inflammatory mediation (56). MMP9 was reported to be associated with neurodegeneration processes including extracellular Aβ degradation, neurons degeneration and neurofibrillary tangles formation (57), thus TIMP1 interacting with MMP9 promoted cell proliferation of glial and enhanced the inflammatory response to eliminate amyloid deposition from AD (56). Meanwhile, neurotoxic Aβ fragment could induce the release of MMP9 and TIMP1, and cause their expression changes, which was correlated with the neurotoxicity process (58). The imbalance of levels between MMP9 and TIMP1 in AD patients was associated with senile plaque homoeostasis and tau oligomer formation in brain regions. James D. Doecke and colleagues

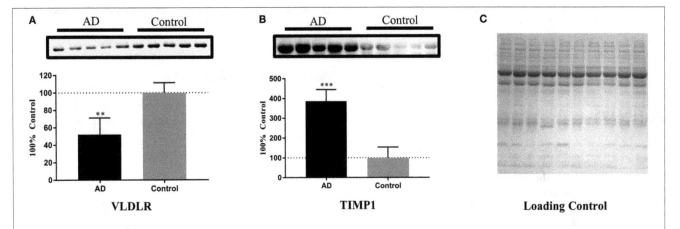

FIGURE 5 | Further validation of the potential protein biomarkers for AD by Western blot analyses. **(A)** The concentration of VLDLR was decreased significantly in AD samples, with **$p < 0.01$ vs. control samples. **(B)** The concentration of TIMP1 was increased significantly in AD samples, with ***$p < 0.001$ vs. control samples. The expression level of protein was normalized by the mean of the controls ($n = 5$), with each bar representing SEM. The upper images of Western blot analysis correspond to the lower histograms of semi-quantification. The statistical results of the data were show as *$p < 0.05$, **$p < 0.01$, ***$p < 0.001$. **(C)** A loading control is presented aiming to verify the normalization of protein amounts.

identified that the level of TIMP1 in plasma of AD was higher than that in healthy controls (34). However, Lorenzl S et al did not observe the level change of TIMP1 in plasma between AD patients and healthy subjects (59). Herein, we found that the level of TIMP1 was significantly up-regulated in AD serums.

VLDLR is an apolipoprotein E receptor involved in synaptic plasticity, learning, and memory (60). It was presented at synaptic compartments, and could alter presynaptic composition and postsynaptic dendritic spine formation through the Ras signaling pathway that is associated in neurodegeneration such as AD (60). Thus, it could be speculated that VLDLR might involve in AD pathogenesis through Ras signaling pathway. Additionally, VLDLR was reported to be one of receptors for AD-related risk factor ApoE (61). ApoE4 was shown to mediate its effects in AD pathogenesis by interfering with Reelin signaling in the brain (62). While Reelin is the major ligand for VLDLR, so it could be speculated that VLDLR might be involved in AD pathogenesis through the ApoE4-Reelin pathway as well. In our study, we found that VLDLR was down-regulated in the brain of AD patients and its encoded protein was predicted and validated with a lower concentration level in blood of AD patients relative to controls.

APLP2, an APP like protein, could bind to synaptic signaling molecules exhibiting synaptogenic activity (63). Furthermore, APLP2 shares essential functions with APP, as it could also interact with proteins Stub1 and CRL4 (CRBN) to facilitate ubiquitination of proteins involved in presynaptic functions and neurodegeneration (64). Herein, we predicted and validated that the encoded protein of APLP2 was down-regulated in the blood of AD patients.

As a whole, this novel biomarker discovery strategy, namely computational prediction combined with experimental verification, provides some potential blood biomarkers for AD. To our knowledge, this is the first report to use such a strategy for AD blood biomarker discovery. Meanwhile, VLDLR is the first time reported here as potential protein biomarker for AD

in blood. In addition, this strategy for biomarker discovery could also be used for discovering biomarkers of other nervous system diseases such as Parkinson's disease. Worth noting, this method provides an effective way to find pathology-associated biomarkers in blood, but there are still some shortages in this strategy that could affect our results. For example, there might be some false positive blood-secretory proteins coming from the computational prediction, so the sensitivity of the blood-secretory protein predictor need to be improved in the future. Additionally, gene expression changes in ADs vs. controls could not accurately reflect their proteins' expression changes, so the predicted proteins need to be validated on large scale blood samples further.

CONCLUSION

A total of 2754 genes were identified differentially expressed in brain tissues of AD, among which 296 genes were predicted to encode blood-secretory proteins. GO enrichment analysis on the predicted blood-secretory proteins suggested that they were associated with AD and might act as candidate protein biomarkers of AD in blood. Furthermore, ten proteins were chosen for validation by ELISA and five proteins (GSN, BDNF, TIMP1, VLDLR, and APLP2) were validated changed significantly in serum samples of AD vs. controls. ROC curves analyses on these five proteins showed that VLDLR and TIMP1 were with more power in distinguishing AD samples from controls. Western blot analyses on VLDLR and TIMP1 were further revealed that they might serve as potential blood biomarkers for AD. Obviously, further studies are required to confirm these findings.

AUTHOR CONTRIBUTIONS

FY, QL, and JN conceived and designed this study. YZ collected data from database and literature. KZ and SX designed and performed the experimental work. FY and LS processed the data and carried out the statistical analysis. YG and AL recruited and diagnosed the patients and provided the blood samples. FY and LS wrote the manuscript. All authors have read and proved the final manuscript.

FUNDING

This work was financially supported by the National Natural Science Foundation of China [grant numbers 31470804, 31771407, 21603147], the Shenzhen Science and Technology Innovation Commission [grant numbers JCYJ20170818102400 688, JCYJ20150529164656093, JCYJ20170412110026229], and the Natural Science Foundation of Guangdong Province [grant number 2015A030313555].

ACKNOWLEDGMENTS

We would thank Dr. Wei Du for some advices on data analyses. Additionally, we would thank assistant researcher Xukun Liu for his help on the Western blot analyses.

REFERENCES

1. Blennow K, de Leon MJ, Zetterberg H. Alzheimer's disease. *Lancet* (2006) 368:387–403. doi: 10.1016/S0140-6736(06)69113-7
2. Inoue K, Tsutsui H, Akatsu H, Hashizume Y, Matsukawa N, Yamamoto T, et al. Metabolic profiling of Alzheimer's disease brains. *Sci Rep.* (2013) 3:2364. doi: 10.1038/srep02364
3. Prince M, Jackson J. *World Alzheimer Report 2009.* Alzheimer's Disease International (2009).
4. Daffner KR. Current approaches to the clinical diagnosis of Alzheimer's disease. In: Scinto LFM, Daffner KR, editors. *Early Diagnosis of Alzheimer's Disease* Totowa, NJ: Humana Press (2000). p. 29–64.
5. Blennow K, Hampel H. CSF markers for incipient Alzheimer's disease. *Lancet Neurol.* (2003) 2:605–13. doi: 10.1016/S1474-4422(03)00530-1
6. Sunderland T, Gur RE, Arnold SE. The use of biomarkers in the elderly: current and future challenges. *Biol Psychiatry* (2005) 58:272–6. doi: 10.1016/j.biopsych.2005.05.016
7. de Almeida SM, Shumaker SD, LeBlanc SK, Delaney P, Marquie-Beck J, Ueland S, et al. Incidence of post-dural puncture headache in research volunteers. *Headache* (2011) 51:1503–10. doi: 10.1111/j.1526-4610.2011.01959.x
8. Ray S, Britschgi M, Herbert C, Takeda-Uchimura Y, Boxer A, Blennow K, et al. Classification and prediction of clinical Alzheimer's diagnosis based on plasma signaling proteins. *Nature Med.* (2007) 13:1359–62. doi: 10.1038/nm1653
9. Liao PC, Yu L, Kuo CC, Lin CJ, Kuo YM. Proteomics analysis of plasma for potential biomarkers in the diagnosis of Alzheimer's disease. *Proteomics Clin Appl.* (2007) 1:506–12. doi: 10.1002/prca.200600684
10. Lovell MA, Markesbery WR. Oxidative damage in mild cognitive impairment and early Alzheimer's disease. *J Neurosci Res.* (2007) 85:3036–40. doi: 10.1002/jnr.21346
11. Pratico D, Clark CM, Lee VM, Trojanowski JQ, Rokach J, FitzGerald GA. Increased 8,12-iso-iPF2alpha-VI in Alzheimer's disease: correlation of a noninvasive index of lipid peroxidation with disease severity. *Ann Neurol.* (2000) 48:809–12. doi: 10.1002/1531-8249(200011)48:5andlt;809::AID-ANA19andgt;3.0.CO;2-9
12. Pratico D, Clark CM, Liun F, Rokach J, Lee VY, Trojanowski JQ. Increase of brain oxidative stress in mild cognitive impairment: a possible predictor of Alzheimer disease. *Arch Neurol.* (2002) 59:972–6. doi: 10.1001/archneur.59.6.972
13. Bantscheff M, Schirle M, Sweetman G, Rick J, Kuster B. Quantitative mass spectrometry in proteomics: a critical review. *Anal Bioanal Chem.* (2007) 389:1017–31. doi: 10.1007/s00216-007-1486-6
14. Edgar R, Domrachev M, Lash AE. Gene expression omnibus: NCBI gene expression and hybridization array data repository. *Nucleic Acids Res.* (2002) 30:207–10. doi: 10.1093/nar/30.1.207
15. Berchtold NC, Cribbs DH, Coleman PD, Rogers J, Head E, Kim R, et al. Gene expression changes in the course of normal brain aging are sexually dimorphic. *Proc Natl Acad Sci USA.* (2008) 105:15605–10. doi: 10.1073/pnas.0806883105
16. Berchtold NC, Coleman PD, Cribbs DH, Rogers J, Gillen DL, Cotman CW. Synaptic genes are extensively downregulated across multiple brain regions in normal human aging and Alzheimer's disease. *Neurobiol Aging* (2013) 34:1653–61. doi: 10.1016/j.neurobiolaging.2012.11.024
17. Liang WS, Dunckley T, Beach TG, Grover A, Mastroeni D, Walker DG, et al. Gene expression profiles in anatomically and functionally distinct regions of the normal aged human brain. *Physiol Genomics* (2007) 28:311–22. doi: 10.1152/physiolgenomics.00208.2006
18. Irizarry RA, Hobbs B, Collin F, Beazer-Barclay YD, Antonellis KJ, Scherf U, et al. Exploration, normalization, and summaries of high density oligonucleotide array probe level data. *Biostatistics* (2003) 4:249–64. doi: 10.1093/biostatistics/4.2.249
19. Massey FJ. The Kolmogorov-Smirnov test for goodness of fit. *J Am Statist Assoc.* (1951) 46:68–78. doi: 10.1080/01621459.1951.10500769
20. Mann HBW, Donald R. On a test of whether one of two random variables is stochastically larger than the other. *Ann Math Statist.* (1947) 18:50–60. doi: 10.1214/aoms/1177730491
21. Benjamini YHY. (1995). Controlling the false discovery rate: a practical and powerful approach to multiple testing. *J Royal Statist Soc.* 57:289–300.
22. Cui J, Liu Q, Puett D, Xu Y. Computational prediction of human proteins that can be secreted into the bloodstream. *Bioinformatics* (2008) 24:2370–5. doi: 10.1093/bioinformatics/btn418
23. Souza BF, Carvalho AP. Gene selection based on multi-class support vector machines and genetic algorithms. *Genet Mol Res.* (2005) 4:599–607.
24. McDonald JH (Ed.). G-test of goodness-of-fit. In: *Handbook of Biological Statistics* (4th edn). Baltimore, MD: Sparky House Publishing (2014). p. 53–8.
25. Fawcett T. An introduction to ROC analysis. *Pattern Recogni Lett.* (2006) 27:861–74. doi: 10.1016/j.patrec.2005.10.010
26. Robin X, Turck N, Hainard A, Tiberti N, Lisacek F, Sanchez JC, et al. pROC: an open-source package for R and S+ to analyze and compare ROC curves. *BMC Bioinformatics* (2011) 12:77. doi: 10.1186/1471-2105-12-77
27. Yao F, Hong X, Li S, Zhang Y, Zhao Q, Du W, et al. Urine-based biomarkers for alzheimer's disease identified through coupling computational and experimental methods. *J Alzheimers Dis.* (2018) 65:421–31. doi: 10.3233/JAD-180261
28. Ruan Q, D'Onofrio G, Sancarlo D, Greco A, Yu Z. Potential fluid biomarkers for pathological brain changes in Alzheimer's disease: implication for the screening of cognitive frailty. *Mol Med Rep.* (2016) 14:3184–98. doi: 10.3892/mmr.2016.5618
29. Zipser BD, Johanson CE, Gonzalez L, Berzin TM, Tavares R, Hulette CM, et al. Microvascular injury and blood-brain barrier leakage in Alzheimer's disease. *Neurobiol Aging* (2007) 28:977–86. doi: 10.1016/j.neurobiolaging.2006.05.016
30. Erickson MA, Banks WA. Blood-brain barrier dysfunction as a cause and consequence of Alzheimer's disease. *J Cereb Blood Flow Metab.* (2013) 33:1500–13. doi: 10.1038/jcbfm.2013.135

31. Guntert A, Campbell J, Saleem M, O'Brien DP, Thompson AJ, Byers HL, et al. Plasma gelsolin is decreased and correlates with rate of decline in Alzheimer's disease. *J Alzheimers Dis.* (2010) 21:585–96. doi: 10.3233/JAD-2010-100279

32. Yu HL. Aberrant profiles of native and oxidized glycoproteins in Alzheimer plasma. *Proteomics* (2004) 3:2240–8. doi: 10.1002/pmic.200300475

33. Ijsselstijn L, Dekker LJM, Stingl C, van der Weiden MM, Hofman A, Kros JM, et al. Serum levels of pregnancy zone protein are elevated in presymptomatic Alzheimer's disease. *J Proteome Res.* (2011) 10:4902–10. doi: 10.1021/pr200270z

34. Doecke JD, Laws SM, Faux NG, Wilson W, Burnham SC, Lam CP, et al. Blood-based protein biomarkers for diagnosis of Alzheimer disease. *Arch Neurol.* (2012) 69:1318–25. doi: 10.1001/archneurol.2012.1282

35. Mhyre TR, Loy R, Tariot PN, Profenno LA, Maguire-Zeiss KA, Zhang D, et al. Proteomic analysis of peripheral leukocytes in Alzheimer's disease patients treated with divalproex sodium. *Neurobiol Aging* (2008) 29:1631–43. doi: 10.1016/j.neurobiolaging.2007.04.004

36. Cutler P, Akuffo EL, Bodnar WM, Briggs DM, Davis JB, Debouck CM, et al. Proteomic identification and early validation of complement 1 inhibitor and pigment epithelium -derived factor: two novel biomarkers of Alzheimer's disease in human plasma. *Proteomics Clini Appl.* (2008) 2:467–77. doi: 10.1002/prca.200780101

37. Wang C, Cui Y, Yang J, Zhang J, Yuan D, Wei Y, et al. Combining serum and urine biomarkers in the early diagnosis of mild cognitive impairment that evolves into Alzheimer's disease in patients with the apolipoprotein E 4 genotype. *Biomarkers* (2015) 20:84–8. doi: 10.3109/1354750X.2014.994036

38. Kim BY, Lee SH, Graham PL, Angelucci F, Lucia A, Pareja-Galeano H, et al. Peripheral brain-derived neurotrophic factor levels in Alzheimer's disease and mild cognitive impairment: a comprehensive systematic review and meta-analysis (2016). *Mol Neurobiol.* 54:7297–311. doi: 10.1007/s12035-016-0192-9

39. Huang DW, Sherman BT, Lempicki RA. Bioinformatics enrichment tools: paths toward the comprehensive functional analysis of large gene lists. *Nucleic Acids Res.* (2009) 37:1–13. doi: 10.1093/nar/gkn923

40. Becker KG, Barnes KC, Bright TJ, Wang SA. The genetic association database. *Nat Genet.* (2004) 36:431–2. doi: 10.1038/ng0504-431

41. Kanehisa M, Goto S. KEGG: Kyoto Encyclopedia of Genes and Genomes. *Nucleic Acids Res.* (2000) 28:27–30. doi: 10.1093/nar/28.1.27

42. Rappaport N, Twik M, Nativ N, Stelzer G, Bahir I, Stein TI, et al. MalaCards: a comprehensive automatically-mined database of human diseases. *Curr Protoc Bioinformatics* (2014) 47, 1 24 1–19. doi: 10.1002/0471250953.bi0124s47

43. Handen A, Ganapathiraju MK. LENS: web-based lens for enrichment and network studies of human proteins. *BMC Med Genomics* (2015) 8 (Suppl. 4):S2. doi: 10.1186/1755-8794-8-S4-S2

44. Padurariu M, Ciobica A, Lefter R, Serban IL, Stefanescu C, Chirita R. The oxidative stress hypothesis in Alzheimer's disease. *Psychiatr Danub.* (2013) 25:401–9.

45. Zimmer ER, Leuzy A, Bhat V, Gauthier S, Rosa-Neto P. *In vivo* tracking of tau pathology using positron emission tomography (PET) molecular imaging in small animals. *Transl Neurodegener.* (2014) 3:6. doi: 10.1186/2047-9158-3-6

46. Zheng L, Roberg K, Jerhammar F, Marcusson J, Terman A. Oxidative stress induces intralysosomal accumulation of Alzheimer amyloid beta-protein in cultured neuroblastoma cells. *Ann N Y Acad Sci.* (2006) 1067:248–51. doi: 10.1196/annals.1354.032

47. Xie AM, Gao J, Xu L, Meng DM. Shared mechanisms of neurodegeneration in Alzheimer's disease and Parkinson's disease. *Biomed Res Int.* (2014) 2014:648740. doi: 10.1155/2014/648740

48. Peng M, Jia JP, Qin W. Plasma gelsolin and matrix metalloproteinase 3 as potential biomarkers for Alzheimer disease. *Neurosci Lett.* (2015) 595:116–21. doi: 10.1016/j.neulet.2015.04.014

49. Shen LM, Liao LP, Chen C, Guo Y, Song DL, Wang Y, et al. Proteomics analysis of blood serums from Alzheimer's disease patients using iTRAQ labeling technology. *J Alzheimers Dis.* (2017) 56:361–78. doi: 10.3233/JAD-160913

50. Ji L, Zhao X, Hua Z. Potential therapeutic implications of gelsolin in Alzheimer's disease. *J Alzheimers Dis.* (2015) 44:13–25. doi: 10.3233/JAD-141548

51. Yang WZ, Chauhan A, Mehta S, Mehta P, Gu F, Chauhan V. Trichostatin A increases the levels of plasma gelsolin and amyloid beta-protein in a transgenic mouse model of Alzheimer's disease. *Life Sci.* (2014) 99:31–6. doi: 10.1016/j.lfs.2014.01.064

52. Acheson A, Conover JC, Fandl JP, Dechiara TM, Russell M, Thadani A, et al. A bdnf autocrine loop in adult sensory neurons prevents cell death. *Nature* (1995) 374:450–3. doi: 10.1038/374450a0

53. Huang EJ, Reichardt LF. Neurotrophins: roles in neuronal development and function. *Ann Rev Neurosci.* (2001) 24:677–736. doi: 10.1146/annurev.neuro.24.1.677

54. Mattson MP. Glutamate and neurotrophic factors in neuronal plasticity and disease. *Ann N Y Acad Sci.* (2008) 1144:97–112. doi: 10.1196/annals.1418.005

55. Braun DJ, Kalinin S, Feinstein DL. Conditional depletion of hippocampal brain-derived neurotrophic factor exacerbates neuropathology in a mouse model of Alzheimer's disease. *ASN Neuro.* (2017) 9:1759091417696161. doi: 10.1177/1759091417696161

56. Hernandez-Guillamon M, Delgado P, Ortega L, Pares M, Rosell A, Garcia-Bonilla L, et al. Neuronal TIMP-1 release accompanies astrocytic MMP-9 secretion and enhances astrocyte proliferation induced by beta-amyloid 25-35 fragment. *J Neurosci Res.* (2009) 87:2115–25. doi: 10.1002/jnr.22034

57. Mroczko B, Koper OM, Groblewska M, Zboch M, Kulczynska-Przybik A, Szmitkowski M. Matrix metalloproteinase-9 (mmp-9) and its tissue inhibitor-1 (timp-1) as biomarkers of alzheimer's disease. *J Alzheimer's Dis.* (2014) 10:P520. doi: 10.1016/j.jalz.2014.05.811

58. Wang XX, Tan MS, Yu JT, Tan L. Matrix metalloproteinases and their multiple roles in Alzheimer's disease. *Biomed Res Int.* (2014) 2014:908636. doi: 10.1155/2014/908636

59. Lorenzl S, Albers DS, Relkin N, Ngyuen T, Hilgenberg SL, Chirichigno J, et al. Increased plasma levels of matrix metalloproteinase-9 in patients with Alzheimer's disease. *Neurochem Int.* (2003) 43:191–6. doi: 10.1016/S0197-0186(03)00004-4

60. DiBattista AM, Dumanis SB, Song JM, Bu G, Weeber E, Rebeck GW, et al. Very low density lipoprotein receptor regulates dendritic spine formation in a RasGRF1/CaMKII dependent manner. *Biochim Biophys Acta* (2015) 1853:904–17. doi: 10.1016/j.bbamcr.2015.01.015

61. Nakamura Y, Yamamoto M, Kumamaru E. Significance of the variant and full-length forms of the very low density lipoprotein receptor in brain. *Brain Res.* (2001) 922:209–15. doi: 10.1016/S0006-8993(01)03170-5

62. Lane-Donovan C, Herz J. The ApoE receptors Vldlr and Apoer2 in central nervous system function and disease. *J Lipid Res.* (2017) 58:1036–43. doi: 10.1194/jlr.R075507

63. Schilling S, Mehr A, Ludewig S, Stephan J, Zimmermann M, August A, et al. APLP1 Is a synaptic cell adhesion molecule, supporting maintenance of dendritic spines and basal synaptic transmission. *J Neurosci.* (2017) 37:5345–65. doi: 10.1523/JNEUROSCI.1875-16.2017

64. Del Prete D, Rice RC, Rajadhyaksha AM, D'Adamio L. Amyloid Precursor Protein (APP) may act as a substrate and a recognition unit for CRL4CRBN and Stub1 E3 ligases facilitating ubiquitination of proteins involved in presynaptic functions and neurodegeneration. *J Biol Chem.* (2016) 291:17209–27. doi: 10.1074/jbc.M116.733626

10

Biomarkers of Neurodegeneration in Autoimmune-Mediated Encephalitis

Peter Körtvelyessy[1,2,3,4]*, Harald Prüss[3,4], Lorenz Thurner[5], Walter Maetzler[6,7,8], Deborah Vittore-Welliong[9], Jörg Schultze-Amberger[10], Hans-Jochen Heinze[1,2,11], Dirk Reinhold[12], Frank Leypoldt[8], Stephan Schreiber[13] and Daniel Bittner[1,2]

[1] Department of Neurology, University Hospital Magdeburg, Magdeburg, Germany, [2] German Center for Neurodegenerative Diseases Magdeburg, Magdeburg, Germany, [3] Department of Neurology, Charité-Universitätsmedizin Berlin, Berlin, Germany, [4] German Center for Neurodegenerative Diseases Berlin, Berlin, Germany, [5] José Carreras Center for Immuno- and Gene Therapy and Internal Medicine I, Saarland University Medical School, Homburg, Germany, [6] Department of Neurodegeneration, Hertie Institute for Clinical Brain Research (HIH), University of Tübingen, Tübingen, Germany, [7] German Center for Neurodegenerative Diseases Tübingen, Tübingen, Germany, [8] Department of Neurology, University Hospital Schleswig-Holstein, Kiel, Germany, [9] Department of Neurology and Epileptology, Universitätsklinikum Tübingen, Universität Tübingen, Tübingen, Germany, [10] Department of Neurology, Median Clinic Kladow, Kladow, Germany, [11] Department of Behavioral Neurology, Leibniz Institute for Neurobiology, Magdeburg, Germany, [12] Department of Immunohistopathology, Institute of Molecular and Clinical Immunology, Magdeburg, Germany, [13] Asklepios Department of Neurology, Brandenburg a.d. Havel, Germany

*Correspondence:
Peter Körtvelyessy
peter.koertvelyessy@med.ovgu.de
,

Progranulin (PGRN), Total-Tau (t-tau), and Neurofilament light chain (NfL) are well known biomarkers of neurodegeneration. The objective of the present study was to investigate whether these parameters represent also biomarkers in autoimmune-mediated Encephalitis (AE) and may give us insights into the pathomechanisms of AE. We retrospectively examined the concentration of PGRN in the cerebrospinal fluid (CSF) and serum of 38 patients suffering from AE in acute phase and/or under treatment. This AE cohort comprises patients with autoantibodies against: NMDAR ($n = 18$ patients), Caspr2 ($n = 8$), Lgi-1 ($n = 10$), GABAB(R) ($n = 1$), and AMPAR ($n = 1$). Additionally, the concentrations of NfL ($n = 25$) and t-tau ($n = 13$) in CSF were measured when possible. Follow up data including MRI were available in 13 patients. Several age-matched cohorts with neurological diseases besides neuroinflammation or neurodegeneration served as control groups. We observed that PGRN was significantly elevated in the CSF of patients with NMDAR-AE in the acute phase, but normalized at follow up under treatment ($p < 0.01$). In the CSF of other patients with AE PGRN was in the range of the CSF levels of control groups. T-tau was highly elevated in the CSF of patients with temporal FLAIR-signal in the MRI and in patients developing a hippocampal sclerosis. NfL was exceptionally high initially in Patients with AE with a paraneoplastic or parainfectious cause and also normalized under treatment. The normalizations of all biomarkers were mirrored in an improvement on the modified Rankin scale. The data suggest that the concentration of PGRN in CSF might be a biomarker for acute NMDAR-AE. Pathological high t-tau levels may indicate a risk for hippocampal sclerosis. The biomarker properties of NfL remain unclear since the levels decrease under treatment, but it could not predict severity of disease in this small cohort. According to our results, we recommend to measure in clinical practice PGRN and t-tau in the CSF of patients with AE.

Keywords: progranulin, neurofilament light chain, NMDAR encephalitis, Lgi-1 encephalitis, Caspr2 encephalitis, tau, autoimmune encephalitis

INTRODUCTION

Since the appearance of antibody-mediated autoimmune encephalopathy (AE) numerous antibodies (ab) have been linked to different clinical symptoms such as limbic encephalitis, faciobrachial dystonic seizures or dementia-like symptoms (1–3). Biomarkers of neurodegeneration mirror certain pathomechanisms of neuronal or axonal loss. The measurement of these biomarkers should bear the potential to provide useful information in everyday clinical life, e.g., to monitor the immunosuppressive therapy in Patients with AE. CSF antibody titres in e.g., contactin-associated-protein-receptor-2 (Caspr2)-AE or Leucin-rich glioma inactivated ptotein-1 (Lgi-1)-AE do not mirror the disease course in a linear way (4, 5). Furthermore, the clinical course in several patients suggests that an antibody titer independent pathomechanism might take place (6–8). The underlying mechanisms causing this dichotomy of clinical symptoms and antibody titer are largely unknown (8). One possible explanation could be the effect of the long survival of plasma cells in the brain (9). The brain-resident plasma cells itself cannot be measured as yet, but the damage possibly caused by autoantibodies should be detected via biomarkers for neuronal and axonal loss such as t-tau, PGRN, and NfL.

Recently, a direct connection between neurodegenerative mechanisms and AE has been detected in AEs mediated by IgLON5 causing an atypical tauopathy (10). Vice versa a correlation between autoimmune diseases and Tar DNA-binding Protein 43 (TDP-43) mediated neurodegeneration in FTD patients has been reported (11). There is also some debate about IgA-NMDAR-Abs and IgM-NMDAR-Abs (3, 12, 13) causing dementia-like symptoms and mimicking neurodegenerative diseases. Histopathological examinations in patients with AE have been focused on the immunological mechanisms triggered and maintained by the antibodies (8) disregarding a systematic research for markers of neurodegeneration so far. Only one case report of a Lgi-1 antibody positive patient presenting some neurodegenerative markers has been reported at autopsy, without witnessing pathological changes in alpha-synuclein, beta-amyloid, or neurofibrillary tangle (14). MRI findings and long-term neuropsychological data also suggest an involvement of the frontal and temporal lobes in the clinical course of the NMDAR-AE and voltage-gated-potassium channel (VGKC)-complex-mediated AE (15–18). Another group has looked at the glial fibrillary acid, NfL and t-tau levels in patients with suspected AE (19). Their group only encompassed four patients with NMDAR-AE and one Lgi-1 patient with most of them having a status epilepticus (SE) before, as SE is known for confounding the protein levels in the CSF (20, 21). They found higher NfL

and t-tau levels in all patients, which is most likely due to the SE before. In pediatric opsoclonus-myoclonus syndrome caused by antibodies with intracellular epitopes, immunosuppressive treatment has shown to decrease the CSF-Neurofilament light chain levels together with a concomitant clinical improvement (22, 23).

Here, we examined concentrations of PGRN, NfL, and t-tau, well-established biomarkers of neurodegeneration, in CSF and serum of 38 patients with antibody positive AE. The aim of this study is to investigate if these proteins are possible biomarkers in Patients with AE. Also, the knowledge about the biomarkers of neurodegeneration CSF-levels may give clues about the pathological mechanisms in these patients.

METHODS
Clinical Cohort

This retrospective study was performed according to the local ethical committees in Berlin, Potsdam, Brandenburg, Magdeburg and Bielefeld, respectively. All patients gave written and informed consent (ethics committee approval number 100/16). We included only patients with a proven AE by clinical symptoms as recommended by Graus et al. (24) and detection of pathological antibodies with extracellular epitopes via indirect immunofluorescence tests. The samples of AE-Patients were collected from April 2013 until October 2017 in Berlin, Potsdam, Tübingen, Bielefeld, and Magdeburg where their samples were initially stored at −80°C and sent to Magdeburg. Every sample was stored in Magdeburg at −80°C and all biomarkers were measured in Magdeburg. All samples were run in duplicate with the mean taken as result. Samples were measured over time and not in a batch.

All patients received a lumbar puncture as part of the diagnostical work up when presenting for the first time on the ward and for antibody titre control in follow up depending on each individual disease course. At least 5 ml up to 13 ml CSF was taken and serum was collected in serum separator tubes and centrifuged at site. Every patient ($n = 38$) suffered from a limbic encephalitis including its variants, e.g., limbic encephalitis together with vegetative and/or peripheral neurological symptoms. All patients improved under immunosuppressive therapy. Treatment comprised methylprednisolone (dosage ranges from 3 g up to 18 g during disease course), cyclophosphamid or rituximab (with a minimum dosage of 2g), plasmapheresis or ivIG. We had no patients with a relapse in this cohort. None of the patients had a status epilepticus before lumbar puncture confounding the biomarker levels because of neuronal and axonal death due to the status epilepticus.

Two patients with other antibodies targeting extracellular epitopes [AMPAR and GABAB(R)] were not considered in the statistical analysis but for **Figure 3** to illustrate the biomarker and MRI timeline an AE patients. See **Table 1** for the different AE cohorts used per biomarker. We had follow up data in 13 patients. All other patients (samples) were categorized into either initial/acute phase or under treatment.

Abbreviations: Ab, Antibody; AD, Alzheimer's disease; AE, Autoimmune mediated Encephalitis; AMPAR, alpha-amino-3-hydroxy-5-methyl-4-isoxazolepropionic acid receptor; Caspr2, Contactin associated protein 2; CSF, cerebrospinal fluid; FTD, Frontotemporal dementia; GABAB(R), Gabaaminobutyrat-B subunit receptor; Lgi1, Leucin-rich glioma inactivated protein1; NMDAR, N-methyl-D-aspartate receptor; NfL, Neurofilament light chain; PGRN, Progranulin; SE, Status Epilepticus; t-tau, T-tau; VGKC, Voltage-gated potassium channel.

TABLE 1 | Epidemiological data.

Biomarker	Antibody	Initial [age/sex]	Follow up [age/sex]
Progranulin	NMDAR	**6** [28.9/6:0]	**17** [27.1/16:1]
	Caspr2	**8** [61.9/2:6]	**5** [67.1/0:5]
	Lgi-1	**7** [69.0/5:2]	**6** [63.2/3:3]
T-Tau	NMDAR	**3** (38.7/3:0)	**3** (38.7/3:0)
	Caspr2	**5** [69.6/0:5]	**5** [69.6/0:5]
	Lgi-1	**3** [63.7/2:1]	**3** [63.7/2:1]
Nfl	NMDAR	**3** (38.7/3:0)*	**13** (30.2/12:0)
VGKC-group {	Caspr2	**6** (68.3/1:5]	**5** [67.1/0:5]
	Lgi-1	**3** [63.7/2:1]	**3** [63.7/2:1]
Control group young	None	**24** [29.9/18:6]	*
Control group old	None	**21** [60.0/9:12]	*

*not part of statistics

sex = female:male

Overview of the single groups tested in this study. Number of patients included in bold, sex and mean age are listed.

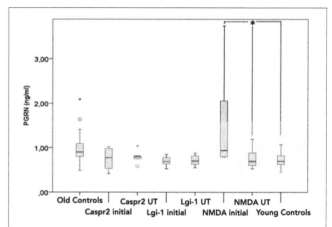

FIGURE 1 | CSF Progranulin levels [pg/ml] in patients with AE ($n = 36$) measured divided by antibody and by phase of disease (initial vs. under treatment). Significant results are marked with a *. Normal range is marked in light red. Line represents the median and the error bars represent the interquartile range. Black points are outliers.

Magdeburg Group

Patients with AE who were identified and treated in Magdeburg ($n = 13$) build a special cohort, because we could e.g., compare serial MRIs to look for AE caused lesions, basic CSF parameters, the outcome with the modified Rankin scale, t-tau, and other biomarker levels in the CSF and ab titer. The modified Rankin scale in this cohort was assessed by two experienced neurologist (PK, DB). Six out of thirteen had a paraneoplastic origin and one patient a postinfectious origin of the AE.

CSF-Neurofilament Light Chain Measurements

We divided the AE cohort into three groups regarding the CSF-NfL measurements in order to be able to perform a sufficient statistical analysis (see **Table 1**). One group with voltage-gated potassium channels (VGKC) mediated AE (comprising the Caspr2 and Lgi-1 patients) subdivided in an "initial" ($n = 9$) and "under treatment," meaning after several immunosuppressive therapies, subgroup ($n = 8$) and one group with NMDA patients under treatment ($n = 13$) (see **Table 1** and **Figure 1**). There were not enough NMDA patients who would fit into an initial/acute phase group ($n = 3$). Therefore, this group could unfortunately not be part of the statistical analysis.

Neurofilament light chain was measured with a commercial ELISA (Umandiagnostics, Sweden, catalogue number 10-7001 CE). The sensitivity of this assay is 31 pg/ml. The cut-off for pathological levels was set at 3523 ng/ml (mean (1823[ng/ml]) + 2 standard deviation (850[ng/ml]) above). Intraessay coefficient of variance is 7.4% and interessay coefficient of variance is 6%. NfL is a stable protein, which can be measured in the CSF even though the sample was on room temperature for up to 8 days (25). Therefore, we could measure NfL in samples not collected at Magdeburg, We used an already established control group at Magdeburg ($n = 34$, mean age = 64.4, CSF-NfL= 1823 ± 850 [ng/ml]) comprising patients with other than neuroinflammatory or neurodegenerative diseases (e.g., headache, suspicion of infection in the CNS etc.).

Total-Tau Measurements

The correct measurement of t-tau due to manufacturer's instructions requires different than standard processing of the CSF samples to create a cell-free sample excluding this parameter from a retrospective study. We yielded t-tau levels only in the Magdeburg group, as t-tau is part of the routine in Magdeburg but not in the other centers involved. Total-Tau levels were determined using a commercially available single-parameter ELISA kit [Innogenetics, Ghent, Belgium, catalogue numbers: 81572 (962-CE) and 81573] established in our routine diagnostical work up. Intraessay coefficient of variance is 13.2% and interessay coefficient of variance is 11.5%. The pathological levels were considered according to the manufacture guidelines.

CSF-Progranulin Measurements

We measured PGRN in CSF and serum of 36 Patients with AE. We divided our AE cohort ($n = 36$) into three groups according to the antibody causing the limbic encephalitis when looking statistically at the CSF-PGRN levels: one Lgi-1 group ($n = 10$, mean age = 69.2), one Caspr2 group ($n = 8$, mean age = 61.9) and a NMDAR group ($n = 18$, mean age = 27.1). These three groups were subdivided into two subgroups respectively one before and one after initiating immunosuppressive therapy (again, called "initial" or "under treatment") (see **Table 1** and **Figure 2**).

A commercial ELISA was performed to determine the levels of PGRN (Human Progranulin ELISA Kit, Mediagnost, Reutlingen, Germany, catalogue number E103) according to the manufacturer's instructions. Intraessay coefficient of variance is 4.4% and interessay coefficient of variance is 8.0%.

We established two control groups for PGRN measurements. Since PRGN levels are age dependent, we build a younger control group ($n = 24$; mean age 29.3 years; 18–40yrs) and one older group ($n = 39$; mean age 66.3 years,

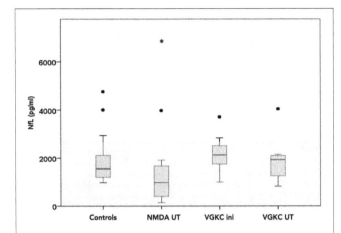

FIGURE 2 | CSF-Neurofilament light chain (NfL) levels divided into three possible groups (NMDA under treatment $n = 14$, VGKC initial $n = 7$ and under treatment $n = 6$) as box plots (number of measurements, $n = 30$). The area in light red marks the normal range. Please note that all levels are inside the normal range. Line represents the median and the error bars represent the interquartile range. White points mean outlier and star extreme outliers.

50–75 years) and correlated it to age. The patients from these control groups had other neurological diseases than neuroinflammatory or neurodegenerative (e.g., acute headache, excluding neuroinflammatory diseases, no epilepsy patients). CSF-PGRN level was considered pathological, when the CSF-PGRN levels per control group were two standard deviation above or below the mean for each control group respectively.

Antibody Detection
Antibody detection was either performed at the antibody laboratory Bielefeld, at the University Hospital Schleswig-Holstein, Department of Neuroimmunology Kiel and Lübeck or at the Institute of Molecular and Clinical Immunology Magdeburg. Standard indirect immunofluorescence tests were performed on antigen-specific transfected Hek293 cells as commercially available and used in clinical routine (EUROIMMUN, Lübeck, Germany, catalogue numbers: FA 112d-1003-6, FA 112d-1003-51, FA 1430-1003-1) for each patient revealing the specific antibody and the titer in CSF and serum.

Statistics
Statistics were calculated by SPSS 21.0 (IBM, Seattle, USA). Since group size and variances were not equal non-parametric tests were applied. For comparison of more than two different groups Kruskal-Wallis test was used with tamhanes *post-hoc* analysis. Group comparison of two groups was analyzed with Mann-Whitney-U test when they were independent and with the Wilcoxon test when the samples were paired to each other. For correlational analysis of serum and CSF PGRN Spearmann-rho correlation was applied. Tests were considered significant when reaching $p < 0.05$. There was no test for outliers applied.

RESULTS
Cohorts
Since the CSF-PGRN level is age-dependent we established a younger control group aged 18–40 years ($n = 24$, CSF-PGRN= 0.72 ± 0.17 ng/ml, Serum-PGRN = 36.4 ng/ml, mean age = 29.3 years) and a control group 50-75 years ($n = 39$, CSF-PGRN = 0.94 ± 0.22 ng/ml, Serum-PGRN = 28.5 ng/ml mean age = 66.3 ± 9.8 years). Spearman correlation statistics revealed a significant correlation between CSF-PGRN and age ($r = 0.275$, $p = 0.02$).

In the Magdeburg group 9/13 had a FLAIR-intense signal in the limbic system on the MRI. Five out of thirteen patients developed a hippocampal sclerosis due to AE (see **Table 2** and **Figure 3**). Every patient with pathologically elevated t-tau levels developed a hippocampal sclerosis. The one patient, who developed a hippocampal sclerosis without elevated t-tau levels but elevated NfL concentrations, was administered after he was already treated and had a hippocampal sclerosis. Therefore the CSF was taken and measured ~8 months after beginning of the AE and treatment. On the contrary only 4 out of 7 patients with pathological NfL levels developed a hippocampal sclerosis. Every marker of neurodegeneration and the modified Rankin scale (mRS) decreased after initializing the immunosuppressive treatment paralleled by a decrease in antibody titre (see **Figure 3** for examples and **Table 2** for the follow up data).

Neurofilament Light Chain
NfL was pathologically high (>3523 pg/ml) in 7/23 patients at different stages of the AE (see **Figures 2, 3** and **Table 2**). Out of these seven patients, four had a paraneoplastic origin of the AE and one a postinfectious origin. Furthermore, 5/7 patients had a FLAIR-intense signal in the limbic areas on the MRI, which normalized during immunosuppressive treatment. This decrease in FLAIR signal was mirrored by a decrease in NfL-levels reaching normal NfL levels during disease course (see **Figure 3** and **Table 2**). Three out of five patients who developed hippocampal sclerosis had elevated CSF-NfL levels additionally to the also elevated t-tau. Solely elevated CSF-NfL was found in 4 patients. We correlated the leukocyte count to the NFL levels in the Magdeburg cohort and found no correlation (Spearmans $r = 0.625$).

There was a trend toward a lower NfL in the NMDA under treatment group (CSF-NfL = 1455 [pg/ml], range 142–6841[pg/ml]) compared to the VGKC under treatment group (CSF-NfL = 2164 [pg/ml], range 821–4039 [pg/ml]) (Mann-Whitney U test $p = 0.052$ Z = -1.941), while there was no difference comparing the VGKC subgroups initial vs. under treatment (Wilcoxon test $p = 0.735$ and Z = -0.338).

Total Tau
Looking at the initial t-tau in our patients (before initiating the treatment) revealed a pathologically high t-tau in 4 patients (see **Table 2**). All 4 patients had MRI-FLAIR intense signals in the temporal lobe/limbic system and subsequently a hippocampal sclerosis. Immunosuppressive treatment did show an effect on

TABLE 2 | Biomarkers in the Magdeburg cohort.

	Antibody	Titer	Age	Year	T-tau	NFlight	CSF-PGRN	Serum-PGRN	Cell count	mRS	Comment
		CSF/Serum	Onset		pg/ml	ng/ml	pg/ml	pg/ml	CSF		
					>370	>3488	<0.54–1.4>	<18–54>	< 4 cells/mm2		
Patient 1	Caspr2	1:128/1:32000	60–65	2013	253	12342	0.76	n.a.	3	5	Temporal FLAIR-intense signal
		none/1:375		2015	133	2152	0.8	32.5	0	3	Paraneoplastic origin
		none /1:128		2015	108	2055	0.61	30.62	1	3	Hippocampal sclerosis
Patient 2	Caspr2	1:64000/1:750000	75–80	2014 #	292	2047	1.02	27.11	13	5	Temporal FLAIR-intense signal
		1:6000/1:96000		2015	213	2123	0.87	30.63	17	1	
Patient 3	Caspr2	1:320/1:3200	70–75	2015 #	367	4536	0.84	21.94	0	1	Normal MRI
		1:320/1:3200		2015 #	328	3580	0.74	22.05	3	1	
Patient 4	Caspr2	1:3200/1:1000	70–75	2016 #	314	3705	0.95	35.18	6	5	Temporal FLAIR-intense signal
		1:10 /1:2000		2016	317	4039	0.82	51.57	2	1	
Patient 5	Caspr2	1:320/1:4000	66–70	2017 #	349	2159	1.01	32.04	5	4	Normal MRI
		1:8/1:1000		2017	375	2586	0.82	43.58	2	0	
Patient 6	Lgi-1	none/1:100	60–65	2015 #	796	2128	0.63	32.97	1	3	Temporal FLAIR-intense signal
		none/1:32		2015	>11	2493	0.54	38.92	0	0	Hippocampal sclerosis
Patient 7	Lg-1	1:2/1:1000	65–70	2017 #	128	993	0.74	19.97	1	3	Paraneoplastic origin
		none/1:320		2017	149	1273	0.73	23	0	0	
Patient 8	Lgi-1	1:2 /1:160	60–65	2017 #	197	1582	0.65	27.33	0	3	Temporal FLAIR-intense signal
		1:20/1:10		2017	161	1233	0.68	30.12	2	0	
Patient 9	NMDA	1:32/1:320	25–30	2010 #	141	n.a.	0.76	29.11	1	5	Paraneoplastic origin
		1:10/1:100		2014	105	390	0.89	33.06	3	1	
		1:1/none		2015	58	553	1.3	n.a.	2	1	
Patient 10	NMDA	1:40/1:80	25–30	2016 #	869	38650	1	23.08	7	5	Temporal FLAIR-intense signal
		1:10/1:5		2016	229	20736	0.71	17.86	6	2	Hippocampal sclerosis
		1:5/1:5		2017	68	6841	0.71	25.43	3	1	Postinfectious origin
Patient 11	NMDA	none/1:10	60–65	2014 #	801	28791	1.53	35.51	96	4	Hippocampal sclerosis
		none/1:10		2014	372	42286	1.19	32.9	43	0	Temporal FLAIR-intense signal
		none/none		2015	192	3975	0.96	35.4	9	0	Paraneoplastic
Patient 12	GABA(B)R	1:320/1:32	50–55	2016 #	135	32029	1.79	37.21	47	5	Paraneoplastic origin
		1:320/1:1		2016	168	21439	1.03	37.5	1	3	Temporal FLAIR-intense signal
		none/1:10		2016	126	3581	0.95	n.a.	1	2	
Patient 13	AMPA	1:32/1:3200	70–75	2014 #	1950	32151	2.47	34.21	43	5	Paraneoplastic origin
		1:8/1:375		2014	1984	20354	1.23	38.22	90	4	Temporal FLAIR-intense signal
		1:1/none		2015	173	2892	0.7	n.a.	3	2	Hippocampal sclerosis
	#		Before treatment								
	n.a.		Not available								

Complete list of all 13 patients in the cohort where follow up data is available including antibody, antibody serum titer, age, year at which the sample has been obtained, Neurofilament light chain (NfL), Total-tau (T-Tau), CSF-Progranulin (PGRN), Serum-Progranulin, cell count, modified Rankin scale (mRS) and comments on MRI abnormalities and putative pathogenesis; n.a., not available; #, timepoint before start of the immunosuppression.

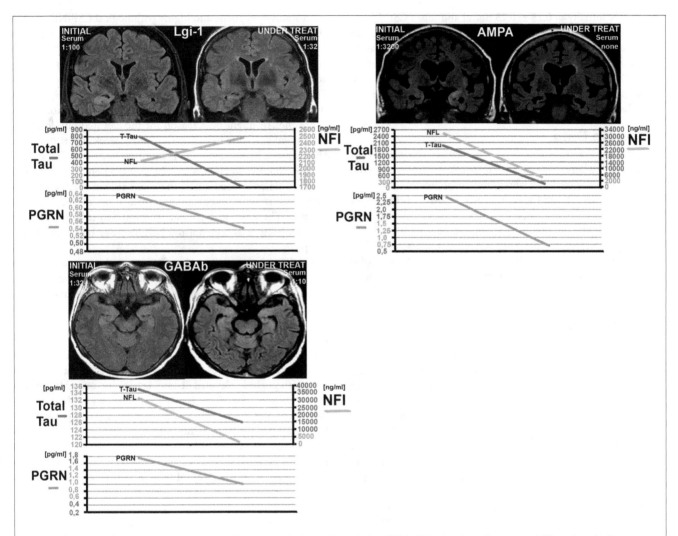

FIGURE 3 | Three examples of patients from the Magdeburg cohort (patient 5, 12, and 13 see **Table 1**) showing the under treatment MRI together with the CSF-Neurofilament light chain (NfL), CSF-Progranulin (PGRN), and Total tau. Normal levels are marked in green at the y-axis and pathological levels are marked in red. Notice the hippocampal sclerosis in the Lgi-1 patient and the complete recovery from the oedema in the GABA(B)R-AE-patient without a clear sign of a hippocampal atrophy. The third patient has a AMPAR-AE. The follow up in this patient shows a severe bilateral hippocampal atrophy. Nevertheless the patient improved over years.

the modified Rankin scale and also resulted in a decrease of t-tau in these patients. The FLAIR signal also decreased in these patients (see **Figure 3**). In the other 8 patients without elevated t-tau levels immunosuppressive therapy had no effect on t-tau levels. A concomitant tumor had no impact at all on the t-tau levels. (see **Table 2**).

Progranulin

The mean CSF-PGRN levels were pathologically high in the initial NMDAR-group (CSF-PGRN=1.55 ± 1.1 ng/ml) reaching significance when compared to the NMDAR under treatment group (Mann-Whitney-U test Z = −2.5 and $p = 0.012$) and also when compared to the age-matched healthy group (Mann-Whitney-U test Z = −2.689 and $p = 0.007$). Serum PGRN levels were inside normal ranges in every AE patient and did not change after immunosuppression (see **Figure S1**). CSF-PGRN and CSF-Serum ratios ranged from 0.01 to 0.1, still CSF-PGRN

is show to originate from the CNS when measured in the CSF (26, 27) We also could not find a correlation between Serum-PGRN and CSF-PGRN in all groups (Spearman-rho coefficient $r = 0.17$, $p = 0.3$) (**Figure S1** in the Supplement).After initiating the immunosuppressive therapy CSF-PGRN dropped to normal levels (CSF-PGRN = 0.75 ± 0.2 ng/ml) in the "under treatment"-group.

Mean CSF-PGRN levels were normal in the Lgi-1 "initial" group (CSF-PGRN = 0.71 ± 0.11 ng/ml) and in the under treatment group (CSF-PGRN = 0.72 ± 0.12 ng/ml) (see **Figure 1**). Comparing these results to the age-matched group revealed significant differences (Kruskal-Wallis test: for "initial" PGRN: $p = 0.009$, $X^2 = 9.4$, for follow-up: $p = 0.04$, $X^2 = 6.3$). There were significantly lower levels in tamhane *post-hoc* in the Patients with AE (Lgi-1 initial vs. control $p = 0.009$ and $p = 0.041$ for the under treatment vs. control) The CSF-PGRN levels in both Caspr2 groups were inside the normal range (mean

CSF-PRGN initially $= 0.75 \pm 0.23$ ng/ml and mean CSF-PGRN under treatment $= 0.8 \pm 0.16$ ng/ml) without significant results when compared to the age-matched controls (Caspr2 initial vs. under treatment $p = 0.35$ and Caspr2 under treatment vs. control $p = 0.92$). There was no difference between the "initial" and the "under treatment" group in the Lgi-1 and Caspr2 cohorts, respectively.

Follow Up Data

In summary, in all cases with an elevated biomarker of neurodegeneration in the CSF a decrease of biomarkers, ab titres, and mRS was observed following immunosuppressive treatment in all patients (see **Table 1** and **Figure 3**) regardless if the origin was postinfectious, paraneoplastic, or cryptogenic. There were two patients with all biomarkers simultaneously elevated. None of these parameters could predict a hippocampal sclerosis for sure on the one hand; on the other hand every patient who developed a sclerosis had either elevated t-tau or NfL levels with t-tau appearing to be more predictive.

DISCUSSION

We could show for the first time that biomarkers of neurodegeneration originating from CNS are mirroring the clinical and probably neuroimmunological course of patients suffering from AE associated with antibodies to extracellular epitopes. CSF-PGRN is elevated in patients with NMDAR-AE during the acute phase. Furthermore, biomarkers of neurodegeneration such as t-tau together with CSF-NfL in Patients with AE might be predictive of the clinical outcome especially for developing a hippocampal sclerosis. The pathologically elevated biomarkers correlated with the mRS, the clinical course and the antibody titre. Besides Progranulin in acute NMDAR-AE, NfL, PGRN and t-tau did not seem to be restricted to one special autoantibody mediated AE. This may be due to the fact that the neuronal and axonal damages in general are mirrored and not the distinct pathomechanisms of each putative pathological autoantibody.

Neurofilament Light Chain

NfL has been proven as an excellent marker of axonal loss (28). It seems very unlikely and there has been no data on whether peripheral tumors such as teratomas nor other neuroendocrine tumors can influence the CSF-NfL levels as possible confounders in our study. The co-occurrence of MRI changes, hippocampal sclerosis, and elevated NfL levels in our Magdeburg cohort is pointing at a pathomechanism causing the edema and subsequently the FLAIR signal resulting in the axonal dysfunction and subsequently increased NfL levels in the CSF. Other than in neurodegenerative diseases such as FTD (29, 30) the axonal loss in AE ceases after initiating sufficient immunosuppressive therapy as seen by the group of Pranzatelli in pediatric patients with opsoclonus-myoclonus syndrome caused by antibodies with intracellular epitopes (22, 23). Constantinescu et al. also measured CSF-NfL in four Patients with NMDAR-AE with AE and one Lgi-1 patient (19). Three NMDA-patients

had a status epilepticus and highly pathological CSF-NFL levels, which has been seen in SE for nearly every marker of neuronal death (20, 21). In our cohort none had a status epilepticus confounding the biomarkers. This is possibly the reason why we found normal CSF-NfL levels in all measured Patients with NMDAR-AE except for the one with postinfectious origin. The meningoencephalitis with subsequent neuronal and axonal loss before the AE might be a reason for the elevated NfL levels in this patient since the infection was only 7 weeks apart from the AE. Our results are also much more in line with the known pathomechanism in NMDAR-AE (31, 32) where only marginal neuronal damage occurs and the main reason for the clinical symptoms is most likely the internalization of the NMDA-receptor. The one Lgi-1 patient (without SE) in the cohort of Constantiescu et al had normal NfL levels as our entire Lgi-1 group.

Total-Tau is a better marker for neuronal death as NfL (see below). However, FLAIR intense signals in the hippocampus as a consequence of disturbances of neuronal membrane function did correlate with NfL levels in our small cohort.

Total-Tau

Total-tau is an excellent marker for neuronal death (21, 33) 4/5 patients who developed a hippocampal sclerosis had pathological elevated t-tau levels in our Magdeburg cohort ($n = 13$). This is well in line with the current concept of the pathomechanisms leading to a sclerosis (34). Although, patient 1 (see **Table 2**) with the Caspr2 AE who was already treated months before admission to Magdeburg had only elevated CSF-NfL and normal t-tau levels and a hippocampal sclerosis (see **Table 2**). Sadly, it was not possible to measure NfL and t-tau levels in this patients initial CSF.

In sum, the measurement of t-tau may be a good marker before treatment decision in suspected autoimmune encephalitis or before deciding on the further immunosuppressive treatment but is limited to laboratories with expertise in measuring t-tau.

Progranulin

PGRN is playing a role in autoimmune mediated diseases such as rheuma or bowel disease or status epilepticus or in suppression of neuroinflammation (30, 35–37) Recently, EpiphrinA2 as a part of the Ephrin receptor kinase has been identified as functional receptor of PGRN and the potential of PGRN phosphorylating and activating the EpiphrinB2 receptor (38) linking it to the dysfunction in the EpiphrinB2 pathway known in AE mediated by autoantibodies against the NMDA-receptor (39, 40). The distribution in the fronto-temporal structures (41), the possible common link with the AE mediated by NMDAR via the EpiphrinA2-EpiphrinB2 pathway and the known role as a mediator in neuroinflammation and autoimmunity makes PGRN an interesting protein in AE.

We detected elevated CSF-PGRN levels in our NMDA-patients with a severe ongoing AE. On the other hand, CSF-PGRN was low in patients suffering from Lgi-1-AE sometimes reaching levels of FTD patients (29) in contrast to Patients with NMDAR-AE and controls. The significance of this low

CSF-PGRN is doubtful because none of the CSF-PGRN levels normalized after initiating the immunosuppressive therapy. Also most CSF-PGRN levels in the patients with Lgi-1-AE were still inside the normal range.

When looking at the t-cell or b-cell specific cytokine patterns in the patient's CSF suffering from NMDAR-AE several groups have seen a massive b-cell predominant cytokine pattern in the beginning especially in CXCL-13 levels (42, 43) and then a decrease in follow up. Also, cytokine pattern associated with t-cell activation were detectable throughout the course of AE without relevant changes. This course in cytokine levels could explain the elevated Progranulin levels in patients having acute NMDAR-AE.

PGRN in Serum and CSF was not elevated in patients with AE due to paraneoplastic origin although PGRN is also known as a tumor marker for certain tumors such as Lymphomas (44) The missing correlation between the serum-PGRN and CSF-PGRN is pointing at a cerebral origin of the CSF-PGRN as already seen in other diseases (26, 27). Overall, this result is probably due to an affection of the CSF-PGRN pathway in acute NMDAR-AE but needs more *in vivo* and *in vitro* experiments to be further examined.

One major limitation of the study is the small sample size in every subgroup tested. This fact is due to the very low numbers of patients with AE overall. Although total numbers are too small to draw a final conclusion the t-tau levels together with the CSF-NFL levels seem to best characterize the stage of neuronal death in the brain. The diagnostic value of NFL levels in the CSF should be evaluated in further studies. Another limitation is that we only had follow up data in 13 patients limiting our knowledge about MRI, mRS, and ab titres. Another limitation of the study is that due to the scarcity of the diseases measurements of the biomarkers could not be done in a batch but on demand.

A larger study should be conducted to further elucidate the correlation of these interesting parameters how they could contribute to therapeutic decisions.

CONCLUSION

NfL, t-tau and PGRN could be potential biomarkers of neuronal or axonal loss in patients suffering from AE. Especially, the Patients with NMDAR-AE have elevated PGRN levels at the acute phase of the AE. This fact further strengthens the hypothesis of a pathological change in the Epiphrin receptor metabolism in NMDAR patients. CSF-PGRN may be a marker for acute NMDA-AE.

Furthermore, we strongly recommend measuring NfL and t-tau in the CSF of every patient with AE although one biomarker for itself could not predict all hippocampal sclerosis in this pilot study. Pathological levels of a biomarker of neurodegeneration should be considered as an on-going AE and may be taken into account when planning further therapy.

AUTHOR CONTRIBUTIONS

PK has access to all the data and takes responsibility for the data, accuracy of the data analysis, and the conduct of the research design or conceptualization of the study and analysis or interpretation of the data and drafting or revising the manuscript for intellectual content; HP and DB: Design and conceptualization of the study; analysis or interpretation of the data; drafting and revising the manuscript for intellectual content; LT: Conceptualization of the study; analysis of the data; drafting the manuscript for intellectual content; DV-W, JS-A, and SS: Conceptualization of the study; drafting the manuscript for intellectual content; WM, DR and FL: Conceptualization of the study; analysis and interpretation of the data; drafting and revising the manuscript for intellectual content; H-JH: Design of the study; drafting the manuscript for intellectual content.

ACKNOWLEDGMENTS

First, we have to thank our patients for the willingness to take part in this study. We have to thank Jeanette Witzke and Kerstin Kaiser at the neurochemical laboratory, Magdeburg for performing the excellent laboratory work. Furthermore, we have to thank Christian Bien at the Mara Epilepsy Center Bielefeld, Germany for laboratory work, samples and comments on the manuscript. We also appreciate the laboratory work of EUROIMMUN, Lübeck, Germany.

REFERENCES

1. Dalmau J, Gleichman AJ, Hughes EG, Rossi JE, Peng X, Lai MS, et al. Anti-NMDA-receptor encephalitis: case series and analysis of the effects of antibodies. *Lancet Neurol.* (2008) 7:1091–8. doi: 10.1016/S1474-4422(08)70224-2
2. Irani SR, Stagg CJ, Schott JM, Rosenthal CR, Schneider SA, Pettingill PR, et al. Faciobrachial dystonic seizures: the influence of immunotherapy on seizure control and prevention of cognitive impairment in a broadening phenotype. *Brain* (2013) 136:3151–62. doi: 10.1093/brain/awt212
3. Doss S, Wandinger KP, Hyman BT, Panzer JA, Synofzik M, Dickerson BB, et al. High prevalence of NMDA receptor IgA/IgM antibodies in different dementia types. *Ann Clin Transl Neurol.* (2014) 1:822–32. doi: 10.1002/acn3.120
4. Malter MP, Frisch C, Schoene-Bake JC, Helmstaedter C, Wandinger KP, Stoecker W, et al. Outcome of limbic encephalitis with VGKC-complex

antibodies: relation to antigenic specificity. *J Neurol.* (2014) 261:1695–705. doi: 10.1007/s00415-014-7408-6

5. van Sonderen A, Petit-Pedrol M, Dalmau J, Titulaer MJ. The value of LGI1, Caspr2 and voltage-gated potassium channel antibodies in encephalitis. *Nat Rev Neurol.* (2017) 13:290–301. doi: 10.1038/nrneurol.2017.43

6. Körtvelyessy P, Bauer J, Stoppel CM, Brück W, Gerth I, Vielhaber S, et al. Complement-associated neuronal loss in a patient with CASPR2 antibody-associated encephalitis. *Neurol Neuroimmunol Neuroinflamm.* (2015) 2:e75. doi: 10.1212/NXI.0000000000000075

7. Taguchi Y, Takashima S, Nukui T, Tanaka K. Reversible "brain atrophy" in anti-NMDA receptor encephalitis. *Intern Med.* (2011) 50:2697. doi: 10.1097/MD.0000000000006776

8. Bien CG, Vincent A, Barnett MH, Becker AJ, Blümcke I, Graus FK, et al. Immunopathology of autoantibody-associated encephalitides: clues for pathogenesis. *Brain* (2012) 135:1622–38. doi: 10.1093/brain/aws082

9. Martinez-Hernandez E, Horvath J, Shiloh-Malawsky Y, Sangha N, Martinez-Lage M, Dalmau J. Analysis of complement and plasma cells in the brain of patients with anti-NMDAR encephalitis. *Neurology* (2011) 77:589–93. doi: 10.1212/WNL.0b013e318228c136

10. Sabater L, Gaig C, Gelpi E, Bataller L, Lewerenz J, Torres-Vega E, et al. A novel non-rapid-eye movement and rapid-eye-movement parasomnia with sleep breathing disorder associated with antibodies to IgLON5: a case series, characterisation of the antigen, and post-mortem study. *Lancet Neurol.* (2014) 13:575–86. doi: 10.1016/S1474-4422(14)70051-1

11. Miller ZA, Rankin KP, Graff-Radford NR, Takada LT, Sturm VE, Cleveland CM, et al. TDP-43 frontotemporal lobar degeneration and autoimmune disease. *J Neurol Neurosurg Psychiatry* (2013) 84:956–62. doi: 10.1136/jnnp-2012-304644

12. Dahm L, Ott C, Steiner J, Stepniak B, Teegen B, Saschenbrecker SC, et al. Seroprevalence of autoantibodies against brain antigens in health and disease. *Ann Neurol.* (2014) 76:82–94. doi: 10.1002/ana.24189

13. Hara M, Martinez-Hernandez E, Ariño H, Armangué T, Spatola M, Petit-Pedrol M, et al. Clinical and pathogenic significance of IgG, IgA, and IgM antibodies against the NMDA receptor. *Neurology* (2018) 90:e1386–94. doi: 10.1212/WNL.0000000000005329

14. Schultze-Amberger J, Pehl D, Stenzel W. LGI-1-positive limbic encephalitis: a clinicopathological study. *J Neurol.* (2012) 259:2478–80. doi: 10.1007/s00415-012-6559-6

15. Wagner J, Witt JA, Helmstaedter C, Malter MP, Weber B, Elger CE. Automated volumetry of the mesiotemporal structures in antibody-associated limbic encephalitis. *J Neurol Neurosurg Psychiatry* (2014) 86:735–42. doi: 10.1136/jnnp-2014-307875

16. Wagner J, Weber B, Elger CE. Early and chronic gray matter volume changes in limbic encephalitis revealed by voxel-based morphometry. *Epilepsia* (2015) 56:754–61. doi: 10.1111/epi.12968

17. Finke C, Kopp UA, Prüss H, Dalmau J, Wandinger KP, Ploner CJ. Cognitive deficits following anti-NMDA receptor encephalitis. *J Neurol Neurosurg Psychiatry* (2012) 83:195–8. doi: 10.1136/jnnp-2011-300411

18. Leypoldt F, Gelderblom M, Schöttle D, Hoffmann S, Wandinger KP. Recovery from severe frontotemporal dysfunction at 3 years after N-methyl-d-aspartic acid (NMDA) receptor antibody encephalitis. *J Clin Neurosci.* (2013) 20:611–3. doi: 10.1016/j.jocn.2012.03.036

19. Constantinescu R, Krýsl D, Bergquist F, Andrén K, Malmeström C, Asztély F, et al. Cerebrospinal fluid markers of neuronal and glial cell damage to monitor disease activity and predict long-term outcome in patients with autoimmune encephalitis. *Eur J Neurol.* (2016) 23:796–806. doi: 10.1111/ene.12942

20. Huchtemann T, Körtvélyessy P, Feistner H, Heinze HJ, Bittner D. Progranulin levels in status epilepticus as a marker of neuronal recovery and neuroprotection. *Epilepsy Behav.* (2015) 49:170–2. doi: 10.1016/j.yebeh.2015.06.022

21. Monti G, Tondelli M, Giovannini G, Bedin R, Nichelli PF, Trenti T, et al. Cerebrospinal fluid tau proteins in status epilepticus. *Epilepsy Behav.* (2015) 49:150–4. doi: 10.1016/j.yebeh.2015.04.030

22. Pranzatelli MR, Tate ED, McGee NR, Verhulst SJ. CSF neurofilament light chain is elevated in OMS (decreasing with immunotherapy) and other pediatric neuroinflammatory disorders. *J Neuroimmunol.* (2014) 266:75–81. doi: 10.1016/j.jneuroim.2013.11.004

23. Pranzatelli MR, McGee NR. Neuroimmunology of OMS and ANNA-1/anti-Hu paraneoplastic syndromes in a child with neuroblastoma. *Neurol Neuroimmunol Neuroinflamm.* (2018) 5:e433. doi: 10.1212/NXI.0000000000000433

24. Graus F, Titulaer MJ, Balu R, Benseler S, Bien CG, Cellucci T, et al. A clinical approach to diagnosis of autoimmune encephalitis. *Lancet Neurol.* (2016) 15:391–404. doi: 10.1016/S1474-4422(15)00401-9

25. Kuhle J, Plattner K, Bestwick JP, Lindberg RL, Ramagopalan SV, Norgren N, et al. A comparative study of CSF neurofilament light and heavy chain protein in MS. *Mult Scler.* (2013) 19:1597–603. doi: 10.1177/1352458513482374

26. Nicholson AM, Finch NA, Thomas CS, Wojtas A, Rutherford NJ, Mielke MM, et al. Progranulin protein levels are differently regulated in plasma and CSF. *Neurology* (2014) 82:1871–8. doi: 10.1212/WNL.0000000000000445

27. Wilke C, Gillardon F, Deuschle C, Dubois E, Hobert MA, Müller vom Hagen J, et al. Serum levels of progranulin do not reflect cerebrospinal fluid levels in neurodegenerative disease. *Curr Alzheimer Res.* (2016) 13:654–62. doi: 10.2174/1567205013666160314151247

28. Steinacker P, Feneberg E, Weishaupt J, Brettschneider J, Tumani H, Andersen PM, et al. Neurofilaments in the diagnosis of motoneuron diseases: a prospective study on 455 patients. *J Neurol Neurosurg Psychiatry* (2016) 87:12–20. doi: 10.1136/jnnp-2015-311387

29. Körtvélyessy P, Gukasjan A, Sweeny-Reed C, Heinze HJ, Thurner L, Bittner DM. Progranulin and Amyloid-β levels: relationship to neuropsychology in frontotemporal and Alzheimer's Disease. *J Alzheimers Dis* (2015) 46:375–80. doi: 10.3233/JAD-150069

30. Kortvelyessy P, Heinze HJ, Prudlo J, Bittner D. CSF biomarkers of neurodegeneration in progressive non-fluent aphasia and other forms of frontotemporal dementia: clues for pathomechanisms? *Front Neurol.* (2018) 9:504. doi: 10.3389/fneur.2018.00504

31. Planagumà J, Leypoldt F, Mannara F, Gutiérrez-Cuesta J, Martín-García E, Aguilar E, et al. Human N-methyl D-aspartate receptor antibodies alter memory and behaviour in mice. *Brain* (2015) 138:94–109. doi: 10.1093/brain/awu310

32. Kreye J, Wenke NK, Chayka M, Leubner J, Murugan R, Maier NB, et al. Human cerebrospinal fluid monoclonal N-methyl-D-aspartate receptor autoantibodies are sufficient for encephalitis pathogenesis. *Brain* (2016) 139:2641–52. doi: 10.1093/brain/aww208

33. Spillantini MG, Goedert M. Tau pathology and neurodegeneration. *Lancet Neurol.* (2013) 12:609–22. doi: 10.1016/S1474-4422(13)70090-5

34. Thom M, Eriksson S, Martinian L, Caboclo LO, McEvoy AW, Duncan JS, et al. Temporal lobe sclerosis associated with hippocampal sclerosis in temporal lobe epilepsy: neuropathological features. *J Neuropathol Exp Neurol.* (2009) 68:928–38. doi: 10.1097/NEN.0b013e3181b05d67

35. Cenik B, Sephton CF, Kutluk Cenik B, Herz J, Yu G. Progranulin: a proteolytically processed protein at the crossroads of inflammation and neurodegeneration. *J Biol Chem.* (2012) 287:32298–306. doi: 10.1074/jbc.R112.399170

36. De Muynck L, Van Damme P. Cellular effects of progranulin in health and disease. *J Mol Neurosci.* (2011) 45:549–60. doi: 10.1007/s12031-011-9553-z

37. Jian J, Li G, Hettinghouse A, Liu C. Progranulin: A key player in autoimmune diseases. *Cytokine* (2016) 101:48–55. doi: 10.1016/j.cyto.2016.08.007

38. Neill T, Buraschi S, Goyal A, Sharpe C, Natkanski E, Schaefer L, et al. EphA2 is a functional receptor for the growth factor progranulin. *J Cell Biol.* (2016) 215:687–703. doi: 10.1083/jcb.201603079

39. Mikasova L, De Rossi P, Bouchet D, Georges F, Rogemond V, Didelot A, et al. Disrupted surface cross-talk between NMDA and Ephrin-B2 receptors in anti-NMDA encephalitis. *Brain* (2012) 135:1606–21. doi: 10.1093/brain/aws092

40. Planagumà J, Haselmann H, Mannara F, Petit-Pedrol M, Grünewald B, Aguilar E, et al. Ephrin-B2 prevents N-methyl-D-aspartate receptor antibody effects on memory and neuroplasticity. *Ann Neurol.* (2016) 80:388–400. doi: 10.1002/ana.24721

41. Daniel R, He Z, Carmichael KP, Halper J, and Bateman A. Cellular localization of gene expression for progranulin. *J Histochem Cytochem.* (2000) 48:999–1009. doi: 10.1177/002215540004800713

42. Liba Z, Kayserova J, Elisak M, Marusic P, Nohejlova H, Hanzalova J, et al. Anti-N-methyl-D-aspartate receptor encephalitis: the clinical course in light of the chemokine and cytokine levels in cerebrospinal fluid. *J Neuroinflammation* (2016) 13:55. doi: 10.1186/s12974-016-0507-9

43. Leypoldt F, Höftberger R, Titulaer MJ, Armangue T, Gresa-Arribas N, Jahn H, et al. Investigations on CXCL13 in Anti-N-Methyl-D-aspartate receptor encephalitis: a potential biomarker of treatment response. *JAMA Neurol* (2014) 72:180–6. doi: 10.1001/jamaneurol.2014.2956

44. Arechavaleta-Velasco F, Perez-Juarez CE, Gerton GL, Diaz-Cueto L. Progranulin and its biological effects in cancer. *Med Oncol.* (2017) 34:194. doi: 10.1007/s12032-017-1054-7

11

Moderate Frequency Resistance and Balance Training do not Improve Freezing of Gait in Parkinson's Disease

Christian Schlenstedt*, Steffen Paschen, Jana Seuthe, Jan Raethjen, Daniela Berg, Walter Maetzler and Günther Deuschl

Department of Neurology, University Hospital Schleswig-Holstein, Christian-Albrechts-University, Kiel, Germany

Correspondence:
Christian Schlenstedt
c.schlenstedt@neurologie.uni-kiel.de

Background and Aim: Individuals with Parkinson's disease (PD) and Freezing of Gait (FOG) have impaired postural control, which relate to the severity of FOG. The aim of this study was to analyze whether a moderate frequency resistance (RT) and balance training (BT), respectively, are effective to diminish FOG.

Methods: This *post-hoc* sub-analysis of a randomized controlled training intervention study of PD patients with and without FOG reports about results from FOG patients. Twelve FOG patients performed RT and 8 BT (training 2x/week, 7 weeks). Testing was performed prior and post intervention. FOG was assessed with the FOG Questionnaire (FOGQ) and with the FOG score of a FOG provoking walking course. Balance performance was evaluated with the Fullerton Advanced Balance (FAB) scale. Tests were conducted by raters blinded to group allocation and assessment time point (only FOG score and FAB scale).

Results: For the FOGQ and FOG score, no significant differences were found within and between the two training groups ($p > 0.05$) and effect sizes for the improvements were small ($r < 0.1$). Groups did not significantly improve in the FAB scale. FOG score changes and FAB scale changes within the RT group showed a trend toward significant negative correlation (Rho $= -0.553$, $p = 0.098$).

Conclusions: Moderate frequency RT and BT was not effective in reducing FOG in this pilot study. The trend toward negative correlation between changes in FOG score and FAB scale suggests an interaction between balance (improvement) and FOG (improvement). Future studies should include larger samples and high frequency interventions to investigate the role of training balance performance to reduce the severity of FOG.

Keywords: freezing, postural control, balance, Parkinson's disease, exercise, training

INTRODUCTION

Freezing of gait (FOG) in Parkinson's disease (PD) is a disabling symptom which is defined as the "brief, episodic absence or marked reduction of forward progression of the feet despite the intention to walk" (1). It has been shown that FOG-specific training interventions, such as cueing, can reduce FOG (2–4). It is however unclear whether non-FOG-specific exercises which target FOG-related deficits also alleviate FOG.

Individuals with PD with FOG (PD + FOG) have postural control deficits (5, 6) and the severity of FOG relates to the degree of postural instability (5). Recently it has been shown that PD+FOG have smaller anticipatory postural adjustments (APAs) when preparing for step initiation compared to patients without FOG (PD-FOG) and that the size of medio-lateral APAs was positively correlated with FOG severity (7). It has been suggested that reducing the size of APA might be a compensatory strategy addressing postural control deficits (7). Further, Plotnik et al. (8) proposed that FOG might be a result of multiple with FOG associated motor impairments such as dynamic postural control, gait asymmetry, and gait variability. According to this framework, FOG might occur if enough of these features deteriorate. It is unclear, whether an improvement of postural control as one of these FOG related features might diminish FOG.

In a recent study we compared resistance training (RT) with balance training (BT) to improve postural control in PD and we showed that RT was beneficial to improve balance performance. This sub-analysis has two aims: first, to test whether RT or BT is effective to reduce the severity of FOG and second, whether an improvement in FOG is related to improved postural control.

MATERIALS AND METHODS

This study is a sub-analysis (only PD + FOG, $N = 20$) of a randomized controlled trial that investigated the efficacy of RT vs. BT to improve postural control in PD ($N = 40$) (9).

Participants

Inclusion criteria were the diagnosis of idiopathic PD as defined by the UK Brain Bank criteria, FOG based on the FOG Questionnaire (10) (FOGQ) (item 3 > 0) and postural instability [Fullerton Advanced Balance (FAB) scale <26 points (11)]. Details about the exclusion criteria are reported in Schlenstedt et al. (9). Individuals had to be on stable medication during the training and assessment periods.

This study was carried out in accordance with the recommendations of Ethik-Kommission, Universitätsklinikum Schleswig-Holstein, Campus Kiel, Arnold-Heller-Straße 3, 24105 Kiel, Germany, with written informed consent from all subjects. All subjects gave written informed consent in accordance with the Declaration of Helsinki. The protocol was approved by the Ethik-Kommission, Universitätsklinikum Schleswig-Holstein, Campus Kiel, Arnold-Heller-Straße 3, 24105 Kiel, Germany.

Randomization and Intervention

Participants were randomized into either RT or BT (7 weeks, 2x/week, 60 min per session) within the original study. There was no stratification for FOG in the original randomization. Training was conducted in groups of 4–5 people. Each session started with a warm-up (10 min) followed by either RT or BT. In brief, RT consisted of lower limb muscle strength exercises and participants' own weight, cuff weights, and elasticated bands were used as resistance. Squats, knee extensions, toe/calf raises, hip abductions, and other exercises were performed [for details see (9)].

BT consisted of static and dynamic postural control tasks. Participants were asked to train their limits of stability by leaning forward/backward/sideward. Reactive postural control was trained by shoulder pulls. One option to reach training progression was the inclusion of unstable surfaces on which the participants had to stand or walk [see Schlenstedt et al. (9) for further details about training progression].

Testing Procedure and Outcome Measures

Participants were tested 1 week prior (PRE) and 1 week post (POST) intervention. Testing was conducted in the ON state of medication at the same time of a day for each participant. Severity of FOG was assessed with the FOGQ (10) and with the FOG score by Ziegler et al. (12). The FOGQ was conducted by an assessor blinded to group allocation. Trials of the FOG score were video-recorded and videos were rated by an independent rater, also blinded to assessment time point and group allocation.

Furthermore, the following tests were included in the analysis: FAB scale (to assess postural control) (11, 13), Unified Parkinson's Disease Rating Scale (UPDRS), and Mini Mental State Examination.

Statistical Analysis

Demographic and baseline differences between groups were analyzed with a Mann-Whitney-U-Test (except for gender: Chi-Square Test). As data were not normally distributed, non-parametric tests were used. A Wilcoxon-Signed-Rank-Test was conducted to analyze the changes from PRE to POST within one group. To compare the different training types, the differences from PRE to POST were calculated and the magnitude of change were compared between the two groups were analyzed with using the Mann-Whitney-U-Test. Effect sizes were calculated ($r = z$-score$/(n)^\wedge 1/2$). We considered effect sizes to be small with $0.1 < r < 0.3$, medium with $0.3 < r < 0.5$ and large with $r > 0.5$ (14). The magnitude of change in FOG severity was correlated [Spearman's rank correlation coefficient [Rho] with the change

TABLE 1 | Participant characteristics.

Variable	Resistance training (n = 12)	Balance training (n = 8)	p-value*
Age (y)	78.3 (5.8)	81.4 (7.3)	0.41
Gender (M/F)	9/3	6/2	1.00
BMI (kg/m²)	27.3 (6.5)	24.5 (3.5)	0.34
Disease duration (y)	11.2 (6.6)	8.4 (7.3)	0.38
HandY stage	2.8 (0.3)	2.9 (0.5)	1.00
UPDRS	43.2 (13.2)	45.8 (9.8)	0.51
UPDRS III	24.3 (10.0)	25.8 (5.7)	0.61
FAB scale	21.1 (4.7)	22.4 (5.2)	0.61
MMSE	27.4 (3.7)	26.2 (4.0)	0.44
LEDD	765 (448)	652 (286)	0.46
FOGQ	12.5 (4.5)	15.3 (3.1)	0.22
FOG score	6.6 (7.2)	5.9 (4.4)	0.92

*Values represent mean (SD) or number. *p-value of Mann-Whitney-U-Test (and Chi-Square-Test for Gender).*

TABLE 2 | Statistical results of the FOGQ and FOG score.

Test	Group	Value	PRE	POST	Within group comparison from PRE to POST		Between group comparison of changes from PRE to POST	
					p-value*	Effect size *r*	*p*-value**	Effect size *r*
FOGQ	RT	Mean (SD)	12.5 (4.5)	12.3 (4.8)	0.878	0.031	0.279	0.255
		Median (Range)	12 (5–20)	13.5 (5–19)				
	BT	Mean (SD)	15.3 (3.1)	17.0 (2.4)	0.136	0.430		
		Median (Range)	16 (10–19)	17.5 (13–19)				
FOG score	RT	Mean (SD)	6.6 (7.2)	6.9 (9.1)	0.833	0.047	0.153	0.347
		Median (Range)	5 (0–22)	3.5 (0–29)				
	BT	Mean (SD)	5.9 (4.4)	8.7 (5.1)	0.105	0.433		
		Median (Range)	6 (0–12)	8 (2–15)				
FAB scale	RT	Mean (SD)	21.1 (4.7)	23.2 (5.0)	0.245	0.336	0.534	0.139
		Median (Range)	22 (10–29)	22.5 (15–34)				
	BT	Mean (SD)	22.4 (5.2)	22.4 (5.7)	1.000	0.000		
		Median (Range)	23.5 (15–27)	25.5 (12–27)				

*p-value of Wilcoxon Signed Rank Test. **p-value of Mann-Whitney-U Test. RT, Resistance Training; BT, Balance Training.

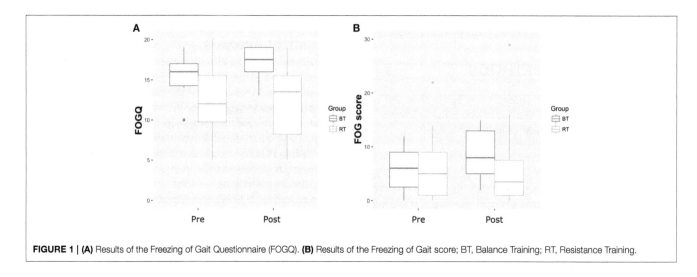

FIGURE 1 | (A) Results of the Freezing of Gait Questionnaire (FOGQ). **(B)** Results of the Freezing of Gait score; BT, Balance Training; RT, Resistance Training.

in balance performance (FAB scale). Level of significance was set at $p < 0.05$. Statistical analysis was performed with R (version 1.1.442) (15).

RESULTS

Table 1 shows the participant characteristics. RT and BT groups neither significantly differed in any demographic variable, nor with regard to severity of FOG. Both training types had no significant effect on FOGQ and FOG score (**Table 2** and **Figure 1**) ($p < 0.05$). The effect sizes for the slight improvements within the RT group were small ($r < 0.1$) (14). Within this sample, the groups did not improve significantly in postural control as measured with the FAB scale ($p < 0.05$). Although statistically not significant within this sample, a large effect was found within the RT group when relating the change in balance performance (FAB scale) with the change in FOG score (Rho $= -0.553$, $p = 0.098$). A similar trend was found when calculating this correlation taken

both groups together ($p = 0.11$, Rho $= -0.4$). A medium effect was found within the BT group ($p = 0.426$, Rho $= 0.361$). Changes in FOGQ was not related to the change in FAB scale (RT: $p = 0.948$; BT: $p = 0.612$). The exclusion of outliers did not relevantly affect our results.

DISCUSSION

We could not show that a moderate frequency RT and BT is effective to diminish FOG in people with PD in the present pilot study. As FOG-specific training interventions such as cueing did indeed show statistically significant reduction in FOG severity (2–4), our study might indirectly supports the hypothesis that exercises specifically designed to target FOG might be more beneficial than non-FOG-specific interventions. We acknowledge that our sample was small and results have to be interpreted cautiously; however, due to the low effect sizes we do not expect reaching significant results with this training protocol even with a larger sample. We rather believe that increasing the intensity and frequency of training is required to see a relevant effect and this has been suggested by other larger trials (16).

As FOG is related to postural control deficits (5, 6) the idea of this project was that improved postural control might lead to a reduction in FOG episodes. In the original study, participants of the RT group significantly improved postural control whereas the group of BT did not. We found a large effect when correlating the change in balance performance with the change in FOG severity within the RT group, indicating that those participants who improved postural control may also benefit with respect to FOG, supporting our hypothesis with respect to study aim II. However, this failed to reach statistical significance within this sample and the subgroup of participants with FOG did not significantly improve their postural control in this sub-analysis. This might be explained by the low training frequency (2x/week) and by the small subsample size, as in the original study on all participants of the RT balance performance improved significantly (9). Thus, the impact of training balance performance on FOG cannot clearly be answered with this study.

The following limitations have to be mentioned: Sample size is small and results therefore have to be interpreted cautiously. This study did not include a non-exercise control group which would give additional information with respect to the training effects.

A moderate frequency RT and BT was not effective to diminish FOG within this small sample. This pilot study might help designing future studies which should include larger samples and higher training frequency to investigate the role of training balance performance to reduce FOG occurrence in PD.

AUTHOR CONTRIBUTIONS

CS: Study design, study conduction, data collection, statistical analysis, and writing of first draft; SP and JS: Data analysis and manuscript critical revision; JR and GD: Study design and manuscript critical revision; DB and WM: Manuscript critical revision.

ACKNOWLEDGMENTS

We thank our participant for donating their time to volunteer. We thank Annika Kruse and Anna Krebs for helping in conducting the training sessions and in data collection. This publication was made possible with support from the Coppenrath-Foundation, Geeste/Groß-Hesepe, Niedersachsen, Germany and Krumme-Stiftung, Eckernförde, Schleswig-Holstein, Germany (Schlenstedt). We acknowledge financial support by Land Schleswig-Holstein within the funding programme Open Access Publikationsfonds.

REFERENCES

1. Giladi N, Nieuwboer A. Understanding and treating freezing of gait in parkinsonism, proposed working definition, and setting the stage. *Mov Disord.* (2008) 23(Suppl. 2):S423–5. doi: 10.1002/mds.21927

2. Fietzek UM, Schroeteler FE, Ziegler K, Zwosta J, Ceballos-Baumann AO. Randomized cross-over trial to investigate the efficacy of a two-week physiotherapy programme with repetitive exercises of cueing to reduce the severity of freezing of gait in patients with Parkinson's disease. *Clin Rehabil.* (2014) 28:902–11. doi: 10.1177/0269215514527299

3. Plotnik M, Shema S, Dorfman M, Gazit E, Brozgol M, Giladi N, et al. A motor learning-based intervention to ameliorate freezing of gait in subjects with Parkinson's disease. *J Neurol.* (2014) 261:1329–39. doi: 10.1007/s00415-014-7347-2

4. Barthel C, Nonnekes J, van Helvert M, Haan R, Janssen A, Delval A, et al. The laser shoes: a new ambulatory device to alleviate freezing of gait in Parkinson disease. *Neurology* (2018) 90:e164–71. doi: 10.1212/WNL.0000000000004795

5. Schlenstedt C, Muthuraman M, Witt K, Weisser B, Fasano A, Deuschl G. Postural control and freezing of gait in Parkinson's disease. *Parkinsonism Relat Disord.* (2016) 24:107–12. doi: 10.1016/j.parkreldis.2015.12.011

6. Bekkers EMJ, Dijkstra BW, Dockx K, Heremans E, Verschueren SMP, Nieuwboer A. Clinical balance scales indicate worse postural control in people with Parkinson's disease who exhibit freezing of gait compared to those who do not: a meta-analysis. *Gait Posture* (2017) 56:134–40. doi: 10.1016/j.gaitpost.2017.05.009

7. Schlenstedt C, Mancini M, Nutt J, Hiller AP, Maetzler W, Deuschl G, et al. Are hypometric anticipatory postural adjustments contributing to freezing of gait in Parkinson's disease? *Front Aging Neurosci.* (2018) 10:36. doi: 10.3389/fnagi.2018.00036

8. Plotnik M, Giladi N, Hausdorff JM. Is freezing of gait in Parkinson's disease a result of multiple gait impairments? Implications for treatment. *Parkinsons Dis.* (2012) 2012:459321. doi: 10.1155/2012/459321

9. Schlenstedt C, Paschen S, Kruse A, Raethjen J, Weisser B, Deuschl G. Resistance versus balance training to improve postural control in Parkinson's disease: a randomized rater blinded controlled study. *PLoS ONE* (2015) 10:e0140584. doi: 10.1371/journal.pone.0140584

10. Giladi N, Tal J, Azulay T, Rascol O, Brooks DJ, Melamed E, et al. Validation of the freezing of gait questionnaire in patients with Parkinson's disease. *Mov Disord.* (2009) 24:655–61. doi: 10.1002/mds.21745

11. Schlenstedt C, Brombacher S, Hartwigsen G, Weisser B, Moller B, Deuschl G. Comparing the fullerton advanced balance scale with the mini-BESTest and Berg Balance Scale to assess postural control in patients with Parkinson disease. *Arch Phys Med Rehabil.* (2015) 96:218–25. doi: 10.1016/j.apmr.2014.09.002

12. Ziegler K, Schroeteler F, Ceballos-Baumann AO, Fietzek UM. A new rating instrument to assess festination and freezing gait in Parkinsonian patients. *Mov Disord.* (2010) 25:1012–8. doi: 10.1002/mds.22993

13. Rose DJ, Lucchese N, Wiersma LD. Development of a multidimensional balance scale for use with functionally independent older adults. *Arch Phys Med Rehabil.* (2006) 87:1478–85. doi: 10.1016/j.apmr.2006.07.263

14. Cohen J. A power primer. *Psychol Bull.* (1992) 112:155–9.

15. Development Core Team. *R: A Language and Environment for Statistical Computing.* Vienna: R Foundation for Statistical Computing (2005).

16. Clarke CE, Patel S, Ives N, Rick CE, Woolley R, Wheatley K, et al. Clinical effectiveness and cost-effectiveness of physiotherapy and occupational therapy versus no therapy in mild to moderate Parkinson's disease: a large pragmatic randomised controlled trial (PD REHAB). *Health Technol Assess.* (2016) 20:1–96. doi: 10.3310/hta 20630

12

HMGB1: A Common Biomarker and Potential Target for TBI, Neuroinflammation, Epilepsy and Cognitive Dysfunction

Yam Nath Paudel[1], Mohd. Farooq Shaikh[1]*, Ayanabha Chakraborti[2], Yatinesh Kumari[1], Ángel Aledo-Serrano[3], Katina Aleksovska[4], Marina Koutsodontis Machado Alvim[5] and Iekhsan Othman[1]

[1] *Neuropharmacology Research Laboratory, Jeffrey Cheah School of Medicine and Health Sciences, Monash University Malaysia, Bandar Sunway, Malaysia,* [2] *Department of Surgery, University of Alabama at Birmingham, Birmingham, AL, United States,* [3] *Department of Neurology, Epilepsy Program, Hospital Ruber Internacional, Madrid, Spain,* [4] *Medical Faculty, Department of Neurology, "Saints Cyril and Methodius" University, Skopje, Macedonia,* [5] *Department of Neurology, Neuroimaging Laboratory, State University of Campinas, Campinas, Brazil*

*Correspondence:
Mohd. Farooq Shaikh
farooq.shaikh@monash.edu

High mobility group box protein 1 (HMGB1) is a ubiquitous nuclear protein released by glia and neurons upon inflammasome activation and activates receptor for advanced glycation end products (RAGE) and toll-like receptor (TLR) 4 on the target cells. HMGB1/TLR4 axis is a key initiator of neuroinflammation. In recent days, more attention has been paid to HMGB1 due to its contribution in traumatic brain injury (TBI), neuroinflammatory conditions, epileptogenesis, and cognitive impairments and has emerged as a novel target for those conditions. Nevertheless, HMGB1 has not been portrayed as a common prognostic biomarker for these HMGB1 mediated pathologies. The current review discusses the contribution of HMGB1/TLR4/RAGE signaling in several brain injury, neuroinflammation mediated disorders, epileptogenesis and cognitive dysfunctions and in the light of available evidence, argued the possibilities of HMGB1 as a common viable biomarker of the above mentioned neurological dysfunctions. Furthermore, the review also addresses the result of preclinical studies focused on HMGB1 targeted therapy by the HMGB1 antagonist in several ranges of HMGB1 mediated conditions and noted an encouraging result. These findings suggest HMGB1 as a potential candidate to be a common biomarker of TBI, neuroinflammation, epileptogenesis, and cognitive dysfunctions which can be used for early prediction and progression of those neurological diseases. Future study should explore toward the translational implication of HMGB1 which can open the windows of opportunities for the development of innovative therapeutics that could prevent several associated HMGB1 mediated pathologies discussed herein.

Keywords: HMGB1, RAGE, TLR4, TBI, epilepsy, neuroinflammation, cognitive dysfunction

HIGHLIGHTS

- The nuclear protein HMGB1 is a mediator for neurological conditions such as TBI, neuroinflammation, epilepsy and cognitive dysfunction.
- HMGB1 could be a common functional biomarker of TBI, neuroinflammation, epileptogenesis and cognitive dysfunction.
- Inhibiting the HMGB1/RAGE/TLR4 signaling axis could be a novel therapeutic strategy against several HMGB1 mediated conditions like TBI, neuroinflammation, epilepsy and cognitive dysfunction.

INTRODUCTION

Epilepsy is a serious neurological condition characterized by spontaneous and recurrent seizures (Liu et al., 2018) affecting people of all ages. Current anti-epileptic drugs (AEDs) only provides symptomatic relief rather than interfering with the disease mechanism, as well as one third of the patients are resistant to AEDs (Ravizza et al., 2017; Walker et al., 2017). Moreover, epilepsy imposes a burden by impacting several aspects of patients and family life. In addition, the burden is intensified due to the ranges of associated comorbidities such as cognitive dysfunctions, anxiety and depression. Hence, the development of novel biomarker which can predict and assess the disease condition as well as patient's outcome of the therapy against epilepsy is an unmet clinical need. As well as there is a pressing need of exploring new therapy against epilepsy which not only retard the seizure precipitation but also minimizes the associated comorbidities. In this regard, HMGB1 has emerged as a novel frontier and mounting number of preclinical studies targeting HMGB1 have been successful in diverse ranges of neurological conditions provoked by inflammatory responses (Wang et al., 2017; Zhao et al., 2017; Andersson et al., 2018).

High mobility group box 1 proteins are a family of DAMPs (Lotze and Tracey, 2005), which are highly conserved non-histone nuclear proteins and contributes to the architecture of chromatin DNA (Baxevanis and Landsman, 1995). HMGB1 acts as an inflammatory cytokine in response to epileptogenic insults (Kaneko et al., 2017). HMGB1 acts as a pathogenic

Abbreviations: AD, Alzheimer's disease; APOE-ε4, Apo lipoprotein E-ε4; BBB, blood–brain barrier; BDNF, brain derived neurotropic factor; BLA, basolateral amygdala; COX-2, cyclooxygenase-2; CREB, CAMP response element binding; CXCR4, chemokine receptor type 4; DAMPs, damage-associated molecular patterns; DNA, deoxyribonucleic acid; EEG, electroencephalogram; GABA, gamma amino butyric acid; GEPRS, genetically epilepsy prone rats; GLUR2, glutamate receptor 2; GRIA2, glutamate receptor ionotropic AMPA 2; HMGB1, high mobility group box 1; IHC, immunohistochemistry; KA, kainic acid; KIR4.1, inwardly rectifying potassium channel 4.1; LTP, long-term potentiation; MiR-129-5p, micro RNA-129-5p; MS, multiple sclerosis; MWM, Morris water maze; NORT, novel object recognition test; PAMPs, pathogen-associated molecular patterns; PD, Parkinson's disease; POCD, post-operative cognitive dysfunction; PRNCs, primary rats neural cells; PRR, pattern recognition receptor; PTZ, pentylenetetrazol; RAGE, receptor for advanced glycation end Products; RAS, retrovirus-associated DNA sequences; ROS, reactive oxygen species; SE, status epilepticus; TBI, traumatic brain injury; TEM, transmission electron microscopy; TGF-β, transforming growth factor-β; TLE, temporal lobe epilepsy; TLR4, toll-like receptor 4; TNF-α, tumor necrosis factor-α.

inflammatory response to mediate ranges of conditions such as epilepsy (Maroso et al., 2010), septic shock (Wang et al., 1999), ischemia (Kim et al., 2006; Wang et al., 2015), TBI (Okuma et al., 2012), PD (Sasaki et al., 2016), AD (Fujita et al., 2016), and MS (Andersson et al., 2008). Structural evaluation of HMGB1 suggests that it exhibits two domains for DNA-binding, known as box A and box B, as well as C-terminal acidic tail comprised of repeating glutamic and aspartic acid residues (Venereau et al., 2016; Aucott et al., 2018b). DAMPs can influence synaptic function in the brain regions such as the hippocampus, which is involved in hyperexcitability and cognitive decline in epilepsy (Ravizza et al., 2017). It has been reported that immediately after neuronal injury, there is a passive release of significant amounts of HMGB1 from the nucleus into the extracellular space (Scaffidi et al., 2002).

High mobility group box 1 has several extracellular receptors such as RAGE, TLR9, TLR4, TLR2, integrin, a-synuclein filaments, proteoglycans, T-cell immunoglobulin and mucin domain (TIM-3), triggering receptor expressed on myeloid cells-1 (TREM1), cluster of differentiation 24 (CD24), C-X-C CXCR4, N-methyl-D-aspartate receptor (NMDAR) (Kang et al., 2014). Among these receptors, RAGE and TLR4 are the only receptors that are extensively studied and reported without doubt (Andersson et al., 2018). HMGB1 initiates several cell responses including inflammation as well as mediate the activation of inflammatory process via binding with RAGE and TLR4 (Bianchi and Manfredi, 2007; Iori et al., 2013). During neuroinflammatory conditions, HMGB1 is actively released by neurons and glia cells upon inflammasome activation and in turn activates at least two PRRs, namely TLR4 and RAGE on target cells (Ravizza et al., 2017). Once released extracellularly, HMGB1 binds to the TLR4 and RAGE expressed by immune cells which leads to nuclear factor kappa-light-chain-enhancer of activated B cells (NF-κB) mediated production of pro-inflammatory cytokines (Iori, 2017). Role of HMGB1 in the development and disease of central nervous system (CNS) has been well described (Fang et al., 2012) where contribution of HMGB1 to the neurogenesis in the early phase of brain development, in neurite extension as well as its dual role in neural development and neurodegeneration is well discussed. HMGB1 promoted neuronal differentiation of adult hippocampal neural progenitors via activation of RAGE/NF-κB suggesting the role of HMGB1 in maintaining and sustaining hippocampal neurogenesis (Meneghini et al., 2013).

A previous study reported HMGB1 translocation as the main culprit for TBI (Li Y. et al., 2017). Recently, HMGB1 has received greater attention for its role in epilepsy (Zhao et al., 2017). It has been hypothesized that HMGB1 might be involved in epileptogenesis, especially through BBB disruption and induction of inflammatory processes though the precise mechanism remains still elusive. Several studies were previously conducted to determine the involvement of HMGB1 in the pathogenesis of epilepsy (Fu et al., 2017). HMGB1 plays a pivotal role in cognitive decline where HMGB1 is supposed to caused disruption of the BBB leading to cognitive deficits in aged rats (He et al., 2012). Interestingly, accumulating evidence suggests that neuroinflammation is highly associated with epilepsy and cognitive dysfunction after TBI and HMGB1 exhibits a key role as an initiator and amplifier of neuroinflammation as well as in neuronal excitation (Frank et al., 2015). Annegers and Coan (2000) suggested that there is a high risk of epilepsy after TBI and epilepsy is associated with neurological comorbidities such as cognitive dysfunction (Pascente et al., 2016; Ravizza et al., 2017).

Treatments based on HMGB1 antagonists via targeting extracellular HMGB1 have generated encouraging results in a wide number of experimental models though the clinical studies are yet to be reported. Anti-HMGB1 monoclonal antibodies (mAbs) have demonstrated beneficial effects on epilepsy and TBI. The therapeutic benefits of anti-HMGB1 mAb on epilepsy have been previously demonstrated in animal model of epilepsy (Fu et al., 2017). Potential neuroprotective effects of HMGB1 has been reported in few studies where anti-HMGB1 mAb prevented intracerebral hemorrhage (ICH)-induced brain injury (Wang et al., 2017).

Interestingly, HMGB1 has been associated with all of the neurological conditions previously outlined (**Figure 1**). Neuroinflammation is the mediator of damage in TBI, epileptogenesis and cognitive decline are the post-TBI events. This makes worth further exploring the HMGB1 and the rationale behind the current review is to explore the potential of HMGB1 as a common biomarker and potential target for several neurological phenotypes discussed in this review. In spite of its proven role in TBI, neuroinflammation, epilepsy and cognitive

decline there has been little interest in exploring HMGB1 as a common target and biomarker for those conditions. The preclinical and clinical evidences discussed herein strengthens HMGB1 to stand as a promising candidate to be the common biomarker and treatment target for the neurological conditions where neuroinflammatory pathway plays a central role. Hence, this review summarizes recent advances and discuss these emerging findings to explore the potential of HMGB1 as a common biomarkers and treatment target which could pave the way in developing therapies with broad application modifying the disease progression.

NEUROINFLAMMATION AS A PRIME DRIVER OF TBI, EPILEPSY AND COGNITIVE DECLINE?

Neuroinflammation is the key component of neuropathology after TBI and contributes to the chronic neurodegeneration and neurological impairments associated with TBI (Kumar and Loane, 2012). This is supported by gene profiling studies which show that genes related to neuroinflammation are upregulated after brain injury (Kobori et al., 2002) and elevated levels of the inflammatory cytokines TNF-α, TGF-β, and IL-1β are expressed after TBI (Morganti-Kossmann et al., 2002; DeKosky et al.,

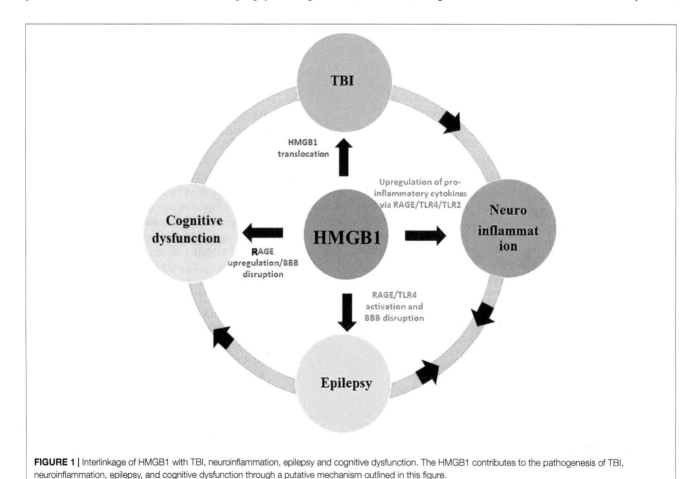

FIGURE 1 | Interlinkage of HMGB1 with TBI, neuroinflammation, epilepsy and cognitive dysfunction. The HMGB1 contributes to the pathogenesis of TBI, neuroinflammation, epilepsy, and cognitive dysfunction through a putative mechanism outlined in this figure.

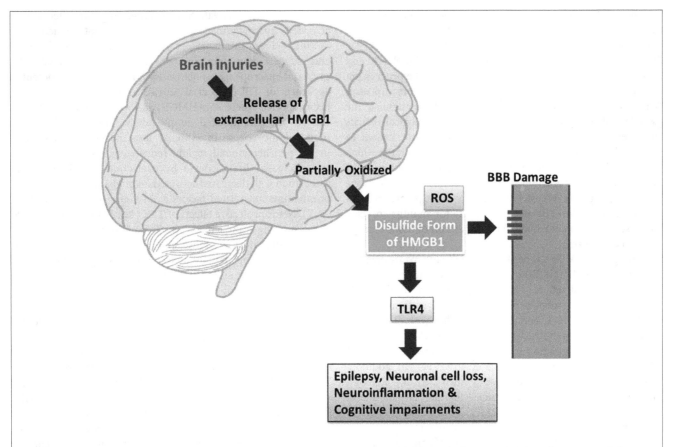

FIGURE 2 | Mechanism of HMGB1 release via brain injury. HMGB1 translocation results from brain injuries and epileptogenesis. Dying cells, neurons and glia are responsible for the release of extracellular HMGB1 which can be partially oxidized. Neuronal excitability is enhanced via the mediation of pro-inflammatory activities through the activation of TLR4 signaling by disulphide HMGB1. The stabilization of HMGB1 in its disulphide form is promoted by the generation of ROS. HMGB1 via activating receptors RAGE and TLR4 leads to neuronal cell loss, neuroinflammation, epilepsy, and cognitive dysfunction (Ravizza et al., 2017).

2013). Several experimental and clinical evidences support the role of inflammatory mediators as the origin of both seizures and epileptogenesis (Vezzani and Granata, 2005; Shimada et al., 2014). Brain inflammation contributes to the generation of individual seizures as well as cell death, which in turn contributes to the development of seizures via activation of inflammatory pathways (Vezzani et al., 2011). Moreover, there is evidence which highlights that inflammation can be a cause as well as consequences of epilepsy (Vezzani et al., 2011).

Traumatic brain injury incites a neuroinflammatory axis in the brain which perpetuates neurodegeneration and increases the chances of initiating epileptogenesis (Webster et al., 2017) However, the probability of developing epilepsy after TBI varies from 4.4% to 53% (Frey, 2003) and becomes more likely with a higher injury severity and a younger age at injury (Barlow et al., 2000). Neuroinflammation is a contributing factor to the pathophysiology of post-TBI epileptogenesis (Riazi et al., 2010). Neuroinflammation can alter the BBB permeability directly via cytokine aided activation of metalloproteinase or via disruption of tight junctions (Gloor et al., 2001; Utech et al., 2009), though the precise mechanism remains elusive. It is worthwhile to note that although neuroinflammation is typically provoked after a series of epileptogenic brain injuries, the proportion of patients

developing the disease is small (Vezzani, 2015). The pivotal role of neuroinflammation in cognitive dysfunction has been reported but the underlying molecular mechanism are not yet known. However, there are insights regarding certain inflammatory pathways underlying hyperexcitability and excitotoxicity that can promote cognitive decline (Vezzani, 2015).

In recent days, research using experimental and clinical models has focused on the pathogenesis of how HMGB1 proteins contributes to TBI, neuroinflammation, epilepsy and cognitive decline. Such research has sought to pave the way to understand how these mechanisms can be interfered to develop therapies for the aforementioned neurological conditions. Moreover, accumulating evidence reported beneficial effects on evaluating anti-HMGB1 mAb and HMGB1 inhibitors against TBI, neuroinflammation, epilepsy, and cognitive decline. We will therefore discuss the outcomes of such experimental and clinical experiments in an individual pattern.

ROLE OF HMGB1 IN TBI

TBI is an insult to the brain through any external mechanical force (Webster et al., 2017), which makes TBI a devastating and intractable cause of worldwide morbidity and mortality. Survivors live the rest of their lives with cognitive, motor, behavioral or speech and language disabilities (Richard et al., 2017). However, the pathophysiology of TBI is still elusive and a tremendous research must be made to explore the progression of neurodegeneration and the ensuing inflammatory processes (Parker et al., 2017). It is currently unavailable to attenuate the pathological process of TBI and improve neurological deficits (Jiang et al., 2018). TBI involves a primary insult known as structural damage due to any external mechanical force which is followed by a secondary injury including a multitude of neuroinflammatory phenomena such as excitotoxicity, oxidative stress and apoptosis (Webster et al., 2017). These processes begin within minute after TBI and can persist for months to years and is suspected to contribute to the expansion of tissue damage (Hinson et al., 2015).

During TBI, HMGB1 is released via the N-methyl D-aspartate receptor subtype 2B (NR2B)-mediated mechanism from necrotic neurons (Richard et al., 2017). HMGB1 mediates sterile inflammation and provokes macrophages and endothelial cells to release TNF-α, IL-1, and IL-6 by binding with RAGE and TLR4. This binding further activates the NF-κB pathway and facilitates the upregulation of HMGB1 and the expression of pro-inflammatory mediators (Gao et al., 2012). In addition, neuroinflammatory processes mainly mediated by activated microglia and astrocytes are crucial for the initiation and progression of TBI (Li D. et al., 2017). TBI induces a series of events including BBB breakdown, brain edema, upregulation of tight junction proteins (TJPs), expression of inflammation related molecules (Yang et al., 2018). TLR4 has been linked with TBI where TLR4 mediates glial phagocytic activity and inflammatory cytokines production (Jiang et al., 2018) and plays an important role in inflammatory response and brain injury (Fang et al., 2013). Once HMGB1 is released into the extracellular settings following TBI, it binds to transmembrane major mediators of the inflammatory response, TLR2, TLR4, and RAGE (Yang et al., 2005). Excessive inflammation resulting from activation of the HMGB1/TLR4 pathway in the brain has been implicated in TBI and ischemia-reperfusion injury (Yang et al., 2011). However, the mechanistic interlinkage between intracellular danger signaling, which involves the nuclear chromatin-binding factor, HMGB1 and inflammatory pathways after TBI is not yet fully understood (Parker et al., 2017). There is an increased understanding that TBI may induce activation of HMGB1/TLR4/RAGE/NF-κB signaling pathway and inflammatory cytokine expression, which would induce and/or aggravate the secondary brain injury where HMGB1 is supposed to implicate a critical role in promoting inflammation and aggravating damage after TBI (Xiangjin et al., 2014) (Figure 2). Several HMGB1 inhibitors have demonstrated protective effect against TBI via inhibiting HMGB1/TLR4/NF-κB pathway activation (Su et al., 2011), and by reducing HMGB1/RAGE interaction (Okuma et al., 2014).

Inhibition of HMGB1 expression and the TLR4/NF-κB pathways exhibits protective effects in animal model of TBI. HMGB1 inhibitors (glycyrrhizic acid) attenuated TBI by inhibiting the classically activated microglia/macrophages

(M1) phenotype activation and promoting the alternatively activated microglia/macrophages (M2) phenotype activation of microglia/macrophages, via the inhibition of HMGB1 and suggest that targeting of HMGB1 to modulate the microglia/macrophage polarization might be a potential approach for TBI (Gao et al., 2018). Similar line of results has been reported where anti-HMGB1 mAb improved neurological deficits in ICH-induced brain injury. Anti-HMGB1 mAb inhibited the release of HMGB1 into the extracellular space in the peri-hematomal region, reduced serum HMGB1 levels and decreased brain edema by protecting BBB integrity, in association with decreased activated microglia and the expression of inflammation-related factors at 24 h after ICH (Wang et al., 2017). Neuroprotective effects of TLR4 knockdown has emerged as a promising approach for TBI. TLR4 knockdown ameliorated neuroinflammatory response and brain injury after TBI and suppressing autophagy induction and astrocyte activation is postulated the main mechanism behind the neuroprotective effects of TLR4 (Jiang et al., 2018). Data obtained from western blot analysis in an experimental study reported the release profile of HMGB1 and RAGE after TBI where HMGB1 was released as soon as 30 min after TBI and a decline in its expression was noted between 1 and 6 h after TBI. However, the expression level of RGAE was elevated at 6 h after TBI and reached its peak after 1 day (Table 1) (Gao et al., 2012). An immunostaining study reported that septic brain injury results in increased HMGB1 cytoplasmic translocation in neurons (Table 1) (Li Y. et al., 2017). A few studies have reported a noteworthy elevation of HMGB1, IL-1β, and TNF-α levels in serum as estimated by an enzyme linked immunosorbent assay (ELISA) kit in an experimentally induced TBI model in rabbits (Mohamed et al., 2017). However, ELISA analysis does not precisely differentiate between release pattern of HMGB1 either by necrosis, or from macrophages and monocytes, or a combination of both (Au et al., 2012).

High mobility group box 1 A-box fragment, an antagonist competing with HMGB1 for receptor binding, significantly ameliorated the BBB breakdown and brain edema induced by controlled cortical impact (CCI), and these effects were associated with the decrease in expressions of inflammation-related factors as well as improved neurological functions (Yang et al., 2018). Ethyl pyruvate (Table 1) (Su et al., 2011) and omega-3 polyunsaturated fatty acid supplementation (Chen et al., 2017b) has demonstrated its effectiveness against TBI via inhibition of the HMGB1/TLR4/NF-κB pathway. Evaluation of anti-HMGB1 mAb therapy against TBI in rats reported that anti-HMGB1 mAb remarkably inhibited fluid percussion-induced brain edema in rats, which was associated with an inhibition of HMGB1 translocation, protection of BBB architecture, downregulation of inflammatory molecule expression, and improvement in motor function (Table 1) (Okuma et al., 2012). Increased inhibition of the expression of HMGB1 signaling axis, with RAGE and TLR4, NF-κB DNA binding and downstream inflammatory cytokines were reported on glycyrrhizin treatment (Okuma et al., 2014).

The literature review ranging from human to animal studies suggests an important association between TBI and increased levels of HMGB1 in serum and cerebrospinal fluid (CSF) (Okuma et al., 2014). In addition, emerging data reported HMGB1

TABLE 1 | Summary of findings reporting HMGB1 in TBI.

S.N.	Intervention	Model	Mechanism	Observations	Reference
1.	HMGB1	Rat	• Inhibition of HMGB1 expression and TLR4/NF-κB pathway	• ↓ Reduced expression of HMGB1 and TLR4 • Improved motor function and lessened brain oedema	Su et al., 2011
2	Anti-HMGB1 mAb	Rat	• Protection against BBB disruption • Inhibition of the inflammatory responses	• Inhibition of translocation of HMGB1, protection of BBB permeability • Downregulation of inflammatory molecule expression • Improvement of motor function	Okuma et al., 2012
3	HMGB1	Rat	• Interference with HMGB1 and RAGE interaction • Inhibition of the expressions of TNF-a, IL-1β, and IL-6	• Inhibited the ↑ in BBB permeability and impairment in motor functions • Inhibition of translocation of HMGB1 in neurons at the site of injury	Okuma et al., 2014
4	Anti-HMGB1 mAb	Rat	• Protecting BBB integrity • ↓ Expression of inflammation-related factors	• ↓ Release of HMGB1 to the extracellular space in the peri-hematomal region • ↓ Serum HMGB1 levels and brain edema through maintaining BBB integrity	Wang et al., 2017
5	HMGB1	Rat	• Downregulation of sepsis-induced RAGE and NF-κBp65 expression	• HMGB1 was ↑ in the cytoplasm via translocation • RAGE and NF-κβ p 65 were up regulated after brain injury • HMGB1 and its signaling transduction have a key role in the pathogenesis of septic brain injury	Li Y. et al., 2017
6	HMGB1	Human	• Targeting HMGB1/RAGE signaling	• HMGB1 disappeared or translocated from the nucleus to the cytoplasm at early stages after TBI • RAGE expression ↑ after TBI	Gao et al., 2012
7	HMGB1	Human	• Activation of microglial TLR4 and the subsequent expression of AQP4	• Peak CSF HMGB1 level in human TBI was within 0–72 h. • HMGB1 released from necrotic neurons through a NR2B-mediated mechanism	Laird et al., 2014

S.N., serial number; ↑, increased; ↓, decreased; HMGB1, high mobility group box 1; TRL4, Toll like receptor 4; RAGE, receptor for advanced glycation end products; NF-κB p 65, nuclear factor kappa-light-chain-enhancer of activated β cells p 65; IL-6, interleukin-6; IL-1β, interleukin-1β; TNF-α, tumor necrosis factor-α; BBB, blood–brain barrier; TBI, traumatic brain injury; CSF, cerebrospinal fluid; MRI, magnetic resonance imaging; ICP, intra-cranial pressure; NR2B, N-methyl D-aspartate receptor subtype 2B; AQP4, astrocytic water channel aquaporin-4.

in the CSF of subarachnoid hemorrhage (SAH) (Nakahara et al., 2009) and in the serum of ICH (Zhou et al., 2010) highlighting as a potential biomarker of neurological outcome. Nevertheless, the clinical output of HMGB1 antagonist against several forms of brain injury is yet to be reported. Similar line of evidence were observed in which HMGB1 is associated with increased levels of intracranial pressure (ICP) in patients and promoted cerebral edema after TBI where the detrimental effects of HMGB1 are mediated through the microglial TLR4 activation and the expression of the astrocytic water channel aquaporin-4 (AQP4) (Richard et al., 2017). HMGB1 plasma levels were reported to increase within 30 min after severe trauma in humans and suggested a correlation between plasma levels

of HMGB1 with early post-traumatic coagulopathy and severe systemic inflammatory response (Cohen et al., 2009). There was a 30-fold increment of plasma HMGB1 levels after trauma, as compared to normal controls during a 1-h period of injury which provides insights regarding the post-injury elevation levels of HMGB1 in human (Peltz et al., 2009) However, the study did not report any correlation between HMGB1 levels and the patients' outcome. Furthermore, a compelling relationship between plasma HMGB1 absorption and the severity of acute TBI was unraveled and correlation between Glasgow Coma Scale score and HMGB1 levels were reported, which can serve as prognostic information in patients with severe TBI (Wang et al., 2012). Higher CSF HMGB1s level are considered as an important biomarker to predict outcome after pediatric TBI (Au et al., 2012).

The pathophysiology behind the complex inflammation cascades secondary to TBI is not yet fully understood. However, resulting injuries and outcomes after TBI have been studied in the past and have suggested HMGB1 to be a major player in disease progression as well as a potential therapeutic target to reduce the injuries and improve outcome following TBI. As well as the current biomarkers of TBI such as glial fibrillary acidic protein (GFAP) and S100B (Vos et al., 2010) are limited by low sensitivity, predictivity, and specificity (Metting et al., 2012). In this regard, due to its profound role in TBI pathology and inflammatory pathways post-TBI, HMGB1 appears to be a promising candidate which can be used as a prognostic marker of TBI. Moreover, downregulating HMGB1/RAGE/TLR4/NF-κB axis might be a novel strategy against TBI which could attenuate the neurological functions as well.

ROLE OF HMGB1 IN NEUROINFLAMMATION AND RELATED PATHOLOGIES

Neuroinflammation is considered as an innate immune responses in the CNS, which is triggered in response to several inflammatory signals such as pathogen infection, injury or trauma, which might ultimately result in neurotoxicity (Streit et al., 2004). Microglia are known as the predominant innate immune cell in the CNS and are thus considered a pivotal mediator of neuroinflammatory processes (Gehrmann et al., 1995). Microglia express TLRs, in particular TLR4 (Ransohoff and Perry, 2009), and are reported to mediate the pro-inflammatory effects of HMGB1 in peripheral innate immune cells (Yang et al., 2010). Disulphide form of HMGB1 (ds-HMGB1) potentiates the microglia pro-inflammatory response to an immune challenge suggesting that acute increases or exposure to ds-HMGB1, as may occur during acute stress or trauma, might induce a primed immune phenotype in the CNS, which may lead to an exacerbated neuroinflammatory response if exposure to a subsequent pro-inflammatory stimulus occurs (Frank et al., 2016). There is an increased understanding that HMGB1 mediates inflammatory and immune reactions in CNS and emerging evidence reveals that HMGB1 plays an essential role in neuroinflammation through receptors such as TLR, RAGE, and NMDAR (Wan et al., 2016). Moreover, HMGB1 induces RAGE and TLR4 mediated neuroinflammation and necrosis after injuries such as lesions in the spinal cord and brain (Fang et al., 2012). HMGB1 mediates inflammation by activating the innate immune receptors during sterile injury, in a similar manner to activation by PAMPs (Yang and Tracey, 2010). The BBB is a special microvessel structure in the CNS, consisting of microvascular endothelial cells sealed by tight junctions. Its permeability is closely related with degeneration, injury and inflammation of the CNS (Huang et al., 2011). Similar line of study shows that damaged BBB correlates directly with neuroinflammation involving microglial activation and reactive astrogliosis, which is associated with increased expression and/or release of HMGB1 (Festoff et al., 2016). In an experiment evaluating the contribution of extracellular, cerebral HMGB1 (in absence of other DAMPs) in its disulphide or fully redox form to neuroinflammation demonstrate that ds-HMGB1 and fully redox HMGB1 (fr-HMGB1) function as pro-inflammatory mediators in the CNS, promoting BBB disruption and cytokine production (Aucott et al., 2018a). Thus, anti-neuroinflammation and maintenance of BBB integrity may be potential targets for neuroprotection (Cheng et al., 2018). Increasing evidence suggests that selective targeting of CNS inflammation is a viable strategy for interfering disease onset or progression for a number of neurodegenerative disorders where neuroinflammation is the key player (Hong et al., 2016). Despite the deteriorating role of neuroinflammation in many neurological diseases, the number of existing anti-inflammatory drugs is quite limited because of insufficient efficacy or undesired side effect (Craft et al., 2005). HMGB1 has emerged has a novel frontiers due to its plausible role in neuroinflammation (Lee et al., 2014) as well as in inflammatory diseases (Harris et al., 2012) where the causal role for HMGB1 in a range of non-degenerative neuroinflammatory conditions has been well reported. Moreover, HMGB1 blocking therapies have proven to be highly beneficial, demonstrating remarkable neuroprotection in several neuroinflammation models (Kim et al., 2006).

Inflachromene (ICM), a microglial inhibitor possessing anti-inflammatory effects via binding with HMGB1 blocks the sequential processes of cytoplasmic localization and extracellular release of HMGBs by perturbing its post-translational modification as well as downregulates pro-inflammatory functions of HMGB and reduces neuronal damage *in vivo* demonstrating its potential against neuroinflammatory diseases (Lee et al., 2014). HMGB1 binds with lipopolysaccharides (LPS) and IL-1 to initiate and synergize TLR4-mediated pro-inflammatory response and immediately after pro-inflammatory stimulation by LPS, TNF-α, IL-1, IL-6, and IL-8, HMGB1 is released from activated monocytes and macrophages (Youn et al., 2008). The regulation of HMGB1 secretion is crucial for the regulation of HMGB1 mediated inflammation and is dependent on various processes such as phosphorylation by calcium-dependent protein kinase C (Oh et al., 2009). HMGB1 acts as a novel pro-inflammatory cytokine-like factor and regulates excitotoxicity-induced acute damage processes and delayed inflammatory mechanisms in the post-ischemic brain of Sprague Dawley (SD) rats (**Table 2**) (Kim et al., 2006). Elevation of HMGB1 in brain was measured in several non-degenerative neuroinflammatory condition such as ethanol exposure (Zou and Crews, 2014), and stress-induced neuroinflammatory priming (Weber et al., 2015). Neuroinflammation contributes to the progression of several neurodegenerative diseases including PD (Tansey and Goldberg, 2010) and AD (Heneka et al., 2015). Blocking the neuroinflammatory pathways in these neurodegenerative diseases will exerts neuroprotection against these diseases. Anti-HMGB1 mAb has inhibited the activation of microglia, prevents BBB breakdown, and inhibit the expression of inflammation cytokines such as IL-1β and IL-6 in an experimental model of PD demonstrating its neuroprotective effects possibly via suppressing neuroinflammation (Sasaki et al.,

TABLE 2 | Summary of findings reporting HMGB1 in neuroinflammation mediated conditions.

S.N.	Intervention	Model	Mechanism	Observation	Reference
1.	HMGB1	Rat	• Delayed inflammatory processes by extracellular HMGB1	• HMGB1 was released during the excitotoxicity-induced acute damaging process • Extracellular HMGB1 provokes inflammatory processes and acts like a novel pro-inflammatory cytokine-like factor	Kim et al., 2006
2	HMGB1	Mice	• Activation of NF-κB and NADPH oxidase by HMGB1 via binding with Mac1	• HMGB1-Mac1-NADPH oxidase signaling cascades connects chronic neuroinflammation and dopaminergic neurodegeneration	Gao et al., 2011
3	HMGB1	Rat	• HMGB1 acted as an early pro-inflammatory cytokine	• HMGB1 released into the cytoplasm soon after ICH • Mediate inflammation during the acute phase of ICH	Lei et al., 2013
4	HMGB1	Rat	• Inflammatory responses produced via HMGB1/TLR4/NF-κB signaling	• HMGB1 ↓ the release of IL-6 and TNF-α • HMGB1 inhibited activation of NF-κB in the developing brain	Tian et al., 2015
5	HMGB1	Rat	• Regulation of age-related priming of the neuroinflammatory responses by HMGB1	• HMGB1was ↑ in aged rodent brains and CSF • Blocking HMGB1 "desensitized" microglia in the aged brain and prevent pathological infection-elicited neuroinflammatory responses	Fonken et al., 2016

S.N., serial number; ↑, increased; ↓, decreased; HMGB1, high mobility group box 1; ICH, intracerebral hemorrhage; Mac1, macrophage antigen complex 1; CSF, cerebrospinal fluid; TNF-α, tumor necrosis factor-α; NF-κB, nuclear factor kappa-light-chain-enhancer of activated B cells; TLR4, Toll like receptor 4; RAGE, receptor for advanced glycation end products; IL-6, interleukin-6; NADPH, nicotinamide adenine dinucleotide phosphate hydrogen.

2016). Glycyrrhizin attenuated neuroinflammation, cognitive deficits, microglial activation related over-expression of pro-inflammatory cytokines in the hippocampus induced by LPS showcasing its therapeutic potential against neurodegenerative diseases like AD (Song et al., 2013).

Multiple sclerosis is an autoimmune-mediated chronic, inflammatory, demyelinating disease of CNS characterized by axonal damage (Compston and Coles, 2008). Experimental autoimmune encephalomyelitis (EAE) is the most reliable experimental model of MS (Miller et al., 2010). HMGB1 is receiving increasing attention in autoimmune disorders including MS. The very first study unraveling the role of HMGB1 in the pathophysiology of MS reported increased numbers of macrophages with cytoplasmic HMGB1 in active lesions (Andersson et al., 2008) and suggest HMGB1 as a novel biomarker of inflammatory demyelinating disease. Several researches has emerged on the base of earlier studies and suggest that the expression and release of HMGB1 are remarkably elevated in several stages of EAE where HMGB1 expression pattern is dynamically changed during the progression of EAE, as well as validated HMGB1 as a key mediator of EAE pathology (Sun et al., 2015). Targeting HMGB1 locally might exhibits therapeutic potential against EAE which can attenuate the disease severity and incidence as well as delayed disease onset time

(Robinson et al., 2013). Neutralization of HMGB1 appears to be a novel strategy against MS as evidenced by an experimental study of MS, where anti-HMGB1 mAb ameliorated clinical severity, reduced CNS pathology, and blocked the production of pro-inflammatory cytokine (Uzawa et al., 2013).

Amyotrophic lateral sclerosis (ALS) is a non-demyelinating neurodegenerative disease characterized by increased neuronal loss and enhanced neuroinflammation, with extensive activation of glial cells and microglia stimulation releasing pro-inflammatory molecules, ROS, and nitric oxide (Ray et al., 2016). Neuroinflammation is postulated as a pathological hallmark of ALS (Lewis et al., 2012), and HMGB1 has been extensively studied in ALS due to its putative involvement in the pathology of ALS which is elusive yet. However, the elevated level of HMGB1 in the spinal cord of transgenic mice (SOD1G93A transgenic mice) were observed and reported that HMGB1 may have a role in the progressive inflammatory and neurodegenerative processes in response to the neurotoxic environment present in the spinal cord of SOD1G93A mice rather than to be involved as a primary event in the motor neuron death (Coco et al., 2007).

Withaferin A in an animal model of HMGB1-induced inflammatory responses suppressed the production of

IL-6, TNF-α and the activation NF-κB by HMGB1 (Lee et al., 2012). HMGB1 acts a pathogenic factor in many inflammatory conditions including experimental arthritis models (Schierbeck et al., 2011). HMGB1 has been observed to be a key mediator of intestinal inflammation in non-alcoholic fatty liver disease (NAFLD) via RAGE and redox signaling (Chandrashekaran et al., 2017). Another study reported that liver inflammation in diabetic mice was improved via regulation of the HMGB1/TLR4/NF-κB signaling pathway (Yin et al., 2018). Taken together, these results clearly highlight HMGB1 as a key mediator in several inflammatory diseases and suggest that HMGB1 exhibits therapeutic potential against these HMGB1 mediated inflammatory disease. Evaluating the ameliorative effects of glycyrrhizin on SAH in a rat model significantly improved neurological scores, reduced HMGB1-positive cells, downregulated mRNA and protein levels of HMGB1, inhibited BBB permeability, and attenuated neuronal cell death and apoptosis after SAH, suggesting it as a promising candidate for brain inflammation (Ieong et al., 2018).

The result obtained from human studies on MS patients corroborated with the experimental studies where HMGB1 and its receptors (RAGE, TLR2, and TLR4) were up-regulated in CSF of MS patients implicating that RAGE, TLR2, and TLR4 actively participate in an inflammatory, innate immune response driving and shaping the ensuing adaptive immune response during MS (Andersson et al., 2008). In clinical studies in patients with ALS, activation of TLR/RAGE signaling pathways were observed as evidenced by the elevated expression of HMGB1 and its receptors in reactive glia in human ALS spinal cord. The activation of these pathways might contribute to the progression of inflammation, resulting in motor neuron injury (Casula et al., 2011). In addition, serum HMGB1 auto antibody (Ab) has been suggested as a biomarker for the diagnosis of ALS and can be used to monitor disease progression (Hwang et al., 2013). High level of HMGB1, IL-6, and IL-17A has been detected in CSF of patients with an anti-NMDA receptor (NMDAR) encephalitis (neuroinflammatory disorder) (Ai et al., 2018), reflecting the underlying neuroinflammatory processes but does not report any precise role of HMGB1 in disease pathology. Clinical study performed on patients with AD and mild cognitive impairment (MCI) observed enhanced BBB permeability by HMGB1 and suggest HMGB1 as a clinical biomarker as well as validates HMGB1 as a non-invasive biomarker of BBB dysfunction and neuroinflammation which can assess the progression of neurodegeneration in AD and MCI patients (Festoff et al., 2016).

On the ground of evidences highlighted above, HMGB1 has been implicated in ranges of neuroinflammatory diseases as well as inflammation mediated disorders and HMGB1 exhibits huge potential to be a reliable biomarker for neuroinflammation related pathologies. On the positive note, beneficial effects of targeting HMGB1 in brain inflammation related pathologies is well documented. Extensive exploration to innovate therapeutic strategy to attenuate uncontrolled neuroinflammation triggered by HMGB1 is a pressing need.

ROLE OF HMGB1 IN EPILEPSY

Epileptogenesis is described as complex structural changes in the brain that convert a normal brain into a brain debilitated by recurrent seizure activity (Sloviter and Bumanglag, 2013). Neurodegeneration (Pitkanen and Lukasiuk, 2009; Reddy, 2013), disruption of BBB (Bar-Klein et al., 2017), the amygdala (Aroniadou-Anderjaska et al., 2008), the glutamatergic system (Aroniadou-Anderjaska et al., 2008), oxidative stress (Ashrafi et al., 2007), and epigenetic modification of DNA (Hauser et al., 1993) are all involved in epileptogenesis and aggravates the process (**Figure 3**).

Due to the lack of disease modifying effect in mainstream AEDs, precise understanding of diseases pathology and developing novel therapeutic approach for epilepsy-related hyperexcitability is a current need. Searching for molecular mediators of epileptogenesis in animal models, much attention has been paid to the potential pathogenic role of HMGB1 in the generation and recurrence of seizures (Kaneko et al., 2017; Yang et al., 2017). In spite of tremendous advancement in research, the pathogenesis of epilepsy is still complex, however, brain inflammation is supposed to play the role (Riazi et al., 2010). There is mounting evidence which report that neuroinflammatory processes in the pathophysiology of seizures/epilepsy and HMGB1 were found to behave like an inflammatory cytokine in response to epileptogenic insults (Kaneko et al., 2017). Glial cells activation has been reported to serve an important role in the development of epilepsy and HMGB1 may mediate microglial activation via the TLR4/NF-κB signaling pathway during seizures (Shi et al., 2018). HMGB1 activates IL-1R/TLR signaling in neurons and has a key role in seizure generation and recurrence via rapid sarcoma family kinases catalyzed phosphorylation of NMDA-NR2B receptors (Vezzani et al., 2012). As well as, HMGB1 serves a key role in epileptogenesis via microglial activation, via TLR4-NF-κB signaling pathway activation (Shi et al., 2018). An array of investigation has reported the role of HMGB1 in seizure but the precise mechanism on how HMGB1 leads to seizure generation is not documented well. HMGB1 released from glia and neurons and its signaling with TLR4 are suggested in generating and perpetuating seizures, the suggestion was based on the anti-convulsant activity of TLR4 inhibitors and Box A, a competitor of endogenous HMGB1 but the study lacks detailed mechanism how HMGB1/TLR4 axis leads to seizure generation (Maroso et al., 2010). Although HMGB1 activates both TLR4 and RAGE, the role of RAGE in seizures is less prominent than that of TLR4 (Iori et al., 2013).

Mesial temporal lobe epilepsy (MTLE) is a most common refractory focal epilepsy syndromes (Palleria et al., 2015) and role of HMGB1 in the pathogenesis of MTLE remains unknown. Experimental MTLE study reported significant upregulation of HMGB1 and TLR4 gene expression in the hippocampi of a rat and correlated this overexpression of HMGB1 and TLR4 to the pathogenesis of MTLE in immature rats (Yang et al., 2017). In addition, the role of HMGB1 and its receptors (RAGE and TLR4), including the pro-inflammatory cytokine IL-1β, in generating and perpetuating seizures is well documented

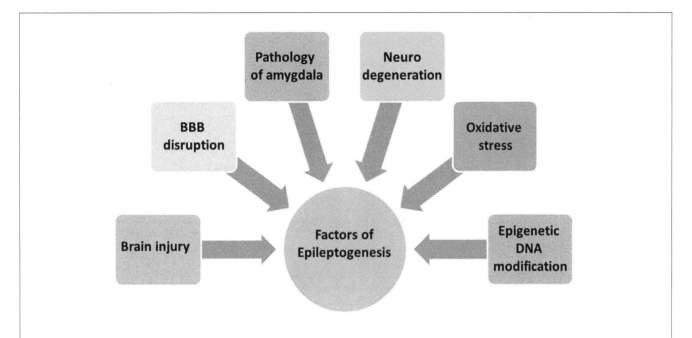

FIGURE 3 | Array of factors contributing to epileptogenesis. Much is unknown about the precise mechanism of epileptogenesis making it difficult to design and develop new therapies. But there is an increased understanding that brain injury, BBB disruption, neurodegeneration, oxidative stress, epigenetic DNA modification and pathology of amygdala contribute and aggravate the epileptogenesis.

(Zaben et al., 2017). Pharmacological and genetic studies on animal and clinical brain specimens showed that translocation and release of HMGB1 occurs in the pathological epileptogenic focus of different type of epilepsy (Maroso et al., 2010; Iori et al., 2013). It is worth noting that HMGB1/TLR4 axis not only reduced seizure frequency and duration, but also accelerated seizure onset, which usually occurs within minutes in kainite and bicuculline-induced seizure models implicating the important role of HMGB1 in the precipitation of the first seizure after a pro-convulsant administration (Maroso et al., 2010). Abnormal extracellular HMGB1 might contribute to the pathophysiology of epilepsy-related hyperexcitability as evidenced by study on PRNCs demonstrate a surge in extracellular HMGB1 approximated seizure initiation, establishing HMGB1 as a key pathophysiological contributor to the onset of epilepsy-related hyperexcitability (**Table 3**) (Kaneko et al., 2017).

TLR4 activation in neurons and astrocytes by HMGB1 proteins is a key mechanism of seizure generation and blocking TLR4 signaling using an antagonist could also reduce the severity of epilepsy (Iori et al., 2013). Investigation on post-surgery patients with intractable epilepsy revealed increased levels of HMGB1, TLR4, RAGE, NF-κB, p65 and inducible nitric oxide synthase (iNOS) in the brain of the epilepsy group as well as increased levels of IL-1, IL-6, TNF-α, TGF-β, and IL-10 in epilepsy patients (Shi et al., 2018).

Targeting HMGB1/TLR4/RAGE signaling for epilepsy has gained more attention in recent years. MicroRNA-129-5p inhibited the development of autoimmune encephalomyelitis (AE)-related epilepsy by HMGB1 expression and inhibiting the TLR4/NF-κB signaling pathway (Liu et al., 2017). HMGB1 and TLR4 antagonists slowed seizure precipitation, prevented

acute and chronic seizure recurrence in C57BL/6 mice as well as reported increased expression of HMGB1 and TLR4 in human epileptogenic tissue, which is similar to a mouse model of chronic seizures and suggest a role for the HMGB1-TLR4 axis in human epilepsy (Maroso et al., 2010). Thus, HMGB1/RAGE/TLR4 signaling might contribute toward the generation and perpetuation of seizures (**Figure 4**) in humans and can be successfully targeted to attain anti-convulsant effects in epilepsies which are resistant to drugs. The expression level of HMGB1 was significantly elevated in the hippocampus and cortex after 24-h in a KA-induced model of SE, which suggests that the HMGB1 protein has a key role in epilepsy (Walker et al., 2014). HMGB1 enhances hypothermia induced seizures and contributes to the pathogenesis of febrile seizure. However, the precise mechanism of HMGB1 in febrile seizures remains unclear (Ito et al., 2017).

Limited data is available regarding evaluation of therapeutic benefits of HMGB1 inhibitors in animal models of epilepsy. However, glycyrrhizin demonstrates neuroprotection against lithium/pilocarpine-induced SE in rats, as well as ameliorates pilocarpine-induced oxidative injury and inflammatory responses via suppressing IL-1β and TNF-α, (González-Reyes et al., 2016) but did not demonstrate anti-epileptic activity. Dynamic changes in HMGB1 expression in the hippocampus of the mouse brain was reported after KA administration and glycyrrhizin exerts neuroprotective but not anti-epileptic effects via suppressing both acute and delayed HMGB1 inductions in the hippocampal cornu ammonis (CA)1 and CA3 region as well as its accumulation in serum (Luo et al., 2014).

Anti-HMGB1 mAb demonstrated an anti-seizure effect as evident by the lack of a disruption on the physical EEG

TABLE 3 | Summary of findings reporting HMGB1 in epilepsy.

S.N.	Intervention	Model	Mechanism	Observations	Reference
1	HMGB1	KA-induced seizure in mice	• Targeting HMGB1/TLR4 axis	• ↑ Frequency of seizure and total duration • Seizure can be ↓ by TLR4 and HMGB1 antagonists	Maroso et al., 2010
2	Anti-HMGB1 mAb	Acute seizure (MES and PTZ); Chronic seizure by KA in mice	• Inhibition of HMGB1 translocation	• ↓ Seizure threshold; ↓ time in tonic–clonic seizures and ↓ death • Delayed onset of generalized seizures; ↓ seizure stage; ↓ incidence of tonic seizures	Zhao et al., 2017
3	Molecular isoforms of HMGB1	Electrically induced Se in rats	• Activation of HMGB1/TLR4 axis	• ↑ level of HMGB1 and its acetylated and disulphide isoforms in blood	Walker et al., 2017
4	HMGB1	Pilocarpine-induced SE in rats	• Regulation of P-gp expression via RAGE/NF-κB inflammatory signaling pathways	• ↓ The expression levels of MDR1A/B mRNA and P-gp protein	Xie et al., 2017
5	HMGB1	KA-induced epilepsy in rats	• Modulation of glutamate metabolism	• ↑ Extracellular HMGB1 suggesting contribution of HMGB1 in epilepsy related hyperexcitability • Translocation of HMGB1 from nucleus to cytosol after KA administration	Kaneko et al., 2017
6	HMGB1	Pilocarpine-induced epilepsy in rats	• Targeting HMGB1 via TLR4/NF-kB signaling pathway	• Inhibit the development of AE-related epilepsy • Suppression of HMGB1 expression • MiR-129-5p mediated TLR4/NF-kB signaling pathway ameliorated AE-related epilepsy	Liu et al., 2017
7	Anti-HMGB1 mAb	Pilocarpine-induced SE in mice	• Inhibition of HMGB1 release and inflammation	• Protection of BBB permeability; ↓ HMGB1 translocation • ↓ Latency and frequency of stage 5 seizures	Fu et al., 2017
8	Molecular isoforms of HMGB1	Human	• Evaluation of HMGB1 isoforms as mechanistic biomarkers of epileptogenesis in sera obtained from epileptic patients	• HMGB1 isoforms in the brain and blood were changed • Expression of disulphide HMGB1 in newly diagnosed epilepsy patients	Walker et al., 2017

S.N., serial number; ↑, increased; ↓, decreased; BBB, blood–brain barrier; Pgp, P-glycoprotein; MES, maximal electroshock seizures; KA, kainic acid; PTZ, pentylenetetrazol; HMGB1, high mobility group box 1; EEG, electroencephalogram; MDR1A/B, multidrug resistance protein 1A/B; RAGE, receptor for advanced glycation end products; NF-κB, nuclear factor kappa-light-chain-enhancer of activated B cells; miR-129-5p, micro RNA-129-5p; qRT-PCR, quantitative real-time polymerase chain reaction; AE, autoimmune encephalitis; mAb, monoclonal antibody; PRNCs, primary rats neural cells.

rhythm and basic physical functions as it prevents the translocation of HMGB1 from nuclei following a seizure. This anti-seizure effect was not observed in TLR4 knockout mice (**Table 3**) (Zhao et al., 2017). Moreover, anti-HMGB1 mAb also demonstrated a disease-modifying anti-epileptogenic effect on epileptogenesis after SE, as evidenced by a reduced seizure frequency and improved cognitive function (Zhao et al., 2017). The minimization of seizure frequency and duration can be achieved by inhibitors of HMGB1 which is supposed

to act via targeting the HMGB1/RAGE/TLR4 axis and retard seizure precipitation via inhibition of HMGB1 translocation, protection of BBB integrity. In a similar line, anti-HMGB1 mAb exhibited inhibitory effects on the BBB leakage and pilocarpine-induced HMGB1 translocation. As well as prevented the BBB permeability and reduced HMGB1 translocation (**Table 3**) (Fu et al., 2017). Zhao et al. (2017) evaluated the anti-epileptic effect of anti-HMGB1 mAb on human brain slices from clinical drug-resistant epilepsy patients (**Table 3**)

HMGB1: A Common Biomarker and Potential Target for TBI, Neuroinflammation, Epilepsy and Cognitive...

107

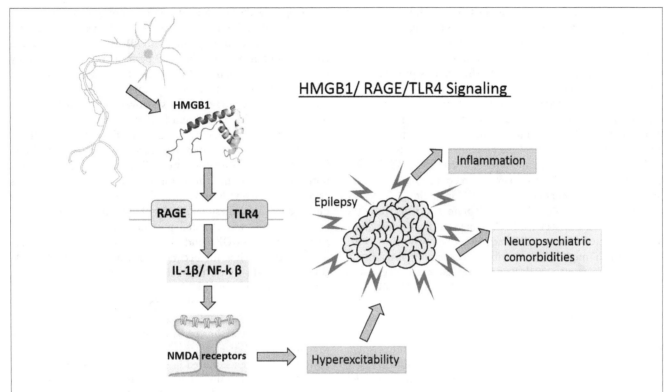

FIGURE 4 | HMGB1/TLR4/RAGE signaling in epilepsy. HMGB1 released from glia and neuronal cells in the CNS, activates its main receptor (TLR4 and RAGE) and contributes to epileptogenesis possibly via BBB disruption and activation of neuroinflammatory pathways.

where anti-HMGB1 mAb binds to HMGB1 and demonstrate long-lasting anti-epileptic properties, which is consistent with the previously estimated long half-time elimination in the brain (Zhang et al., 2011).

Extensive research highlights the putative role of HMGB1 in seizure generation, increased expression level of HMGB1 in epileptic brain (Chen et al., 2015) retardation of seizure precipitation by HMGB1 inhibitors (Zhao et al., 2017) implicating that HMGB1 is involved in all aspect from seizure generation to seizure retardation making HMGB1 as a strong candidate to be a reliable biomarkers for epileptogenesis. Moreover, the prevailing prognostic markers for seizure recurrence and seizure remission in patients diagnosed with epilepsy are solely based on supplementary factors including age, seizure type, EEG, and MRI, but are limited in their accuracy (Ravizza et al., 2017). Earlier study recommended HMGB1 isoforms as a mechanistic biomarkers for epileptogenesis where they investigate the value of blood HMGB1 in predicting epilepsy development as well as differentiating epileptogenic from non-epileptogenic rats after SE (Walker et al., 2017). HMGB1 as a biomarker of epileptogenesis will eventually provide a deeper insight on the normal biologic processes, pathogenic processes, or responses to an exposure or intervention, including therapeutic interventions with broad applications that are clinically able to arrest disease progression or to improve its clinical course. Moreover, precise understanding of mechanistic pathway on how HMGB1 induce seizure via inflammatory signaling will play a vital role in designing new therapies targeting inflammatory

pathways to minimize seizures. However, the association between HMGB1 and seizure needs further exploration. Overall findings suggest that blocking the HMGB1/TLR4/RAGE regulatory axis may represent a novel method for treating epilepsy.

ROLE OF HMGB1 IN COGNITIVE DYSFUNCTION

Cognition refers to a collection of cognitive phenomenon such as learning and memory, attention, executive function, consciousness, and language (McAfoose and Baune, 2009). Cognitive dysfunction is among the most prevalent and debilitating features highly associated with epilepsy (de Krom, 2006), PD (Kalia, 2018), AD (Elgh et al., 2006). The precise mechanism of cognitive dysfunction is not well understood, though there is an increased understanding about chronic activation of cytokine-dependent inflammatory signaling contributing to neuronal dysfunctions manifesting as cognitive deficits (Cunningham and Sanderson, 2008). In addition, increased brain cytokine signaling impairs learning and memory (Dantzer et al., 2008). Moreover, neuroinflammation has been reported to cause memory impairments as evidenced by an experimental study where LPS administration cause memory impairment via inducing neuroinflammation (Lee et al., 2008). Several study has been reported where cognitive impairment has been ameliorated via alleviating neuroinflammation (Ganai and Husain, 2018).

The main focus of the topic is HMGB1, which is an initiator and amplifier of neuroinflammatory process. HMGB1 has been implicated in impairing memory via mediating RAGE and TLR4 (Mazarati et al., 2011) however, the exact mechanism of HMGB1 in cognitive decline is limited. HMGB1 exhibits pro-excitatory effects in the hippocampus by elevating the phosphorylation of NR2B-NMDA receptors (Maroso et al., 2010), and thus increasing the receptor calcium channel conductance (Viviani et al., 2003). NR2B-containing NMDA receptors prevent cell surface expression of the GluR1 subunit of the α-amino-3-hydroxy-5-methyl-4-isoxazole propionic acid (AMPA) receptor (Kim et al., 2005), which has a key role in both synaptic plasticity and memory (Sanderson et al., 2008), including the NORT (Schiapparelli et al., 2006). In the adult brain, NR2B decreases the span of retrovirus-associated DNA sequences (Ras)/extracellular signal-regulated kinases (ERK) activation pathway (Kim et al., 2005), which might also contribute to memory impairment (Weeber and Sweatt, 2002). Remarkably, the same mechanism that modulates the seizure-facilitating effect of HMGB1 (i.e., the activation of NR2B-containing NMDA receptor) might be simultaneously involved in facilitating learning deficits. Recombinant HMGB1 impaired memory encoding in wild type (WT), TLR4 knockout and RAGE knockout animals, but no effect was observed either on memory consolidation, nor retrieval. Moreover, memory deficits was not exhibited on TLR4 knockout nor RAGE knockout mice *per se*. Blockade of TLR4 in RAGE knockout mice using *Rhodobacter sphaeroides* LPS attenuated the memory function impaired by HMGB1(Mazarati et al., 2011). The upregulation of microglia and systemic HMGB1 levels were correlated with cognitive dysfunction (Terrando et al., 2010). IL-1 modulation has been implicated to ameliorate LPS-induced cognitive dysfunction, however, IL-1 blockade ameliorated cognitive decline by reducing microglia without affecting HMGB1 (Terrando et al., 2010).

Plausible detrimental effects of HMGB1 on memory may have broad clinical implications. In an experimental model of chronic cerebral hypoperfusion (CCH), HMGB1 neutralization attenuates hippocampal neuronal death and cognitive impairment where anti-HMGB1 neutralizing Ab exerts long-time positive effects on hippocampal CA1 neuronal survival and cognitive abilities in the chronic phase of CCH as well as preserves BBB integrity, and suppresses hippocampal glial activation, pro-inflammatory cytokine production (Hei et al., 2018). Anti-HMGB1 mAb has ameliorated the symptoms and phenotype of AD in an experimental model where mAb against HMGB1 completely rescued cognitive impairment in a mouse model via inhibiting neurite degeneration even in the presence of amyloid beta (Aβ) plaques. The recovery in the memory impairment was evidenced by Y-maze test (Fujita et al., 2016).

Post-operative cognitive dysfunction is probably the most frequent type of postoperative cognitive impairment and the pathophysiology of POCD remains incompletely understood (Grape et al., 2012). HMGB1 has been extensively studied against POCD. Possible role of neuroinflammation mediated by HMGB1, RAGE, and S100B (a class of DAMPs) was hypothesized in the pathophysiology of POCD, however, the relationship between HMGB1 or S100B or RAGE signaling and cognitive dysfunction was not completely confirmed (Li et al., 2013). HMGB1 and RAGE levels were remarkably upregulated after surgery and HMGB1 is supposed to cause cognitive decline via breaking BBB permeability, however, study did not conclude either BBB is disrupted after surgery and relationship between HMGB1 and cognitive decline cannot be ascertained as the study did not selectively block HMGB1 using mAb (He et al., 2012). Administration of endogenous HMGB1 proteins produced cognitive decline in mice and neutralized HMGB1 mAb ameliorated cognitive decline and inhibited the inflammatory response after tibial surgery, suggesting a initiating role for this mediator in POCD (**Table 4**) (Vacas et al., 2014). As well as clinical data obtained from patients undergoing gastrointestinal surgery showed that serum HMGB1 and IL-6 levels was elevated post-surgery, and the increased post-operative HMGB1 and IL-6 levels were associated with the cognitive decline the occurs 1-week post-surgery (**Table 4**) (Lin et al., 2014). Oral pretreatment of glycyrrhizin inhibited HMGB1 cytosolic expression, alleviates the surgery-Induced HMGB1 upregulation in the hippocampus of the mice and attenuated the severity of post-operative memory impairment, as evidenced by the shorter swimming latency and distance in MWM trials (Chen et al., 2017a). The therapeutic benefits of HMGB1 have been explored in sepsis survivors where HMGB1 mediates cognitive dysfunction in a murine model of severe sepsis survivors (Chavan et al., 2012). Administration of neutralizing anti-HMGB mAb to survivors, beginning 1 week after the onset of peritonitis, significantly ameliorate memory impairments and brain pathology.

Cognitive decline induced by epilepsy is supported by number of previous studies (Kundap et al., 2017). Earlier studies documented selective deficits in memory encoding in TLE (Schwarze et al., 2009). The plausible role of HMGB1 in epilepsy induced cognitive dysfunction has not yet been reported, though administration of anti-HMGB1 mAb in mice delayed epilepsy onset as well as ameliorated cognitive functions (Zhao et al., 2017). However, the precise role of HMGB1 protein in epielpsy induced cognitive dysfunction has not yet been reported. In order to obtain a precise understanding, it is necessary to perform a longitudinal studies to investigate the levels of HMGB1 in epileptic animal models and concurrently undertake behavioral studies to assess the cognitive function of the animals and evaluate the expression pattern of HMGB1 throughout the study.

There are very few clinical studies that have been conducted till date regarding the effectiveness of anti-HMGB1 mAb on ameliorating cognitive dysfunction in patients. Foo et al. (2017) earlier reported that an interaction between HMGB1 and APOE-ε4 is associated with cortical thinning in MCI. This interaction was observed by studying genomic DNA extracted from peripheral blood and the plasma HMGB1 was measured with an ELISA kit (**Table 4**) (Foo et al., 2017). In human brain slice studies obtained from surgical resection of clinical drug-resistant epilepsy patients, anti-HMGB1 mAb demonstrated an attenuation of cognitive function as well as a disease-modifying anti-epileptogenesis effect, which is indicated by reduction in seizure frequency (Zhao et al., 2017).

TABLE 4 | Summary of findings reporting HMGB1 in cognitive dysfunction.

S.N.	Intervention	Model	Mechanism	Observation	Reference
1	HMGB1	Mice	• Activation of inflammatory pathways by stimulating RAGE and TLR4	• ↑ Brain levels of HMGB1 induce cognitive abnormalities and are mediated by either TLR4 or RAGE.	Mazarati et al., 2011
2	HMGB1	Mice	• Activation and trafficking of circulating bone marrow-derived macrophages to the brain	• POCD can be prevented by minimizing the effects of HMGB1 • A neutralizing antibody to HMGB1 protein reduced memory dysfunction	Vacas et al., 2014
3	HMGB1	Mice	• Neuroinflammation mediated by HMGB1 and RAGE	• Expression of HMGB1, RAGE and NF-κB p6 ↑ after surgery. • HMGB1 and RAGE signaling modulate the hippocampal inflammatory response	Koeth et al., 2013
4	HMGB1	Rat	• HMGB1 and RAGE signaling	• HMGB1 and RAGE ↑ in the hippocampus of operated animals • HMGB1 interrupt and regulate the inflammatory response associated with the pathogenesis of POCD	He et al., 2012
5	HMGB1	Human	• Interaction between APOE-ε4 and HMGB1	• HMGB1 showed an association with ↓ cortical thickness • APOE-ε4 and HMGB1 are responsible for extensive cortical thinning in MCI.	Foo et al., 2017
6	HMGB1	Human	• POCD induced via inflammatory response	• HMGB1, IL-6 levels ↑ in patients after surgery • Elevated levels of HMGB1, IL-6 might be associated with cognitive dysfunctions after surgery	Lin et al., 2014

S.N., serial number; ↑, increased; ↓, decreased; HMGB1, high mobility group box 1; TRL4, toll like receptor 4; RAGE, receptor for advanced glycation end products; NF-κB, nuclear factor kappa-light-chain-enhancer of activated B cells; TEM, transmission electron microscopy; IHC, immunohistochemistry; MCI, mild cognitive impairments; APOE-ε4, Apo lipoprotein E ε4; IL-6, interleukin-6; POCD, post-operative cognitive dysfunctions.

HMGB1: TRANSLATIONAL IMPLICATION

Recent investigation shed more light on multiple roles of HMGB1 in a diverse range of pathologies such as brain injury, epilepsy, and neuroinflammation and cognitive decline. Treatments based on HMGB1 antagonists via targeting extracellular HMGB1 have generated encouraging results in a wide number of experimental models of aforementioned HMGB1 mediated pathologies, though the clinical studies are yet to be reported. However, complex biology of HMGB1 has not been fully understood yet and there is a notion that association between HMGB1 and brain injury, epilepsy, neuroinflammation mediated pathologies and cognitive decline requires deeper exploration, as the precise mechanism of on how HMGB1 mediates these neurological conditions are yet to be well documented. Despite of that, the identification of HMGB1 inhibitors results in significant experimental and clinical interest. Moreover, HMGB1 as a common biomarker of TBI, neuroinflammation, epileptogenesis and cognitive decline might be instrumental in assessing the disease progression, early prediction of disease as well

as evaluating patient's response to therapy. Translational implication of HMGB1 will be a paradigm shift, which will not only overcome the limitation of currently available AEDs, improve the cognitive decline as well. Moreover, via inhibiting the neuroinflammatory pathways HMGB1 can ameliorate several brain injuries and neuroinflammation mediated pathologies. More precisely, inhibiting HMGB1/RAGE/TLR4 pathway represents a promising approach which can interfere with disease progression in epileptogenesis, neuroinflammatory disease, several forms of brain injury as well as memory impairment. The focus of the topic is TBI, neuroinflammation, epilepsy and cognitive decline, however, blocking HMGB1 might achieves significant neuroprotection in several forms of neurodegenerative disorders where neuroinflammation plays a crucial role. Future strategy should be focused on exploring several HMGB1 antagonist which can efficiently interact with the main HMGB1-receptor, RAGE, acting as competitive antagonists of HMGB1, such as recombinant box A (the truncated N-terminal domain of HMGB1) or S100P-derived RAGE peptide (Musumeci et al., 2014).

SUMMARY OF FINDINGS AND CONCLUSION

Neuroinflammation has been implicated in ranges of neurological disorders such as TBI, epilepsy and memory impairment. HMGB1 being the mediator of neuroinflammation has been reported to play crucial role in TBI, neuroinflammatory diseases and epileptogenesis via an unknown mechanism. As well as elevated level of HMGB1 in serum and CSF has been observed in these neuroinflammation mediated pathologies. These strengthens the rationale of our study in suggesting HMGB1 as a common biomarker in TBI, neuroinflammation, epilepsy and cognitive decline. Biomarker discovery together with investigations into novel therapeutic candidates would give a noteworthy headway in the treatment of TBI, epilepsy, memory impairment and neuroinflammation via acting on its mechanistic pathway rather than symptomatic control. In current review, an attempt was made to connect the dots between HMGB1 and its putative role in several forms of brain injury, neuroinflammation mediated conditions, epilepsy and cognitive decline using preclinical and clinical evidence.

Several important limitations regarding the topic should not be ruled out, such as feasibility and viability issues in making HMGB1 a common functional biomarker for neuroinflammation mediated pathologies discussed herein. Can inhibiting HMGB1/RAGE/TLR4 axis be a common target for these neurological conditions? Can therapeutic outcomes obtained from experimental evidence regarding the role of HMGB1 in all these neurological conditions be easily translated into clinical settings? These are the concerns that remains unsolved as more experimental data are yet to come.

Despite accumulating scientific evidence of HMGB1 in the neuroinflammation mediated conditions discussed in current review, no attempt has been made in portraying HMGB1 as common biomarker and target for these HMGB1 mediated neurological conditions. We suggest, HMGB1 proteins can be considered as a promising non-invasive, common biomarker of TBI, neuroinflammation, epilepsy and cognitive dysfunction as it meets many criteria to stand as a common biomarker. It is relatively stable in blood and can be rapidly and inexpensively measured in blood. Moreover, changes in the total HMGB1 levels in the brain during neurological conditions discussed herein, can be mirrored in the blood.

As a concluding remark, drawing evidence from earlier preclinical and clinical studies, the current review advances the concept of positioning HMGB1 as common functional biomarker that can significantly improve risk assessment, diagnosis and monitoring of the neurological diseases discussed in this review. As well as HMGB1 can emerge as a novel avenues against TBI, neuroinflammation, epilepsy and cognitive deficits which acts by blocking the neuroinflammatory pathway.

AUTHOR CONTRIBUTIONS

YP and MS carried out literature review, conceptualized, designed and drafted the manuscript. AC, YK, ÁA-S, KA, MA and IO provided critical revisions and contributed to the final manuscript. YK also designed the figures. All authors read and approved the final manuscript.

ACKNOWLEDGMENTS

We would like to thank Mr. Vineet Mehta, Ph.D., Jaypee University of Information Technology, India for his contribution in assessing manuscript. In addition, we are also thankful to Brandon Choo Kar Meng, Charlotte Squier, and Uday Praful Kundap, Monash University Malaysia for their effort in proof reading the manuscript.

REFERENCES

1. Ai, P., Zhang, X., Xie, Z., Liu, G., Liu, X., Pan, S., et al. (2018). The HMGB1 is increased in CSF of patients with an Anti-NMDAR encephalitis. *Acta Neurol. Scand.* 137, 277–282. doi: 10.1111/ane.12850
2. Andersson, Å., Covacu, R., Sunnemark, D., Danilov, A. I., Bianco, A., Khademi, M., et al. (2008). Pivotal advance: HMGB1 expression in active lesions of human and experimental multiple sclerosis. *J. Leukoc. Biol.* 84, 1248–1255. doi: 10.1189/ jlb.1207844
3. Andersson, U., Yang, H., and Harris, H. (2018). Extracellular HMGB1 as a therapeutic target in inflammatory diseases. *Expert Opin. Ther. Targets* 22, 263–277. doi: 10.1080/14728222.2018.1439924
4. Annegers, J. F., and Coan, S. P. (2000). The risks of epilepsy after traumatic brain injury. *Seizure* 9, 453–457. doi: 10.1053/seiz.2000.0458
5. Aroniadou-Anderjaska, V., Fritsch, B., Qashu, F., and Braga, M. F. (2008). Pathology and pathophysiology of the amygdala in epileptogenesis and epilepsy. *Epilepsy Res.* 78, 102–116. doi: 10.1016/j.eplepsyres.2007.11.011
6. Ashrafi, M. R., Shams, S., Nouri, M., Mohseni, M., Shabanian, R., Yekaninejad,
7. M. S., et al. (2007). A probable causative factor for an old problem: selenium and glutathione peroxidase appear to play important roles in epilepsy pathogenesis. *Epilepsia* 48, 1750–1755. doi: 10.1111/j.1528-1167.2007.01143.x
8. Au, A. K., Aneja, R. K., Bell, M. J., Bayir, H., Feldman, K., Adelson, P. D., et al. (2012). Cerebrospinal fluid levels of high-mobility group box 1 and cytochrome C predict outcome after pediatric traumatic brain injury. *J. Neurotrauma* 29, 2013–2021. doi: 10.1089/neu.2011.2171
9. Aucott, H., Lundberg, J., Salo, H., Klevenvall, L., Damberg, P., Ottosson, L., et al. (2018a). Neuroinflammation in response to intracerebral injections of different HMGB1 redox isoforms. *J. Innate Immun.* 10, 215–227. doi: 10.1159/0004 87056
10. Aucott, H., Sowinska, A., Harris, H. E., and Lundback, P. (2018b). Ligation of free HMGB1 to TLR2 in the absence of ligand is negatively regulated by the C-terminal tail domain. *Mol. Med.* 24:19. doi: 10.1186/s10020-018-0021-x
11. Bar-Klein, G., Lublinsky, S., Kamintsky, L., Noyman, I., Veksler, R., Dalipaj, H., et al. (2017). Imaging blood–brain barrier dysfunction as a biomarker for epileptogenesis. *Brain* 140, 1692–1705. doi: 10.1093/brain/awx073
12. Barlow, K. M., Spowart, J. J., and Minns, R. A. (2000). Early posttraumatic seizures in non-accidental head injury: relation to outcome. *Dev. Med. Child Neurol.* 42, 591–594. doi: 10.1017/S0012162200001110
13. Baxevanis, A. D., and Landsman, D. (1995). The HMG-1 box protein family: classification and functional relationships. *Nucleic Acids Res.* 23, 1604–1613. doi: 10.1093/nar/23.9.1604
14. Bianchi, M. E., and Manfredi, A. A. (2007). High-mobility group box 1 (HMGB1) protein at the crossroads between innate and adaptive immunity. *Immunol. Rev.* 220, 35–46. doi: 10.1111/j.1600-065X.2007.00574.x
15. Casula, M., Iyer, A., Spliet, W., Anink, J., Steentjes, K., Sta, M., et al. (2011). Toll-like receptor signaling in amyotrophic lateral sclerosis spinal cord tissue. *Neuroscience* 179, 233–243. doi: 10.1016/j.neuroscience.2011.02.001

16. Chandrashekaran, V., Seth, R. K., Dattaroy, D., Alhasson, F., Ziolenka, J., Carson, J., et al. (2017). HMGB1-RAGE pathway drives peroxynitrite signaling-induced IBD-like inflammation in murine nonalcoholic fatty liver disease. *rDX bIO* 13, 8–19. doi: 10.1016/j.redox.2017.05.005

17. Chavan, S. S., Huerta, P. T., Robbiati, S., Valdes-Ferrer, S. I., Ochani, M., Dancho, M., et al. (2012). HMGB1 mediates cognitive impairment in sepsis survivors. *Mol. Med.* 18, 930–937. doi: 10.2119/molmed.2012.00195

18. Chen, X., Hua, H.-P., Liang, L., and Liu, L.-J. (2017a). The oral pretreatment of glycyrrhizin prevents surgery-induced cognitive impairment in aged mice by reducing neuroinflammation and alzheimer's-related pathology via HMGB1 inhibition. *J. Mol. Neurosci.* 63, 385–395. doi: 10.1007/s12031-017-0989-7

19. Chen, X., Wu, S., Chen, C., Xie, B., Fang, Z., Hu, W., et al. (2017b). Omega-3 polyunsaturated fatty acid supplementation attenuates microglial-induced inflammation by inhibiting the HMGB1/TLR4/NF-κB pathway following experimental traumatic brain injury. *J. Neuroinflamm.* 14:143. doi: 10.1186/s12974-017-0917-3

20. Chen, Y., Huang, X.-J., Yu, N., Xie, Y., Zhang, K., Wen, F., et al. (2015). HMGB1 contributes to the expression of P-glycoprotein in mouse epileptic brain through toll-like receptor 4 and receptor for advanced glycation end products. *PLoS One* 10:e0140918. doi: 10.1371/journal.pone.014 0918

21. Cheng, X., Yang, Y.-L., Yang, H., Wang, Y.-H., and Du, G.-H. (2018). Kaempferol alleviates LPS-induced neuroinflammation and BBB dysfunction in mice via inhibiting HMGB1 release and down-regulating TLR4/MyD88 pathway. *Int. Immunopharmacol.* 56, 29–35. doi: 10.1016/j.intimp.2018.01.002

22. Coco, D. L., Veglianese, P., Allievi, E., and Bendotti, C. (2007). Distribution and cellular localization of high mobility group box protein 1 (HMGB1) in the spinal cord of a transgenic mouse model of ALS. *Neurosci. Lett.* 412, 73–77. doi: 10.1016/j.neulet.2006.10.063

23. Cohen, M. J., Brohi, K., Calfee, C. S., Rahn, P., Chesebro, B. B., Christiaans, S. C., et al. (2009). Early release of high mobility group box nuclear protein 1 after severe trauma in humans: role of injury severity and tissue hypoperfusion. *Crit. Care* 13:R174. doi: 10.1186/cc8152

24. Compston, A., and Coles, A. (2008). Multiple sclerosis. *Lancet* 372, 1502–1517. doi: 10.1016/S0140-6736(08)61620-7

25. Craft, J. M., Watterson, D. M., and Van Eldik, L. J. (2005). Neuroinflammation: a potential therapeutic target. *Expert Opin. Ther. Targets* 9, 887–900. doi: 10.1517/ 14728222.9.5.887

26. Cunningham, C., and Sanderson, D. J. (2008). Malaise in the water maze: untangling the effects of LPS and IL-1β on learning and memory. *Brain Behav. Immun.* 22, 1117–1127. doi: 10.1016/j.bbi.2008.05.007

27. Dantzer, R., O'Connor, J. C., Freund, G. G., Johnson, R. W., and Kelley, K. W. (2008). From inflammation to sickness and depression: when the immune system subjugates the brain. *Nat. Rev. Neurosci.* 9:46. doi: 10.1038/nrn2297

28. de Krom, M. (2006). Cognitive dysfunction in epilepsy. *Seizure-Eur. J. Epilepsy* 15, 264–266. doi: 10.1016/j.seizure.2006.02.020

29. DeKosky, S. T., Blennow, K., Ikonomovic, M. D., and Gandy, S. (2013). Acute and chronic traumatic encephalopathies: pathogenesis and biomarkers. *Nat. Rev. Neurol.* 9, 192–200. doi: 10.1038/nrneurol.2013.36

30. Elgh, E., Åstot, A. L., Fagerlund, M., Eriksson, S., Olsson, T., and Näsman, B. (2006). Cognitive dysfunction, hippocampal atrophy and glucocorticoid feedback in Alzheimer's disease. *Biol. Psychiatry* 59, 155–161. doi: 10.1016/j.biopsych.2005. 06.017

31. Fang, H., Wang, P.-F., Zhou, Y., Wang, Y.-C., and Yang, Q.-W. (2013). Toll-like receptor 4 signaling in intracerebral hemorrhage-induced inflammation and injury. *J. Neuroinflamm.* 10:794. doi: 10.1186/1742-2094-10-27

32. Fang, P., Schachner, M., and Shen, Y. Q. (2012). HMGB1 in development and diseases of the central nervous system. *Mol. Neurobiol.* 45, 499–506. doi: 10. 1007/s12035-012-8264-y

33. Festoff, B. W., Sajja, R. K., van Dreden, P., and Cucullo, L. (2016). HMGB1 and thrombin mediate the blood-brain barrier dysfunction acting as biomarkers of neuroinflammation and progression to neurodegeneration in Alzheimer's disease. *J. Neuroinflamm.* 13:194. doi: 10.1186/s12974-016-0670-z

34. Fonken, L. K., Frank, M. G., Kitt, M. M., D'Angelo, H. M., Norden, D. M., Weber, M. D., et al. (2016). The alarmin HMGB1 mediates age-induced neuroinflammatory priming. *J. Neurosci.* 36, 7946–7956. doi: 10.1523/JNEUROSCI.1161-16.2016

35. Foo, H., Ng, K. P., Tan, J., Lim, L., Chander, R. J., Yong, T. T., et al. (2017). Interaction between APOE-ε4 and HMGB1 is associated with widespread cortical thinning in mild cognitive impairment. *J. Neurol. Neurosurg. Psychiatry* 2017:315869.

36. Frank, M. G., Weber, M. D., Fonken, L. K., Hershman, S. A., Watkins, L. R., and Maier, S. F. (2016). The redox state of the alarmin HMGB1 is a pivotal factor in neuroinflammatory and microglial priming: a role for the NLRP3 inflammasome. *Brain Behav. Immun.* 55, 215–224. doi: 10.1016/j.bbi.2015. 10.009

37. Frank, M. G., Weber, M. D., Watkins, L. R., and Maier, S. F. (2015). Stress sounds the alarmin: the role of the danger-associated molecular pattern HMGB1 in stress-induced neuroinflammatory priming. *Brain Behav. Immun.* 48, 1–7. doi: 10.1016/j.bbi.2015.03.010

38. Frey, L. C. (2003). Epidemiology of posttraumatic epilepsy: a critical review. *Epilepsia* 44 (Suppl 10), 11–17. doi: 10.1046/j.1528-1157.44.s10.4.x

39. Fu, L., Liu, K., Wake, H., Teshigawara, K., Yoshino, T., Takahashi, H., et al. (2017). Therapeutic effects of anti-HMGB1 monoclonal antibody on pilocarpine-induced status epilepticus in mice. *Sci. Rep.* 7:1179. doi: 10.1038/s41598-017-01325-y

40. Fujita, K., Motoki, K., Tagawa, K., Chen, X., Hama, H., Nakajima, K., et al. (2016). HMGB1, a pathogenic molecule that induces neurite degeneration via TLR4-MARCKS, is a potential therapeutic target for Alzheimer's disease. *Sci. Rep.* 6:31895. doi: 10.1038/srep31895

41. Ganai, A. A., and Husain, M. (2018). Genistein alleviates neuroinflammation and restores cognitive function in rat model of hepatic encephalopathy: underlying mechanisms. *Mol. Neurobiol.* 55, 1762–1772. doi: 10.1007/s12035-017-0454-1

42. Gao, H.-M., Zhou, H., Zhang, F., Wilson, B. C., Kam, W., and Hong, J.-S. (2011). HMGB1 acts on microglia Mac1 to mediate chronic neuroinflammation that drives progressive neurodegeneration. *J. Neurosci.* 31, 1081–1092. doi: 10.1523/ JNEUROSCI.3732-10.2011

43. Gao, T., Chen, Z., Chen, H., Yuan, H., Wang, Y., Peng, X., et al. (2018). Inhibition of HMGB1 mediates neuroprotection of traumatic brain injury by modulating the microglia/macrophage polarization. *Biochem. Biophys. Res. Commun.* 497, 430–436. doi: 10.1016/j.bbrc.2018.02.102

44. Gao, T. L., Yuan, X. T., Yang, D., Dai, H. L., Wang, W. J., Peng, X., et al. (2012). Expression of HMGB1 and RAGE in rat and human brains after traumatic brain injury. *J. Trauma Acute Care Surg.* 72, 643–649. doi: 10.1097/ TA.0b013e31823c54a6

45. Gehrmann, J., Matsumoto, Y., and Kreutzberg, G. W. (1995). Microglia: intrinsic immuneffector cell of the brain. *Brain Res. Rev.* 20, 269–287. doi: 10.1016/0165- 0173(94)00015-H

46. Gloor, S. M., Wachtel, M., Bolliger, M. F., Ishihara, H., Landmann, R., and Frei, K. (2001). Molecular and cellular permeability control at the blood–brain barrier. *Brain Res. Rev.* 36, 258–264. doi: 10.1016/S0165-0173(01)00102-3

47. González-Reyes, S., Santillán-Cigales, J. J., Jiménez-Osorio, A. S., Pedraza-Chaverri, J., and Guevara-Guzmán, R. (2016). Glycyrrhizin ameliorates oxidative stress and inflammation in hippocampus and olfactory bulb in lithium/pilocarpine-induced status epilepticus in rats. *Epilepsy Res.* 126, 126–133. doi: 10.1016/j.eplepsyres.2016.07.007

48. Grape, S., Ravussin, P., Rossi, A., Kern, C., and Steiner, L. (2012). Postoperative cognitive dysfunction. *Trends Anaesth. Crit. Care* 2, 98–103. doi: 10.1016/j.tacc. 2012.02.002

49. Harris, H. E., Andersson, U., and Pisetsky, D. S. (2012). HMGB1: a multifunctional alarmin driving autoimmune and inflammatory disease. *Nat. Rev. Rheumatol.* 8:195. doi: 10.1038/nrrheum.2011.222

50. Hauser, W. A., Annegers, J. F., and Kurland, L. T. (1993). Incidence of epilepsy and unprovoked seizures in Rochester, Minnesota: 1935–1984. *Epilepsia* 34, 453–458. doi: 10.1111/j.1528-1157.1993.tb02586.x

51. He, H. J., Wang, Y., Le, Y., Duan, K. M., Yan, X. B., Liao, Q., et al. (2012). Surgery upregulates high mobility group box-1 and disrupts the blood-brain barrier causing cognitive dysfunction in aged rats. *CNS Neurosci. Therap.* 18, 994–1002. doi: 10.1111/cns.12018

52. Hei, Y., Chen, R., Yi, X., Long, Q., Gao, D., and Liu, W. (2018). HMGB1 neutralization attenuates hippocampal neuronal death and cognitive impairment in rats with chronic cerebral hypoperfusion via suppressing inflammatory responses and oxidative stress. *Neuroscience* 383, 150–159. doi: 10.1016/j.neuroscience.2018.05.010

53. Heneka, M. T., Carson, M. J., El Khoury, J., Landreth, G. E., Brosseron, F., Feinstein, D. L., et al. (2015). Neuroinflammation in Alzheimer's disease. *Lancet Neurol.* 14, 388–405. doi: 10.1016/S1474-4422(15)70016-5

54. Hinson, H. E., Rowell, S., and Schreiber, M. (2015). Clinical evidence of inflammation driving secondary brain injury: a systematic review. *J. Trauma Acute Care Surg.* 78, 184–191. doi: 10.1097/TA.00000000000 00468

55. Hong, H., Kim, B. S., and Im, H.-I. (2016). Pathophysiological role

of neuroinflammation in neurodegenerative diseases and psychiatric disorders. *Int. Neurourol. J.* 20(Suppl. 1), S2. doi: 10.5213/inj.1632604.302

56. Huang, W., András, I. E., Rha, G. B., Hennig, B., and Toborek, M. (2011). PPARα and PPARγ protect against HIV-1-induced MMP-9 overexpression via caveolae-associated ERK and Akt signaling. *FASEB J.* 25, 3979–3988. doi: 10. 1096/fj.11-188607

57. Hwang, C.-S., Liu, G.-T., Chang, M. D.-T., Liao, I.-L., and Chang, H.-T. (2013). Elevated serum autoantibody against high mobility group box 1 as a potent surrogate biomarker for amyotrophic lateral sclerosis. *Neurobiol. Dis.* 58, 13–18. doi: 10.1016/j.nbd.2013.04.013

58. Ieong, C., Sun, H., Wang, Q., and Ma, J. (2018). Glycyrrhizin suppresses the expressions of HMGB1 and ameliorates inflammative effect after acute subarachnoid hemorrhage in rat model. *J. Clin. Neurosci.* 47, 278–284. doi: 10.1016/j.jocn.2017.10.034

59. Iori, V. (2017). *Epigenetic and Pharmacological Targeting of Neuroinflammation as Novel Therapeutic Interventions for epilepsy.* Ph.D. thesis, Faculty of Medicine (AMC-UvA), Amsterdam.

60. Iori, V., Maroso, M., Rizzi, M., Iyer, A. M., Vertemara, R., Carli, M., et al. (2013). Receptor for advanced glycation endproducts is upregulated in temporal lobe epilepsy and contributes to experimental seizures. *Neurobiol. Dis.* 58, 102–114. doi: 10.1016/j.nbd.2013.03.006

61. Ito, M., Takahashi, H., Yano, H., Shimizu, Y. I., Yano, Y., Ishizaki, Y., et al. (2017). High mobility group box 1 enhances hyperthermia-induced seizures and secondary epilepsy associated with prolonged hyperthermia-induced seizures in developing rats. *Metab. Brain Dis.* 32, 2095–2104. doi: 10.1007/s11011-017- 0103-4

62. Jiang, H., Wang, Y., Liang, X., Xing, X., Xu, X., and Zhou, C. (2018). Toll- like receptor 4 knockdown attenuates brain damage and neuroinflammation after traumatic brain injury via inhibiting neuronal autophagy and astrocyte activation. *Cell Mol. Neurobiol.* 38, 1009–1019. doi: 10.1007/s10571-017- 0570-5

63. Kalia, L. V. (2018). Biomarkers for cognitive dysfunction in Parkinson's disease. *Parkinsonism Relat. Disord.* 46, S19–S23. doi: 10.1016/j.parkreldis.2017.07.023 Kaneko, Y., Pappas, C., Malapira, T., Vale, F. L., Tajiri, N., and Borlongan, C. V.

64. (2017). Extracellular HMGB1 modulates glutamate metabolism associated with kainic acid-induced epilepsy-like hyperactivity in primary rat neural cells. *Cell Physiol. Biochem.* 41, 947–959. doi: 10.1159/000460513

65. Kang, R., Chen, R., Zhang, Q., Hou, W., Wu, S., Cao, L., et al. (2014). HMGB1 in health and disease. *Mol. Aspects Med.* 40, 1–116. doi: 10.1016/j.mam.2014. 05.001

66. Kim, J. B., Choi, J. S., Yu, Y. M., Nam, K., Piao, C. S., Kim, S. W., et al. (2006). HMGB1, a novel cytokine-like mediator linking acute neuronal death and delayed neuroinflammation in the postischemic brain. *J. Neurosci.* 26, 6413–6421. doi: 10.1523/JNEUROSCI.3815-05.2006

67. Kim, M. J., Dunah, A. W., Wang, Y. T., and Sheng, M. (2005). Differential roles of NR2A-and NR2B-containing NMDA receptors in Ras-ERK signaling and AMPA receptor trafficking. *Neuron* 46, 745–760. doi: 10.1016/j.neuron.2005. 04.031

68. Kobori, N., Clifton, G. L., and Dash, P. (2002). Altered expression of novel genes in the cerebral cortex following experimental brain injury. *Brain Res. Mol. Brain Res.* 104, 148–158. doi: 10.1016/S0169-328X(02)00331-5

69. Koeth, R. A., Wang, Z., Levison, B. S., Buffa, J. A., Org, E., Sheehy, B. T., et al. (2013). Intestinal microbiota metabolism of L-carnitine, a nutrient in red meat, promotes atherosclerosis. *Nat. Med.* 19:576. doi: 10.1038/nm. 3145

70. Kumar, A., and Loane, D. J. (2012). Neuroinflammation after traumatic brain injury: opportunities for therapeutic intervention. *Brain Behav. Immun.* 26, 1191–1201. doi: 10.1016/j.bbi.2012.06.008

71. Kundap, U. P., Kumari, Y., Othman, I., and Shaikh, M. (2017). Zebrafish as a model for epilepsy-induced cognitive dysfunction: a pharmacological, biochemical and behavioral approach. *Front. Pharmacol.* 8:515. doi: 10.3389/fphar.2017. 00515

72. Laird, M. D., Shields, J. S., Sukumari-Ramesh, S., Kimbler, D. E., Fessler, R. D., Shakir, B., et al. (2014). High mobility group box protein-1 promotes cerebral edema after traumatic brain injury via activation of toll-like receptor 4. *Glia* 62, 26–38. doi: 10.1002/glia.22581

73. Lee, J. W., Lee, Y. K., Yuk, D. Y., Choi, D. Y., Ban, S. B., Oh, K. W., et al. (2008). Neuro-inflammation induced by lipopolysaccharide causes cognitive impairment through enhancement of beta-amyloid generation. *J. Neuroinflamm.* 5:37. doi: 10.1186/1742-2094-5-37

74. Lee, S., Nam, Y., Koo, J. Y., Lim, D., Park, J., Ock, J., et al. (2014). A small molecule binding HMGB1 and HMGB2 inhibits microglia-

mediated neuroinflammation. *Nat. Chem. Biol.* 10:1055. doi: 10.1038/nchembio.1669

75. Lee, W., Kim, T. H., Ku, S.-K., Min, K.-J., Lee, H.-S., Kwon, T. K., et al. (2012). Barrier protective effects of withaferin A in HMGB1-induced inflammatory responses in both cellular and animal models. *Toxicol. Appl. Pharmacol.* 262, 91–98. doi: 10.1016/j.taap.2012.04.025

76. Lei, C., Lin, S., Zhang, C., Tao, W., Dong, W., Hao, Z., et al. (2013). High- mobility group box1 protein promotes neuroinflammation after intracerebral hemorrhage in rats. *Neuroscience* 228, 190–199. doi: 10.1016/j.neuroscience. 2012.10.023

77. Lewis, C.-A., Manning, J., Rossi, F., and Krieger, C. (2012). The neuroinflammatory response in ALS: the roles of microglia and T cells. *Neurol. Res. Int.* 2012:803701. doi: 10.1155/2012/803701

78. Li, D., Liu, N., Zhao, H.-H., Zhang, X., Kawano, H., Liu, L., et al. (2017). Interactions between Sirt1 and MAPKs regulate astrocyte activation induced by brain injury in vitro and in vivo. *J. Neuroinflamm.* 14:67. doi: 10.1186/s12974- 017-0841-6

79. Li, Y., Li, X., Qu, Y., Huang, J., Zhu, T., Zhao, F., et al. (2017). Role of HMGB1 translocation to neuronal nucleus in rat model with septic brain injury. *Neurosci. Lett.* 645, 90–96. doi: 10.1016/j.neulet.2016.11.047

80. Li, R. L., Zhang, Z. Z., Peng, M., Wu, Y., Zhang, J. J., Wang, C. Y., et al. (2013). Postoperative impairment of cognitive function in old mice: a possible role for neuroinflammation mediated by HMGB1, S100B, and RAGE. *J. Surg. Res.* 185, 815–824. doi: 10.1016/j.jss.2013.06.043

81. Lin, G. X., Wang, T., Chen, M. H., Hu, Z. H., and Ouyang, W. (2014). Serum high-mobility group box 1 protein correlates with cognitive decline after gastrointestinal surgery. *Acta Anaesthesiol. Scand.* 58, 668–674. doi: 10.1111/ aas.12320

82. Liu, A.-H., Wu, Y.-T., and Wang, Y.-P. (2017). MicroRNA-129-5p inhibits the development of autoimmune encephalomyelitis-related epilepsy by targeting HMGB1 through the TLR4/NF-kB signaling pathway. *Brain Res. Bull.* 132, 139–149. doi: 10.1016/j.brainresbull.2017.05.004

83. Liu, Z., Yang, C., Meng, X., Li, Z., Lv, C., and Cao, P. (2018). Neuroprotection of edaravone on the hippocampus of kainate-induced epilepsy rats through Nrf2/HO-1 pathway. *Neurochem. Int.* 112, 159–165. doi: 10.1016/j.neuint.2017. 07.001

84. Lotze, M. T., and Tracey, K. J. (2005). High-mobility group box 1 protein (HMGB1): nuclear weapon in the immune arsenal. *Nat. Rev. Immunol.* 5, 331–342. doi: 10.1038/nri1594

85. Luo, L., Jin, Y., Kim, I.-D., and Lee, J.-K. (2014). Glycyrrhizin suppresses HMGB1 inductions in the hippocampus and subsequent accumulation in serum of a kainic acid-induced seizure mouse model. *Cell. Mol. Neurobiol.* 34, 987–997. doi: 10.1007/s10571-014-0075-4

86. Maroso, M., Balosso, S., Ravizza, T., Liu, J., Aronica, E., Iyer, A. M., et al. (2010). Toll-like receptor 4 and high-mobility group box-1 are involved in ictogenesis and can be targeted to reduce seizures. *Nat. Med.* 16:413. doi: 10.1038/nm. 2127

87. Mazarati, A., Maroso, M., Iori, V., Vezzani, A., and Carli, M. (2011). High-mobility group box-1 impairs memory in mice through both toll-like receptor 4 and receptor for advanced glycation end products. *Exp. Neurol.* 232, 143–148. doi: 10.1016/j.expneurol.2011.08.012

88. McAfoose, J., and Baune, B. (2009). Evidence for a cytokine model of cognitive function. *Neurosci. Biobehav. Rev.* 33, 355–366. doi: 10.1016/j.neubiorev.2008. 10.005

89. Meneghini, V., Bortolotto, V., Francese, M. T., Dellarole, A., Carraro, L., Terzieva, S., et al. (2013). High-mobility group box-1 protein and β-amyloid oligomers promote neuronal differentiation of adult hippocampal neural progenitors via receptor for advanced glycation end products/nuclear factor- κB axis: relevance for Alzheimer's disease. *J. Neurosci.* 33, 6047–6059. doi: 10.1523/JNEUROSCI.2052-12.2013

90. Metting, Z., Wilczak, N., Rodiger, L., Schaaf, J., and Van Der Naalt, J. (2012). GFAP and S100B in the acute phase of mild traumatic brain injury. *Neurology* 78, 1428–1433. doi: 10.1212/WNL.0b013e318253d5c7

91. Miller, S. D., Karpus, W. J., and Davidson, T. S. (2010). Experimental autoimmune encephalomyelitis in the mouse. *Curr. Protoc. Immunol.* 88, 15.11.11–15.11.20. doi: 10.1002/0471142735.im1501s88

92. Mohamed, A., Elbohi, K., Sharkawy, N., and Hassan, M. (2017). Biochemical and apoptotic biomarkers as indicators of time elapsed since death in experimentally induced traumatic brain injury. *SM J. Forensic Res. Criminol.* 1:1010.

93. Morganti-Kossmann, M. C., Rancan, M., Stahel, P. F., and Kossmann, T. (2002). Inflammatory response in acute traumatic brain injury: a double-edged sword. *Curr. Opin. Crit. Care* 8, 101–105. doi: 10.1097/00075198-200204000-00002

94. Musumeci, D., Roviello, G. N., and Montesarchio, D. (2014). An overview on HMGB1 inhibitors as potential therapeutic agents in HMGB1-related pathologies. *Pharmacol. Therap.* 141, 347–357. doi: 10.1016/j.pharmthera.2013. 11.001

95. Nakahara, T., Tsuruta, R., Kaneko, T., Yamashita, S., Fujita, M., Kasaoka, S., et al. (2009). High-mobility group box 1 protein in CSF of patients with subarachnoid hemorrhage. *Neurocrit. Care* 11:362. doi: 10.1007/s12028-009-9276-y

96. Oh, Y. J., Youn, J. H., Ji, Y., Lee, S. E., Lim, K. J., Choi, J. E., et al. (2009). HMGB1 is phosphorylated by classical protein kinase C and is secreted by a calcium- dependent mechanism. *J. Immunol.* 182, 5800–5809. doi: 10.4049/jimmunol. 0801873

97. Okuma, Y., Liu, K., Wake, H., Liu, R., Nishimura, Y., Hui, Z., et al. (2014). Glycyrrhizin inhibits traumatic brain injury by reducing HMGB1–RAGE interaction. *Neuropharmacology* 85, 18–26. doi: 10.1016/j.neuropharm.2014. 05.007

98. Okuma, Y., Liu, K., Wake, H., Zhang, J., Maruo, T., Yoshino, T., et al. (2012). Anti- high mobility group box-1 antibody therapy for traumatic brain injury. *Ann. Neurol.* 72, 373–384. doi: 10.1002/ana.23602

99. Palleria, C., Coppola, A., Citraro, R., Del Gaudio, L., Striano, S., De Sarro, G., et al. (2015). Perspectives on treatment options for mesial temporal lobe epilepsy with hippocampal sclerosis. *Exp. Opin. Pharmacother.* 16, 2355–2371. doi: 10. 1517/14656566.2015.1084504

100. Parker, T. M., Nguyen, A. H., Rabang, J. R., Patil, A. A., and Agrawal, D. K. (2017). The danger zone: systematic review of the role of HMGB1 danger signalling in traumatic brain injury. *Brain Inj.* 31, 2–8. doi: 10.1080/02699052.2016.1217045 Pascente, R., Frigerio, F., Rizzi, M., Porcu, L., Boido, M., Davids, J., et al. (2016). Cognitive deficits and brain myo-Inositol are early biomarkers of epileptogenesis in a rat model of epilepsy. *Neurobiol. Dis.* 93, 146–155. doi: 10.1016/j.nbd.2016.05.001

101. Peltz, E. D., Moore, E. E., Eckels, P. C., Damle, S. S., Tsuruta, Y., Johnson, J. L., et al. (2009). HMGB1 is markedly elevated within 6 hours of mechanical trauma in humans. *Shock (Augusta, GA)* 32, 17. doi: 10.1097/SHK.0b013e3181997173

102. Pitkanen, A., and Lukasiuk, K. (2009). Molecular and cellular basis of epileptogenesis in symptomatic epilepsy. *Epilepsy Behav.* 14(Suppl. 1), 16–25. doi: 10.1016/j.yebeh.2008.09.023

103. Ransohoff, R. M., and Perry, V. H. (2009). Microglial physiology: unique stimuli, specialized responses. *Annu. Rev. Immunol.* 27, 119–145. doi: 10.1146/annurev. immunol.021908.132528

104. Ravizza, T., Terrone, G., Salamone, A., Frigerio, F., Balosso, S., Antoine, D. J., et al. (2017). High mobility group box 1 is a novel pathogenic factor and a mechanistic biomarker for epilepsy. *Brain Behav. Immun.* 72, 14–21. doi: 10.1016/j.bbi.2017.10.008

105. Ray, R., Juranek, J. K., and Rai, V. (2016). RAGE axis in neuroinflammation, neurodegeneration and its emerging role in the pathogenesis of amyotrophic lateral sclerosis. *Neurosci. Biobehav. Rev.* 62, 48–55. doi: 10.1016/j.neubiorev. 2015.12.006

106. Reddy, D. S. (2013). Neuroendocrine aspects of catamenial epilepsy. *Horm. Behav.* 63, 254–266. doi: 10.1016/j.yhbeh.2012.04.016

107. Riazi, K., Galic, M. A., and Pittman, Q. J. (2010). Contributions of peripheral inflammation to seizure susceptibility: cytokines and brain excitability. *Epilepsy Res.* 89, 34–42. doi: 10.1016/j.eplepsyres.2009.09.004

108. Richard, S. A., Min, W., Su, Z., and Xu, H. (2017). High mobility group box 1 and traumatic brain injury. *J. Behav. Brain Sci.* 7:50. doi: 10.4236/jbbs.2017.72006

109. Robinson, A. P., Caldis, M. W., Harp, C. T., Goings, G. E., and Miller, S. D. (2013). High-mobility group box 1 protein (HMGB1) neutralization ameliorates experimental autoimmune encephalomyelitis. *J. Autoimmun.* 43, 32–43. doi: 10.1016/j.jaut.2013.02.005

110. Sanderson, D. J., Good, M. A., Seeburg, P. H., Sprengel, R., Rawlins, J. N., and Bannerman, D. M. (2008). The role of the GluR-A (GluR1) AMPA receptor subunit in learning and memory. *Prog. Brain Res.* 169, 159–178. doi: 10.1016/ S0079-6123(07)00009-X

111. Sasaki, T., Liu, K., Agari, T., Yasuhara, T., Morimoto, J., Okazaki, M., et al. (2016). Anti-high mobility group box 1 antibody exerts neuroprotection in a rat model of Parkinson's disease. *Exp. Neurol.* 275(Pt 1), 220–231. doi: 10.1016/ j.expneurol.2015.11.003

112. Scaffidi, P., Misteli, T., and Bianchi, M. E. (2002). Release of chromatin protein HMGB1 by necrotic cells triggers inflammation. *Nature* 418, 191–195. doi: 10.1038/nature00858

113. Schiapparelli, L., Simon, A., Del Rio, J., and Frechilla, D. (2006). Opposing effects of AMPA and 5-HT 1A receptor blockade on passive avoidance and object recognition performance: correlation with AMPA receptor subunit expression in rat hippocampus. *Neuropharmacology* 50, 897–907. doi: 10.1016/ j.neuropharm.2006.02.005

114. Schierbeck, H., Lundback, P., Palmblad, K., Klevenvall, L., Erlandsson-Harris, H., Andersson, U., et al. (2011). Monoclonal anti-HMGB1 (high mobility group box chromosomal protein 1) antibody protection in two experimental arthritis models. *Mol. Med.* 17, 1039–1044. doi: 10.2119/molmed.2010. 00264

115. Schwarze, U., Hahn, C., Bengner, T., Stodieck, S., Buchel, C., and Sommer, T. (2009). Enhanced activity during associative encoding in the affected hippocampus in right temporal lobe epilepsy patients. *Brain Res.* 1297, 112–117. doi: 10.1016/j.brainres.2009.08.036

116. Shi, Y., Zhang, L., Teng, J., and Miao, W. (2018). HMGB1 mediates microglia activation via the TLR4/NF-κB pathway in coriaria lactone induced epilepsy. *Mol. Med. Rep.* 17, 5125–5131. doi: 10.3892/mmr.2018.8485

117. Shimada, T., Takemiya, T., Sugiura, H., and Yamagata, K. (2014). Role of inflammatory mediators in the pathogenesis of epilepsy. *Mediat. Inflamm.* 2014:901902. doi: 10.1155/2014/901902

118. Sloviter, R. S., and Bumanglag, A. V. (2013). Defining "epileptogenesis" and identifying "antiepileptogenic targets" in animal models of acquired temporal lobe epilepsy is not as simple as it might seem. *Neuropharmacology* 69, 3–15. doi: 10.1016/j.neuropharm.2012.01.022

119. Song, J.-H., Lee, J.-W., Shim, B., Lee, C.-Y., Choi, S., Kang, C., et al. (2013). Glycyrrhizin alleviates neuroinflammation and memory deficit induced by systemic lipopolysaccharide treatment in mice. *Molecules* 18, 15788–15803. doi: 10.3390/molecules181215788

120. Streit, W. J., Mrak, R. E., and Griffin, W. S. T. (2004). Microglia and neuroinflammation: a pathological perspective. *J. Neuroinflamm.* 1:14.

121. Su, X., Wang, H., Zhao, J., Pan, H., and Mao, L. (2011). Beneficial effects of ethyl pyruvate through inhibiting high-mobility group box 1 expression and TLR4/NF-B pathway after traumatic brain injury in the rat. *Mediat. Inflamm.* 2011:807142. doi: 10.1155/2011/807142

122. Sun, Y., Chen, H., Dai, J., Zou, H., Gao, M., Wu, H., et al. (2015). HMGB1 expression patterns during the progression of experimental autoimmune encephalomyelitis. *J. Neuroimmunol.* 280, 29–35. doi: 10.1016/j.jneuroim.2015. 02.005

123. Tansey, M. G., and Goldberg, M. S. (2010). Neuroinflammation in Parkinson's disease: its role in neuronal death and implications for therapeutic intervention. *Neurobiol. Dis.* 37, 510–518. doi: 10.1016/j.nbd.2009.11.004

124. Terrando, N., Rei Fidalgo, A., Vizcaychipi, M., Cibelli, M., Ma, D., Monaco, C., et al. (2010). The impact of IL-1 modulation on the development of lipopolysaccharide-induced cognitive dysfunction. *Crit. Care* 14:R88. doi: 10. 1186/cc9019

125. Tian, J., Dai, H., Deng, Y., Zhang, J., Li, Y., Zhou, J., et al. (2015). The effect of HMGB1 on sub-toxic chlorpyrifos exposure-induced neuroinflammation in amygdala of neonatal rats. *Toxicology* 338, 95–103. doi: 10.1016/j.tox.2015.10.010

126. Utech, M., Mennigen, R., and Bruewer, M. (2009). Endocytosis and recycling of tight junction proteins in inflammation. *BioMed. Res. Int.* 2010:484987.

127. Uzawa, A., Mori, M., Taniguchi, J., Masuda, S., Muto, M., and Kuwabara, S. (2013). Anti-high mobility group box 1 monoclonal antibody ameliorates experimental autoimmune encephalomyelitis. *Clin. Exp. Immunol.* 172, 37–43. doi: 10.1111/ cei.12036

128. Vacas, S., Degos, V., Tracey, K. J., and Maze, M. (2014). High-mobility group box 1 protein initiates postoperative cognitive decline by engaging bone marrow–derived macrophages. *Anesthesiology* 120, 1160–1167. doi: 10.1097/ ALN.0000000000000045

129. Venereau, E., De Leo, F., Mezzapelle, R., Careccia, G., Musco, G., and Bianchi, M. E. (2016). HMGB1 as biomarker and drug target. *Pharmacol. Res.* 111, 534–544. doi: 10.1016/j.phrs.2016.06.031

130. Vezzani, A. (2015). Anti-inflammatory drugs in epilepsy: does it impact epileptogenesis? *Exp. Opin. Drug Saf.* 14, 583–592. doi: 10.1517/14740338.2015. 1010508

131. Vezzani, A., Auvin, S., Ravizza, T., and Aronica, E. (2012). "Glia-neuronal interactions in ictogenesis and epileptogenesis: role of inflammatory mediators," in *SourceJasper's Basic Mechanisms of the Epilepsies [Internet]*, 4th Edn, eds J. L. Noebels, M. Avoli, M. A. Rogawski, R. W. Olsen, and A. V. Delgado-Escueta (Bethesda, MD: National Center for Biotechnology Information).

132. Vezzani, A., French, J., Bartfai, T., and Baram, T. Z. (2011). The role of inflammation in epilepsy. *Nat. Rev. Neurol.* 7, 31–40. doi: 10.1038/nrneurol. 2010.178

133. Vezzani, A., and Granata, T. (2005). Brain inflammation in epilepsy: experimental and clinical evidence. *Epilepsia* 46, 1724–1743. doi: 10.1111/j.1528-1167.2005. 00298.x

134. Viviani, B., Bartesaghi, S., Gardoni, F., Vezzani, A., Behrens, M., Bartfai, T., et al. (2003). Interleukin-1β enhances NMDA receptor-mediated intracellular calcium increase through activation of the Src family of kinases. *J. Neurosci.* 23, 8692–8700. doi: 10.1523/JNEUROSCI.23-25-08692.2003

135. Vos, P., Jacobs, B., Andriessen, T., Lamers, K., Borm, G., Beems, T., et al. (2010). GFAP and S100B are biomarkers of traumatic brain injury An observational cohort study. *Neurology* 75, 1786–1793. doi: 10.1212/WNL.0b013e3181fd62d2 Walker, L., Tse, K., Ricci, E., Thippeswamy, T., Sills, G. J., White, S. H., et al. (2014). High mobility group box 1 in the inflammatory pathogenesis of epilepsy: profiling circulating levels after experimental and clinical seizures. *Lancet* 383:S105. doi: 10.1016/S0140-6736(14)60368-8

136. Walker, L. E., Frigerio, F., Ravizza, T., Ricci, E., Tse, K., Jenkins, R. E., et al. (2017). Molecular isoforms of high-mobility group box 1 are mechanistic biomarkers for epilepsy. *J. Clin. Invest.* 127, 2118–2132. doi: 10.1172/JCI 92001

137. Wan, W., Cao, L., Khanabdali, R., Kalionis, B., Tai, X., and Xia, S. (2016). The emerging role of HMGB1 in neuropathic pain: a potential therapeutic target for neuroinflammation. *J. Immunol. Res.* 2016, 1–9. doi: 10.1155/2016/643 0423

138. Wang, D., Liu, K., Wake, H., Teshigawara, K., Mori, S., and Nishibori, M. (2017). Anti-high mobility group box-1 (HMGB1) antibody inhibits hemorrhage- induced brain injury and improved neurological deficits in rats. *Sci. Rep.* 7:46243. doi: 10.1038/srep46243

139. Wang, H., Bloom, O., Zhang, M., Vishnubhakat, J. M., Ombrellino, M., Che, J., et al. (1999). HMG-1 as a late mediator of endotoxin lethality in mice. *Science* 285, 248–251. doi: 10.1126/science.285.5425.248

140. Wang, J., Hu, X., Xie, J., Xu, W., and Jiang, H. (2015). Beta-1-adrenergic receptors mediate Nrf2-HO-1-HMGB1 axis regulation to attenuate hypoxia/reoxygenation-induced cardiomyocytes injury in vitro. *Cell Physiol. Biochem.* 35, 767–777. doi: 10.1159/000369736

141. Wang, K. Y., Yu, G. F., Zhang, Z. Y., Huang, Q., and Dong, X. Q. (2012). Plasma high-mobility group box 1 levels and prediction of outcome in patients with traumatic brain injury. *Clin. Chim. Acta* 413, 1737–1741. doi: 10.1016/j.cca. 2012.07.002

142. Weber, M. D., Frank, M. G., Tracey, K. J., Watkins, L. R., and Maier, S. F. (2015). Stress induces the danger-associated molecular pattern HMGB-1 in the hippocampus of male Sprague Dawley rats: a priming stimulus of microglia and the NLRP3 inflammasome. *J. Neurosci.* 35, 316–324. doi: 10.1523/JNEUROSCI. 3561-14.2015

143. Webster, K. M., Sun, M., Crack, P., O'Brien, T. J., Shultz, S. R., and Semple, B. D. (2017). Inflammation in epileptogenesis after traumatic brain injury. *J. Neuroinflamm.* 14:10. doi: 10.1186/s12974-016-0786-1

144. Weeber, E. J., and Sweatt, J. D. (2002). Molecular neurobiology of human cognition. *Neuron* 33, 845–848. doi: 10.1016/S0896-6273(02)00634-7

145. Xiangjin, G., Jin, X., Banyou, M., Gong, C., Peiyuan, G., Dong, W., et al. (2014). Effect of glycyrrhizin on traumatic brain injury in rats and its mechanism. *Chin. J. Traumatol* 17, 1–7.

146. Xie, Y., Yu, N., Chen, Y., Zhang, K., Ma, H. Y., and Di, Q. (2017). HMGB1 regulates P-glycoprotein expression in status epilepticus rat brains via the RAGE/NF- κB signaling pathway. *Mol. Med. Rep.* 16, 1691–1700. doi: 10.3892/mmr.2017. 6772

147. Yang, H., Hreggvidsdottir, H. S., Palmblad, K., Wang, H., Ochani, M., Li, J., et al. (2010). A critical cysteine is required for HMGB1 binding to Toll-like receptor 4 and activation of macrophage cytokine release. *Proc. Natl. Acad. Sci. U.S.A.* 107, 11942–11947. doi: 10.1073/pnas.1003893107

148. Yang, H., and Tracey, K. J. (2010). Targeting HMGB1 in inflammation. *Biochim. Biophys. Acta* 1799, 149–156. doi: 10.1016/j.bbagrm.2009.11.019

149. Yang, H., Wang, H., Czura, C. J., and Tracey, K. J. (2005). The cytokine activity of HMGB1. *J. Leukoc. Biol.* 78, 1–8. doi: 10.1189/jlb.1104648

150. Yang, L., Wang, F., Yang, L., Yuan, Y., Chen, Y., Zhang, G., et al. (2018). HMGB1 a-box reverses brain edema and deterioration of neurological function in a traumatic brain injury mouse model. *Cell. Physiol. Biochem.* 46, 2532–2542. doi: 10.1159/000489659

151. Yang, Q.-W., Lu, F.-L., Zhou, Y., Wang, L., Zhong, Q., Lin, S., et al. (2011). HMBG1 mediates ischemia—Reperfusion injury by TRIF-adaptor independent toll-like receptor 4 signaling. *J. Cereb. Blood Flow Metab.* 31, 593–605. doi: 10.1038/ jcbfm.2010.129

152. Yang, W., Li, J., Shang, Y., Zhao, L., Wang, M., Shi, J., et al. (2017). HMGB1-TLR4 axis plays a regulatory role in the pathogenesis of mesial temporal lobe epilepsy in immature rat model and children via the p38MAPK

153. signaling pathway. *Neurochem. Res.* 42, 1179–1190. doi: 10.1007/s11064-016- 2153-0

153. Yin, H., Huang, L., Ouyang, T., and Chen, L. (2018). Baicalein improves liver inflammation in diabetic db/db mice by regulating HMGB1/TLR4/NF-κB signaling pathway. *Int. Immunopharmacol.* 55, 55–62. doi: 10.1016/j.intimp. 2017.12.002

154. Youn, J. H., Oh, Y. J., Kim, E. S., Choi, J. E., and Shin, J. S. (2008). High mobility group box 1 protein binding to lipopolysaccharide facilitates transfer of lipopolysaccharide to CD14 and enhances lipopolysaccharide-mediated TNF-alpha production in human monocytes. *J. Immunol.* 180, 5067–5074. doi: 10.4049/jimmunol.180.7.5067

155. Zaben, M., Haan, N., Asharouf, F., Di Pietro, V., Khan, D., Ahmed, A., et al. (2017). Role of proinflammatory cytokines in the inhibition of hippocampal neurogenesis in mesial temporal lobe epilepsy. *Lancet* 389:S105. doi: 10.1016/ S0140-6736(17)30501-9

156. Zhang, J., Takahashi, H. K., Liu, K., Wake, H., Liu, R., Maruo, T., et al. (2011). Anti-high mobility group box-1 monoclonal antibody protects the blood– brain barrier from ischemia-induced disruption in rats. *Stroke* 42, 1420–1428. doi: 10.1161/STROKEAHA.110.598334

157. Zhao, J., Wang, Y., Xu, C., Liu, K., Wang, Y., Chen, L., et al. (2017). Therapeutic potential of an anti-high mobility group box-1 monoclonal antibody in epilepsy. *Brain Behav. Immun.* 64, 308–319. doi: 10.1016/j.bbi.2017.02.002

158. Zhou, Y., Xiong, K.-L., Lin, S., Zhong, Q., Lu, F.-L., Liang, H., et al. (2010). Elevation of high-mobility group protein box-1 in serum correlates with severity of acute intracerebral hemorrhage. *Mediat. Inflamm.* 2010:142458. doi: 10.1155/2010/142458

159. Zou, J. Y., and Crews, F. T. (2014). Release of neuronal HMGB1 by ethanol through decreased HDAC activity activates brain neuroimmune signaling. *PLoS One* 9:e87915. doi: 10.1371/journal.pone.0087915

13

An Assay to Determine Mechanisms of Rapid Autoantibody-Induced Neurotransmitter Receptor Endocytosis and Vesicular Trafficking in Autoimmune Encephalitis

Elsie Amedonu[1,2], Christoph Brenker[3], Sumanta Barman[4], Julian A. Schreiber[1], Sebastian Becker[1], Stefan Peischard[1], Nathalie Strutz-Seebohm[1], Christine Strippel[2], Andre Dik[2], Hans-Peter Hartung[4], Thomas Budde[5], Heinz Wiendl[2], Timo Strünker[3], Bernhard Wünsch[6], Norbert Goebels[4], Sven G. Meuth[2], Guiscard Seebohm[1] and Nico Melzer[2]*

[1] Myocellular Electrophysiology and Molecular Biology, Institute for Genetics of Heart Diseases, University of Muenster, Muenster, Germany, [2] Department of Neurology, University of Muenster, Muenster, Germany, [3] Centre of Reproductive Medicine and Andrology, University of Muenster, Muenster, Germany, [4] Department of Neurology, Universitätsklinikum and Center for Neurology and Neuropsychiatry LVR Klinikum, Heinrich Heine University Duesseldorf, Duesseldorf, Germany, [5] Institute for Physiology I, University of Muenster, Muenster, Germany, [6] Institute for Pharmaceutical and Medical Chemistry, University of Muenster, Muenster, Germany

*Correspondence:
Nico Melzer
nico.melzer@ukmuenster.de

N-Methyl-D-aspartate (NMDA) receptors (NMDARs) are among the most important excitatory neurotransmitter receptors in the human brain. Autoantibodies to the human NMDAR cause the most frequent form of autoimmune encephalitis involving autoantibody-mediated receptor cross-linking and subsequent internalization of the antibody-receptor complex. This has been deemed to represent the predominant antibody effector mechanism depleting the NMDAR from the synaptic and extra-synaptic neuronal cell membrane. To assess in detail the molecular mechanisms of autoantibody-induced NMDAR endocytosis, vesicular trafficking, and exocytosis we transiently co-expressed rat GluN1-1a-EGFP and GluN2B-ECFP alone or together with scaffolding postsynaptic density protein 95 (PSD-95), wild-type (WT), or dominant-negative (DN) mutant Ras-related in brain (RAB) proteins (RAB5WT, RAB5DN, RAB11WT, RAB11DN) in HEK 293T cells. The cells were incubated with a pH-rhodamine-labeled human recombinant monoclonal GluN1 IgG1 autoantibody (GluN1-aAb$^{pH-rhod}$) genetically engineered from clonally expanded intrathecal plasma cells from a patient with anti-NMDAR encephalitis, and the pH-rhodamine fluorescence was tracked over time. We show that due to the acidic luminal pH, internalization of the NMDAR-autoantibody complex into endosomes and lysosomes increases the pH-rhodamine fluorescence. The increase in fluorescence allows for mechanistic assessment of endocytosis, vesicular trafficking in these vesicular compartments, and exocytosis of the NMDAR-autoantibody complex under steady state conditions. Using this method, we demonstrate a role for PSD-95 in stabilization of NMDARs in the cell membrane in the presence of GluN1-aAb$^{pH-rhod}$, while RAB proteins did not exert a significant effect on vertical trafficking of the internalized NMDAR autoantibody complex in this heterologous expression system. This novel assay allows to unravel molecular mechanisms of autoantibody-induced receptor internalization and to study novel small-scale specific molecular-based therapies for autoimmune encephalitis syndromes.

Keywords: autoimmune encephalitis, N-Methyl-D-aspartate receptors, cross-linking, endocytosis, vesicular trafficking, exocytosis, autoantibodies

INTRODUCTION

Most of the glutamatergic signaling mechanisms in the central nervous system (CNS) rely on the binding of this neurotransmitter (NT) to specific glutamate receptors (GluRs). Ionotropic ligand-gated ion channels (iGluRs) and metabotropic G protein-coupled receptors (mGluRs) mediate fast and slow glutamatergic excitatory synaptic transmission at synapses between neuronal axons and dendrites (1). The iGluRs include the slow, modulatory N-Methyl-D-aspartate receptors (NMDARs), the fast α-Amino-3-hydroxy-5-methyl-4-isoxazolepropionic acid receptors (AMPARs) (2), and the Kainate receptors (KARs), which typically do not contribute to baseline synaptic transmission.

Functional adult neuronal NMDARs are hetero-tetrameric complexes, formed predominantly by two GluN1 and two GluN2 subunits (3). The subunits share a similar membrane topology, i.e., four transmembrane domains (M1–M4), a reentrant membrane loop between M3 and M4 domains, and long extracellular N- and intracellular C-termini (relatively short for GluN1) (4). Hallmarks of NMDARs include voltage-sensitive block by extracellular Mg^{2+}, slow current kinetics, and high Ca^{2+} permeability (1). Thereby, NMDARs serve a crucial function in synaptic plasticity (expressed as a change in receptor number and functional properties), learning, and memory. These processes start with the release of glutamate from presynaptic axon terminals and the subsequent binding together with the co-agonist glycine mainly to postsynaptic NMDARs. Postsynaptic NMDARs, in turn, are associated with and regulated by several proteins that together constitute the postsynaptic density (PSD), an elaborate complex of interlinked proteins and elements of the cytoskeleton.

Neuronal glutamate receptor trafficking is a multi-step process that involves protein synthesis at the dendritic tree of the postsynaptic neuron, receptor subunit quality control and

assemblage in the endoplasmic reticulum (ER), processing in the Golgi apparatus (GA), vesicular packaging in the Golgi complex (GC), subsequent *vertical trafficking* to the neuronal cell surface membrane and anchorage at the PSD, *lateral trafficking* into and out of the PSD, as well as the internalization (endocytosis), subsequent neuronal surface membrane reinsertion (exocytosis) carried out by endosomes (*vertical trafficking*) or degradation carried out by lysosomes (5). At each step of the trafficking process, NMDARs associate with specific partner proteins that allow for their maturation and/or transportation (4).

Glutamate receptors are major targets in autoimmune encephalitis syndromes (6, 7), in which autoantibodies of the immunoglobulin (Ig) G type target iGluRs like NMDARs (8) and AMPARs (9) as well as mGluRs like metabotropic glutamate receptor 1 (mGluR1) (10) and 5 (mGluR5) (11). These autoantibodies disrupt receptor function, cross-link receptors leading to internalization of the antibody-receptor complex (9, 12–15), and activate complement depending on the autoantibody, its IgG subclass, and the complement concentration in the cerebrospinal fluid.

NMDAR autoantibodies are of the IgG 1 or 3 subtypes and can directly affect the gating of the receptor (16). Residues N^{368}/G^{369} in the extracellular domain of the GluN1 subunit of NMDARs may form part of the immunodominant binding region for IgG on the receptor molecule. In single-channel recordings, antibody binding to the receptor instantly caused more frequent openings and prolonged open times of the receptor (16). Moreover, NMDAR autoantibodies caused selective and reversible decrease in postsynaptic surface density and synaptic anchoring of NMDAR in both glutamatergic and GABAergic rat hippocampal neurons by disrupting the interaction of NMDAR with Ephrin-B2 receptors (17), followed by selective NMDAR cross-linking and internalization (13, 14). Consistently, NMDAR antibodies selectively decreased NMDAR-mediated miniature excitatory post-synaptic currents (mEPSCs) without affecting AMPAR-mediated mEPSCs in cultured rat hippocampal neurons (13).

In cultured rat hippocampal neurons, once internalized, antibody-bound NMDAR traffic through recycling endosomes and lysosomes, but do not induce compensatory changes in glutamate receptor gene expression (14). The internalized antibody-receptor complexes co-localize rather with RAB11-positive recycling endosomes than with Lamp1-positive lysosomes suggesting subsequent recycling and exocytosis (14). The process of NMDAR internalization plateaus after 12 h, reaching a steady state that persists throughout the duration of the antibody treatment (14), likely reflecting a state of equilibrium between the rate of receptor internalization and the

Abbreviations: AMPA, α-Amino-3-hydroxy-5-methyl-4-isoxazolepropionic acid; AMPAR, α-Amino-3-hydroxy-5-methyl-4-isoxazolepropionic acid receptor; CNS, central nervous system; DMEM, Dulbecco's modified Eagle's medium; DN, dominant-negative; ECFP, enhanced cyan fluorescent protein; EE, early endosomes; EGFP, enhanced green fluorescent protein; ER, endoplasmic reticulum; FBS, fetal bovine serum; GluN1-aAb$^{pH-rhod}$, pH-rhodamine-labeled human recombinant monoclonal GluN1 IgG1 autoantibody; GA, Golgi apparatus; GC, Golgi complex; GluR, glutamate receptors; Ig, immunoglobulin; iGluR, ionotropic glutamate receptor; KAR, kainate receptor; NEAA, non-essential amino acids; NMDA, N-Methyl-D-aspartate; NMDAR, N-Methyl-D-aspartate receptor; NT, neurotransmitter; mEPSCs, miniature excitatory post-synaptic currents; mGluR, metabotropic G-protein coupled receptor; PSD-95, postsynaptic density protein 95; RAB, Ras-related in brain; RE, recycling endosomes; RV, recycling vesicle; WT, wild-type.

rate of receptor (re-)insertion from different compartments into the surface membrane (14).

Probably due to the lack of blood-brain barrier disruption in NMDAR encephalitis and subsequent lack of relevant complement concentrations in the cerebrospinal fluid, as well as internalization of NMDAR together with the autoantibodies, no complement depositions or major neuronal loss could be detected in biopsy specimens of patients with NMDAR encephalitis, despite large numbers of intracerebral autoantibody-secreting plasma cells (18, 19). Indeed, fully reversible impairment of behavior and memory occurs in mice receiving passive intrathecal transfer of NMDAR autoantibodies (20, 21) that is prevented by co-application of ephrin (22).

The effects on receptor-mediated currents are rather small in heterologous expression systems and do not allow for mechanistic studies on autoantibody-induced neurotransmitter receptor internalization and trafficking in anti-NMDAR encephalitis and other forms of autoimmune encephalitis (21). Thus, the aim of this study was to develop an assay suitable to study in molecular detail the mechanism of autoantibody-induced NMDAR endocytosis, vesicular trafficking, and exocytosis and potentially to study novel small-scale specific molecular-based therapies for autoimmune encephalitis syndromes.

MATERIALS AND METHODS

Construction of NMDAR Expression Vectors

NMDAR constructs were kindly provided by Prof. Michael Hollmann, Receptor Biochemistry, Faculty of Chemistry and Biochemistry, Ruhr University Bochum, Germany. cDNAs encoding the rat GluN1-1a and GluN2B NMDAR subunits were sub-cloned into the pEGFP-N1 and pECFP-N1 mammalian expression vectors, respectively. To allow for the visualization of the subunits, enhanced cyan fluorescent protein (ECFP), and enhanced green fluorescent protein (EGFP) were inserted in-frame at the N-terminus of the subunits. The subunit-containing plasmids were amplified via growth in E. coli followed by purification based on a modified alkaline lysis procedure (QIAGEN Miniprep kit).

The generation of PSD-95 as well as WT and DN RAB5 and RAB11 expression vector constructs has been described elsewhere (5, 23).

HEK 293T Cell Co-transfection

HEK 293T cells were cultured in growth media comprising high-glucose Dulbecco's modified Eagle's medium (DMEM) supplemented with 10% fetal bovine serum (FBS), non-essential amino acids (NEAA), Pen-Strep, and 2 mM glutamine. Two days prior to transfection, exponentially growing cells were seeded on poly-D-lysine-coated glass bottom 96-well-plates to a density of approximately 5.0–8.0×10^5/well. Two hours prior to co-transfection, the culture medium was replaced with fresh culture medium. HEK 293T cells were then transiently co-transfected with the cDNAs (0.25 μg GluN1-1a-EGFP and 0.25 μg GluN2B-ECFP) encoding the NMDAR subunits as well as

PSD-95, or WT, or DN RAB proteins using the FuGene HD (Promega Corporations) transfection technique according to manufacturer's instructions or left untransfected. 24 h post co-transfection, cells were seeded onto poly-D-lysine-coated glass bottom 96-well-plates. Confocal laser-scanning microscopy was used to quantify cell-surface NMDAR density (×63 glycerol objective; TCS-SP5 Leica- Microsystems, Germany).

pH-rhodamine Labeling of a Human Recombinant Monoclonal GluN1 Autoantibody

Generation of a recombinant human monoclonal GluN1 autoantibody (GluN1-aAb) engineered from clonally expanded intrathecal plasma cells of a patient with anti-NMDAR encephalitis has recently been described (21). Labeling of GluN1-aAb was performed using a pHrodo™ Red Microscale Labeling Kit (Thermofisher Scientific) according to the recommendations of the supplier. Briefly, 100 μL of GluN1-aAb solution (1 mg/mL in PBS) were transferred to a "component D" containing reaction tube and supplemented with 10 μL of 1M sodium bicarbonate. pHrodo red succinimidyl ester was dissolved in 10 μL of DMSO. From the resulting solution, 0.70 μL (as calculated according to the equation 1 of the labeling kit's protocol) was added to the reaction tube containing the pH-adjusted GluN1-aAb. This reaction mixture was incubated for 15 min at RT to allow conjugation. For separation from unbound dye, the reaction mix was spun through a resin-containing column (provided with the kit) at 1,000 g for 5 min. The purified pH-rhodo red labeled GluN1-aAb (GluN1-aAb$^{\text{pH−rhod}}$) was recovered from the collection tube and stored aliquoted at −20°C, while unbound dye remained in the resin.

Co-incubation of GluN1-aAb$^{\text{pH-rhod}}$ With HEK 293T Cells Expressing GluN1-1a-EGFP/GluN2B-ECFP NMDARs and Fluorescence Intensity Analysis

The rhodamine fluorophore possesses a well-known pH- and temperature-dependent fluorescence quantum yield (24), which decreases linearly as pH and temperature increases (25). These physicochemical properties needed to be considered in our experimental setting.

Untransfected or co-transfected HEK 293T cells from the same 96-well-plate were incubated with GluN1-aAb$^{\text{pH−rhod}}$ at a concentration of 4 μg/ml in phosphate-buffered saline (PBS, pH 7.4) for 2 min. After that, unbound GluN1-aAb$^{\text{pH−rhod}}$ was washed-out by superfusing 96-wells with PBS to yield cell-bound GluN1-aAb$^{\text{pH−rhod}}$ fluorescence. Wells on the same 96-well-plate without cells incubated with GluN1-aAb$^{\text{pH−rhod}}$ at a concentration of 4 μg/ml in PBS without wash-off served as control. All incubations were conducted at 4°C on ice to prevent endocytosis prior to recordings.

Subsequently, fluorescence of GluN1-EGFP and GluN1-aAb$^{\text{pH−rhod}}$ was excited at 480 and 520 nm and detected at 510 nm (confocal imaging) and 580 nm (plate reader), respectively, verifying GluN1-1a-EGFP expression and presence of the GluN1-aAb-bound rhodamine fluorescence (GluN1-aAb$^{pH-rhod}$).

Subsequently, the temperature was increased rapidly from 4 to 30°C to allow for endocytosis, and pH-rhodamine-fluorescence was repetitively excited at 520 nm and the emission was detected at 580 nm. The overall pH-rhodamine fluorescence decreased exponentially with time reaching a steady state after approximately 500 s mainly reflecting the known temperature-dependent fluorescence quantum yield of rhodamine under all experimental conditions.

The steady state pH-rhodamine-fluorescence intensity at 580 nm after 500 s of HEK 293T cells expressing GluN1-1a-EGFP/GluN2B-ECFP NMDARs was significantly higher compared to untransfected HEK 293T cells and served as a cumulative measure of endocytosis of GluN1-aAb$^{pH-rhod}$ bound to the NMDAR with subsequent acidification within endosomes and/or lysosomes and exocytosis. This allowed for mechanistic studies in HEK 293T cells expressing GluN1-1a-EGFP/GluN2B-ECFP NMDARs co-transfected with scaffolding protein PSD-95 as well as RAB5WT and RAB5DN (mediating vesicle endocytosis) and RAB11WT or RAB11DN (mediating vesicle exocytosis).

Statistical Analysis

Data was analyzed using Origin 9 (OriginLab Corporation). One-way ANOVA followed by multiple pair-wise comparisons with Bonferroni's *post-hoc* correction was used to statistically analyze differences in fluorescence intensity; $p \leq 0.05$ were considered as significant; data in figures were expressed as mean ± SEM. All experiments were performed in triplicates.

RESULTS

To assess in detail the molecular mechanisms of NMDAR autoantibody-induced NMDAR endocytosis, vesicular trafficking, and exocytosis we transiently expressed rat GluN1-1a-EGFP and GluN2B-ECFP alone or together with PSD-95 or with WT- or DN-mutant RAB proteins (RAB5WT, RAB5DN, RAB11WT, RAB11DN) in HEK 293T cells. As a control, HEK 293T cells were left untransfected.

The cells were incubated with a pH-rhodamine-labeled human recombinant monoclonal GluN1 IgG1 autoantibody [GluN1-aAb$^{pH-rhod}$, (21)].

We surmised that the pH-rhodamine fluorescence is increased during the ensuing internalization of the NMDAR-autoantibody complex, due to the acidic luminal pH of endosomes and lysosomes. This might allow for mechanistic assessment of endocytosis, vesicular trafficking in both vesicular compartments and exocytosis of the NMDAR-autoantibody complex (for assay design see **Figure 1**).

In a first set of experiments, HEK 293T cells were transiently co-transfected only with rat GluN1-1a-EGFP and GluN2B-ECFP or left untransfected. After 2 days, expression of fluorescently labeled NMDARs was verified using confocal laser-scanning microscopy. About 70–80% of the cells expressed GluN1-1a-EGFP as subunit putatively targeted by the GluN1-aAb$^{pH-rhod}$ (**Figure 2A**) and GluN2B-ECFP (data not shown). Longer

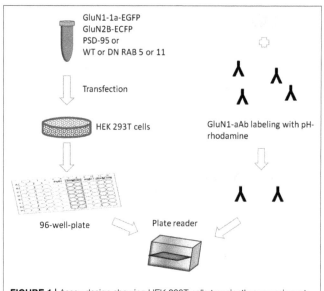

FIGURE 1 | Assay design showing HEK 293T cells transiently expressing rat GluN1-1a-EGFP/GluN2B-ECFP incubated with GluN1-aAb$^{pH-rhod}$ in 96-well-plates under variable conditions in parallel.

expression times or higher amounts of NMDAR-cDNA for transfections decreased expression levels, supposedly due to cytotoxic effects of pronounced overexpression of NMDARs.

Next, GluN1-1a-EGFP- and GluN2B-ECFP-transfected and untransfected cultured cells were incubated with GluN1-aAb$^{pH-rhod}$. The incubation was performed at 4°C to stop ongoing endocytosis. After that, unbound GluN1-aAb$^{pH-rhod}$ was washed-off. As a control, wells without cells were incubated with GluN1-aAb$^{pH-rhod}$ without wash-off.

Subsequently, GluN1-1a-EGFP and GluN1-aAb$^{pH-rhod}$ fluorescence was excited at 480 nm and 520 nm and measured at 510 and 580 nm, respectively, verifying GluN1-1a-EGFP expression of transfected but not untransfected cells and presence of the GluN1-aAb-bound rhodamine fluorescence (GluN1-aAb$^{pH-rhod}$, **Figure 2B**).

The plate was subsequently transferred to a fluorescence plate reader for time-resolved detection of the pH-rhodamine fluorescence intensity at 30°C. The temperature was increased rapidly from 4–30°C to start endocytosis, and pH-rhodamine-fluorescence was repetitively excited at 520 nm and the emission was detected at 580 nm. The overall rhodamine fluorescence at 580 nm decreased exponentially with time, reaching a steady state after approximately 500 s (**Figure 3B**) mainly reflecting the known temperature-dependent fluorescence quantum yield of rhodamine (24–26) under all experimental conditions.

Of note, the fluorescence-spectrum did not change over time (**Figure 3A**), illustrating that pH-rhodamine fluorescence was detected throughout the experiments. Moreover, steady-state fluorescence intensities of empty wells without wash-off of GluN1-aAb$^{pH-rhod}$ were much larger than those of wells with HEK 293T cells illustrating the known background fluorescence of pH rhodamine at neutral pH of 7.4 in PBS (roughly 1/3 of the maximal fluorescence at acidic pH of 4.0) and thus the necessity of the washing step (**Figure 3B**).

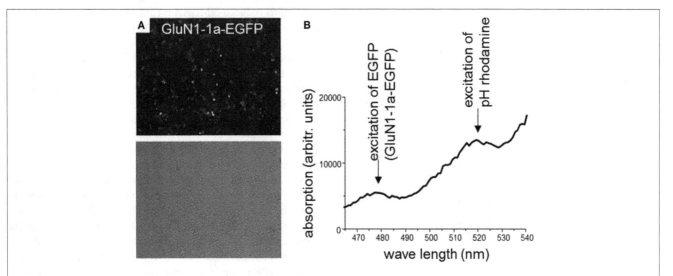

FIGURE 2 | **(A)** HEK 293T cells co-expressing rat GluN1-1a-EGFP and GluN2B-ECFP. 2 days after transfection, expression of fluorescently labeled NMDARs was verified using confocal laser-scanning microscopy. About 70–80% of the cells expressed GluN1-1a-EGFP as subunit putatively targeted by the GluN1-aAb$^{pH-rhod}$ (upper panel) and GluN2B-ECFP (data not shown). Light microscopy demonstrates typical cell densities (lower panel). **(B)** Binding of GluN1-aAb$^{pH-rhod}$ to the NMDAR subunits as determined by the plate reader experiment. HEK 293T cells expressing GluN1-1a-EGFP/GluN2B-ECFP were incubated with GluN1-aAb$^{pH-rhod}$ on ice in 96-well-plates. GluN1-1a-EGFP and GluN1-aAb$^{pH-rhod}$ fluorescence was excited at wavelengths of 480 nm and 520 nm and emission measured at wavelengths of 510 and 580 nm, respectively, verifying the GluN1-1a-EGFP expression and the binding of GluN1-aAb$^{pH-rhod}$.

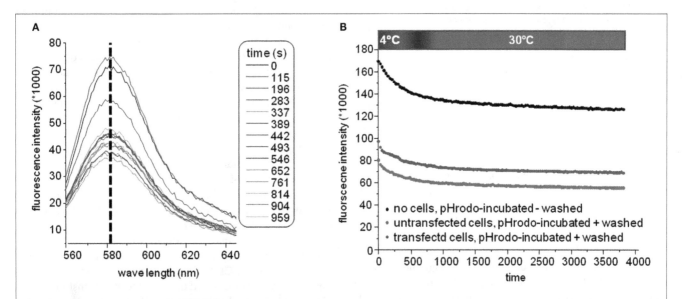

FIGURE 3 | **(A)** Spectra of the GluN1-aAb$^{pH-rhod}$ fluorescence. The overall fluorescence at 580 nm decreased over time reaching a steady state after approximately 500 s mainly reflecting the known temperature-dependent fluorescence quantum yield of rhodamine (24–26) elicited by elevating the temperature for 4–30°C at the beginning of the experiment under all experimental conditions. During this decay, the excitation spectrum did not shift/change indicating that indeed pH-rhodamine-fluorescence was detected throughout the whole experiment. **(B)** Representative time-dependent traces of the GluN1-aAb$^{pH-rhod}$ fluorescence without wash-off of the unbound GluN1-aAb$^{pH-rhod}$ in PBS at pH 7.4 (black trace) and after wash-off of unbound GluN1-aAb$^{pH-rhod}$ in wells seeded with HEK 293T cells expressing GluN1-1a-EGFP/GluN2B-ECFP (blue trace) or untransfected HEK 293T cells (red trace). The steady state pH-rhodamine-fluorescence intensity at 580 nm after 500 s of HEK 293T cells expressing GluN1-1a-EGFP/GluN2B-ECFP NMDARs was significantly higher compared to the background fluorescence of untransfected HEK 293T cells and served as a cumulative measure of endocytosis of GluN1-aAb$^{pH-rhod}$ bound to the NMDAR with subsequent acidification within endosomes and/or lysosomes and exocytosis.

The steady state pH-rhodamine-fluorescence intensity at 580 nm after 500 s of HEK 293T cells expressing GluN1-1a-EGFP/GluN2B-ECFP NMDARs was significantly higher compared to the background fluorescence of untransfected HEK 293T cells (**Figure 4**) and served as a cumulative measure of endocytosis of GluN1-aAb$^{pH-rhod}$ bound to the NMDAR with

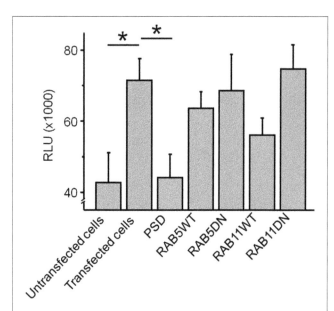

FIGURE 4 | The co-expression of GluN1-1a-EGFP/GluN2B-ECFP NMDARs with the scaffolding protein PSD-95 significantly reduced the cumulative steady state pH-rhodamine-fluorescence intensity at 580 nm after 500 s toward background levels of untransfected HEK 293T cells. In contrast, co-transfection with RAB5WT or RAB5DN (mediating/inhibiting endocytosis) or RAB11 WT or RABDN (mediating/inhibiting exocytosis) did not significantly affect the cumulative steady state pH-rhodamine-fluorescence intensity at 580 nm after 500 s in this heterologous expression system. One-way ANOVA followed by multiple pair-wise comparisons with Bonferroni's post-hoc correction was used to statistically analyze differences in fluorescence intensity; $p \leq 0.05$ were considered as significant (*); data are expressed as mean ± SEM. All experiments were performed in triplicates.

subsequent acidification within endosomes and/or lysosomes and exocytosis. This allowed for mechanistic studies in HEK 293T cells expressing GluN1-1a-EGFP/GluN2B-ECFP NMDARs co-transfected with scaffolding protein PSD-95 as well as WT and DN RAB5 (mediating vesicle endocytosis) and RAB11 (mediating vesicle exocytosis).

The co-expression of GluN1-1a-EGFP/GluN2B-ECFP NMDARs with the scaffolding protein PSD-95 significantly reduced the cumulative steady state pH-rhodamine-fluorescence intensity at 580 nm after 500 s toward background levels of untransfected HEK 293T cells (**Figure 4**). In contrast, co-transfection with RAB5WT or RAB5DN (mediating/inhibiting endocytosis) or RAB11 WT or RABDN (mediating/inhibiting exocytosis) did not significantly affect the cumulative steady state pH-rhodamine-fluorescence intensity at 580 nm after 500 s in this heterologous expression system (**Figure 4**).

DISCUSSION

NMDARs are among the most important excitatory receptors in the human brain. NMDAR autoantibodies cause encephalitis by binding to NMDARs, transducing conformational changes and subsequent endocytosis (21, 27). Recently, we showed that pre-incubation for an hour of a recombinant human monoclonal GluN1 autoantibody engineered from clonally expanded intrathecal plasma cells of a patient with anti-NMDAR

encephalitis reduced NMDAR-mediated currents recorded from *Xenopus laevis* oocytes by about 20% (21). This result is similar to previous results in *Xenopus laevis* oocytes, showing a time-dependent inhibition of steady-state NMDAR-mediated currents of about 30% within 16 min upon exposure to dialysed sera of patients with anti-NMDAR encephalitis (28). To record NMDAR-mediated currents *in Xenopus laevis* oocytes (and other heterologous expression systems), it is required to use Ca^{2+}-free media to block current inactivation (29). This might explain the rather small antibody-mediated action in oocytes (and probably other heterologous expression systems) compared to the pronounced effects on NMDAR expression on neuronal cell surface *in vitro*, *ex vivo*, and on memory impairment *in vivo* in mice. The Ca^{2+}-free recording conditions may cause conformational changes of the NMDAR induced by binding of the antibody or modulate antibody binding itself and thus diminish subsequent receptor cross-linking and internalization.

These effects on receptor-mediated currents in *Xenopus laevis* oocytes (and other heterologous expression systems) do not allow for further mechanistic studies on autoantibody-induced neurotransmitter receptor internalization and trafficking in anti-NMDAR encephalitis and other forms of autoimmune encephalitis (30). Thus, the aim of this study was to develop an assay suitable for this kind of study.

We used a pH-rhodamine labeled single recombinant human GluN1 IgG1 autoantibody [GluN1-aAb$^{pH-rhod}$, (21)]. This monoclonal autoantibody has previously been shown to evoke all effects of natural NMDAR autoantibodies contained in cerebrospinal fluid of patients with anti-NMDAR encephalitis *in vitro* and *in vivo* (21).

We tested the effects of GluN1-aAb$^{pH-rhod}$ incubation on NMDAR endocytosis, trafficking, and exocytosis mechanisms in HEK 293T cells co-transfected with EGFP-tagged GluN1-1a and ECFP-tagged GluN2B subunits alone or together with PSD-95 or WT- or DN-mutant RAB 5 (mediating endocytosis) and 11 (mediating exocytosis) proteins.

Endocytosis, intracellular trafficking, and exocytosis of the antibody-receptor complex is mediated by transporting vesicles with acidic luminal pH. Thus, we took advantage of this fact, as we found that the use of the steady state GluN1-aAb$^{pH-rhod}$ fluorescence in HEK 293T cells expressing GluN1-1a-EGFP/GluN2B-ECFP NMDARs was significantly higher compared to the background fluorescence of untransfected HEK 293T cells. Thus, this steady state fluorescence served as a cumulative measure of endocytosis of GluN1-aAb$^{pH-rhod}$ bound to the NMDAR with subsequent acidification within endosomes and/or lysosomes and exocytosis.

Using this approach we could demonstrate a role for PSD-95 for stabilization of NMDAR in the cell membrane in the presence of NMDAR autoantibodies. This suggests that autoantibody-induced depletion from the cell membrane predominantly affects extra-synaptic NMDARs not associated with PSD-95 and to a lesser extent synaptic NMDARs. This finding is consistent with the notion that autoantibodies through dissociation from clustering ephrinB2 receptors lead to lateral diffusion of synaptic NMDARs within the neuronal cell membrane out to the synapse where they become cross-linked and internalized as extra-synaptic NMDARs (17, 31). Cell membrane stabilization of synaptic NMDARs [displaying pro-survival functions (32)] and internalization of extra-synaptic NMDARs [displaying cell-death promoting functions (32)] is further consistent with the lack of overt neurodegeneration in NMDAR encephalitis despite excitotoxic excessive extracellular levels of glutamate (33–35).

Endocytosis, intracellular trafficking and exocytosis are under the guidance of small G-proteins of the RAB type. The use of functional WT and DN mutants has been previously successful in identification of intracellular trafficking pathways of glutamate receptors (36). We found that co-transfection with WT or DN RAB5 (mediating/inhibiting endocytosis) did not affect the cumulative steady state GluN1-aAb$^{pH-rhod}$ fluorescence intensity, whereas the cumulative steady state GluN1-aAb$^{pH-rhod}$ fluorescence intensity was tentatively lowered by co-transfection with WT RAB11 (mediating exocytosis) and tentatively augmented by co-transfection with RAB11DN (inhibiting exocytosis) compared to expression of NMDARs alone. This lack of overt effects of RAB proteins on endocytosis, trafficking and exocytosis of the antibody-receptor complex in our assay is probably due to the overlay by the temperature-dependent fluorescence decrease the amplitude of which is roughly as large as the steady state amplitude of the pH-dependent fluorescence increase upon internalization of the antibody-receptor complex. These opposing effects hinder detailed kinetic analysis of the autoantibody-induced vertical trafficking of the NMDAR performed here.

Hence, given the necessity of washing-off unbound GluN1-aAb$^{pH-rhod}$ and halting trafficking during that time by lowering the temperature due to the residual rhodamie fluorescence at pH 7.4 in PBS, the use of fluorophores (that inevitably are also concordantly temperature-sensitive) with an optimized pH-dependence i.e., no fluorescence at physiological pH of 7.4 might be better suited for our assay. They would enable synchronic adding of the labeled antibody to the cells cultured in PBS at pH 7.4 at constant temperature of 30°C and thus time-resolved tracking of fluorescence increase upon antibody-receptor internalization.

Taken together, we demonstrate a role for PSD-95 for stabilization of NMDAR in the cell membrane of HEK 293T cells in the presence of NMDAR autoantibodies, while RAB proteins did not exert a significant effect on vertical trafficking of the internalized NMDAR autoantibody complex in this heterologous expression system.

Our assay should be sensitive enough to study novel small-scale specific molecular-based therapies for autoimmune encephalitis that may become feasible as follows:

1) Autoantibody binding to the GluN1 subunit and subsequent induction of conformational changes in the NMDAR could be blocked by antibody fragments, for example. However, with existence of a multitude of autoantibody epitopes within the NMDAR, this approach may not be successful.
2) The autoantibody binding-induced conformational changes within the NMDAR. Small molecule allosteric modulators have recently been developed (5, 37, 38). Potentially, these compounds may be used to block the conformational changes induced by GluN1-aAb$^{pH-rhod}$ binding and thus inhibit internalization.

3) Inhibition of the GluN1-aAb$^{pH-rhod}$-induced internalization. To achieve this, general cellular trafficking pathways have to be blocked. It is questionable if such an approach can be tolerated by patients and would not cause severe side effects.

Taking these considerations into account, development and use of small molecule allosteric modulators may represent a group of drug candidates for anti-NMDAR encephalitis and other forms of autoimmune encephalitis. Evidenced by the relatively robust novel assay, they may be used to screen for compounds that block autoantibody-induced NMDAR cross-linking and internalization. This should always be accompanied by NMDAR stabilization within the synapse to avoid accumulation of NMDAR at extra-synaptic sides of the cell membrane potentially promoting excitotoxic cell death in NMDAR encephalitis.

Therefore, screening results obtained with our assay in HEK 293T overexpressing NMDAR should always be validated using super-resolution microscopy in cultured living neurons and brain slices exhibiting physiological expression levels and subcellular localization of NMDARs.

CONCLUSION

This novel assay allows to unravel molecular mechanisms of autoantibody-induced receptor internalization and to study novel small-scale specific molecular-based therapies for autoimmune encephalitis syndromes.

AUTHOR CONTRIBUTIONS

CS and AD: collected patient samples under the supervision of HW, SM, and NM; SBa and NG: performed the synthesis and pH-rhodamine labeling of GluN1-aAb$^{pH-rhod}$; EA, SBe, SP, and JS: performed the transfection, immunocytochemistry, and confocal microscopy with the HEK 293T cells; EA, CB, and TS: together with TB, NS-S, GS, and NM performed incubation of transfected HEK 293T cells with GluN1-aAb$^{pH-rhod}$ and data analysis; H-PH, BW, SM, GS, and NM: designed and supervised the project; EA, SM, GS, and NM: wrote the first draft of the manuscript. All authors contributed to and approved the final version of the manuscript.

FUNDING

This work was supported by the German Research Foundation (DFG, INST 2105/27-1 to SM), the German Academic Exchange Service (DAAD-MoE postgraduate scholarship to EA), the Walter und Ilse-Rose-Stiftung (to H-PH), the Forschungskommission of the Heinrich-Heine-University Düsseldorf, Germany (to NG) and the Bundesministerium für Bildung und Forschung (BMBF 031A232 to NG).

ACKNOWLEDGMENTS

We thank Prof. Michael Hollmann, Receptor Biochemistry, Faculty of Chemistry and Biochemistry, Ruhr University Bochum, Germany for providing the NMDAR constructs used in this study, and Christina Burhoi, Institute for Genetics of Heart Diseases (IfGH), University of Muenster, Germany, for excellent technical assistance.

REFERENCES

1. Traynelis SF, Wollmuth LP, Mcbain CJ, Menniti FS, Vance KM, Ogden KK, et al. Glutamate receptor ion channels: structure, regulation, and function. *Pharmacol Rev.* (2010) 62:405–96. doi: 10.1124/pr.109.002451

2. Hollmann M, Heinemann S. Cloned glutamate receptors. *Annu Rev Neurosci.* (1994) 17:31–108. doi: 10.1146/annurev.ne.17.030194.000335

3. Dingledine R, Borges K, Bowie D, Traynelis SF. The glutamate receptor ion channels. *Pharmacol Rev.* (1999) 51:7–61.

4. Petralia RS, Al-Hallaq RA, Wenthold RJ. Trafficking and targeting of NMDA receptors. In: Van Dongen AM, editor. *Biology of the NMDA Receptor.* Boca Raton, FL: CRC Press/Taylor & Francis (2009).

5. Seebohm G, Neumann S, Theiss C, Novkovic T, Hill EV, Tavare JM, et al. Identification of a novel signaling pathway and its relevance for GluA1 recycling. *PLoS ONE.* (2012) 7:e33889. doi: 10.1371/journal.pone.0033889

6. Melzer N, Meuth SG, Wiendl H. Paraneoplastic and non-paraneoplastic autoimmunity to neurons in the central nervous system. *J Neurol.* (2013) 260:1215–33. doi: 10.1007/s00415-012-6657-5

7. Graus F, Titulaer MJ, Balu R, Benseler S, Bien CG, Cellucci T, et al. A clinical approach to diagnosis of autoimmune encephalitis. *Lancet Neurol.* (2016) 15:391–404. doi: 10.1016/S1474-4422(15)00401-9

8. Dalmau J, Gleichman AJ, Hughes EG, Rossi JE, Peng X, Lai M, et al. Anti-NMDA-receptor encephalitis: case series and analysis of the effects of antibodies. *Lancet Neurol.* (2008) 7:1091–8. doi: 10.1016/S1474-4422(08)70224-2

9. Lai M, Hughes EG, Peng X, Zhou L, Gleichman AJ, Shu H, et al. AMPA receptor antibodies in limbic encephalitis alter synaptic receptor location. *Ann Neurol.* (2009) 65:424–34. doi: 10.1002/ana.21589

10. Sillevis Smitt P, Kinoshita A, De Leeuw B, Moll W, Coesmans M, Jaarsma D, et al. Paraneoplastic cerebellar ataxia due to autoantibodies against a glutamate receptor. *N Engl J Med.* (2000) 342:21–7. doi: 10.1056/NEJM200001063420104

11. Lancaster E, Martinez-Hernandez E, Titulaer MJ, Boulos M, Weaver S, Antoine JC, et al. Antibodies to metabotropic glutamate receptor 5 in the Ophelia syndrome. *Neurology.* (2011) 77:1698–701. doi: 10.1212/WNL.0b013e3182364a44

12. Coesmans M, Smitt PA, Linden DJ, Shigemoto R, Hirano T, Yamakawa Y, et al. Mechanisms underlying cerebellar motor deficits due to mGluR1-autoantibodies. *Ann Neurol.* (2003) 53:325–36. doi: 10.1002/ana.10451

13. Hughes EG, Peng X, Gleichman AJ, Lai M, Zhou L, Tsou R, et al. Cellular and synaptic mechanisms of anti-NMDA receptor encephalitis. *J Neurosci.* (2010) 30:5866–75. doi: 10.1523/JNEUROSCI.0167-10.2010

14. Moscato EH, Peng X, Jain A, Parsons TD, Dalmau J, Balice-Gordon RJ. Acute mechanisms underlying antibody effects in anti-N-methyl-D-aspartate receptor encephalitis. *Ann Neurol.* (2014) 76:108–19. doi: 10.1002/ana.24195

15. Peng X, Hughes EG, Moscato EH, Parsons TD, Dalmau J, Balice-Gordon RJ. Cellular plasticity induced by anti-alpha-amino-3-hydroxy-5-methyl-4-isoxazolepropionic acid (AMPA) receptor encephalitis antibodies. *Ann Neurol.* (2015) 77:381–98. doi: 10.1002/ana.24293

16. Gleichman AJ, Spruce LA, Dalmau J, Seeholzer SH, Lynch DR. Anti-NMDA receptor encephalitis antibody binding is dependent on amino acid identity of a small region within the GluN1 amino terminal domain. *J Neurosci.* (2012) 32:11082–94. doi: 10.1523/JNEUROSCI.0064-12.2012

17. Mikasova L, De Rossi P, Bouchet D, Georges F, Rogemond V, Didelot A, et al. Disrupted surface cross-talk between NMDA and Ephrin-B2 receptors in anti-NMDA encephalitis. *Brain.* (2012) 135:1606–21. doi: 10.1093/brain/aws092

18. Martinez-Hernandez E, Horvath J, Shiloh-Malawsky Y, Sangha N, Martinez-Lage M, Dalmau J. Analysis of complement and plasma cells in the brain of patients with anti-NMDAR encephalitis. *Neurology.* (2011) 77:589–93. doi: 10.1212/WNL.0b013e318228c136

19. Bien CG, Vincent A, Barnett MH, Becker AJ, Blumcke I, Graus F, et al. Immunopathology of autoantibody-associated encephalitides: clues for pathogenesis. *Brain.* (2012) 135:1622–38. doi: 10.1093/brain/aws082

20. Planaguma J, Leypoldt F, Mannara F, Gutierrez-Cuesta J, Martin-Garcia E, Aguilar E, et al. Human N-methyl D-aspartate receptor antibodies alter memory and behaviour in mice. *Brain.* (2015) 138:94–109. doi: 10.1093/brain/awu310

21. Malviya M, Barman S, Golombeck KS, Planaguma J, Mannara F, Strutz-Seebohm N, et al. NMDAR encephalitis: passive transfer from man to mouse by a recombinant antibody. *Ann Clin Transl Neurol.* (2017) 4:768–83. doi: 10.1002/acn3.444

22. Planaguma J, Haselmann H, Mannara F, Petit-Pedrol M, Grunewald B, Aguilar E, et al. Ephrin-B2 prevents N-methyl-D-aspartate receptor antibody effects on memory and neuroplasticity. *Ann Neurol.* (2016) 80:388–400. doi: 10.1002/ana.24721

23. Seebohm G, Strutz-Seebohm N, Birkin R, Dell G, Bucci C, Spinosa MR, et al. Regulation of endocytic recycling of KCNQ1/KCNE1 potassium channels. *Circ Res.* (2007) 100:686–92. doi: 10.1161/01.RES.0000260250.83824.8f

24. Ferguson J, Mau AWH. Spontaneous and stimulated emission from dyes. Spectroscopy of the neutral molecules of acridine orange, proflavine, and rhodamine B. *Aust J Chem.* (1973) 26:1617–24. doi: 10.1071/CH9731617

25. Kubin RF, Fletcher AN. Fluorescence quantum yields of some rhodamine dyes. *J Lumin.* (1982) 27:455–62. doi: 10.1016/0022-2313(82)90045-X

26. Moreau D, Lefort C, Burke R, Leveque P, O'connor RP. Rhodamine B as an optical thermometer in cells focally exposed to infrared laser light or nanosecond pulsed electric fields. *Biomed Opt Express.* (2015) 6:4105–17. doi: 10.1364/BOE.6.004105

27. Kreye J, Wenke NK, Chayka M, Leubner J, Murugan R, Maier N, et al. Human cerebrospinal fluid monoclonal N-methyl-D-aspartate receptor autoantibodies are sufficient for encephalitis pathogenesis. *Brain.* (2016) 139:2641–52. doi: 10.1093/brain/aww208

28. Castillo-Gomez E, Oliveira B, Tapken D, Bertrand S, Klein-Schmidt C, Pan H, et al. All naturally occurring autoantibodies against the NMDA receptor subunit NR1 have pathogenic potential irrespective of epitope and immunoglobulin class. *Mol Psychiatry.* (2017) 22:1776–84. doi: 10.1038/mp.2016.125

29. Levitan IB. It is calmodulin after all! Mediator of the calcium modulation of multiple ion channels. *Neuron.* (1999) 22:645–8. doi: 10.1016/S0896-6273(00)80722-9

30. Crisp SJ, Kullmann DM, Vincent A. Autoimmune synaptopathies. *Nat Rev Neurosci.* (2016) 17:103–17. doi: 10.1038/nrn.2015.27

31. Jezequel J, Johansson EM, Dupuis JP, Rogemond V, Grea H, Kellermayer B, et al. Dynamic disorganization of synaptic NMDA receptors triggered by autoantibodies from psychotic patients. *Nat Commun.* (2017) 8:1791. doi: 10.1038/s41467-017-01700-3

32. Hardingham GE, Bading H. Synaptic versus extrasynaptic NMDA receptor signalling: implications for neurodegenerative disorders. *Nat Rev Neurosci.* (2010) 11:682–96. doi: 10.1038/nrn2911

33. Melzer N, Biela A, Fahlke C. Glutamate modifies ion conduction and voltage-dependent gating of excitatory amino acid transporter-associated anion channels. *J Biol Chem.* (2003) 278:50112–9. doi: 10.1074/jbc.M307990200

34. Melzer N, Torres-Salazar D, Fahlke C. A dynamic switch between inhibitory and excitatory currents in a neuronal glutamate transporter. *Proc Natl Acad Sci USA.* (2005) 102:19214–8. doi: 10.1073/pnas.0508837103

35. Manto M, Dalmau J, Didelot A, Rogemond V, Honnorat J. *In vivo* effects of antibodies from patients with anti-NMDA receptor encephalitis: further evidence of synaptic glutamatergic dysfunction. *Orphanet J Rare Dis.* (2010) 5:31. doi: 10.1186/1750-1172-5-31

36. Seebohm G, Piccini I, Strutz-Seebohm N. Paving the way to understand autoantibody-mediated epilepsy on the molecular level. *Front Neurol.* (2015) 6:149. doi: 10.3389/fneur.2015.00149

37. Dey S, Temme L, Schreiber JA, Schepmann D, Frehland B, Lehmkuhl K, et al. Deconstruction - reconstruction approach to analyze the essential structural elements of tetrahydro-3-benzazepine-based antagonists of GluN2B subunit containing NMDA receptors. *Eur J Med Chem.* (2017) 138:552–64. doi: 10.1016/j.ejmech.2017.06.068

38. Gawaskar S, Temme L, Schreiber JA, Schepmann D, Bonifazi A, Robaa D, et al. Design, synthesis, pharmacological evaluation and docking studies of GluN2B-selective NMDA receptor antagonists with a Benzo[7]annulen-7-amine Scaffold. *Chem Med Chem.* (2017) 12:1212–22. doi: 10.1002/cmdc.201700311

14

Induction of Osmolyte Pathways in Skeletal Muscle Inflammation: Novel Biomarkers for Myositis

Boel De Paepe[1]*, Jana Zschüntzsch[2], Tea Šokčević[1], Joachim Weis[3], Jens Schmidt[2†] and Jan L. De Bleecker[1†]

[1] Department of Neurology and Neuromuscular Reference Center, Ghent University Hospital, Ghent, Belgium, [2] Department of Neurology, University Medical Center Göttingen, Göttingen, Germany, [3] Institute for Neuropathology, Reinisch-Westfälische Technische Hochschule Aachen University Hospital, Aachen, Germany

*Correspondence:
Boel De Paepe
boel.depaepe@ugent.be

[†] These authors have contributed equally to this work

We recently identified osmolyte accumulators as novel biomarkers for chronic skeletal muscle inflammation and weakness, but their precise involvement in inflammatory myopathies remains elusive. In the current study, we demonstrate in vitro that, in myoblasts and myotubes exposed to pro-inflammatory cytokines or increased salt concentration, mRNA levels of the osmolyte carriers SLC5A3, SLC6A6, SLC6A12, and AKR1B1 enzyme can be upregulated. Induction of SLC6A12 and AKR1B1 was confirmed at the protein level using immunofluorescence and Western blotting. Gene silencing by specific siRNAs revealed that these factors were vital for muscle cells under hyperosmotic conditions. Pro-inflammatory cytokines activated mitogen-activated protein kinases, nuclear factor κB as well as nuclear factor of activated T-cells 5 mRNA expression. In muscle biopsies from patients with polymyositis or sporadic inclusion body myositis, osmolyte pathway activation was observed in regenerating muscle fibers. In addition, the osmolyte carriers SLC5A3 and SLC6A12 localized to subsets of immune cells, most notably to the endomysial macrophages and T-cells. Collectively, this study unveiled that muscle cells respond to osmotic and inflammatory stress by osmolyte pathway activation, likely orchestrating general protection of the tissue. Moreover, pro-inflammatory properties are attributed to SLC5A3 and SLC6A12 in auto-aggressive macrophages and T-cells in inflamed skeletal muscle.

Keywords: inflammatory myopathy, osmotic stress, inflammatory stress, osmolytes, muscle regeneration

INTRODUCTION

The idiopathic inflammatory myopathies represent a diverse group of autoimmune muscle diseases. The main disease entities recognized today are dermatomyositis (DM), polymyositis (PM), sporadic inclusion body myositis (IBM), immune-mediated necrotizing myopathy (IMNM), anti-synthetase syndrome, and unspecific myositis, each of which possess distinct clinical and myopathological characteristics (1–5). DM patients develop complement-mediated blood vessel destruction, perimysial inflammation and perifascicular muscle fiber atrophy (6). PM and IBM are characterized by invasion of nonnecrotic muscle fibers by auto-aggressive cytotoxic T-cells and macrophages, with inflammation building up mostly at endomysial sites (7). In IBM muscle fibers, additional degenerative phenomena occur, with rimmed vacuoles and inclusions that contain aggregates of ectopic proteins (8), a process that is presumed to follow inflammation (9). IMNM represents 3 subdivisions according to serologic characteristics: anti-3-hydroxy-3-methylglutaryl-coenzyme A reductase myopathy, signal recognition particle myopathy, and myositis-specific autoantibody negative IMNM (10). Many of the immunopathogenic mechanisms underlying the inflammatory myopathies remain poorly understood, hampering the development of successful therapies that suit the different patient subtypes.

Muscle is a highly adaptive and dynamic tissue capable of increasing its mass in response to exercise and of restoring damage caused by injury via processes that require hypertrophy and regeneration, respectively. In addition, cells possess a universal ability to adapt to changing osmotic conditions, a feature essential for their survival, allowing active anticipation toward perturbations in volume and disrupted cellular homeostasis. A complex intracellular mixture of interacting osmolytes regulates osmotic pressure, which takes shape through the synthesis and/or import of osmo-active compounds in cells (11). The solute carrier family (SLC) contains several salt-dependent membrane transport proteins involved in the selective import of extracellular constituents: (i) the sodium-myoinositol cotransporter SLC5A3, (ii) the high-affinity taurine transporter SLC6A6, and (iii) the betaine and γ-amino-n-butyric acid (GABA) transporter SLC6A12. AKR1B1 is an aldose reductase that catalyzes the intracellular conversion of glucose to sorbitol. In a joint effort, these osmoprotective constituents represent a universal tool for mammalian cells, and their accumulators can be ubiquitously expressed throughout human tissues. The central regulator of osmolyte pathway gene expression is the transcription factor nuclear factor of activated T-cells 5 (NFAT5), also termed tonicity enhancer-binding protein (12).

Several observations allowed us to speculate NFAT5-inducible pathways might be involved in the inflammatory myopathies. Firstly, the NFAT5 pathway participates in muscle development and regeneration, by regulating the differentiation of immature myoblasts to mature multinucleated myotubes (13). NFAT5 levels have been shown to increase in the regenerating fibers of mice exposed to experimental muscle tissue injury (14), attributing the transcription factor a role in countering disease-inflicted muscle tissue damage. Secondly, the NFAT5 pathway has been firmly linked to nuclear factor κB (NFκB) activity (15), the latter a key regulator of inflammatory diseases in general and the inflammatory myopathies in particular (16). NFAT5 and NFκB share multiple molecular targets (17), many of which are involved in the immunopathogeneses of inflammatory

myopathy including CCL2, also termed monocyte chemo-attractant protein-1 (MCP-1) (18), lymphotoxin β (LTβ) (19), tumor necrosis factor α (TNFα) (20), inducible nitric oxide synthase (iNOS) (21), and heat shock protein family of 70kd (HSP70) (22). Thirdly, NFAT5-downstream osmolyte pathways are potent activators of cytotoxic activities of immune cells and could therefore be implicated in human autoimmune disease. In addition, dietary salt is determinant to T-cell differentiation, by direct activation of glycogen synthase kinase 1 (GSK-1) and subsequent Interleukin 23 receptor stabilization, which enforces the type 17 helper T-cell (Th17), a T-cell phenotype associated with autoimmune disease (23).

We recently were the first to describe upregulation of the osmolyte accumulators SLC5A3, SLC6A6 and AKR1B1 in muscle tissues from myositis patients (24), and described NFAT5 expression in myoblasts in culture (25), yet the precise role osmolyte pathways play in disease mechanisms remained unexplored. With this study, we aim to substantiate and functionally connect these biomarkers with muscle inflammation. We set up in vitro muscle cell models to investigate osmolyte pathway member expression, using both the human rhabdomyosarcoma CCL-136 cell line and normal primary human myotubes. In addition, we investigated their possible signaling routes, which involves the upstream transcription factors NFκB and NFAT5, and the mitogen-activated protein kinases (MAPKs). We confronted this in vitro evidence with findings in muscle biopsies from patients diagnosed with inflammatory myopathies.

METHODS

Cell Cultures

Human rhabdomyosarcoma CCL-136 cells (ATCC, Manassas, VA) were kept in Dulbecco's modified Eagle medium (DMEM) supplemented with 10% fetal calf serum (Biochrom, Berlin, Germany) and 1% L-glutamine (ThermoFisher Scientific, Waltham, MA). Human muscle cell cultures originated from muscle biopsies taken from healthy patients needing knee surgery, obtained with patient consent and approved by the local ethics committee. Biopsies were minced and trypsinized. Fragments were seeded in DMEM with pyruvate, high glucose and L-glutamine, supplemented with penicillin, streptomycin and 10% fetal calf serum (ThermoFisher Scientific). Cells were cultured for 2 periods of ∼ 3 weeks during which CD56+ cells were purified twice with magnetic separation MiniMACS columns using the supplier's standard protocol (Miltenyi Biotec, Bergisch Gladbach, Germany). Myotubes were obtained by allowing cells to differentiate for approximately 5 days in DMEM medium supplemented with penicillin, streptomycin and 2% horse serum (ThermoFisher Scientific). **Supplementary Figure S1** illustrates a representative culture of differentiated myotubes, showing aligned multinucleate muscle cells. All cells were kept in culture wells or chamber slides at 37°C in a humified atmosphere containing 5% CO_2. Conditions for cytokine stimulation were as determined earlier (26), being 30 ng/ml TNFα, 300 u/ml Interferon γ (IFNγ), 20 ng/ml Interleukin 1β (IL1β) (R and D Systems, Minneapolis, MN), or

---

Abbreviations: AKR1B1, aldose reductase; DM, dermatomyositis; dMyHC, developmental myosin heavy chain; ERK, extracellular signal-regulated kinase; GAPDH, glyceraldehyde-3-phosphate dehydrogenase; GSK-3α/β, glycogen synthase kinase 3α/β; HSP70, heat shock protein family of 70kd; IBM, sporadic inclusion body myositis; IFNγ, Interferon γ; IL1β, Interleukin 1β; IMNM, immune-mediated necrotizing myopathy; iNOS, inducible nitric oxide synthase; LTβ, lymphotoxin β; MAPK, mitogen-activated protein kinase; MCP-1, monocyte chemo-attractant protein-1; MSK2, mitogen- and stress-activated kinase 2; NFAT5, nuclear factor of activated T-cells 5; NFκB, nuclear factor κB; PM, polymyositis; siRNA, silencing RNA; SLC5A3, solute carrier sodium-myoinositol cotransporter; SLC6A6, solute carrier taurine transporter; SLC6A12, solute carrier betaine and γ-amino-n-butyric acid (GABA) transporter; Th17, Interleukin 17-producing T-cells; TNFα, tumor necrosis factor α.

double combinations. Hyperosmotic conditions were created by supplementing the culture medium with 25–150 mM of added NaCl. Higher concentrations of NaCl lead to complete cell death within 24 h.

Quantitative Reverse Transcription PCR

RNA was prepared from cells cultured in 12-well culture plates, using the RNeasy Mini kit and according to the manufacturer's specifications (Qiagen, Hilden, Germany). RNA concentration was measured with a Nanodrop 1000 (ThermoFisher Scientific). cDNA was prepared from 200 ng of RNA with SuperScript II reverse transcriptase, 500 ng/µl oligo dTs, 0.1 M DTT, and 10 mM dNTPs each (Invitrogen, Darmstadt, Germany). cDNA was quantified through PCR reaction with Taqman Gene Expression Master mix (Applied Biosystems, Foster City, CA), using 6-carboxy-fluorescein-labeled probes and specific primers for: SLC5A3, Hs00272857 _s1; SLC6A6, Hs00161778_m1; SLC6A12, HS00758246_ m1; AKR1B1, Hs00739326_m1; NFAT5, Hs00232437_m1; MAPK14, Hs01051152_m1; RELA, Hs00153294_m1; NFKB1, Hs00765730_m1; NFKB2, Hs01028901_g1; glyceraldehyde-3-phosphate dehydrogenase (GAPDH), Hs99999905_m1 (Applied Biosystems). Reactions were run in triplicate, following the standard cycle protocol on a 7500 Real Time PCR System, and analyzed with software version 2.0.6. (Applied Biosystems). Data was presented as $\Delta\Delta$Ct fold-changes compared to the expression levels in untreated cells, with GAPDH as an internal housekeeping gene standard.

Immunofluorescent Cytostaining

Cells cultured on glass chamber slides were fixed with ice-cold acetone and blocked in phosphate buffered saline with 10% bovine serum albumin and 10% goat serum for 1 h at room temperature. Immunofluorescent detection was carried out for 1 h at room temperature with commercially available antibodies: mouse (4 µg/ml, sc-514024, SantaCruz Biotechnology, Santa Cruz, CA) and rabbit (10 µg/ml, nbp188641, Novus Biologicals, Abingdon, UK) anti-SLC6A12; rabbit (2 µg/ml, sc-33219, SantaCruz Biotechnology) and goat (1 µg/ml, sc-17732, SantaCruz Biotechnology) anti-AKR1B1; mouse anti-developmental myosin heavy chain (dMyHC) (40 µg/ml, RMMy2/9D2, Leica Biosystems, Nussloch, Germany). The corresponding Alexa594—and Alexa488-labeled secondary antibodies (ThermoFisher Scientific) were added. After mounting in Fluoromount G (Southern Biotech, Alabama, USA), digital photography was performed on a Zeiss Axiophot microscope (Zeiss, Goettingen, Germany). Pictures were taken by a cooled CCD digital camera (Retiga 1300, Qimaging, Burnaby, BC, Canada) and visualized with ImageProPlus software (MediaCybernetics, Bethesda, MD).

Immunofluorescent Histostaining

For localization studies in muscle tissues, 8 µm cryostat sections were cut from frozen muscle biopsies obtained from patients without muscle abnormalities ($n = 10$), inflammatory myopathies ($n = 28$), and disease controls diagnosed with muscular dystrophy ($n = 8$; for pathological information

consult **Supplementary Table S1**). Diagnosis of the disease subgroups PM ($n = 4$), IBM ($n = 9$), DM ($n = 9$), and IMNM ($n = 6$) were based upon clinical and myopathological criteria (27). Diagnosis of PM was reserved to patients with nonnecrotic invaded muscle fibers present in the biopsy that had subsequently responded to immunosuppressive therapy. Sections were fixed in ice-cold acetone and treated with blocking solution containing 5% donkey serum, 10% heat-inactivated human serum and 2% bovine serum albumine in phosphate buffered saline. Incubations with primary antibodies were carried out in the same solution: 4 µg/ml rabbit polyclonal anti-SLC5A3 (NBP1-02399, Novusbio); 4 µg/ml mouse monoclonal anti-SLC6A6 (E10, SantaCruz Biotechnology); 6 µg/ml rabbit polyclonal anti-SLC6A12 (HPA034973; Merck, Kenilworth, NJ); 1 µg/ml goat polyclonal anti-AKR1B1 (N20, SantaCruz Biotechnology). Immune cell subtypes and muscle tissue constituents were visualized through double staining as described (18). Satellite cells were visualized with goat anti-Pax3/7 (1 µg/ml, sc-7748, SantaCruz Biotechnology). To allow double staining of macrophages with mouse monoclonal antibodies, FITC labeled anti-CD68 (Agilent, Santa Clara, CA) was applied. Secondary antibodies were used labeled with CY3 (Jackson ImmunoResearch Laboratories, West Grove, PA) and AlexaFluor488 (ThermoFisher Scientific). Slides were mounted with Fluoromount (Southern Biotech) and visualized with a fluorescence microscope (Zeiss). Conventional semi-quantitative scoring of staining intensity was performed by three non-blinded independent observers. Negative control studies consisted of the omission of primary antibody and the substitution by non-immune IgGs. Positive control tissues for checking immunodetection were cultured Hela cells (SLC6A6), frozen sections containing kidney medulla (SLC5A3, SLC6A12), and Jurkat cells (AKR1B1).

Western Blotting

Cells cultured in 12-well culture plates were lysed in Ripa buffer (50 mM Tris-HCl, 150 mM NaCl, 2.5% Na-deoxycholate, 2.5% NP40, 0.1% sodium dodecyl sulfate pH 7.4) with a protease inhibitor cocktail added (Roche, Indianapolis, IN) and centrifuged for 5 min at 13000 rpm. The supernatant was collected and protein concentrations were determined following a Bradford procedure (Bio-Rad protein assay, Hercules, CA) with bovine serum albumine standard solutions, measured in triplicates on the Infinite M200Pro and analyzed with Magellan 7.2 software (Tecan, Mannedorf, Switzerland). 60 µg protein samples were dissolved in Laemli buffer, boiled for 2 min, separated by 12% sodium dodecyl sulfate-polyacrylamide gelelectrophoresis, and transferred to a nitrocellulose membrane (Schleicher and Schuell, Dassel, Germany). Membranes were blocked with 5% bovine serum albumine for 1 h at 4°C and incubated overnight at 4°C with 2 µg/ml mouse anti-SLC6A12 (sc-514024, SantaCruz Biotechnology), 4 h at room temperature with 2 µg/ml goat anti-AKR1B1 (sc-17732, SantaCruz Biotechnology), and 1 h at room temperature with 0.7 µg/ml mouse anti-GAPDH (Sp210-Ag14; Abcam, Cambridge, UK). All incubations were done in tris-buffered saline buffer containing 0.05% Tween20.

Appropriate horseradish peroxidase-conjugated secondary antibodies (Jackson ImmunoResearch, West Grove, PA) were added for 1 h at room temperature. The chemiluminescent signal was generated with the Pierce Western blotting substrate (ThermoFisher Scientific), visualized with the Fusion FX, and quantified with Vision Capt software, with background noise filtering using a rolling-ball algorithm (Vilber Lourmat, Eberhardzell, Germany).

Protein Phosphorylation Profiling

Protein phosphorylation patterns were determined in extracts obtained from cultured myotubes, using the Proteome Profiler human phosphor-mitogen activated protein kinase (MAPK) antibody array according to the manufacturer's specifications (Bio-Techne, Abingdon, United Kingdom). Briefly, array membranes were incubated overnight at 4°C with lysate containing 200 µg of cellular protein, detection conditions were as described in the western blotting section. Protein densities were quantified, relative to phosphorylated Akt2, as the calculated mean of duplicate spots per protein, using Image Studio 5.2 software (Li-Cor Biosciences, Cambridge, UK).

Knockdown Studies

Pools of three target-specific 19–25 nucleotide silencing RNAs (siRNAs), purchased from SantaCruz Biotechnology, were used: siRNA SLS5A3 (sc-44516), siRNA SLC6A12 (sc-95904), and siRNA AKR1B1 (sc-37119). 50% confluent CCL-136 cells and myotube cultures were changed to 500 µl X-Vivo15 medium (Sartorius, Goettingen, Germany), to which 3 µl of lipofectamine (ThermoFisher) and 100 nM siRNA had been added. After 5 h, an extra 200 µl of X-Vivo15 was added, which in treated cells contained cytokines to a final well concentration of 20 ng/ml IL1β+300 u/ml IFNγ, or 50 mM added NaCl. Cells were assayed 26 h after addition of the siRNAs. Live and dead cells were visualized using the ReadyProbes cell viability imaging blue/green kit (ThermoFisher) according to the manufacturer's specifications. Using a fluorescence microscope, a minimum of 50 cells (blue) was counted per condition, determining the amount of dead cells (green). Afterwards, cell cultures were stained with hematoxylin and eosin according to standard procedures, dehydrated, mounted, and interpreted under a light microscope. Efficiency of knockdown was evaluated at the mRNA level using quantitative reverse transcription PCR, following the method described above. From controls and siRNA-treated CCL-136 cells seeded in 12-well culture plates, protein samples were prepared for electrophoresis by adding lithium dodecyl sulfate sample buffer and reducing agent (Invitrogen, Carlsbad, CA, USA) and boiling for 3 min. Samples were loaded onto 10% bis-tris gels, with prestained markers alongside to determine the molecular weight of protein bands. Proteins were transferred to nitrocellulose membranes by electroblotting, and incubated with 2 µg/ml mouse anti-SLC6A12 (sc-514024), 2 µg/ml goat anti-AKR1B1 (sc-17732), or mouse anti-β actin (sc-47778) (SantaCruz Biotechnology) for 4 h at room temperature on a rocking platform. Immunoreaction was visualized using the chromogenic Western Breeze kit according to the manufacturer's specifications (Invitrogen).

Compliance With Ethical Standards

Human experimentation presented in the study was approved by the Ghent University Hospital Ethics Committee (EC-UZG-#B670201316956) and adhered to privacy regulations (CBPL-BEL-#HM003039095). Written informed consent was obtained from all individual participants included in the study, and all procedures were in accordance with the Declaration of Helsinki.

RESULTS

mRNA Quantification in Cultured Muscle Cells

In CCL-136 cells, expression levels of osmolyte pathway members were determined in cells treated with pro-inflammatory cytokines or added NaCl for 24 h (**Table 1**). In general, a moderate increase of expression was shown for SLC5A3, SLC6A6, SLC6A12, and AKR1B1 when cells were treated with cytokines. The strongest response was a 10-fold increase of SLC5A3 mRNA expression in IL1β+TNFα-treated cells. Hyperosmotic conditions also induced osmolyte pathway expression, with 100 mM of added NaCl leading to a 179-fold increase of SLC6A12, and increasing NFAT5 expression 2.5-fold. MAPK14 levels were 2-fold increased in both IFNγ+TNFα- and 50 mM NaCl-treated cells. Highest levels of RelA, NFkB1 and NFkB2 could be achieved with pro-inflammatory cytokine mixtures, though NFkB1 and NFkB2 expression also responded to added NaCl.

Primary human myotubes treated for 24 h with cytokines or added NaCl showed induction of osmolyte pathway mRNA levels (**Table 2**). For SLC5A3 and AKR1B1, the strongest induction could be achieved with added NaCl; SLC6A6 and SLC6A12 were most strongly induced by pro-inflammatory cytokine mixtures. NFAT5 expression was influenced by both cytokines and increased salt concentrations, but reached higher expression levels with IFNγ+IL1β (4,5-fold) than with 125 mM NaCl (3-fold). MAPK14 expression levels were found increased 2-fold in myotubes treated with IL1β and with 125 mM NaCl. The expression of NFκB subunits was most strongly induced by treatment with pro-inflammatory cytokines. Nonetheless, 25 mM added NaCl increased NFkB1 expression 8,5-fold. In myotubes treated for longer periods, added NaCl lead to continuously increasing SLC5A3, SLC6A12 and AKR1B1 expression levels over time, culminating in levels all exceeding 200-fold at time point 72 h (**Table 3**). In addition, prolonged salt treatment lead to a time-dependent increase of NFAT5 and MAPK14 expression levels, reaching a maximum of 9-fold (NFAT5) and 18-fold (MAPK14). In contrast, the single pulse of pro-inflammatory cytokines resulted in highest expression levels after 24 h, with levels nearing normal after 72 h.

Immunofluorescent Protein Localization Studies in Cultured Muscle Cells

Immunofluorescent staining of CCL-136 cells (**Figure 1A**) confirmed the induction of SLC6A12 and AKR1B1 expression after 24 h of treatment with pro-inflammatory cytokines and

TABLE 1 | Messenger RNA levels in cultured CCL-136 cells treated for 24 h.

	Cytokines						Added NaCl			
	IFNγ	IL1β	TNFα	IFNγ+IL1β	IFNγ+TNFα	IL1β+TNFα	25 mM	50 mM	75 mM	100 mM
SLC5A3	1	1.1	1.3	2.1	4.6	10.3	0.6	0.5	1.9	3.4
SLC6A6	0.5	0.7	0.8	1.4	1.5	4.3	0.9	1.1	1.2	1.5
SLC6A12	1.7	2	1	3.4	3.8	1.2	1.6	7.7	9	178.7
AKR1B1	1.4	2.3	1.9	1.9	1.6	1.7	1.4	2.1	2.4	5.6
NFAT5	1.1	0.3	0.5	1.4	1.7	1	1.4	4.1	0.8	2.5
MAPK14	0.7	0.8	0.8	1.4	1.9	1.4	1.1	2	0.9	1.3
RELA	0.9	1.2	0.9	1.8	1.7	0.5	0.9	0.8	0.9	1.2
NFkB1	1	1.2	1	6	0.5	3.8	1.5	2.9	1.2	1.9
NFkB2	1.3	1.5	2.7	3.3	12.9	1	1.2	2.3	1.5	1.1

Fold changes compared to untreated cells, normalized to glyceraldehyde 3-phosphate dehydrogenase expression levels, were obtained through quantitative reverse transcription PCR and calculated as $2^{-\Delta\Delta Ct}$ (mean of three given). Fold changes >2 green; >5 yellow; >10 orange; >100 red.

TABLE 2 | Messenger RNA levels in cultured normal human myotubes treated for 24 h.

	Cytokines						Added NaCl					
	IFNγ	IL1β	TNFα	IFNγ+IL1β	IFNγ+TNFα	IL1β+TNFα	25 mM	50 mM	75 mM	100 mM	125 mM	150 mM
SLC5A3	2.6	5.8	2.5	2.4	1.4	1.9	1.4	2.1	3.6	13	13.9	5
SLC6A6	1.2	1.9	2.9	3.9	2.2	3.1	1.1	1.9	1.8	1.9	1.8	0.4
SLC6A12	21.3	2.1	1.4	177.7	229.2	3.8	2.1	5.9	7.3	32.4	47.9	9.6
AKR1B1	1.5	6.6	3.7	7.5	5.6	4.9	10.7	3.5	4.7	6.9	8.1	2.5
NFAT5	1.4	4.4	1.6	4.5	2.2	2	0.8	1.6	1.3	2.2	3	0.6
MAPK14	1	1.9	1.1	0.6	0.4	0.9	1.4	1.3	1	1.6	1.9	0.6
RELA	2.1	2	1.4	25.3	18.4	4.2	0.8	1.1	1.2	1.1	1.2	0.5
NFkB1	1.5	1.3	0.8	6.8	3.6	2.6	8.7	0.7	0.7	0.6	1.3	0.7
NFkB2	1.2	4.7	2.7	20.5	4	8.4	0.1	1.3	1.2	0.8	1	0.3

Fold changes compared to untreated cells, normalized to glyceraldehyde 3-phosphate dehydrogenase expression levels, were obtained through quantitative reverse transcription PCR and calculated as $2^{-\Delta\Delta Ct}$ (mean of three given). Fold changes >2 green; >5 yellow; >10 orange; >100 red.

added NaCl at the protein level and showed similar staining patterns with the two different sets of primary antibodies.

Myotubes immunostaining (**Figure 1B**) showed increases of SLC6A12 in response to cytokines at the 48 h time point, with levels declining again at time point 72 h. For AKR1B1, high levels were detected following cytokine stimulation from 24 h onward, compared to the low levels observed in untreated myotubes. A growth-inhibitory effect of hyperosmotic conditions was observed in myotubes, which became conspicuous from the 48 h time point on. NaCl-treatment disfavored differentiation into multinucleate elongated muscle cells, as was assayed with dMyHC staining (**Supplementary Figure S1**). Evaluation of hematoxylin&eosin stains confirmed that salt treatment affected cell morphology and growth, reducing cell elongation and disfavoring multinucleate myotubes.

Protein Quantification and Phosphorylation Patterns of Human Myotubes

SLC6A12 protein levels were below the detection limit in untreated normal myotubes, but SLC6A12 protein could readily be shown in myotubes treated with IL1β+TNFα for 48 h and 72 h (**Figure 2A**). SLC6A12 and AKR1B1 protein levels were found to

increase in a time- and dose-dependent manner when myotubes were exposed to 25 and 50 mM of added NaCl (**Figure 2B**). The expression levels with the higher doses of NaCl already reached a maximum at the 48 h time-point (**Table 4**).

Protein phosphorylation patterns of MAPKs showed that the strongest signals in the array were the phosphorylated forms of Akt2 (S474) and heat shock protein 27 (HSP27) (S78, S82) (**Supplementary Figure S2**). Akt2 and HSP27 activation was prominent in untreated and cytokine-treated myotubes alike. The most notable influence of 24 h IFNγ+IL1β treatment was an increase in phosphorylation of mitogen- and stress-activated kinase 2 (MSK2) (S360) 3-fold and MAPK3 (T202, Y204) 2.5-fold. In addition, levels of phosphorylated glycogen synthase kinase 3α/β (GSK-3α/β) (S9, S21), MAPK12 (T183, Y185), and MAPK13 (T180, Y182) were increased 2-fold.

Knockdown Studies in Cultured Muscle Cells

Both in CCL-136 cells and in primary healthy myotubes, 50 mM of added NaCl decreased cell densities in both siSCL6A12— and siAKR1B1-treated cells at the 24 h time point, while this regimen did not harm growth of siSLC5A3-treated muscle

TABLE 3 | Messenger RNA levels in cultured normal human myotubes treated with cytokines or added NaCl for up to 3 days.

	IFNγ+IL1β			IFNγ+TNFα			100 mM NaCl		
	24 h	48 h	72 h	24 h	48 h	72 h	24 h	48 h	72 h
SLC5A3	1	0.4	0.2	1	0.6	0.5	10.8	5.8	240.7
SLC6A12	19.1	4.9	1	14.5	13	2.5	43	50.9	2 × 10exp8
AKR1B1	2.4	1.3	0.9	1.7	1.9	1.1	7	27.4	528.8
NFAT5	0.8	0.3	0.04	0.8	0.9	0.3	1.4	3.8	9.4
MAPK14	0.9	0.4	0.3	0.6	0.6	0.6	1.1	1.6	17.8

Fold changes compared to untreated cells, normalized to glyceraldehyde 3-phosphate dehydrogenase expression levels, were obtained through quantitative reverse transcription PCR and calculated as $2^{-\Delta\Delta Ct}$ (mean of three given). Fold changes >2 green; >5 yellow; >10 orange; >100 red.

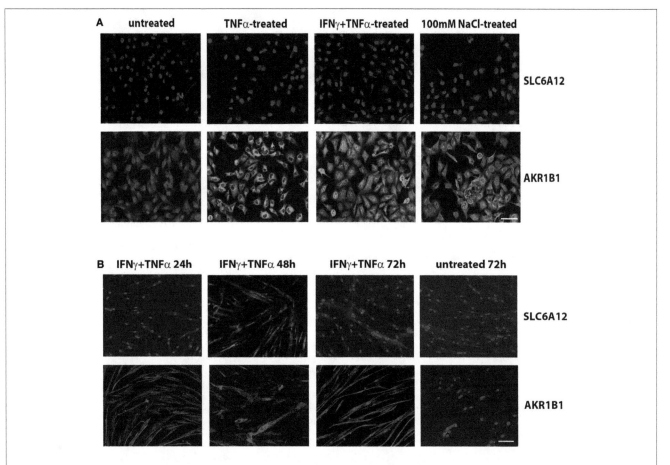

FIGURE 1 | Immunofluorescent cytostaining. **(A)** Staining with mouse anti-SLC6A12 (AlexaFluor 594, red) and rabbit anti-AKR1B1 (AlexaFluor488, green) in CCL-136 cells after 24 h treatment. Untreated control cells shows low levels of SLC6A12 and AKR1B1. Treatment with 30 ng/ml TNFα markedly increases AKR1B1 levels. Treatment with 300 u/ml IFNγ and 30 ng/ml TNFα strongly increases both SLC6A12 levels and AKR1B1 protein levels. Addition of 100 mM NaCl to the medium also increases both SLC6A12 and AKR1B1 protein expression. **(B)** Staining with rabbit anti-SLC6A12 (AlexaFluor 488, green) and goat anti-AKR1B1 (AlexaFluor594, red) in cultured healthy human myotubes at different time points. Myotubes treated with 300 u/ml IFNγ and 30 ng/ml TNFα display low levels of SLC6A12 that is increased at the 48 h time point. Levels return back to constitutive low levels after 72 h, with staining levels similar to those in untreated cells. Staining for AKR1B1 shows continuously high levels between 24 and 72 h. In untreated cells, AKR1B1 expression levels are substantially lower. Scale bar = 50 μm.

cells (**Figure 3A**). Treatment with pro-inflammatory cytokines on the other hand, combined with knockdown of individual osmolyte pathway members, did not cause significant effects on myotube viability, with percentages of dead cells in untreated vs. cytokine-treated cells respectively: 1% vs. 7% (vehicle), 11% vs. 25% (siSLC6A12), 33% vs. 15% (siAKR1B1), and 0% vs. 4%

(siSLC5A3). For silencing procedures, efficiency of knockdown was evaluated in CCL-136 cells (calculated as ΔCt siRNA-treated cells minus ΔCt of the vehicle control) detecting 16% (siSLC5A3), 59% (siSLC6A12), and 6% (siAKR1B1) of residual mRNA expression. Western blotting corroborated efficient AKR1B1 knockdown at the protein level but did not show a

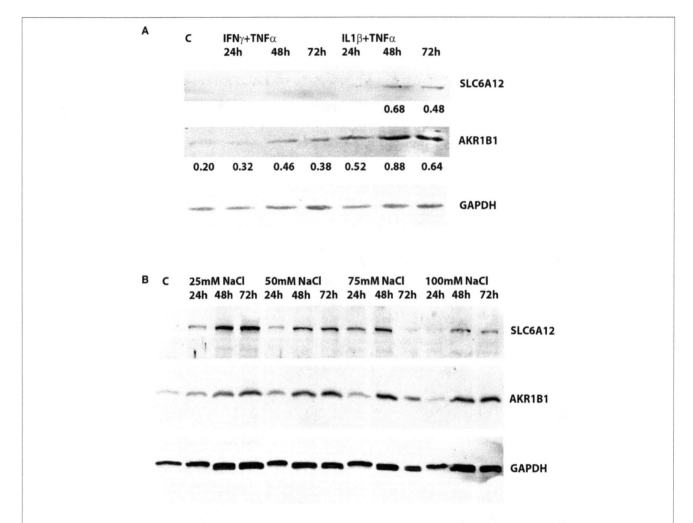

FIGURE 2 | Western blotting of protein extracts preepared from cultured normal human myotubes. **(A)** SLC6A12 and AKR1B1 protein levels in myotubes treated with cytokine mixtures. SLC6A12 and AKR1B1 proteins are visualized in control cells (C) and in cells treated for 24 h-48 h-72 h with either 300 u/ml IFNγ+30 ng/ml TNFα, or 20 ng/ml IL1β+30 ng/ml TNFα. SLC6A12 is undetectable in untreated- and in 300 u/ml IFNγ+30 ng/ml TNFα-treated cells, but is induced by treatment with 20 ng/ml IL1β+30 ng/ml TNFα from the 48 h time point on. Low constitutive levels of AKR1B1 in control cells are increased in myotubes treated with both cytokine mixtures, peaking at the 48 h time point. Relative protein densities of AKR1B1, normalized using glyceraldehyde 3-phosphate dehydrogenase (GAPDH) levels as an internal standard, have been indicated. **(B)** SLC6A12 and AKR1B1 protein levels in myotubes treated with added NaCl. Protein bands for SLC6A12 and AKR1B1, and the internal standard glyceraldehyde 3-phosphate dehydrogenase (GAPDH), are given in an untreated control (C) and in cells treated with different concentrations of added NaCl. A time-dependent increase is observed in cells treated with 25 and 50 mM added NaCl, while more elevated NaCl concentrations show the highest levels at the 48 h timepoint. The corresponding relative protein densities are listed in **Table 4**.

substantial reduction of SLC6A12 protein levels (**Figure 3B**). We could not quantify SLC5A3 protein in muscle samples using western blots, as we were unsuccessful in detecting SLC5A3 in the corresponding positive control samples using rabbit (nbp102399, NovusBiologicals) and goat (sc-23142, SantaCruz Biotechnology) antibodies.

Immunolocalization Studies in Muscle Tissues From Inflammatory Myopathy Patients

Confirming our earlier descriptive myopathological results on SLC5A3, SLC6A6, and AKR1B1 expression (24), we found these factors upregulated in regenerating muscle fibers

present in biopsies in this new cohort of inflammatory myopathy patients. We now also add SLC6A12 to the regenerating muscle fiber's repertory of increased osmolyte accumulators (**Figure 4**). High osmolyte pathway member expression contrasted with the low levels present in muscle fibers in biopsies from healthy subjects. In tissues from muscular dystrophy patients, the SLC6A12 muscle fiber staining pattern was similar to inflammatory myopathies, with diffuse staining mostly in small regenerating CD56 positive muscle fibers and discontinuous sarcolemmal staining in subsets of CD56 negative muscle fibers (**Supplementary Figure S3**). We verified that this did not represent adjacent satellite cells and observed no co-localization with Pax3/7 staining.

TABLE 4 | Protein densities in cultured normal human myotubes treated with added NaCl for varying periods of time.

	Untreated	25 mM NaCl			50 mM NaCl			75 mM NaCl			100 mM NaCl		
		24 h	48 h	72 h	24 h	48 h	72 h	24 h	48 h	72 h	24 h	48 h	72 h
SLC6A12	0.001	0.097	0.264	**0.297**	0.139	0.180	**0.198**	0.154	**0.217**	0.131	0.112	**0.115**	0.094
AKR1B1	0.192	0.202	0.210	**0.347**	0.336	0.377	**0.437**	0.281	**0.436**	0.347	0.209	**0.278**	0.263

*Protein densities of western blots (shown in **Figure 2**) were normalized using glyceraldehyde 3-phosphate dehydrogenase levels. Highest protein expression levels per time point have been highlighted.*

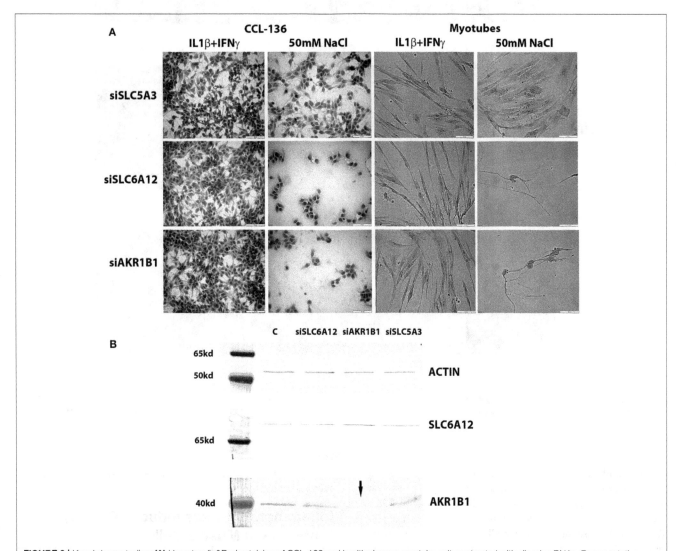

FIGURE 3 | Knockdown studies. **(A)** Hematoxylin&Eosin staining of CCL-136 and healthy human myotube cultures treated with silencing RNAs. Representative images are shown of cell cultures exposed to 300 u/ml IFNγ+20 ng/ml IL1β or to 50 mM of added NaCl. Culture densities decrease substantially in siSLC6A12- and siAKR1B1-treated cultures challenged with 50 mM of added NaCl, both in CCL-136 cells and in normal human myotubes. Addition of siSLC5A3 does not apparently inhibit cell growth, only resulting in mildly reduced densities of CCL-136 cells which could equally be observed in controls treated with 50 mM NaCl. Scale bar = 100 μm. **(B)** Western blots visualizing SLC6A12 and AKR1B1 protein in CCL-136 cells treated with silencing RNAs. The severe reduction of the AKR1B1 protein band in siAKR1B1-treated cells (arrow) shows the efficiency of expression knockdown. C represents the control sample, and equal loading is shown by β-actin protein bands.

SLC5A3 and SLC6A12 were expressed by inflammatory cells in inflammatory myopathy muscle biopsies (**Figure 4**). SLC6A12 was detected in subsets of the endomysial CD68+ cells surrounding muscle fibers in PM and IBM tissues. In comparison, only a small minority of tissue-infiltrating CD68+ cells in DM and in muscular dystrophy tissues were SLC6A12

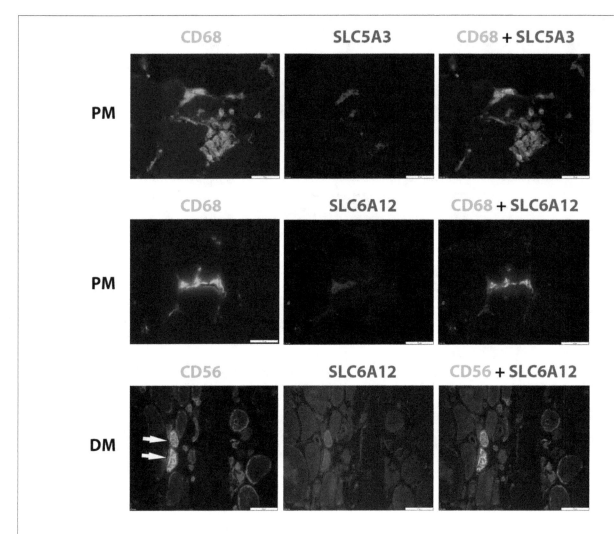

FIGURE 4 | Immunofluorescent histostaining. Staining of SLC6A12 and AKR1B1 in muscle sections from patients diagnosed with inflammatory myopathy. Polymyositis (PM): A subset of CD68+ cells (AlexaFluor488, green), representing mostly M1 phenotype macrophages, express SLC5A3 and SLC6A12 (CY3, red). Dermatomyositis (DM): Two small regenerating muscle fibers (arrows), identified as strongly positive for CD56 (AlexaFluor488, green), express high levels of SLC6A12 protein (CY3, red). Scale bar =50 μm.

positive, and the more sparse inflammatory cells observed in IMNM tissues were SLC6A12 negative. SLC6A12 was rarely observed in the CD8+ T-cells of PM and IBM tissues. SLC5A3 on the other hand, could be detected in a substantial part of CD3+ T-cells, with most non-invading CD8+ T-cells being negative while CD8+ cells actively invading nonnecrotic muscle fibers in PM and IBM were often strongly positive. The majority of CD68+ cells, and part of the CD206+ cells were also SLC5A3 positive. In contrast, inflammatory cells were invariably AKR1B1 and SLC6A6 negative in all muscle tissues tested.

DISCUSSION

Our earlier studies had identified osmolyte pathway members as biomarkers for inflammatory myopathies, yet the pathogenic routes behind their elevated expression remained unknown. The present study offers further context and allows us to speculate on the underlying mechanisms.

Inflammatory Stress Induces Osmolyte Pathways in Muscle Cells

We here report that, in addition to increased NaCl concentrations, pro-inflammatory cytokines can induce osmolyte pathways in muscle cells in an *in vitro* setting. In response to osmotic stress, normal primary myotubes displayed a continuous increase of SLC5A3, SLC6A12, and AKR1B1 mRNA expression levels over time, while single cytokine pulse led to highest mRNA levels after 24 h, steadily decreasing afterwards and returning to near-normal levels at the 72 h time point. Immunocytochemical staining and western blotting experiments confirmed the transient induction pattern of SLC6A12 at the protein level. We cannot rule out fast cytokine degradation in the culture medium, yet this is unlikely as many have reported prolonged effects by single pulse cytokine treatments over several days (28–30). Using silencing techniques, we showed that compromising osmolyte accumulator expression negatively influenced cell growth only when muscle cells faced hyperosmotic conditions. We produced strongest evidence for AKR1B1, for which the knockdown regimen severely reduced AKR1B1 protein levels, yet did not compromise growth when myoblasts and myotubes were challenged with pro-inflammatory cytokines. Based upon this data, we speculate on different levels of importance of the osmolyte pathway dependent upon the challenges muscle cells face: osmolytes being essential protectors against osmotic stress while having a less vital yet regulatory role in the response to inflammatory stress. Our observations would need to be confirmed and analyzed further with knockdown combinations, as an important additional facet is the degree of redundancy of function displayed by the different osmolyte pathway members. In evidence, only SLC5A3 deficiency represents a lethal murine phenotype (31), with knockout of AKR1B1, SLC6A6, and SLC6A12 resulting in viable mice suffering from limited defects in renal function (32–34). The compensatory role of remaining osmolytes when activity of single pathway members is compromised, has long been confirmed in kidney cells (35).

Transcription factors NFκB and NFAT5 represent key regulators of cell's responses to inflammatory stress on the one hand and osmotic stress on the other hand. Not surprisingly therefore, pro-inflammatory cytokines were the most potent inducers of RelA, NFkB1, NFkB2 expression in muscle cells. However, we did observe some effects of NaCl-treatment on NFκB expression levels and, vice versa, NFAT5 expression responded to pro-inflammatory cytokines. Thus, muscle cells' responses to inflammatory and osmotic stress appear not separately regulated via NFκB and NFAT5, respectively.

The MAP kinases, a large family of Ser/Thr kinases that translate cell surface signals to the nucleus, play a crucial role in inflammation (36), which led us to study their involvement in muscle cells' responses to pro-inflammatory cytokines. We found Akt2 and HSP27 were most heavily phosphorylated in myotube cultures, but their activation was unaltered in response to inflammatory cytokines. Akt signaling influences muscle development and regeneration, affecting either initiation (Akt1) or maturation (Akt2) of myotubes (37). HSP27 is also associated with myotube differentiation and was found absent from myoblasts (38). The strong activation of Akt2 and HSP27 we observed in our *in vitro* model fits with the differentiated stage of the myotubes we studied in our experiments. The MAPKs of the p38 subgroup have been put forward as complex regulators of osmolyte pathways, through their hypertonicity-induced phosphorylation, and have been implicated in inflammatory disease (39). Our study found MAPK14 mRNA expression increased up to 2-fold by pro-inflammatory cytokines, and we observe increased phosphorylation of MAPK12 and MAPK13 in human primary myotubes treated for 24 h with IL1β+IFNγ. Of the extracellular signal-regulated kinases (ERK) on the other hand, we observed increased phosphorylation of MAPK3 (ERK1) in IL-1β+IFN-γ-treated myotubes. This is in line with our recent study that showed cytokines induce ERK1/2 phosphorylation,

which subsequently leads to protein deposition and autophagy in muscle cell cultures (40). We propose that the 24 h response of muscle cells to pro-inflammatory cytokines may thus be regulated primarily via such phosphorylation-driven activation of residential MAPKs. Muscle cells exposed to osmotic stress for prolonged periods appear to require extra measures for their protection, culminating in 18-fold (MAPK14) and 9-fold (NFAT5) increases in expression levels.

Osmolyte Pathways Are Activated in Regenerating Muscle Cells

Osmolytes are known regulators of skeletal muscle development, with the involvement of taurine and betaine already described in most detail. Taurine is essential for skeletal muscle buildup, and knockout mice lacking its transporter SLC6A6 display severe structural defects (41) and exercise intolerance (42). The trimethylglycine betaine appears also important for proper muscle functioning, although SLC6A12 knockout mice have been reported to develop only mild myopathy (34). Betaine promotes muscle fiber differentiation and myotube size (43) via stimulation of the mechanistic target of rapamycin pathway (44) and disturbed osmolyte balances have been implicated in muscle disease. Taurine levels were significantly reduced in muscle from myositis patients compared to healthy controls (45), while in urine on the other hand both taurine and betaine levels were increased in patients (46). In the murine Duchenne muscular dystrophy model, taurine content of muscle was low, mostly early in disease progression, and a reduction of its transporter SLC6A6 was observed (47). Yet, in the canine golden retriever muscular dystrophy model, muscle levels of taurine and SLC6A6 were 1.5- and 20-fold increased (48) compared to healthy dogs, pointing to possible differences between species and/or at different disease stages. Our localization studies revealed strong increases of osmolyte accumulators in small regenerating fibers. Possibly, protein replacement and refolding during the regeneration process are chaperoned by osmolytes, the latter aiding protection of functional protein conformations (49).

Subsets of Muscle-Infiltrating Inflammatory Cells Express SLC5A3 and SLC6A12

In addition to the muscle cells' general and dynamic repertory of osmolyte accumulators, we found two osmolyte pathway members, SLC5A3 and SLC6A12, selectively expressed in subsets of macrophages and T-cells infiltrating skeletal muscle. Interestingly, we observed an association with active invasion of nonnecrotic muscle fibers, a phenomenon typically observed in PM and IBM muscle tissues (50), which fits with current notions of how osmolytes behave as potent cytotoxic regulators. Cytotoxic macrophages have been shown to accumulate betaine, myoinositol and taurine as compatible organic osmolytes in response to osmotic stress, via MAPK-regulated upregulation of osmolyte transporters (51, 52). It is well known that macrophages have versatile functionalities, with a spectrum stretching out between the classical inflammatory M1 phenotype, to the alternative anti-inflammatory, tissue repair-oriented

M2 phenotype (53). Significantly higher levels of AKR1B1 mRNA and protein have been reported in M1 macrophages compared with M2-polarized macrophages (54). The upstream transcription factor NFAT5 is enhanced by the M1-promoting pro-inflammatory and hypoxic conditions associated with autoimmune diseases, which is particularly suggested to regulate the chemokine MCP-1 and subsequent synovial macrophage survival in rheumatoid arthritis (55). We found a subset of CD68+ cells, regarded as representing mostly M1 macrophages, to express SLC5A3 and SLC6A12, most prominently in PM and IBM tissues. In addition to macrophages, T-cells have also been shown to engage NFAT5-regulated pathways in their development and activation (56) and, in accordance, we found SLC5A3 and SLC6A12 expression in a minority of T-cells. In helper T-cells (Th-cells), salt-induced NFAT5 activity promotes their differentiation into Interleukin 17-producing Th-cells (Th17-cells) (57). This is relevant to inflammatory myopathy, as IL-17 induces and maintains chronic inflammation, and Th17-cells represent a pathogenic subset of T-cells associated with inflammatory myopathy (58).

CONCLUSIONS

The expression of osmolyte pathway members extends to human tissues that normally are not exposed to hypertonicity, which has led to the assumption that these factors have additional more versatile functions. In this respect, they have been put forward as biomarkers for inflammation (59) and tumor metastasis (60). The data we presented here points to a general role for osmolyte accumulation, via AKR1B1, SLC5A3, SLC6A6, and SLC6A12 upregulation, in muscle cells challenged by inflammatory stress, presumably in an attempt to stabilize protein function in sight of the changed proteome during regeneration. In addition, our data suggest an individual inflammatory role for SLC5A3 and SLC6A12 as potential regulators of the myocytotoxicity displayed

by muscle tissue-infiltrating auto-aggressive immune cells. The data we offer further adds to the complexity of inflammatory myopathy immunopathogeneses, broadening our understanding of this heterogeneous group of diseases.

AUTHOR CONTRIBUTIONS

BD conceived, designed, and executed the study. JW and JD analyzed patient data and material. BD, JZ, and TŠ carried out experiments and analyzed the data. BD drafted the manuscript, which was critically revised by JZ, JS, and JD.

FUNDING

BD is recipient of a research grant from the Association Belge contre les Maladies neuro-Musculaires (ABMM), aides à la recherche 2018. JD received confined sponsoring by CAF DCF. The international cooperation this work entailed, was supported by mobility grants from the Research Foundation—Flanders (FWO), German Academic Exchange Service (DAAD), the International Federation of Medical Students' Associations SCORE research exchange program, and the U4 university network OSMYO.

ACKNOWLEDGMENTS

We graciously thank the patients for their participation in this study, and thank Iris Iben and Sophie D'hose for skilful technical support.

REFERENCES

1. Dalakas MC. Inflammatory muscle diseases. N Eng J Med. (2015) 372:1734–47. doi: 10.1056/NEJMra1402225
2. Mammen AL. Statin-associated autoimmune myopathy. N Eng J Med. (2016) 374:664–9. doi: 10.1056/NEJMra1515161
3. Uruha A, Suzuki S, Suzuki N, Nishino I. Perifascicular necrosis in anti-synthetase syndrome beyond anti-Jo-1. Brain (2016) 139:e50. doi: 10.1093/brain/aww125
4. Malik A, Hayat G, Kalia JS, Guzman MA. Idiopathic inflammatory myopathies: clinical approach and management. Front Neurol. (2016) 7:e64. doi: 10.3389/fneur.2016.00064
5. Allenbach Y, Benveniste O, Goebel HH, Stenzel W. Integrated classification of inflammatory myopathies. Neuropathol Appl Neurobiol. (2017) 43:62–81. doi: 10.1111/nan.12380
6. Lahoria R, Selcen D, Engel AG. Microvascular alterations and the role of complement in dermatomyositis. Brain (2016) 139:1891–903. doi: 10.1093/brain/aww122
7. Dalakas MC. Pathogenesis and therapies of immune-mediated myopathies. Autoimm Rev. (2011) 11:203–6. doi: 10.1016/j.autrev.2011.05.013
8. Askanas V, Engel WK. Molecular pathology and pathogenesis of inclusion-body myositis. Microsc Res Tech. (2005) 67:114–20. doi: 10.1002/jemt.20186
9. Benveniste O, Stenzel W, Hilton-Jones D, Sandri M, Boyer O, van Engelen BGM. Amyloid deposits and inflammatory infiltrates in sporadic inclusion body myositis: the inflammatory egg comes before the degenerative chicken. Acta Neuropathol. (2015) 129:611–24. doi: 10.1007/s00401-015-1384-5
10. Allenbach Y, Mammen AL, Benveniste O, Stenzel W, on behalf of the Immune-Mediated Necrotizing Myopathies Working Group. 224th ENMC International Workshop: Clinico-sero-pathological classification of immune-mediated necrotizing myopathies Zandvoort, The Netherlands, 14–16 October. Neuromuscul Disord. (2017) 28:87–99. doi: 10.1016/j.nmd.2017.09.016
11. Warepam M, Singh LR. Osmolyte mixtures have different effects than individual osmolytes on protein folding and functional activity. Arch Biochem Biophys. (2015) 573:77–83. doi: 10.1016/j.abb.2015.03.017
12. Cheung CY, Ko BCB. NFAT5 in cellular adaptation to hypertonic stress-regulations and functional significance. J Mol Signal. (2013) 8:5. doi: 10.1186/1750-2187-8-5
13. Abbott KL, Friday BB, Thaloor D, Murphy TJ, Pavlath GK. Activation and cellular localization of the cyclosporine A-sensitive transcription factor NF-AT in skeletal muscle cells. Mol Biol Cell (1998) 9:2905–16. doi: 10.1091/mbc.9.10.2905

14. O'Connor RS, Mills ST, Jones KA, Ho SN, Pavlath GK. A combinatorial role for NFAT5 in both myoblast migration and differentiation during skeletal muscle myogenesis. *J Cell Sci.* (2007) 120:149–59. doi: 10.1242/jcs.03307

15. Roth I, Leroy V, Moo Kwon H, Martin PY, Feraille E, Hasler U. Osmoprotective transcription factor NFAT5/TonEBP modulates nuclear factor-kB activity. *Mol Biol Cell* (2010) 21:3459–74. doi: 10.1091/mbc.E10-02-0133

16. Creus KK, De Paepe B, De Bleecker JL. Idiopathic inflammatory myopathies and the classical NF-kappaB complex: current insights and implications for therapy. *Autoimm Rev.* (2009) 8:627–31. doi: 10.1016/j.autrev.2009.02.026

17. De Paepe B. A recipe for myositis: nuclear factor kB and nuclear factor of activated T-cells transcription factor pathways spiced up by cytokines. *AIMS All Immunol.* (2017) 1:31–42. doi: 10.3934/Allergy.2017.1.31

18. De Bleecker J, De Paepe B, Vanwalleghem IE, Schröder JM. Differential expression of chemokines in inflammatory myopathies. *Neurology* (2002) 58:1779–85. doi: 10.1212/WNL.58.12.1779

19. Creus KK, De Paepe B, Weis J, De Bleecker JL. The multifaceted character of lymphotoxin b in inflammatory myopathies and muscular dystrophies. *Neuromuscul Disord.* (2012) 22:712–9. doi: 10.1016/j.nmd.2012.04.012

20. De Bleecker JL, Meire VI, Declercq W, Van Aken EH. Immunolocalization of tumor necrosis factor-alpha and its receptors in inflammatory myopathies. *Neurmuscul Disord.* (1999) 9:239–46. doi: 10.1016/S0960-8966(98)00126-6

21. De Paepe, Racz GZ, Schröder JM, De Bleecker JL. Expression and distribution of the nitric oxide synthases in idiopathic inflammatory myopathies. *Acta Neuropathol.* (2004) 108:37–42. doi: 10.1007/s00401-004-0859-6

22. De Paepe B, Creus KK, Weis J, De Bleecker JL. Heat shock protein families 70 and 90 in Duchenne muscular dystrophy and inflammatory myopathy: Balancing muscle protection and destruction. *Neuromuscul Disord.* (2012) 22:26–33. doi: 10.1016/j.nmd.2011.07.007

23. Van der Meer JW, Netea MG. A salty taste to autoimmunity. *N Engl J Med.* (2013) 368:2520–1. doi: 10.1056/NEJMcibr1303292

24. De Paepe B, Martin JJ, Herbelet S, Jimenez-Mallebrera C, Iglesias E, Jou C, et al. Activation of osmolyte pathways in inflammatory myopathy and Duchenne muscular dystrophy points to osmotic regulation as a contributing pathogenic mechanism. *Lab Invest.* (2016) 96:872–84. doi: 10.1038/labinvest.2016.68

25. Herbelet S, De Vlieghere E, Gonçalves A, De Paepe B, Schmidt K, Nys E, et al. Localization and expression of nuclear factor of activated T-cells 5 in myoblasts exposed to pro-inflammatory cytokines or hyperosmolar stress and in biopsies from myositis patients, *Front Physiol.* (2018) 9:e126. doi: 10.3389/fphys.2018.00126

26. Schmidt J, Barthel K, Zschüntzsch J, Muth IE, Swindle EJ, Hombach A, et al. Nitric oxide stress in sporadic inclusion body myositis muscle fibres: inhibition of inducible nitric oxide synthase prevents interleukin-1β-induced accumulation of β-amyloid and cell death. *Brain* (2012) 135:1102–14. doi: 10.1093/brain/aws046

27. De Bleecker JL, De Paepe B, Aronica E, de Visser M, ENMC Myositis Muscle Biopsy Study Group, Amato A. 205th ENMC International Workshop: Pathology diagnosis of idiopathic inflammatory myopathies Part II 28–30 March 2014, Naarden, The Netherlands. *Neuromuscul Disord.* (2015) 25:268–72. doi: 10.1016/j.nmd.2014.12.001

28. Michaelis D, Goebels N, Hohlfeld R. Constitutive and cytokine-induced expression of human leukocyte antigens and cell adhesion molecules by human myotubes. *Am J Pathol.* (1993) 143:1142–9.

29. Liu CJ, Wang H, Zhao Z, Yu S, Lu YB, Meyer J, et al. MyoD-dependent induction during myoblast differentiation of p204, a protein also inducible by interferon. *Mol Cell Biol.* (2000) 20:7024–36. doi: 10.1128/MCB.20.18.7024-7036.2000

30. Langen RC, Schols AM, Kelders MC, Wouters EF, Janssen-Heininger YM. Inflammatory cytokines inhibit myogenic differentiation through activation of nuclear factor-kappa B. *FASEB J* (2001) 15:1169–80. doi: 10.1096/fj.00-0463

31. Buccafusca R, Venditti CP, Kenyon LC, Johanson RA, Van Bockstaele E, Ren J, et al. Characterization of the null murine sodium/myo-inositol cotransporter 1 (Smit1 or Slc5a3) phenotype: myo-inositol rescue is independent of expression of its cognate mitochondrial ribosomal protein subunit 6 (Mrps6) gene and of phosphatidylinositol levels in neonatal brain. *Mol Genet Metab.* (2008) 95:81–95. doi: 10.1016/j.ymgme.2008.05.008

32. Aida K, Ikegishi Y, Chen J, Tawata M, Ito S, Maeda S, et al. Disruption of aldose reductase gene (Akr1b1) causes defect in urinary concentrating ability and divalent cation homeostasis. *Biochem Biophys Res Commun.* (2000) 277:281–6. doi: 10.1006/bbrc.2000.3648

33. Huang DY, Boini KM, Lang PA, Grahammer F, Duszenko M, Heller-Stilb B, et al. Impaired ability to increase water excretion in mice lacking the taurine transporter gene TAUT. *Eur J Physiol.* (2006) 451:668–77. doi: 10.1007/s00424-005-1499-y

34. Lehre AC, Rowley NM, Zhou Y, Holmseth S, Guo C, Holen T, et al. Deletion of the betaine-GABA transporter (BGT1; slmc6a12) gene does not affect seizure thresholds of adult mice. *Epilepsy Res.* (2011) 95:70–81. doi: 10.1016/j.eplepsyres.2011.02.014

35. Moriyama TA, Garcia-Perez A, Olson A, Burg MB. Intracellular betaine substitutes for sorbitol in protecting renal medullary cells from hypertonicity. *Am J Physiol.* (1991) 260:F494–7. doi: 10.1152/ajprenal.1991.260.4.F494

36. Dong C, Davis RJ, Flavell RA. Map kinases in the immune reponse. *Annu Rev Immunol.* (2002) 20:55–72. doi: 10.1146/annurev.immunol.20.091301.131133

37. Rotwein P, Wilson EM. Distinct actions of Akt1 and Akt2 in skeletal muscle differentiation. *J Cell Physiol.* (2009) 219:503–11. doi: 10.1002/jcp.21692

38. Dubinska-Magiera M, Jablonska J, Saczko J, Kulbacka J, Kagla T, Daczewska M. Contribution of small heat shock proteins to muscle development. *FEBS Lett.* (2014) 588:517–30. doi: 10.1016/j.febslet.2014.01.005

39. Waetzig GH, Seegert D, Rosenstiel P, Nikolaus S, Schreiber S. p38 mitogen-activated protein kinase is activated and linked to TNF-alpha signaling in inflammatory bowel disease. *J Immunol.* (2002) 168:5342–51. doi: 10.4049/jimmunol.168.10.5342

40. Schmidt K, Wienken M, Keller CW, Balcarek P, Munz C, Schmidt J. IL-1β-induced accumulation of amyloid: macrophagy in skeletal muscle depends on ERK. *Mediat Inflamm.* (2017) 2017:e5470831. doi: 10.1155/2017/5470831

41. Ito T, Kimura Y, Uozumi Y, Takai M, Muraoka S, Matsuda T, et al. Taurine depletion caused by knocking out the taurine transporter gene leads to cardiomyopathy with cardiac atrophy. *J Mol Cell Cardiol.* (2008) 44:927–37. doi: 10.1016/j.yjmcc.2008.03.001

42. Warskulat U, Heller-Stilb B, Germann E, Zilles K, Haas H, Lang F, et al. Phenotype of the taurine transporter knockout mouse. *Methods Enzymol.* (2007) 428:439–58. doi: 10.1016/S0076-6879(07)28025-5

43. Senesi P, Luzi L, Montesano A, Mazzocchi N, Terruzzi I. Betaine supplement enhances skeletal muscle differentiation in murine myoblasts via IGF-1 signaling activation. *J Translat Med.* (2013) 11:e174. doi: 10.1186/1479-5876-11-174

44. Huang QC, Xu ZR, Han XY, Li WF. Changes in hormones, growth factor and lipid metabolism in finishing pigs fed betaine. *Livestock Sci.* (2006) 105:78–85. doi: 10.1016/j.livsci.2006.04.031

45. Stuerenburg HJ, Stangneth B, Schoser BG. Age related profiles of free amino acids in human skeletal muscle. *Neuroendocrinol Lett.* (2006) 27:133–6.

46. Chung YL, Wassif WS, Bell JD, Huley M, Scott DL. Urinary levels of creatine and other metabolites in the assessment of polymyositis and dermatomyositis. *Rheumatology* (2003) 42:298–303. doi: 10.1093/rheumatology/keg084

47. Terrill JR, Grounds MD, Arthur PG. Taurine deficiency, synthesis and transport in the mdx mouse model for Duchenne Muscular Dystrophy. *Int J Biochem Cell Biol.* (2015) 66:141–8. doi: 10.1016/j.biocel.2015.07.016

48. Terrill JR, Duong MN, Turner R, Le Guiner C, Boyatzis A, Kettle AJ, et al. Levels of inflammation and oxidative stress, and a role for taurine in dystropathology of the Golden Retriever Muscular Dystrophy dog model for Duchenne Muscular Dystrophy. *Redox Biol.* (2016) 9:276–86. doi: 10.1016/j.redox.2016.08.016

49. Khan SH, Ahmad N, Ahmad F, Kumar R. Naturally occurring organic osmolytes: from cell physiology to disease prevention. *IUBMB Life* (2010) 62:891–5. doi: 10.1002/iub.406

50. De Paepe B, De Bleecker JL. The nonnecrotic invaded muscle fibers of polymyositis and sporadic inclusion body myositis: on the interplay of chemokines and stress proteins. *Neurosci Lett.* (2013) 535:18–23. doi: 10.1016/j.neulet.2012.11.064

51. Warskulat U, Zhang F, Häussinger D. Taurine is an osmolyte in rat liver macrophages (Kupffer cells). *J Hepatol.* (1997) 26:1340–7. doi: 10.1016/S0168-8278(97)80470-9

52. Denkert C, Warskulat U, Hensel F, Häussinger D. Osmolyte strategy in human monocytes and macrophages: involvement of p38MAPK

in hyperosmotic induction of betaine and myoinositol transporters. *Arch Biochem Biophys.* (1998) 354:172–80. doi: 10.1006/abbi. 1998.0661

53. Mantovani A, Sica A, Sozzani S, Allavena P, Vecchi A, Locati M. The chemokine system in diverse forms of macrophage activation and polarization. *Trends Immunol.* (2004) 25:677–86. doi: 10.1016/j.it.2004. 09.015

54. Erbel C, Rupp G, Domschke G, Linden F, Akhavanpoor M, Doesch AO, et al. Differential regulation of aldose reductase expression during macrophage polarization depends on hyperglycemia. *Innate Immun.* (2016) 22:230–7. doi: 10.1177/1753425916632053

55. Choi S, You S, Kim D, Choi SY, Kwon HM, Kim HS, et al. Transcription factor NFAT5 promotes macrophage survival in rheumatoid arthritis. *J Clin Invest.* (2017) 127:954–69. doi: 10.1172/JCI87880

56. Trama J, Go WY, Ho SN. The osmoprotective function of the NFAT5 transcription factor in T cell development and activation. *J Immunol.* (2002) 169:5477–88. doi: 10.4049/jimmunol.169.10.5477

57. Kleinewietfeld M, Manzel A, Totze J, Kvakan H, Yosef N, Linker RA, et al. Sodium chloride drives autoimmune disease by the induction of pathogenic TH17 cells. *Nature* (2013) 496:518–22. doi: 10.1038/nature 11868

58. Tournadre A, Miossec P. Interleukin-17 in inflammatory myopathies. *Curr Rheumatol Rep.* (2012) 14:252–6. doi: 10.1007/s11926-012-0242-x

59. Trama J, Lu Q, Hawley RG, Ho SN. The NFAT-related protein NFATL1 (TonEBP/NFAT5) is induced upon T cell activation in a calcineurin-dependent manner. *J Immunol.* (2000) 165:4884–94. doi: 10.4049/jimmunol.165.9.4884

60. Jauliac S, Lopez-Rodriguez C, Shaw LM, Brown LF, Rao A, Toker A. The role of NFAT transcription factors in integrin-mediated carcinoma invasion. *Nat Cell Biol.* (2002) 4:540–4. doi: 10.1038/ncb816

15

Neurofilament Light Chain: Blood Biomarker of Neonatal Neuronal Injury

Antoinette Depoorter[1]*[†], Roland P. Neumann[2†], Christian Barro[3], Urs Fisch[3], Peter Weber[1], Jens Kuhle[3] and Sven Wellmann[2]

[1] Department of Neuropediatrics and Developmental Medicine, University Children's Hospital Basel, University of Basel, Basel, Switzerland, [2] Department of Neonatology, University Children's Hospital Basel, University of Basel, Basel, Switzerland, [3] Neurologic Clinic and Policlinic, Departments of Medicine, Biomedicine and Clinical Research, University Hospital Basel, University of Basel, Basel, Switzerland

*Correspondence:
Antoinette Depoorter
antoinette.depoorter@ukbb.ch

[†] *These authors have contributed equally to this work*

Background: Neurofilament light chain (NfL) is a highly promising biomarker of neuroaxonal injury that has mainly been studied in adult neurodegenerative disease. Its involvement in neonatal disease remains largely unknown. Our aim was to establish NfL plasma concentrations in preterm and term infants in the first week of life.

Methods: Plasma NfL was measured by single molecule array immunoassay in two neonatal cohorts: cohort 1 contained 203 term and preterm infants, median gestational age (GA) 37.9 weeks (interquartile range [IQR] 31.9–39.4), in whom venous and arterial umbilical cord blood was sampled at birth and venous blood at day of life (DOL) 3; cohort 2 contained 98 preterm infants, median GA 29.3 weeks (IQR 26.9–30.6), in whom venous blood was sampled at DOL 7.

Results: Median NfL concentrations in venous blood increased significantly from birth (18.2 pg/mL [IQR 12.8–30.8, cohort 1]) to DOL 3 (50.9 pg/mL [41.3–100, cohort 1]) and DOL 7 (126 pg/mL [78.8–225, cohort 2]) ($p < 0.001$). In both cohorts NfL correlated inversely with birth weight (BW, Spearman's rho −0.403, $p < 0.001$, cohort 1; R −0.525, $p < 0.001$, cohort 2) and GA (R −0.271, $p < 0.001$, cohort 1; R −0.487, $p < 0.001$, cohort 2). Additional significant correlations were found for maternal age at delivery, preeclampsia, delivery mode, 5-min Apgar, duration of oxygen supplementation, sepsis, and brain damage (intraventricular hemorrhage or periventricular leukomalacia). Multivariable logistic regression analysis identified the independent predictors of NfL in cohort 1 as BW (beta = −0.297, $p = 0.003$), delivery mode (beta = 0.237, $p = 0.001$) and preeclampsia (beta = 0.183, $p = 0.022$) and in cohort 2 as BW (beta = −0.385, $p = 0.001$) and brain damage (beta = 0.222, $p = 0.015$).

Conclusion: Neonatal NfL levels correlate inversely with maturity and BW, increase during the first days of life, and relate to brain injury factors such as intraventricular hemorrhage and periventricular leukomalacia, and also to vaginal delivery.

Keywords: cerebral injury, neuropathology, biomarker, infant, parturition, prematurity

INTRODUCTION

As direct access to the central nervous system (CNS) is almost impossible, neuronal biomarkers have been investigated for decades in order to improve early diagnostics, monitor disease progression and optimize care. Neurofilaments (Nf) are highly specific major neuronal scaffolding proteins comprising 4 subunits: the triplet of Nf light chain (NfL), Nf medium chain, and Nf heavy chain (NfH), and α-internexin in the CNS, or peripherin in the peripheral nervous system (1). Acute or chronic neuronal damage, including traumatic brain injury, stroke, dementia and multiple sclerosis, releases Nf fragments into the cerebrospinal fluid and eventually the blood compartment (2–6). Recent advances using highly sensitive single molecule array (Simoa) immunoassay have improved NfL detection, particularly in peripheral blood, making it a promising and readily accessible biomarker for neuroaxonal injury (7).

Whereas, circulating Nf has been extensively characterized in adults and older children with neurologic disease, data in infants and particularly newborns are sparse. One study reported raised serum NfH in children older than 6 months with febrile seizures lasting >30 min, suggesting that prolonged seizures cause some degree of neuronal damage (8). Plasma NfH in newborns with hypoxic-ischemic encephalopathy (HIE) was also higher than in healthy neonates (9, 10). Moreover, NfL levels in infants undergoing therapeutic hypothermia for HIE were significantly higher in those with unfavorable vs. favorable brain magnetic resonance imaging (MRI) outcome (11). As for mode of delivery, serum NfH levels at day of life (DOL) 2 in a small cohort of newborns did not differ between those born vaginally and those born by cesarean section (12).

Given the potential of Nf in adults with acute or chronic CNS damage and promising results in infants with HIE, we aimed to measure NfL levels by Simoa in two cohorts of preterm and term neonates in umbilical cord blood at birth and in venous blood a few days after birth.

MATERIALS AND METHODS
Study Participants

The study was based on data and blood samples prospectively collected from two neonatal cohorts. Cohort 1 comprised data and blood samples from 203 preterm and term neonates, median gestational age (GA) 37.9 weeks (interquartile range [IQR] 31.9–39.4), born and cared for at the University Hospitals of Zurich and Basel, Switzerland. More specifically, it comprised 89 preterm infants (GA < 37 weeks), including 52 with GA < 32 weeks, and 114 term infants (GA ≥ 37 weeks). The study was approved by the institutional review boards of both university hospitals (Ethikkommission beider Basel, EKBB07/09, Kantonale Ethikkommission Zurich, KEK08/09). Cohort 2 comprised data and blood samples from 98 very preterm neonates (GA < 32 weeks), median GA 29.3 weeks (IQR 26.9–30.6), born and cared

Abbreviations: Nf, Neurofilament; NfL, Neurofilament Light Chain; GA, Gestational Age; BW, Birth Weight; DOL, Day of Life; MPT, Moderate Preterm and Term.

for at the University Hospital of Basel, Switzerland. The study was approved by the institutional review board (Ethikkommission beider Basel, EK233/13) and was carried out in accordance with the declaration of Helsinki. Written informed consent was obtained from the parents prior to enrollment.

Clinical Characteristics (Table 1)

Details of pregnancy (presence/absence of preeclampsia, amniotic infection, preterm labor, maternal age, premature rupture of membranes), delivery (umbilical artery pH, delivery modality), birth (GA, BW, sex, 5- and 10-min Apgar scores), and postnatal course to discharge home (presence/absence of sepsis and/or necrotizing enterocolitis, ultrasound brain damage with periventricular intraventricular hemorrhage [PIVH] or periventricular leukomalacia [PVL], duration of oxygen) were collected from the charts. Definitions of clinical characteristics, including preeclampsia, clinical chorioamnionitis, PIVH, and PVL, have been described previously (13), based on standardized definitions of the Swiss Neonatal Network.

Sample Preparation and Assessment of NfL

In cohort 1, venous blood (0.5 mL) was collected from the umbilical cord at birth (n = 185) and simultaneously with mandatory neonatal metabolic screening at DOL 3 (n = 39); 68 paired umbilical arterial samples were also collected at birth. In cohort 2, venous blood was collected with diagnostic blood samples at DOL 7 (n = 98). All samples were handled according to standard operating procedures for blood sampling in EDTA tubes, subsequent sample transfer to the central laboratory service, centrifugation, preparation of aliquots, and storage at −80°C until batch-wise analysis as described previously (14). Assay technicians were blinded to clinical information and pregnancy outcome.

NfL levels were measured by Simoa immunoassay using capture monoclonal antibody (mAB) 47:3 and biotinylated detector mAB 2:1 (UmanDiagnostics, Umea, Sweden), as previously described (15). Calibrators (neat) and serum samples (1:4 dilution) were measured in duplicate. Bovine lyophilized NfL was obtained from UmanDiagnostics. Calibrators ranged from 0 to 2,000 pg/mL. Batch-prepared calibrators were stored at −80°C. Intra- and interassay variabilities were < 10%; the few samples with intra-assay coefficients of variation >20% were remeasured.

Data Analysis

Statistical analyses were performed using SPSS for Windows version 24 (IBM) and included descriptive statistics, Spearman's rank-order correlation analyses and multiple linear regressions (MLR) using NfL as dependent variable. NfL variables were log10 transformed for the correlations and MLR. The independent variables included for MLR were based on significant correlations and significant non-parametric univariate analyses such as the Mann-Whitney U (2 levels) and Kruskal-Wallis tests (>2 levels). For cohort 1 these variables were: BW, 5-min Apgar, delivery mode (3 levels), preeclampsia, sepsis, and oxygen duration. For cohort 2 they were: BW, 5-min Apgar, sex, brain damage, sepsis, amniotic infection, and oxygen duration. Due to collinearity between BW and GA, we used only BW in MLR, where it showed stronger correlation with NfL than GA.

RESULTS

Baseline NfL Levels

In cohort 1 overall median venous NfL concentrations were 18.2 pg/mL (IQR 12.8–30.8) at birth and 50.9 pg/mL (41.3–100.1) at DOL 3; in cohort 2 they were 128.5 pg/mL (78.8–224.8) at DOL 7.

We split cohort 1 into a very preterm group (GA < 32 weeks; $n = 52$) and a moderate preterm and term (MPT) group (GA ≥ 32 weeks; $n = 151$) with fewer prematurity complications ($n = 1$ in our sample). This also enabled us to compare the first group with cohort 2. NfL levels were significantly higher in very preterm infants than in the MPT group at birth (median 32.5 pg/mL, $n = 47$ vs. 15.3 pg/mL, $n = 138$; $p < 0.001$), but not at DOL 3 (median 48.5 pg/mL, $n = 16$ vs. 51.4 pg/mL, $n = 23$; $p = 0.668$). Moreover, levels increased significantly from birth to DOL 3 in both the very preterm and MPT groups (median 32.5 vs. 48.5 pg/mL, $p = 0.002$; and median 15.3 vs. 51.4 pg/mL, $p < 0.001$), and from DOL 3 to DOL 7 in the very preterm group (median 48.5 vs. 128.5 pg/mL, $p = 0.001$) (**Table 2**). This increase was confirmed in cohort 1 when comparing paired samples from same infants (MPT group $n = 16$, very preterm group $n = 11$) at birth and DOL 3 (median 18.2 pg/mL vs. 49.4 pg/mL). Out of these, only in 2 very preterm infants NfL levels remained unchanged, in all other infants they increased from birth until DOL 3. Paired umbilical cord arterial and venous plasma were closely related ($R = 0.875$, $p < 0.001$). Given this close correlation and the greater number of subjects ($n = 185$), we performed all further analyses using the venous blood samples collected at birth.

NfL and Perinatal Characteristics in Cohort 1

Venous cord blood at birth correlated negatively with BW ($R = -0.403$, $p < 0.001$, **Figure 1**), GA ($R = -0.271$, $p < 0.001$), 5-min Apgar ($R = -0.295$, $p < 0.001$), and 10-min Apgar ($R = -0.363$, $p < 0.001$). In contrast, levels correlated positively with oxygen duration ($R = 0.333$, $p < 0.001$) and delivery mode ($R = 0.156$, p = 0.034).

Presence of preeclampsia (31.0 pg/mL vs. 16.2, $p < 0.001$) and sepsis (32.6 pg/mL vs. 17.85, $p = 0.033$) were associated with higher NfL levels.

In the MPT group NfL levels at birth were significantly higher in infants delivered vaginally than by primary or secondary cesarean section (21.8 vs. 13.9 and 14.4 pg/mL; $p = 0.002$) (**Figure 2**). This was not the case in the very preterm group, presumably due to the few vaginal deliveries ($n = 5$ vs. $n = 47$ cesarean sections). At DOL 3 there was no significant difference ($p = 0.07$) in NfL levels between birth modalities except for vaginal delivery vs. cesarean section (110 pg/mL, $n = 8$ vs. 48.7 pg/mL, $n = 31$; $p = 0.031$).

MLR testing for the best independent predictors of NfL levels at birth used BW, 5-min Apgar, delivery mode, preeclampsia, sepsis and oxygen duration as explanatory variables. The model

TABLE 1 | Descriptive statistics.

	Cohort 1 $n = 203$		Cohort 2 $n = 98$
	Moderate Preterm and Term (≥32 weeks GA) $n = 151$	Very preterm (< 32 weeks GA) $n = 52$	Very preterm (< 32 weeks GA) $n = 98$
NEONATAL CHARACTERISTICS			
GA (weeks)	38.3 (37.0–40.0)	30.1 (28.3–31.3)	29.3 (26.9–30.6)
BW (g)	3270 (2710–3630)	1360 (1063–1463)	1145 (788–1413)
Sex (male, %)	87 (57.6)	25 (48.1)	52 (53.1)
Brain damage (%)	1 (0.7)	10 (19.2)	12 (12.2)
O₂ duration (days)	0	4 (1–15.8)	2.38 (0.05–22.8)
pH umbilical artery	7.30 (7.26–7.33)	7.32 (7.29–7.37)	7.32 (7.28–7.36)
NEC (%)	0	0	3 (3.1)
Sepsis (%)	0	11 (21.2)	13 (13.3)
5-min Apgar	9 (9–9)	7 (5.25–8)	7 (6–8)
Death (%)	0	6 (11.5)	2 (2.0)
MATERNAL CHARACTERISTICS			
Age (years)	32 (29–36)	33 (28.3–36.0)	33 (29–36)
Amniotic infection (%)	5 (3.3)	13(25)	20 (20.4)
Preeclampsia (%)	16 (10.6)	20 (38.5)	16 (16.3)
PROM (%)	14 (9.3)	14 (26.9)	28 (28.6)
DM (%):			
Primary CS	76 (50.3)	26 (50)	27 (27.6)
Secondary CS	29 (19.2)	21 (40.4)	59 (60.2)
VD	46 (30.5)	5 (9.6)	12 (12.2)

GA, gestational age; BW, birth weight; BD, brain damage (PIVH and/or PVL); NEC, necrotizing enterocolitis; PROM, premature rupture of membranes; DM, delivery mode; CS, cesarean section; VD, vaginal delivery. GA, BW, O₂ duration, Apgar, pH and maternal age are presented as median and interquartile range.

was significant ($F_{(6, 176)} = 8.655$, $p < 0.001$), explaining around 23% of NfL variance ($R^2 = 0.228$). The predictors were BW (beta $= -0.297$, $p = 0.003$), delivery mode (beta $= 0.237$, $p = 0.001$), and preeclampsia (beta $= 0.183$, $p = 0.022$).

NfL and Perinatal Characteristics in Cohort 2

NfL at DOL 7 correlated negatively with the main neonatal characteristics such as BW ($R = -0.525$, $p < 0.001$, **Figure 1**), GA ($R = -0.487$, $p < 0.001$), and 5- and 10-min Apgar ($R = -0.247$, $p = 0.014$; $R = -0.228$, $p = 0.024$). Correlation was positive with oxygen duration ($R = 0.358$, $p < 0.001$) and maternal age ($R = 0.353$, $p < 0.001$).

Brain damage (211.5 pg/mL vs. 123, $p = 0.002$) and sepsis (184 pg/mL vs. 124.5, $p = 0.020$) were associated with higher NfL levels. Delivery mode had no significant impact ($p = 0.624$).

MLR analysis of cohort 2 used BW, 5-min Apgar, sex, brain damage, sepsis, amniotic infection, and oxygen duration as explanatory variables. The regression model explained around 37% of NfL variance ($R^2 = 0.366$, $F_{(7, 89)} = 7.331$, $p < 0.001$). Only BW (beta $= -0.385$, $p = 0.001$) and brain damage (beta $= 0.222$, $p = 0.015$) contributed significantly to predicting NfL (**Figure 2**).

DISCUSSION

Neuronal injury marker NfL has proved a sensitive and specific biomarker in adult peripheral blood, serving as a promising adjunct to monitoring and decision-making in acute and chronic neurologic disease (16, 17). Our study provides a first insight into neonatal NfL levels in term and preterm infants. The major findings are that NfL levels increase over the first few days of life, relate inversely to prematurity and BW, and identify BW, delivery mode, preeclampsia and brain damage as independent predictors.

NfL levels at birth in MPT infants resemble those in healthy adults (15). By DOL 3 they rise to the levels seen in adults with neurodegenerative disease such as multiple sclerosis (15). At DOL 7 in very preterm infants NfL levels are in the range of asphyxiated neonates at DOL 4 (11).

The main influencers of NfL in both cohorts were BW and maturity: birth and neonatal levels were both higher in low BW infants (**Figure 1**), perhaps because brain vulnerability to neuronal injury increases with prematurity. Alternatively, high NfL levels in preterm infants might be due to high neuronal

turnover in general, with the much higher postnatal levels at DOL 3 and DOL 7 (**Figure 2**) simply reflecting a neuronal stress reaction to birth, as in healthy term neonates.

Preterm infants are at risk for perinatal brain damage, in particular PIVH and PVL (18). In our sample those with evidence of brain damage had significantly higher NfL levels than those without (**Figure 2**). Brain damage leads directly to neuronal injury, to a degree objectifiable by NfL: levels are higher in asphyxiated neonates with unfavorable brain MRI outcome (11). As in adults, cerebrovascular accident results in immediately higher NfL levels (19), compared to the more gradual neuronal damage seen in neurodegenerative disease (20).

In addition to a direct effect of brain damage, we identified two other stressors that increase NfL, namely delivery mode and preeclampsia. Levels were higher in infants delivered vaginally than by cesarean section (**Figure 2**), suggesting greater neuronal injury and confirming vaginal delivery as one of life's strongest stressors, causing incommensurable release of various fetal stress hormones (21). Preeclampsia, a pregnancy-specific syndrome defined by high blood pressure and other morbidities (22), was the additional stressor, raising NfL levels at birth even after adjustment for BW and GA. Our finding is consistent with the recent report of raised NfL levels in women with preeclampsia (23). Maternal hypertension is closely linked to placental insufficiency which compromises fetal perfusion and may cause cardiovascular disease later in life (24). Our data indicate that preeclampsia involves a risk of neuronal damage in the unborn child.

While the main source of NfL is considered to be the central nervous system, peripheral damage may contribute to increased NfL values as well, as recently revealed by studies on peripheral neuropathies (25, 26). Increased blood levels of the muscle enzyme creatine kinase in newborn infants after vaginal deliveries compared to cesarean sections have been reported (27). They support the notion that increased NfL in these babies may result, at least in part, from peripheral neuronal damage. However, data on the central nervous system biomarker S100 B measured in the maternal serum and cord blood show clearly increased S100B values after vaginal delivery compared to cesarean section (28). It has been shown previously that

TABLE 2 | Cohort neurofilament light chain concentrations at birth and at days of life (DOL) 3 and 7.

Cohort	Neurofilament light chain concentrations (pg/mL)			
	Birth (arterial)	Birth (venous)	DOL 3 (venous)	DOL 7 (venous)
1: Very preterm group (GA < 32 weeks) n = 52		32.5 (17.6–52.5) n = 47	48.5 (37.6–138) n = 16	
1: Moderate Preterm and Term group (GA ≥32 weeks) n = 151	17.7 (12.4–25.4) n = 68	15.3 (12.2–23.9) n = 138	51.4 (41.4–86.4) n = 23	
2: Very preterm group (GA < 32 weeks) n = 98				126 (78.8–225) n = 98

Median and interquartile range. GA, gestational age.

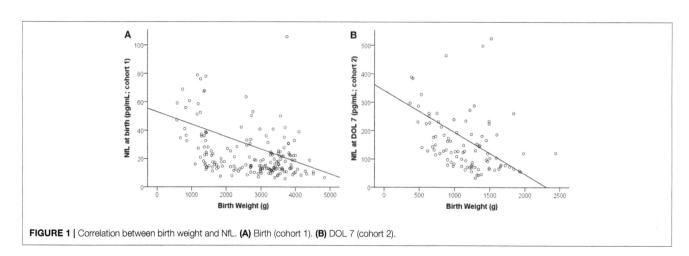

FIGURE 1 | Correlation between birth weight and NfL. **(A)** Birth (cohort 1). **(B)** DOL 7 (cohort 2).

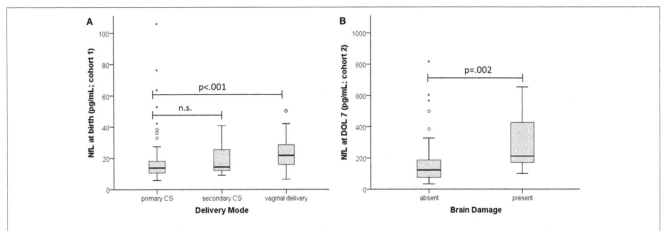

FIGURE 2 | Effect of delivery mode and brain damage on NfL. **(A)** NfL at birth in infants with GA ≥ 32 weeks (cohort 1). **(B)** NfL at DOL 7 (cohort 2). Absent, no brain damage; present, PIVH and/or PVL. Boxplots are presented with median and IQR. The * are extreme outliers.

extracranial sources of S100B do not affect serum levels (29). Taken together, the findings of Schulpis KH et al. corroborate our data that increased levels of the neuronal injury markers S100B and NfL might be caused by the compression on the fetus' brain during delivery.

Further, S100B levels in neonates with HIE exceeded those in healthy controls, proportionately to disease severity and worse outcome (30). Although S100B levels decreased overall from DOL 1 through DOL 9 (31), levels in preterm and term neonatal saliva followed a pattern similar to NfL, being higher in preterm than in term infants and correlating negatively with GA (32). Nerve growth factor (NGF) is a neurotrophic factor involved in brain development and neuroplasticity following brain damage. Unlike NfL, NGF levels in maternal and cord plasma are lower in preterm than in term deliveries (33).

To date the metabolism of NfL in cerebrospinal fluid (CSF) and blood is largely unknown, ways of elimination or protein degradation have not been described. One study examined the influence of blood brain barrier permeability and blood NfL levels. In this study there was no correlation between serum NfL concentration and CSF/serum albumin ratio (34).

Study limitations include the relatively few subjects sampled at DOL 3, which may account for the non-significant difference between very preterm and MPT infants at DOL 3. In the first week of life there is an apparent increase in NfL levels, but in the absence of data points post-DOL 7, the subsequent profile of NfL requires elucidation in further studies. Nor can we exclude other confounders that might influence and explain NfL. Cognitive outcome studies will need to confirm the use of NfL as a predictive biomarker of brain damage and eventual neurodevelopmental deficit. Such early biomarkers are sorely needed to complement ultrasound or MRI in conditions such as PVL (18). In addition, future studies may explore NfL together with other potentially promising biomarkers of brain

damage (35). More generally, research is required to explore and disentangle the causes of the high degree of neuronal injury in the preterm brain.

CONCLUSION

This study provides an initial insight into neuronal injury marker NfL in term and preterm infants. Levels increase through the first week of life. They relate inversely to GA and BW and are higher in brain injury. Obstetric parameters such as delivery mode and preeclampsia also raise NfL levels. Our study supports the use of NfL in neonates to help us understand the factors leading to neuroaxonal injury and how we might monitor and prevent them.

AUTHOR CONTRIBUTIONS

SW and UF designed the study. SW and RN collected the data. JK and CB assayed the serum samples. AD analyzed the data and wrote the manuscript together with SW and PW. All authors provided critical feedback and helped to improve the manuscript.

ACKNOWLEDGMENTS

This research is funded by the Swiss National Science Foundation (320030_169848) and the Gottfried und Julia Bangerter-Rhyner-Stiftung, Bern, Switzerland.

REFERENCES

1. Yuan A, Rao MV, Veeranna, Nixon RA. Neurofilaments and neurofilament proteins in health and disease. *Cold Spring Harbor Perspect Biol.* (2017) 9:a018309. doi: 10.1101/cshperspect.a018309

2. Shahim P, Zetterberg H, Tegner Y, Blennow K. Serum neurofilament light as a biomarker for mild traumatic brain injury in contact sports. *Neurology* (2017) 88:1788–94. doi: 10.1212/WNL.0000000000003912

3. Rohrer JD, Woollacott IO, Dick KM, Brotherhood E, Gordon E, Fellows A, et al. Serum neurofilament light chain protein is a measure of disease intensity in frontotemporal dementia. *Neurology* (2016) 87:1329–36. doi: 10.1212/WNL.0000000000003154

4. De Marchis GM, Katan M, Barro C, Fladt J, Traenka C, Seiffge DJ, et al. Serum neurofilament light chain in patients with acute cerebrovascular events. *Eur J Neurol.* (2018) 25:562–8. doi: 10.1111/ene.13554

5. Mattsson N, Andreasson U, Zetterberg H, Blennow K, Alzheimer's Disease Neuroimaging Initiative. Association of plasma neurofilament light with neurodegeneration in patients with Alzheimer disease. *JAMA Neurol.* (2017) 74:557–66. doi: 10.1001/jamaneurol.2016.6117

6. Barro C, Benkert P, Disanto G, Tsagkas C, Amann M, Naegelin Y, et al. Serum neurofilament as a predictor of disease worsening and brain and spinal cord atrophy in multiple sclerosis. *Brain* (2018) 141:2382–91. doi: 10.1093/brain/awy154

7. Kuhle J, Barro C, Andreasson U, Derfuss T, Lindberg R, Sandelius A, et al. Comparison of three analytical platforms for quantification of the neurofilament light chain in blood samples: ELISA, electrochemiluminescence immunoassay and Simoa. *Clin Chem Lab Med.* (2016) 54:1655–61. doi: 10.1515/cclm-2015-1195

8. Matsushige T, Inoue H, Fukunaga S, Hasegawa S, Okuda M, Ichiyama T. Serum neurofilament concentrations in children with prolonged febrile seizures. *J Neurol Sci.* (2012) 321:39–42. doi: 10.1016/j.jns.2012.07.043

9. Douglas-Escobar M, Yang C, Bennett J, Shuster J, Theriaque D, Leibovici A, et al. A pilot study of novel biomarkers in neonates with hypoxic-ischemic encephalopathy. *Pediatr Res.* (2010) 68:531–6. doi: 10.1203/PDR.0b013e3181f85a03

10. Toorell H, Zetterberg H, Blennow K, Savman K, Hagberg H. Increase of neuronal injury markers Tau and neurofilament light proteins in umbilical blood after intrapartum asphyxia. *J Matern Fetal Neonatal Med.* (2018) 31:2468–72. doi: 10.1080/14767058.2017.1344964

11. Shah DK, Ponnusamy V, Evanson J, Kapellou O, Ekitzidou G, Gupta N, et al. Raised plasma neurofilament light protein levels are associated with abnormal MRI outcomes in newborns undergoing therapeutic hypothermia. *Front Neurol.* (2018) 9:86. doi: 10.3389/fneur.2018.00086

12. Morel AA, Bailey SM, Shaw G, Mally P, Malhotra SP. Measurement of novel biomarkers of neuronal injury and cerebral oxygenation after routine vaginal delivery versus cesarean section in term infants. *J Perinat Med.* (2014) 42:705–9. doi: 10.1515/jpm-2014-0274

13. Schlapbach LJ, Ersch J, Adams M, Bernet V, Bucher HU, Latal B. Impact of chorioamnionitis and preeclampsia on neurodevelopmental outcome in preterm infants below 32 weeks gestational age. *Acta Paediatr.* (2010) 99:1504–9. doi: 10.1111/j.1651-2227.2010.01861.x

14. Wellmann S, Benzing J, Cippa G, Admaty D, Creutzfeldt R, Mieth RA, et al. High copeptin concentrations in umbilical cord blood after vaginal delivery and birth acidosis. *J Clin Endocrinol Metabol.* (2010) 95:5091–6. doi: 10.1210/jc.2010-1331

15. Disanto G, Barro C, Benkert P, Naegelin Y, Schadelin S, Giardiello A, et al. Serum neurofilament light: a biomarker of neuronal damage in multiple sclerosis. *Ann Neurol.* (2017) 81:857–70. doi: 10.1002/ana.24954

16. Blennow K. A review of fluid biomarkers for Alzheimer's disease: moving from CSF to blood. *Neurol Ther.* (2017) 6 (Suppl. 1):15–24. doi: 10.1007/s40120-017-0073-9

17. Barro C, Leocani L, Leppert D, Comi G, Kappos L, Kuhle J. Fluid biomarker and electrophysiological outcome measures for progressive MS trials. *Mult Scler.* (2017) 23:1600–13. doi: 10.1177/1352458517732844

18. Volpe JJ. Brain injury in premature infants: a complex amalgam of destructive and developmental disturbances. *Lancet Neurol.* (2009) 8:110–24. doi: 10.1016/S1474-4422(08)70294-1

19. Gattringer T, Pinter D, Enzinger C, Seifert-Held T, Kneihsl M, Fandler S, et al. Serum neurofilament light is sensitive to active cerebral small vessel disease. *Neurology* (2017) 89:2108–14. doi: 10.1212/WNL.0000000000004645

20. Byrne LM, Rodrigues FB, Blennow K, Durr A, Leavitt BR, Roos RAC, et al. Neurofilament light protein in blood as a potential biomarker of neurodegeneration in Huntington's disease: a retrospective cohort analysis. *Lancet Neurol.* (2017) 16:601–9. doi: 10.1016/S1474-4422(17)30124-2

21. Evers KS, Wellmann S. Arginine vasopressin and copeptin in perinatology. *Front Pediatr.* (2016) 4:75. doi: 10.3389/fped.2016.00075

22. Steegers EA, von Dadelszen P, Duvekot JJ, Pijnenborg R. Pre-eclampsia. *Lancet* (2010) 376(9741):631–44. doi: 10.1016/S0140-6736(10)60279-6

23. Evers KS, Atkinson A, Barro C, Fisch U, Pfister M, Huhn EA, et al. Neurofilament as neuronal injury blood marker in preeclampsia. *Hypertension* (2018) 71:1178–84. doi: 10.1161/HYPERTENSIONAHA.117.10314

24. Paauw ND, van Rijn BB, Lely AT, Joles JA. Pregnancy as a critical window for blood pressure regulation in mother and child: programming and reprogramming. *Acta Physiol.* (2017) 219:241–59. doi: 10.1111/apha.12702

25. Meregalli C, Fumagalli G, Alberti P, Canta A, Carozzi VA, Chiorazzi A, et al. Neurofilament light chain as disease biomarker in a rodent model of chemotherapy induced peripheral neuropathy. *Exp Neurol.* (2018) 307:129–32. doi: 10.1016/j.expneurol.2018.06.005

26. Sandelius A, Zetterberg H, Blennow K, Adiutori R, Malaspina A, Laura M, et al. Plasma neurofilament light chain concentration in the inherited peripheral neuropathies. *Neurology* (2018) 90:e518–e24. doi: 10.1212/WNL.0000000000004932

27. Jedeikin R, Makela SK, Shennan AT, Rowe RD, Ellis G. Creatine kinase isoenzymes in serum from cord blood and the blood of healthy full-term infants during the first three postnatal days. *Clin Chem.* (1982) 28:317–22.

28. Schulpis KH, Margeli A, Akalestos A, Vlachos GD, Partsinevelos GA, Papastamataki M, et al. Effects of mode of delivery on maternal-neonatal plasma antioxidant status and on protein S100B serum concentrations. *Scand J Clin Lab Invest.* (2006) 66:733–42. doi: 10.1080/00365510600977737

29. Pham N, Fazio V, Cucullo L, Teng Q, Biberthaler P, Bazarian JJ, et al. Extracranial sources of S100B do not affect serum levels. *PLoS ONE* (2010) 5:e12691. doi: 10.1371/journal.pone.0012691

30. Zaigham M, Lundberg F, Olofsson P. Protein S100B in umbilical cord blood as a potential biomarker of hypoxic-ischemic encephalopathy in asphyxiated newborns. *Early Hum Dev.* (2017) 112:48–53. doi: 10.1016/j.earlhumdev.2017.07.015

31. Pei XM, Gao R, Zhang GY, Lin L, Wan SM, Qiu SQ. [Effects of erythropoietin on serum NSE and S-100B levels in neonates with hypoxic-ischemic encephalopathy]. *Chin J Contemp Pediatr.* (2014) 16:705–8. doi: 10.7499/j.issn.1008-8830.2014.07.010

32. Gazzolo D, Lituania M, Bruschettini M, Ciotti S, Sacchi R, Serra G, et al. S100B protein levels in saliva: correlation with gestational age in normal term and preterm newborns. *Clin Biochem.* (2005) 38:229–33. doi: 10.1016/j.clinbiochem.2004.12.006

33. Dhobale M, Mehendale S, Pisal H, Nimbargi V, Joshi S. Reduced maternal and cord nerve growth factor levels in preterm deliveries. *Int J Dev Neurosci.* (2012) 30:99–103. doi: 10.1016/j.ijdevneu.2011.12.007

34. Kalm M, Bostrom M, Sandelius A, Eriksson Y, Ek CJ, Blennow K, et al. Serum concentrations of the axonal injury marker neurofilament light protein are not influenced by blood-brain barrier permeability. *Brain Res.* (2017) 1668:12–9. doi: 10.1016/j.brainres.2017.05.011

35. Graham EM, Everett AD, Delpech JC, Northington FJ. Blood biomarkers for evaluation of perinatal encephalopathy: state of the art. *Curr Opin Pediatr.* (2018) 30:199–203. doi: 10.1097/MOP.0000000000000591

16

Predictors for Therapy Response to Intrathecal Corticosteroid Therapy in Multiple Sclerosis

Katja Vohl, Alexander Duscha, Barbara Gisevius, Johannes Kaisler, Ralf Gold and Aiden Haghikia*

Department of Neurology, Ruhr-University Bochum, St. Josef-Hospital, Bochum, Germany

*Correspondence:
Aiden Haghikia
aiden.haghikia@rub.de

Objective: The autoimmune disease Multiple Sclerosis (MS) represents a heterogeneous disease pattern with an individual course that may lead to permanent disability. In addition to immuno-modulating therapies patients benefit from symptomatic approaches like intrathecal corticosteroid therapy (ICT), which is frequently applied in a growing number of centers in Germany. ICT reduces spasticity, which elongates patient's walking distance and speed, thus improves quality of life.

Methods: In our study we set out to investigate cerebrospinal fluid (CSF) parameters and clinical predictors for response to ICT. Therefore, we analyzed 811 CSF samples collected from 354 patients over a time period of 12 years. Patients who received ICT were divided in two groups (improving or active group) depending on their EDSS-progress. As control groups we analyzed data of ICT naïve patients, who were divided in the two groups as well. Additionally we observed the clinical progress after receiving ICT by comparison of patients in both groups.

Results: The results showed clinical data had a significant influence on the probability to benefit from ICT. The probability (shown by Odds Ratio of 1.77–2.43) to belong to the improving group in contrast to the active group is significantly ($p < 0.0001$) higher at later stages of disease with early disease onset (<35 years, OR = 2.43) and higher EDSS at timepoint of ICT-initiation (EDSS > 6, OR = 2.06). Additionally, we observed lower CSF cell counts (6.68 ± 1.37 µl) and lower total CSF protein (412 ± 18.25 mg/l) of patients who responded to ICT compared to patients who did not ($p < 0.05$). In the control group no significant differences were revealed. Furthermore analyses of our data revealed patients belonging to the improving group reach an EDSS of 6 after ICT-initiation less often than patients of the active group (after 13 years 39.8% in the improving group, 67.8% in the active group).

Conclusion: Our study implies two relevant messages: (i) although the study was not designed to prospectively assess clinical data, in this cohort no severe side effects were observed under ICT; (ii) disease onset, EDSS, CSF cell count, and total protein may serve as predictive markers for therapy response.

Keywords: multiple sclerosis, disease progression, intrathecal corticosteroid therapy, clinical predictor, cerebrospinal fluid

INTRODUCTION

Multiple Sclerosis (MS) is one of the most common non-traumatic neurological diseases of young adults (1). Besides the immunological component of MS, axonal damage is a pathological hallmark of disease, which causes permanent disability (2). Despite already existing and approved immuno-modulating therapies for MS, chronic disability, and disease progression caused by neurodegeneration still pose a therapeutic challenge. More than 80% of patients afflicted by MS suffer from spasticity during disease, subsequently leading to critical impairment of daily life routine in 30% of these patients (3), i.e., reduced or diminished walking ability. After insufficient response to first-line (oral) antispastic therapies, intrathecal corticosteroid therapy (ICT) is an adjuvant option to reduce permanent disability (3). Several studies have previously shown the efficacy of ICT in various cohorts (3, 4). ICT can reduce the Expanded Disability Status Scale (EDSS), elongates walking distance and increases walking speed (3). Moreover, ICT improves effectively neuropathic pain which is caused by disease activity (5). In summary, ICT is stated as a safe and effective option for the reduction of disability (6). Additionally, ICT has a beneficial impact on bladder function (3) and generally improves quality of life in responsive patients. Thus, ICT is a promising option to slow down disease progression and reduce permanent disability. However, aside from the clinical improvement no stratifying markers for therapy response/non-response are available so far. Hence, the aim of our study was to identify possible CSF markers that may predict the individual response to ICT. CSF, due to its proximity to MS pathomechanism, has been shown to be a suitable biocompartment, e.g., for epigenetic markers (7), that is usually not affected by systemic metabolic processes derived from the peripheral blood (8).

In our department, we have established (4, 5) and performed ICT for decades. Patients usually receive a cumulative dose of 40–200 mg triamcinolone-acetonide (Volon A) via 1–3 injections (every other day) every 3 months on average in an individualized manner (9). With this study we addressed the following questions: (I) Are there any differences in standard CSF parameters to distinguish between response and non-response to ICT?; and (II) which clinical parameters indicate a beneficial response to ICT?

METHODS

Retrospective data from patients assessed during clinical routine at the Department of Neurology of the Ruhr-University Bochum, St. Josef-Hospital since 2005 were considered for analysis. CSF analysis for possible surrogate markers was approved by the ethics committee of the Department of Medicine at the Ruhr-University Bochum (registration number 4493-12). The mean observation period per patient comprised to 2.58 ± 2.51 years. The distribution of the observation intervals is shown

Abbreviations: MS, Multiple Sclerosis; ICT, intrathecal corticosteroid therapy; EDSS, Expanded Disability Status Scale; CSF, cerebrospinal fluid; RRMS, relapsing remitting MS; SPMS, secondary progressive MS; PPMS, primary progressive MS.

in **Table 1**. We analyzed a total of 811 CSF samples from 354 different patients. All study patients had been diagnosed with MS according to the McDonald criteria (10) including all different disease subtypes, i.e., relapsing remitting (RR), secondary progressive (SP), and primary progressive (PP). Only those patients who had been unstable with other MS medication for at least 6 months and showed insufficient response to oral first line antispastic therapies received ICT. Written and informed consent of all patients was obtained before initiation of ICT. We screened 206 patients (with 508 CSF analyzed samples) who had received ICT at least at one time point, and 148 patients (with 303 CSF analyses) who had been ICT naïve. Patients and CSF values were included in this study fulfilling the mentioned criteria. Patients were followed longitudinally for their EDSS as well as their CSF.

CSF assessment and analysis were performed once before the first ICT injection and afterwards as follow up during longitudinal ICT. Lumbar punctures of patients, who did not receive ICT, were part of diagnostic routine, for instance reevaluation of diagnosis or verification of the conversion of oligoclonal bands. Triamcinolon (40–80 mg) was injected directly into the CSF under sterile conditions using an atraumatic needle (4).

Patients were divided into two groups depending on their respective clinical progress mirrored by individual EDSS (11). EDSS was collected routinely in our department, thus it is possible to monitor patient's disability progression retrospectively over a long period of time as it was essential in our study. We defined two groups based on the ratio of first determined EDSS and the mean of all following respective EDSS of the same patient ≥1: improving group—patients, whose EDSS remained stable or decreased over time <1: active group—patients, whose EDSS increased over time.

Due to the retrospective character of our study, the evaluation of the EDSS in standardized time intervals was not possible. However, the EDSS assessment prior to the first ICT-injection was evaluated in a time range of 1.2 ± 0.24 years, the EDSS

TABLE 1 | Observation Interval of ICT patients; number of values and patients of the observation intervals.

Observation interval	Number of patients	Number of CSF values
Less than 1 year	6	26
1–2 years	93	127
2–3 years	50	75
3–4 years	37	50
4–5 years	34	54
5–6 years	31	66
6–7 years	18	51
7–8 years	15	47
8–9 years	22	81
9–10 years	20	72
10–11 years	11	63
11–12 years	10	51
More than 12 years	7	48

post ICT-injection was evaluated in a time range of 1.68 ± 0.26 years. By definition we excluded patients of whom only one EDSS value was available during the observation period, which leads to an impediment for a definitive group assignment. Hence, for final assessment we included 157 patients with 446 CSF samples who received ICT, and additionally 103 patients with 213 CSF analyses who were ICT naïve. Detailed demographic information of patients is shown in **Table 2**. We compared these two groups separately for patients who received ICT and patients who were ICT naïve, because of the retrospective vs. cross sectional character of data used for the study. Statistical analysis for CSF parameters of these subgroups was performed by Mann-Whitney-U-test, after Kolmogorov–Smirnov-Test had ruled out Gaussian distribution. Therefore, we included all baseline data of CSF of all patients included in the improving or active group to represent the long-term changes. Additionally we analyzed the patients mean cell count to show patient's intrapersonal cell count value dependent on individual disease progress and activity. To examine clinical parameters of patients we used fisher's exact test. For the examination of clinical parameters, we defined specific ranges of these parameters: age range at diagnosis and manifestation were set up to 35 years based on epidemiological data suggesting a transition age of RRMS to SPMS at 33 years (12). We stratified EDSS in below and above EDSS 6 (13, 14).

Kaplan Maier analysis was performed for evaluating risk of disease progression, i.e., disease progression defined as EDSS increase above 6 over time for both ICT receiving groups; statistical analysis was performed by log-rank (Mantel-Cox) test. All statistical data in figures are shown with mean $\pm$ SEM, following p were considered as statistically significant: $p < 0.05$, $p < 0.001$, and $p < 0.0001$.

Additionally, we evaluated the effect of patient specific MS medication in combination with or without ICT, i.e., established

immuno-modulating therapies used in MS like interferon-beta, glatiramer acetate, fingolimod, dimethylfumarat, azathioprine, mitoxantrone, and natalizumab.

RESULTS
CSF Analyses of ICT Patients

Analyzed data of patients who received ICT showed a significant lower absolute cell count in the CSF in the improving group (6.68 ± 1.37 µl) when compared to the active group (9.206 ± 2.39 µl; $p = 0.04416$; **Figure 1A**). This result was confirmed by observation of the individual patient's mean cell count. Also in this analysis the improving group significantly ($p = 0.0221$) showed a lower cell count mean (7.20 ± 3.41 µl) in comparison to the active group (10.82 ± 3.18 µl; **Figure 1B**). The amount of total protein in the CSF was significantly lower in the improving group ($p = 0.0014$, improving group 412 ± 18.25 mg/l vs. active group 462.4 ± 14.04 mg/l; **Figure 1C**). Separately analyzed data of ICT naïve MS-patients did not display significant differences neither in cell count nor in total protein between improving and active group (**Figures 1A–C**).We detected no significant differences in other standardized CSF parameters including erythrocytes count, glucose, lactate, albumin, and IgG (data not shown).

In addition, we investigated whether patient's individual MS medication had an effect on the specific response to ICT. Therefore, we observed the different immune-modulating therapy options of patients receiving ICT based on their assignment for active and improving group. Since patients only received ICT when they were not stable for at least 6 months with other MS medication, the results confirmed that the effects of ICT were not significantly influenced by the specific MS medication (data not shown).

TABLE 2 | Demographic parameters of MS patients; demographic data separated for patients with or without ICT and for improving and active group; [a]in years (mean $\pm$ SD); RRMS, relapsing remitting multiple sclerosis; SPMS, secondary progressive multiple sclerosis; PPMS, primary progressive multiple sclerosis; n, number of patients; f, female; m, male.

			n	Sex	Current age[a]	Age at diagnosis[a]	Disease duration[a]
No intrathecal corticosteroid therapy	Improving group		51	f = 33; m = 18	51.98 ± 11.62	36.18 ± 13.65	15.8 ± 10.48
		RRMS	27	f = 20; m = 7	46.78 ± 11.55	35.7 ± 13.76	11.07 ± 7.67
		SPMS	20	f = 12; m = 8	57.8 ± 8.77	34.65 ± 13.59	23.15 ± 10.69
		PPMS	4	f = 1; m = 3	58 ± 9.42	47 ± 10.89	11 ± 2.16
	Active group		52	f = 30; m = 22	54.13 ± 10.5	37.46 ± 10.16	16.67 ± 8.49
		RRMS	9	f = 3; m = 6	40.11 ± 14.41	29.33 ± 10.56	10.78 ± 6.36
		SPMS	39	f = 26; m = 13	56.85 ± 6.79	38.23 ± 9.19	18.62 ± 8.52
		PPMS	4	f = 1; m = 3	59.25 ± 3.86	48.25 ± 5.19	11 ± 1.41
Intrathecal corticosteroid therapy	Improving group		72	f = 45; m = 27	51.42 ± 10.57	38.42 ± 10.65	13 ± 8.15
		RRMS	35	f = 22: m = 13	46.66 ± 10.19	37.0 ± 11.2	9.66 ± 6.24
		SPMS	31	f = 19; m = 12	57.29 ± 8.2	39.81 ± 10.43	17.48 ± 8.45
		PPMS	6	f = 4; m = 2	48.83 ± 9.83	39.5 ± 8.76	9.33 ± 5.65
	Active group		85	f = 55; m = 30	54.54 ± 10.98	36.52 ± 10.21	18.02 ± 7.86
		RRMS	14	f = 9; m = 5	44.43 ± 12.11	28.14 ± 11.41	16.29 ± 8.79
		SPMS	62	f = 40; m = 22	56.08 ± 8.81	36.85 ± 8.26	19.23 ± 7.13
		PPMS	9	f = 6; m = 3	59.67 ± 14.46	47.22 ± 10.50	12.44 ± 9.15

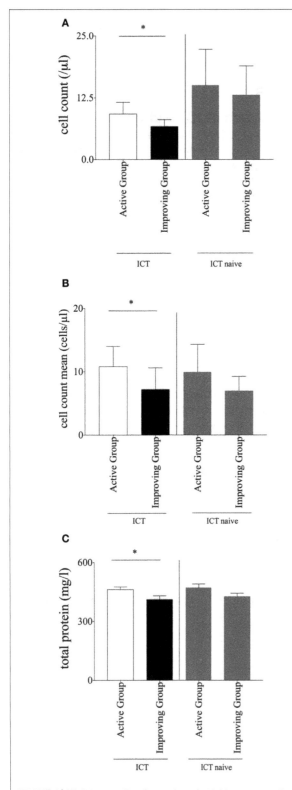

FIGURE 1 | (A) Cell count. Baseline cerebrospinal fluid parameter cell count of multiple sclerosis patients within intrathecal corticosteroid therapy (ICT) compared between the subgroups; separate comparison of multiple sclerosis patients without ICT between the two subgroups; Mann–Whitney-*U*-test, mean with SEM, *n* (improving group ICT) = 172, *n* (active group ICT) = 310, *(Continued)*

FIGURE 1 | *n* (improving group ICT naïve) = 88, *n* (active group ICT naïve) = 137; **p* = 0.0442. **(B)** Cell count mean. Mean of cerebrospinal fluid parameter cell count of multiple sclerosis patients within ICT compared between the subgroups; separate comparison of multiple sclerosis patients without ICT between the two subgroups; Mann–Whitney-*U*-test, mean with SEM, *n* (improving group ICT) = 76, *n* (active group ICT) = 59, *n* (improving group ICT naïve) = 46, *n* (active group ICT naïve) = 47; **p* = 0.0221. **(C)** Total protein. Baseline cerebrospinal fluid parameter total protein of multiple sclerosis patients within ICT compared between the subgroups; separate comparison of multiple sclerosis patients without ICT between the two subgroups; Mann-Whitney-U-test, mean with SEM; *n* (improving group ICT) = 155, *n* (active group ICT) = 282, *n* (improving group ICT naïve) = 88, *n* (active group ICT naïve) = 137; **p* = 0.0014.

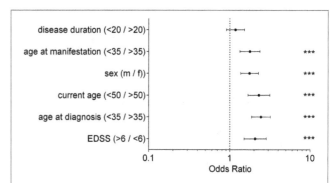

FIGURE 2 | Clinical Parameter; Odds Ratio for each clinical parameter of patients receiving ICT between improving group and active group; fisher's exact test, ****p* < 0.0001; disease duration (*p* = 0.2383); disease duration/current age/age at manifestation/age at diagnosis in years; EDSS, expanded disability status scale; m, male; f, female.

Clinical Parameters for a Response to ICT

The analysis of clinical data revealed that an EDSS > 6 at the first injection of ICT correlated with an increased probability to benefit from ICT (OR = 2.06; 95% CI from 1.5 to 1.75; *p* < 0.0001). Additionally, patients below age of 35 years at first diagnosis of MS benefited most from ICT. In contrast to patients older than 35 years, the probability to belong to the improving group was more than twice as high (OR = 2.43, 95% CI from 1.86 to 3.18, *p* < 0.0001). We found similar results for the individual age at first manifestation of the disease (OR = 1.77, 95% CI from 1.33 to 2.36; *p* < 0.0001).The results showed that an age <50 years currently receiving ICT was accompanied with an increased probability to belong to the improving group (OR = 2.29, 95% CI from 1.68 to 3.14; *p* < 0.0001). Examining the influence of the patients' sex regarding therapy response, male patients responded with a higher probability to ICT than female patients (OR = 1.79, 95% CI from 1.36 to 2.27; *p* < 0.0001). We observed no significant difference between the analyzed groups when assessing disease duration before the start of ICT (OR = 1.18, 95% CI from 0.91 to 1.52; *p* < 0.0001). Results are displayed in **Figure 2**.

Time to Reach EDSS 6

We compared both, the improving and the active group of patients receiving ICT in respect to the time of reaching an EDSS of 6. 13 years after first injection of ICT 39.8% of patients in

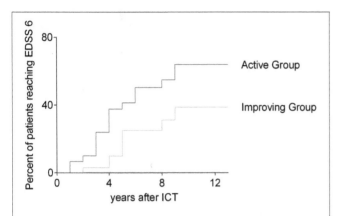

FIGURE 3 | Time to reach EDSS 6; survival curves before reaching an EDSS of 6; all analyzed patients receiving ICT; comparing improving group and active group, Kaplan–Meier survival analysis; log-rank (Mantel-Cox) test, $p = 0.0357$; ICT, intrathecal corticosteroid therapy; EDSS, expanded disability status scale.

the improving group reached an EDSS of 6, whereas 67.8% of patients belonging to the active group reached an EDSS of 6 [$p = 0.0357$; log rank (Mantel-Cox) test]. The results are shown in **Figure 3**.

DISCUSSION

Effective treatment of MS disease progression is one of the major unmet needs in the field of MS therapy. Several studies have demonstrated the safety and efficacy of ICT in MS (3, 4). However, based on its mode of application ICT is not widely used outside German-speaking countries. Also due its invasive nature of application a placebo/sham controlled randomized trial would be un-ethical. The diagnostic value of CSF analysis, however, is being increasingly appreciated even in the age of revised McDonald criteria (10). Our study comprised a cohort of over 200 MS patients with ICT and additionally 148 MS patients without ICT, whose datasets were collected over a time period of 12 years. The weakness of the study is its retrospective nature. However, we could demonstrate a significantly lower level of total protein and cell count in the CSF of patients responding to ICT in a large longitudinally assessed cohort. In

accordance with previous studies (3, 15) no severe side effects were observed. Nonetheless, a marker—ideally derived from neurological laboratory routine diagnostic like CSF cell number or total protein—that stratifies responders and non-responders to ICT, may help to assign patients to this therapy. In accordance with previous studies we could stratify clinical data for a positive therapy response to ICT (16).

Our data suggest that patients benefit most from ICT, when (i) diagnosis (and manifestation) was at a younger age (below 35 years of age); (ii) they are younger than 50 years while receiving ICT; (iii) their EDSS is higher than 6 at start of ICT; (iv) when they are male.

CSF analysis is used to exclude differential diagnosis (17) and the standard CSF values are considered as not useful as markers for disease progression or therapy response (8, 18, 19). Among other immunological effects, systemic glucocorticosteroid application has been shown to decrease the number of leucocytes in CSF and to stabilize the blood-brain-barrier (20–22). It is suggested, that low numbers of CSF cells could indicate a beneficial effect on MS progression (20, 23). Furthermore, a dysfunction of the blood-brain-barrier implies a modified expression and secretion of potentially inflammatory mediators in the CSF, e.g., cytokines (24). ICT is an adjuvant option to reduce spasticity and improve patient's motor disabilities, i.e., elongation of walking distance (4). Furthermore, our retrospective data suggest that ICT may have a positive impact on disability progression.

However, the main weakness of this study is its retrospective nature, particularly regarding the clinical data. Hence, the decision whether ICT is used or not is based on an individual risk and benefit assessment. Our data point to a CSF standard assessment, that may serve as a potential tool of predicting therapy response in context of ICT.

AUTHOR CONTRIBUTIONS

KV and AD conducted and analyzed the data and wrote the manuscript. BG and JK assessed CSF and edited the manuscript. RG designed the study and edited the manuscript. AH designed and supervised the study, analyzed the data, and edited the manuscript.

REFERENCES

1. Haghikia A, Hohlfeld R, Gold R, Fugger L. Therapies for multiple sclerosis: translational achievements and outstanding needs. *Trends Mol Med*. (2013) 19:309–19. doi: 10.1016/j.molmed.2013.03.004
2. Duddy M, Haghikia A, Cocco E, Eggers C, Drulovic J, Carmona O, et al. Managing MS in a changing treatment landscape. *J Neurol*. (2011) 258:728–39. doi: 10.1007/s00415-011-6009-x
3. Kamin F, Rommer PS, Abu-Mugheisib M, Koehler W, Hoffmann F, Winkelmann A, et al. Effects of intrathecal triamincinolone-acetonide treatment in MS patients with therapy-resistant spasticity. *Spinal Cord* (2015) 53:109–13. doi: 10.1038/sc.2014.155
4. Hoffmann V, Kuhn W, Schimrigk S, Islamova S, Hellwig K, Lukas C, et al. Repeat intrathecal triamcinolone acetonide application is

beneficial in progressive MS patients. *Eur J Neurol*. (2006) 13:72–6. doi: 10.1111/j.1468-1331.2006.01145.x
5. Hellwig K, Lukas C, Brune N, Schimrigk S, Przuntek H, Muller T. Repeat intrathecal triamcinolone acetonide application reduces acute occurring painful dysesthesia in patients with relapsing remitting multiple sclerosis. *Sci World J*. (2006) 6:460–5. doi: 10.1100/tsw.2006.86
6. Muller T. Role of intraspinal steroid application in patients with multiple sclerosis. *Expert Rev Neurother*. (2009) 9:1279–87. doi: 10.1586/ern.09.60
7. Haghikia A, Haghikia A, Hellwig K, Baraniskin A, Holzmann A, Decard BF, et al. Regulated microRNAs in the CSF of patients with multiple sclerosis: a case-control study. *Neurology* (2012) 79:2166–70. doi: 10.1212/WNL.0b013e3182759621
8. Tumani H, Hartung HP, Hemmer B, Teunissen C, Deisenhammer F, Giovannoni G, et al. Cerebrospinal fluid biomarkers in multiple sclerosis. *Neurobiol Dis*. (2009) 35:117–27. doi: 10.1016/j.nbd.2009.04.010

9. Rommer PS, Kamin F, Petzold A, Tumani H, Abu-Mugheisib M, Koehler W, et al. Effects of repeated intrathecal triamcinolone-acetonide application on cerebrospinal fluid biomarkers of axonal damage and glial activity in multiple sclerosis patients. *Mol Diagn Ther.* (2014) 18:631–7. doi: 10.1007/s40291-014-0114-3

10. Thompson AJ, Banwell BL, Barkhof F, Carroll WM, Coetzee T, Comi G, et al. Diagnosis of multiple sclerosis: 2017 revisions of the McDonald criteria. *Lancet Neurol.* (2018) 17:162–73. doi: 10.1016/S1474-4422(17)30470-2

11. Kurtzke JF. Rating neurologic impairment in multiple sclerosis: an expanded disability status scale (EDSS). *Neurology* (1983) 33:1444–52. doi: 10.1212/WNL.33.11.1444

12. Skoog B, Tedeholm H, Runmarker B, Oden A, Andersen O. Continuous prediction of secondary progression in the individual course of multiple sclerosis. *Mult Scler Relat Disord.* (2014) 3:584–92. doi: 10.1016/j.msard.2014.04.004

13. Skoog B, Runmarker B, Winblad S, Ekholm S, Andersen O. A representative cohort of patients with non-progressive multiple sclerosis at the age of normal life expectancy. *Brain* (2012) 135(Pt 3):900–11. doi: 10.1093/brain/awr336

14. Alroughani R, Akhtar S, Ahmed S, Behbehani R, Al-Hashel J. Is time to reach EDSS 6.0 faster in patients with late-onset versus young-onset multiple sclerosis? *PLoS ONE* (2016) 11:e0165846. doi: 10.1371/journal.pone.0165846

15. Hoffmann V, Schimrigk S, Islamova S, Hellwig K, Lukas C, Brune N, et al. Efficacy and safety of repeated intrathecal triamcinolone acetonide application in progressive multiple sclerosis patients. *J Neurol Sci.* (2003) 211:81–4. doi: 10.1016/S0022-510X(03)00060-1

16. Lukas C, Bellenberg B, Hahn HK, Rexilius J, Drescher R, Hellwig K, et al. Benefit of repetitive intrathecal triamcinolone acetonide therapy in predominantly spinal multiple sclerosis: prediction by upper spinal cord atrophy. *Ther Adv Neurol Disord.* (2009) 2:42–9. doi: 10.1177/1756285609343480

17. Deisenhammer F, Bartos A, Egg R, Gilhus NE, Giovannoni G, Rauer S, et al. Guidelines on routine cerebrospinal fluid analysis. Report from an EFNS task force. *Eur J Neurol.* (2006) 13:913–22. doi: 10.1111/j.1468-1331.2006.01493.x

18. Walker RW, Thompson EJ, McDonald WI. Cerebrospinal fluid in multiple sclerosis: relationships between immunoglobulins, leucocytes and clinical features. *J Neurol.* (1985) 232:250–9. doi: 10.1007/BF00313789

19. Awad A, Hemmer B, Hartung HP, Kieseier B, Bennett JL, Stuve O. Analyses of cerebrospinal fluid in the diagnosis and monitoring of multiple sclerosis. *J Neuroimmunol.* (2010) 219:1–7. doi: 10.1016/j.jneuroim.2009.09.002

20. Rocchelli B, Poloni M, Mazzarello P, Piccolo G, Delodovici M, Pinelli P. Intrathecal methylprednisolone acetate in multiple sclerosis treatment: effect on the blood-CSF barrier and on the intrathecal IgG production. *Ital J Neurol Sci.* (1982) 3:119–26. doi: 10.1007/BF02043943

21. Rosenberg GA, Dencoff JE, Correa N Jr, Reiners M, Ford CC. Effect of steroids on CSF matrix metalloproteinases in multiple sclerosis: relation to blood-brain barrier injury. *Neurology* (1996) 46:1626–32. doi: 10.1212/WNL.46.6.1626

22. Salvador E, Shityakov S, Forster C. Glucocorticoids and endothelial cell barrier function. *Cell Tissue Res.* (2014) 355:597–605. doi: 10.1007/s00441-013-1762-z

23. Marinangeli F, Ciccozzi A, Donatelli F, Paladini A, Varrassi G. Clinical use of spinal or epidural steroids. *Minerva Anestesiol.* (2002) 68:613–20.

24. McLean BN, Zeman AZ, Barnes D, Thompson EJ. Patterns of blood-brain barrier impairment and clinical features in multiple sclerosis. *J Neurol Neurosurg Psychiatr.* (1993) 56:356–60. doi: 10.1136/jnnp.56.4.356

17

Serum Inflammatory Profile for the Discrimination of Clinical Subtypes in Parkinson's Disease

Rezzak Yilmaz[1†], Antonio P. Strafella[2,3,4,5,6,7†], Alice Bernard[8†], Claudia Schulte[8,9], Lieneke van den Heuvel[3,4], Nicole Schneiderhan-Marra[10], Thomas Knorpp[10], Thomas O. Joos[10], Frank Leypoldt[1,11], Johanna Geritz[1], Clint Hansen[1], Sebastian Heinzel[1], Anja Apel[8,9], Thomas Gasser[8,9], Anthony E. Lang[2,3,4,7,12], Daniela Berg[1,8,9], Walter Maetzler[1,8,9†] and Connie Marras[3,4†]*

[1] Department of Neurology, Christian-Albrechts-University of Kiel, Kiel, Germany, [2] Institute of Medical Science, University of Toronto, Toronto, ON, Canada, [3] Edmond J Safra Program in Parkinson's Disease and the Morton and Gloria Shulman Movement Disorders Clinic, University of Toronto, Toronto, ON, Canada, [4] Division of Neurology, Department of Medicine, University of Toronto, Toronto, ON, Canada, [5] Research Imaging Centre, Centre for Addiction and Mental Health, Toronto, ON, Canada, [6] Division of Brain, Imaging and Behaviour-Systems Neuroscience, Toronto Western Research Institute, University Hospital Network, University of Toronto, Toronto, ON, Canada, [7] Krembil Brain Institute, University Health Network, Toronto, ON, Canada, [8] Department of Neurodegeneration, Hertie Institute for Clinical Brain Research, University of Tübingen, Tübingen, Germany, [9] German Center for Neurodegenerative Diseases (DZNE), Tübingen, Germany, [10] Natural and Medical Sciences Institute (NMI) at the University of Tübingen, Reutlingen, Germany, [11] Neuroimmunology, Institute of Clinical Chemistry, University Hospital Schleswig-Holstein, Kiel, Germany, [12] Tanz Centre for Research in Neurodegenerative Diseases, University of Toronto, Toronto, ON, Canada

Correspondence:
Johanna Geritz
j.geritz@neurologie.uni-kiel.de

[†] *These authors have contributed equally to this work*

Background: Blood levels of immune markers have been proposed to discriminate patients with Parkinson's disease (PD) from controls. However, differences between clinical PD subgroups regarding these markers still need to be identified.

Objective: To investigate whether clinical phenotypes can be predicted by the assessment of immune marker profiles in the serum of PD patients.

Methods: Phenotypes of clinical PD from Tübingen, Germany ($n = 145$) and Toronto, Canada ($n = 90$) were defined regarding clinical subtype, disease onset, severity, and progression as well as presence of cognitive and/or autonomic dysfunction. A panel of serum immune markers was assessed using principal component analysis (PCA) and regression models to define the marker(s) that were associated with clinical phenotypes after adjusting for potential confounders. Findings of both centers were compared for validation. Further, a [18F] FEPPA-PET was performed in a group of patients with high and low values of candidate markers for the assessment of *in vivo* brain microglial activation.

Results: Overall, serum immune markers did not cluster to define a pro/anti-inflammatory profile in PCA. Out of 25 markers only IL-12p40 showed a trend to discriminate between PD subgroups in both cohorts which could not be replicated by [18F] FEPPA-PET.

Conclusions: Assessment of cytokines in serum does not reliably differentiate clinical PD subtypes. Accompanying subtype-irrelevant inflammation in PD, dual activity, and lack of specificity of the immune markers, the complex function of microglia, probable effects of treatment, disease stage, and progression on inflammation as well as current technical limitations may limit the usefulness of serum immune markers for the differentiation of subtypes.

Keywords: Parkinson's inflammation, Parkinson subtypes, immune markers, interleukins, cytokines

INTRODUCTION

Parkinson's disease (PD) is one the most frequent movement disorders affecting about 2–3% of the aging population (1). It has been estimated that the number of people with PD will double by 2030, indicating a progressive increase in the socio-economic burden in the near future (1). For this reason, understanding the underlying neurodegeneration is vital and the development of disease modifying therapies is urgently needed.

The pathological process which eventually leads to both a progressive loss of dopaminergic neurons of the substantia nigra and more widespread neurodegeneration in PD has been associated with neuronal inflammation (1, 2). It has been shown that accumulation of extracellular alpha-synuclein (α-syn) facilitates microglia activation, which further promotes production of immune markers, nitric oxide, and reactive oxygen species. It is proposed that this process may lead to nigral cell death. Within this context, pro-inflammatory cytokines produced by the microglia are responsible for the activation of the neighboring inactive glial cells and thus magnify the inflammation. In addition they attach to surface cytokine receptors of the dopaminergic cells and trigger apoptosis (3). This mechanism may provoke protein misfolding and thus create a vicious cycle (1). Evidence for inflammation has been demonstrated in PD animal models (4) as well as in PD patients in genetic (5, 6), imaging (7), CSF (8, 9), and postmortem studies (10, 11).

PD shows considerable variability with regard to age of onset, clinical manifestations, and disease progression which may indicate pathophysiological heterogeneity. The extent that inflammatory processes differ and potentially contribute to clinical PD subtypes has not been elucidated. Detection of a clinical PD phenotype that associates with an inflammatory profile would be critical in terms of outlining the contribution of the immunologic mechanisms to the underlying pathology, understanding the diversity in issues such as drug-response, or disease progression as well as formulating disease modifying strategies. For this reason, we set out to determine the clinical phenotype that correlates with the presence or absence of an inflammatory profile by extensive clinical phenotyping of PD patients and exploratory analysis of inflammatory markers. The results were validated by the assessment of a separate PD cohort and further evaluated by assessing microglial activation *in vivo* using [18F] FEPPA-PET.

MATERIALS AND METHODS

The current study has been designed as a collaborative project between the German Center for Neurodegenerative Diseases (DZNE), Tübingen, Germany and the University Health Network, Toronto, Canada which was supported by the Centers of Excellence in Neurodegeneration (CoEN) initiative.

Study Design

In this cross-sectional study, two separate prospectively assessed cohorts of PD patients from the centers of Tübingen and Toronto were analyzed independently. In each center, patients were grouped according to their clinical phenotypes (see methods below) and then compared with regard to serum inflammatory markers in order to define a clinical PD phenotype associated with inflammation. Then, the findings of both centers were compared for validation. In case of an agreement between two centers regarding the inflammatory markers that differ between clinical phenotypes, [18F] FEPPA-PET imaging was subsequently performed on a subset of patients to further validate the relevance of the inflammatory marker.

The study was approved by the ethics committees of the Medical Faculties of the University of Tübingen and the University Health Network, Toronto. All procedures were in accordance with the Declaration of Helsinki and a written informed consent was obtained from all participants.

Patients and Clinical Assessments

Participants older than 40 years fulfilling the criteria for idiopathic PD according to the UK Brain Bank Criteria were recruited from the neurology department of University Hospital of Tübingen, Germany, and from the Morton and Gloria Shulman Movement Disorders Clinic of Toronto Western Hospital, Toronto, Canada. Demographic data and detailed PD history including disease onset and duration, medication, presence of wearing off or motor fluctuations, and accompanying non-motor symptoms were collected. Motor performance in the "on" medication state and the disease severity were assessed by the Movement Disorders Society-Unified Parkinson's Disease Rating Scale (MDS-UPDRS) part-III and Hoehn and Yahr Scale (H&Y), respectively. Cognitive performance and autonomic dysfunction were assessed using the Montreal Cognitive Assessment (MoCa) and by Scales for Outcomes in Parkinson's disease—Autonomic (SCOPA-AUT), respectively. Patients with a C-reactive protein (CRP) value above 1.0 mg/dl were excluded from the study based on the assumption that these individuals may have an acute infection that could influence

TABLE 1 | Methods of comparison for PD subtypes (n for Tübingen/Toronto cohort).

Method-1[13]	n	Method-2	n	Method-3[15]	n	Method-4[12,14]	n
Young onset	31/23	Young onset and slow progression	45/31	Benign motor	37/16	Benign motor	50/35
Non-tremor dominant	44/20	Late onset and fast progression	38/17	Benign motor with cognitive/autonomic impairment	26/22	Benign motor with cognitive impairment	15/14
Tremor dominant	24/19	–		Poor motor with cognitive/autonomic impairment	56/12	Poor motor with cognitive impairment	37/15
Rapid progression	32/8	–		–		–	

the levels of the collected inflammation markers. All included PD patients were categorized into different groups with regard to their disease onset, severity or progression rate, autonomic, and cognitive status. Based on the previously published cluster analyses defining PD subtypes (12–15), four different methods of subtype classification were constructed. Each method resulted in 2–4 groups with each group representing a clinically defined PD subtype (**Table 1**). Within these subtypes, "young onset" was defined by an age of onset of <55 or <60 years in method 1 and 2, respectively. Motor subtyping (tremor dominant or non-tremor dominant) of the groups was selected by evaluating the tremor and postural instability and gait disorder (PIGD) scores of MDS-UPDRS part-III. Disease progression was defined by dividing the MDS-UPDRS part-III scores by disease duration. Cognitive or autonomic impairment were defined by Montreal Cognitive Assessment (MoCA) score lower than 26 and Scales for Outcomes in Parkinson's Disease-Autonomic (SCOPA-AUT) equal to or lower than 16, respectively. The details of the group definitions are explained in the **Supplementary Table 1**.

Biomaterial Collection

The following panel of immune markers composed of pro- or anti-inflammatory cytokines as well as neuroprotective trophic factors were assessed from the blood samples of the PD patients: TNF-α, TNF-β, IL-1α, IL-2, IL-3, IL-4, IL-5, IL-7, IL-8, IL-10, IL-12p40, IL-12p70, IL-13, IL-15, IL-16, IL-18, Brain-derived neurotrophic factor (BDNF), Epithelial Neutrophil Activating Peptide (ENA78), granulocyte-macrophage colony-stimulating factor (GM-CSF), lymphotactin, macrophage-derived chemokine (MDC), macrophage inflammatory protein-1β (MIP-1β), monocyte chemotactic protein-1 (MCP-1), stem cell factor (SCF), thrombopoetin (TPO). In both centers, storing and analyses of biomaterial were performed by means of standard operating procedures using the kit components of the multiplexed immunoassay by Myriad RBM, Austin, TX, USA. Blood samples of Toronto were obtained according to the protocol and were sent frozen to Tübingen for the analyses. The Tübingen samples were also frozen before the analysis in order to allow the comparability. Analysis of the serum inflammatory marker levels was performed using the Luminex 100/200 instrument and data were interpreted using the software developed and provided by Myriad RBM. Details of the serum inflammatory marker analysis are given elsewhere (16).

[18F] FEPPA-PET Imaging

Assessment of the *in vivo* brain microglial activation using a [18F] FEPPA-PET imaging was planned as a further validation step given that immune markers that discriminate PD groups were detected in both cohorts. A subgroup of patients from the Toronto cohort that underwent [18F] FEPPA-PET to assess microglial activation were categorized according to values of the cytokines of interest being lower or higher than the 50th percentile of the entire group undergoing PET imaging. [18F] FEPPA-PET images were preprocessed and region of interests (ROI) were automatically generated using in-house software, ROMI (17). In brief, ROMI fits a standard template of ROIs to an individual proton density (PD)-weighted MR image based on the probability of white matter, gray matter, and cerebrospinal fluid. The individual MR images were then co-registered to each summed [18F] FEPPA-PET image using the normalized mutual information algorithm so that individual refined ROI template can be transferred to the PET image space to generate the time activity curve for each ROI. Our a priori ROIs included cortical as well as subcortical brain regions such as frontal and temporal lobes, cingulate cortex, occipital lobe, insula, cerebellum, thalamus, and striatum. Total distribution volume (V_T), of the radioligand concentration in the ROI was measured taking into consideration rs6791 polymorphism binding affinity. The effect of age on the tissue volume was taken into account by partial volume effect correction (PVEC) method. PET scans were obtained with a high resolution PET/CT, Siemens-Biograph HiRez XVI (Siemens Molecular Imaging, Knoxville, TN, U.S.A.).

Statistics

The collected serum inflammatory markers were compared between the groups of each method with an exploratory approach in both cohorts. Statistical analyses were designed in two steps. First, a principal component analysis (PCA) was performed in the Tübingen (main) cohort with a bigger sample size to identify the cytokines that form a pro- or anti-inflammatory immune profile (factor) that could discriminate groups of PD. As the data could not be reduced to factors which convincingly represent the marker profiles (see results), binomial (for Method-2) and multinomial logistic regression analyses (For Methods-1,3, and 4) were performed for each immune marker in the Tübingen and the Toronto cohort in order to explore the predictive effect of an individual immune marker. Subtype was defined as the dependent variable, and the immune marker as the predictor variable with age, sex, disease duration or levodopa equivalent

TABLE 2 | Demographic characteristics of both cohorts.

	Tübingen (n = 145)	Toronto (n = 90)
Age [years], mean (SD)	67 (9)	62 (9)
Male sex [%]	66	70
Disease duration [years], mean (SD)	6.5 (4.0)	7.7 (4.5)
H&Y Stage (0-5), mean	2.3	1.8
LEDD [mg/day], mean (SD)	626 (407)	539 (482)
MDS-UPDRS part-III, mean (SD)	28.4 (12.5)	21.1 (10.3)
MoCA, mean (SD)	26 (3.3)	26.1 (2.6)
SCOPA-AUT, mean (SD)	14.3 (7.8)	13.4 (7)

H&Y, Hoehn & Yahr; LEDD, Levodopa equivalent daily dose, MDS-UPDRS, Movement Disorders Society - Unified Parkinson's Disease Rating Scale; MoCA, Montreal Cognitive Assessment; SCOPA-AUT, Scales for Outcomes in Parkinson's Disease - Autonomic.

daily dose (LEDD) as covariates which were added to the model according to the group definition. For example, in Method-2, age, and disease duration were not added to the model since the groups were defined according to these variables. Some cytokines were dichotomized at the median value when the data did not fit into the regression model.

As 13 group comparisons were performed for each immune marker (6 group comparisons for method-1, one for 2, and three for method-3 and 4), alpha value was corrected as $p < 0.05/13 = 0.0038$ for each cytokine (18). A trend in the data was defined as $p < 0.05$. The results from both cohorts were compared in order to see whether the effect from the Tübingen cohort (main cohort with a larger sample size) was verified by the second (Toronto) cohort. Inclusion of a second cohort in the study for the confirmation of the results was performed to reduce the risk of type-1 error, and only significant results from both centers were considered definitive. For the [18F] FEPPA-PET two-group analysis an independent samples t-test was performed also corrected for multiple comparison. SPSS Statistics 22.0.0 (SPSS Ltd., Chicago IL) was used for statistical analyses.

RESULTS

A total of 145 PD patients from Tübingen and 90 from Toronto were included in the analysis. 14 patients were excluded due to elevated CRP. Demographic data are shown in **Table 2**. IL-12p70 and GM-CSF from Toronto, and IL-2 and lymphotactin from both cohorts were excluded since more than 95% of patients had cytokine levels below analytical limit.

Principal Component Analysis (PCA)

In the Tübingen cohort, a PCA was conducted on serum inflammatory markers with oblique (related) rotation (oblimin) and elimination of factor loadings <0.4. The Kaiser–Meyer–Olkin measure of sampling adequacy was 0.81, verifying the adequacy of the sample size for the analysis. Bartlett's test of sphericity [chi-square(253) = 2125.5, $p < 0.001$] indicated that correlations between items were sufficiently large for PCA. Six components had eigenvalues over Kaiser's criterion of 1 and in combination explained 67% of the variance

(**Supplementary Table 2**). It was found that Factor-1, which has the highest loading (28%), included pro-inflammatory cytokines as well as IL-13 which is an anti-inflammatory cytokine. Likewise, Factor 5 included both pro- (IL-15) and anti-inflammatory (IL-4, IL-10) cytokines. According to the markers that gather on the same factors, a clear separation between pro- and anti-inflammatory marker profiles could not be achieved with PCA (**Figure 1, Supplementary Table 2**).

Logistic Regression Analyses

In the Tübingen cohort, IL-1α and IL-3 (at median), and in Toronto cohort IL-1α, IL-12p40 (at median), IL-3 and IL-5 (as >0) were dichotomized to better fit in the model. None of the analyzed cytokines from either cohort reached significance ($p < 0.0038$) with regard to subtype membership prediction except for BDNF in the Toronto cohort ($p < 0.003$), which could not be confirmed in the Tübingen cohort. Some other cytokines showed a tendency ($p < 0.05$) for group separation. In some markers, a significant confounding effect of age or LEDD (not gender and disease duration) was detected which was inconsistent between cohorts. Comparison of the results in both cohorts is presented in **Supplementary Table 3**.

Out of all cytokines analyzed, only IL-12p40 showed a trend toward significance in both cohorts for distinguishing the "Benign motor" from the "Poor motor with cognitive impairment" group (Method-4, **Supplementary Table 3**). In the Tübingen cohort, lower values of IL-12p40 were associated with the "Poor motor with cognitive impairment" group against "Benign motor" group independent from the effects of age, sex, disease duration, and LEDD [Nagelkerke R^2 23%, B = −3.8, $p = 0.03$, Exp(B) = 0.02]. Likewise, the Toronto cohort showed that individuals with a high IL-12p40 value were less likely to be in the "Poor motor with cognitive impairment" group compared to the "Benign motor" group [Nagelkerke R^2=35%, B = −2.16, $p = 0.02$, Exp(B) = 0.12] (**Supplementary Figure 1**). Details of logistic regression results of other cytokines are given in the **Supplementary Table 4**.

[18F] FEPPA-PET Imaging

A [18F] FEPPA-PET imaging from 8 regions of brain was performed for IL12-p40, since it was the only (trend toward an) effect that could be replicated in the second cohort. Eighteen participants from Toronto were divided into two groups according to the lower and upper half of IL-12p40 values. Individuals in both groups showed a mixture of clinical phenotypes. No significant difference was detected between individuals with high or low values of IL-12p40 regarding the microglial activation from different regions of the brain ($p > 0.10$) (**Figure 2**). Details of the statistical analysis of brain regions are shown in **Supplementary Table 5**.

DISCUSSION

In this study, we compared serum immune markers in PD patients with different clinical subtypes in two independent cohorts. The results show that our assessment of serum immune

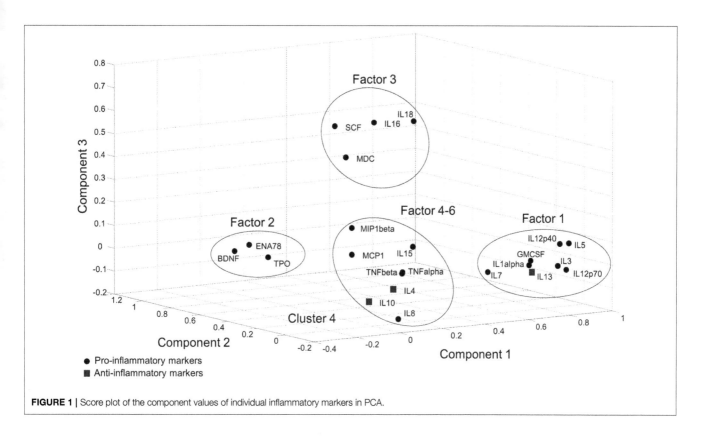

FIGURE 1 | Score plot of the component values of individual inflammatory markers in PCA.

markers, based on the current state of the art of technology, does not sufficiently discriminate clinical subgroups of PD.

Assessing immune marker levels in blood is easily accessible, and therefore has been frequently used to investigate the differences between PD patients and healthy controls. Although there are variations in study design, analysis technology, and findings in these studies (19), peripheral levels of some immune markers seem to be increased in PD patients indicating an ongoing inflammatory process that may trigger or at least accompany neurodegeneration (19). Some of these studies additionally investigated correlations between marker levels and several clinical characteristics such as motor worsening, disease severity, and non-motor status (20–23). Although the results are inconclusive, a further question was raised whether a substantial increase in already existing inflammation may be associated with non-motor features such as autonomic disturbances or dementia. To date, few studies have focused on relationships with non-motor features as the primary outcome. In a 3-year longitudinal study, William-Gray et al. reported that a pro-inflammatory immune marker profile predicted disease progression and correlated with Mini-Mental State Examination scores (24). In another study, Brockmann et al. separated PD patients with LRRK2 mutations according to the presence of non-motor symptoms and found that some pro-inflammatory marker levels were higher in the subgroup with a greater non-motor burden (16).

Contrary to these results, we failed to find an association with these disease specific features. Although some markers showed a trend ($p < 0.05$), no clear finding could be extracted

from the results of both cohorts for separating subtypes. On this basis, it can be argued that a direct or linear association between serum marker levels and symptom profile is unlikely in a complex disorder like PD, which is comprised of a variety of motor, autonomic, cognitive, psychiatric, and sensory symptoms from distinct domains with different onset and progression rates. Besides, studies investigating immune markers in blood samples for a relatively regional neurodegeneration of the central nervous system have important limitations. For example, these immune markers are not specific for neuroinflammation and a co-existing systemic inflammation/infection should be taken into account which was considered only in few of the studies (22, 24). Perhaps even a subclinical infection which cannot be easily ruled out could compromise the results. In our study, we have excluded patients with CRP >1.0 mg/dl at least to rule out clinically relevant infections, but we can still not be entirely sure whether the results were biased by an unknown systemic or regional inflammatory process. Therefore, even if an increase in serum immune markers was detected, this increase may not be indicative of neuroinflammation related to the CNS pathogenesis of PD but rather another overlapping comorbidity such as a metabolic syndrome, rheumatic disease, or another accompanying inflammatory process (e.g., via dysphagia and consecutive subtle pulmonary infection, via urinary symptoms with consecutive infection) secondary to PD since these patients are relatively prone to systemic infections (25).

Immune markers may also have both pro- and anti-inflammatory functions according to the stage of inflammation. Accumulating evidence shows that some of the cytokines, even

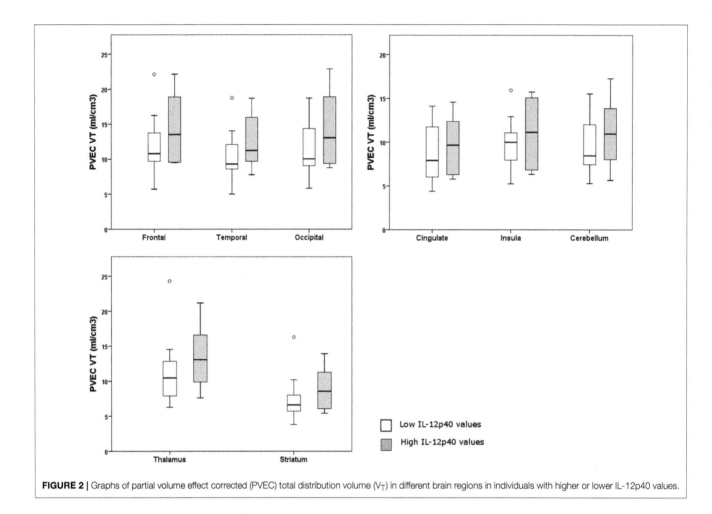

FIGURE 2 | Graphs of partial volume effect corrected (PVEC) total distribution volume (V$_T$) in different brain regions in individuals with higher or lower IL-12p40 values.

the well-known pro-inflammatory cytokines such as TNF-α, IFN-δ, or IL-6 may have a dual function (26–29), which supports the idea that functional distinction of cytokines as pro- or anti-inflammatory is too simplistic and may not adequately describe the actual inflammatory landscape (30). In our study, we found a trend for IL-12p40 to be decreased in more affected PD patients in both cohorts. This result is in line with recent literature about IL-12p40 in Alzheimer disease (31). Alternatively, although IL-12p40 is primarily a pro-inflammatory marker, it can also stimulate an immunosuppressive response when only slightly increased (32), supporting the dual-function hypothesis. This dual function of the cytokines may have prevented the clear separation of factor loadings in our PCA analysis which was also observed in William-Gray et al. (24). In both studies, the component with a pro-inflammatory profile also included anti-inflammatory cytokines indicating that these immune markers act closely in a complex network and cannot be used to determine a PD subgroup.

The levels of serum immune markers are also affected by a variety of factors such as nutrition (33), body mass index (34), sleep (35), smoking (36), thyroid hormone levels (37), exercise (38, 39), drinking coffee (40, 41), frailty (42), or depression (43, 44), and thus can be considered to be non-specific. These factors could have contributed to the negative outcome of this

study. They may also explain the controversial literature that exists for levels of IL-15 (45, 46), IL-6 (47–49), TNF-α (49, 50), IL-10 (32, 51) in association with PD occurrence, TNF-α in association with cognitive scores (20, 52), and IL-6 with UPDRS (24, 53), cognition (20, 54), and depression scores (22, 48) in PD patients. Similarly, results are also conflicting in Alzheimer's disease (55). Considering that all these factors that can hardly be controlled, results from such studies should be interpreted with appropriate caution.

Moreover, intrinsic factors such as treatment and disease progression may contribute to the high variability of immune markers. Little is known about the effect of antiparkinsonian treatment on ongoing inflammation. Several reports have shown that dopamine may have some effect on the immune response (56, 57). Based on these findings, the effect of treatment on immune markers was investigated in some studies (45, 46) or has been taken into account by adding LEDD in the regression model as a confounder (including our study), but not all studies have done this (20, 52). Furthermore, over the course of the progressive disease, the inflammation rate and therefore the blood level of markers may vary since the inflammatory response may modify itself due to the changes in the amount of cells alive, receptor count, or accumulation of α-syn (58). Diversity in the inflammatory response in different brain regions, and up/downregulations in mRNA expression of pro-inflammatory markers between early and late Braak stages have been demonstrated (59). Besides, activation of microglia by α-syn may result in upregulation of both toxic and neuroprotective activity of the microglia (60), further contributing to the limitations in the interpretation of immune markers in PD.

Limitations of the current study have to be mentioned. Eliminating patients with a serum CRP level >1 may have affected our results i.e., may party explain the non-significant results. The serum levels of other positive or negative acute-phase proteins such as procalcitonin, alpha-1 antitrypsin, albumin, or ferritin could also have been alternatively considered for a better detection of individuals with an acute infection. Moreover, we have only considered age, sex, disease duration, and LEDD as potential confounders. Other above mentioned factors such as body mass index, exercise, sleep, smoking, anti-inflammatory drug usage as well as potential comorbidities such as rheumatic or cardiovascular diseases were not taken into account. The possible distortion of results during the transport of frozen blood samples from Toronto and the cross-sectional study-design are also limitations. On the other hand, comparison of the findings in two independent and prospectively assessed cohorts, and although with a small sample, PET imaging are the strengths of the present study. Considering the lack of convincing associations in either cohort, and considering the ambiguous results from previous literature, we conclude that immune mechanisms in PD are far more complex than previously thought. Future longitudinal studies should include strictly designed grouping and confounder assessments to reveal whether specific inflammatory backgrounds are associated with and potentially account for clinical diversity in PD.

AUTHOR CONTRIBUTIONS

AS, TG, AL, DB, WM, and CM conceived the research project. RY, AB, AA, TG, AL, SH, DB, WM, and CM organized the research project. AS, AB, CS, LvdH, NS-M, TK, TJ, TG, AL, DB, WM, and CM executed the research project. RY, AB, LvdH, FL, JG, WM, and CM designed the statistical analysis. RY, AS, SH, and AA executed the statistical analysis. RY and CH wrote the first draft in the manuscript preparation. All authors reviewed and critiqued the statistical analysis and manuscript preparation.

FUNDING

Funding of this research was provided by the German Center for Neurodegenerative Diseases (DZNE) and the Canadian Institutes of Health Research (INE 117891), through CoEN initiative (www.coen.org). We acknowledge financial support by Land Schleswig-Holstein within the funding programme Open Access Publikationsfonds.

REFERENCES

1. Poewe W, Seppi K, Tanner CM, Halliday GM, Brundin P, Volkmann J, et al. Parkinson disease. *Nat Rev Dis Prim.* (2017) 3:17013. doi: 10.1038/nrdp.2017.13
2. Tufekci KU, Meuwissen R, Genc S, Genc K. Inflammation in Parkinson's Disease. In: R. Donev, Editor, *Advances in Protein Chemistry and Structural Biology.* Oxford: Elsevier (2012). p. 69–132.
3. Vila M, Jackson-Lewis V, Guégan C, Wu DC, Teismann P, Choi DK, et al. The role of glial cells in Parkinson's disease. *Curr Opin Neurol.* (2001) 14:483–9.
4. Gao HM, Jiang J, Wilson B, Zhang W, Hong JS, Liu B. Microglial activation-mediated delayed and progressive degeneration of rat nigral dopaminergic neurons: relevance to Parkinson's disease. *J Neurochem.* (2002) 81:1285–97. doi: 10.1046/j.1471-4159.2002.00928.x
5. Saiki M, Baker A, Williams-Gray CH, Foltynie T, Goodman RS, Taylor CJ, et al. Association of the human leucocyte antigen region with susceptibility to Parkinson's disease. *J Neurol Neurosurg Psychiatry* (2010) 81:890–1. doi: 10.1136/jnnp.2008.162883
6. Greggio E, Civiero L, Bisaglia M, Bubacco L. Parkinson's disease and immune system: is the culprit LRRKing in the periphery? *J Neuroinflammation* (2012) 9:94. doi: 10.1186/1742-2094-9-94
7. Ouchi Y, Yoshikawa E, Sekine Y, Futatsubashi M, Kanno T, Ogusu T, et al. Microglial activation and dopamine terminal loss in early Parkinson's disease. *Ann Neurol.* (2005) 57:168–75. doi: 10.1002/ana.20338
8. Zhang J, Sokal I, Peskind ER, Quinn JF, Jankovic J, Kenney C, et al. CSF multianalyte profile distinguishes Alzheimer and Parkinson diseases. *Am J Clin Pathol.* (2008) 129:526–9. doi: 10.1309/W01Y0B80 8EMEH12L

9. Mogi M, Harada M, Narabayashi H, Inagaki H, Minami M, Nagatsu T. Interleukin (IL)-1 beta, IL-2, IL-4, IL-6, and transforming growth factor-alpha levels are elevated in ventricular cerebrospinal fluid in juvenile parkinsonism and Parkinson's disease. *Neurosci Lett.* (1996) 211:13–6. doi: 10.1016/0304-3940(96)12706-3
10. Imamura K, Hishikawa N, Sawada M, Nagatsu T, Yoshida M, Hashizume Y. Distribution of major histocompatibility complex class II-positive microglia and cytokine profile of Parkinson's disease brains. *Acta Neuropathol.* (2003) 106:518–26. doi: 10.1007/s00401-003-0766-2
11. Mogi M, Togari A, Kondo T, Mizuno Y, Komure O, Kuno S, et al. Caspase activities and tumor necrosis factor receptor R1 (p55) level are elevated in the substantia nigra from Parkinsonian brain. *J Neural Transm.* (2000) 107:335–41. doi: 10.1007/s007020050028
12. Graham JM, Sagar HJ. A data-driven approach to the study of heterogeneity in idiopathic Parkinson's disease: identification of three distinct subtypes. *Mov Disord.* (1999) 14:10–20.
13. Lewis SJ, Foltynie T, Blackwell AD, Robbins TW, Owen AM, Barker RA. Heterogeneity of Parkinson's disease in the early clinical stages using a data driven approach. *J Neurol Neurosurg Psychiatry* (2005) 76:343–8. doi: 10.1136/jnnp.2003.033530
14. Dujardin K, Leentjens AF, Langlois C, Moonen AJ, Duits AA, Carette AS, et al. The spectrum of cognitive disorders in Parkinson's disease: a data-driven approach. *Mov Disord.* (2013) 28:183–9. doi: 10.1002/mds.25311
15. Fereshtehnejad SM, Romenets SR, Anang JB, Latreille V, Gagnon JF, Postuma RB. New clinical subtypes of parkinson disease and their longitudinal progression. *JAMA Neurol.* (2015) 72:863–73. doi: 10.1001/jamaneurol.2015.0703
16. Brockmann K, Schulte C, Schneiderhan-Marra N, Apel A, Pont-Sunyer C, Vilas D, et al. Inflammatory profile discriminates clinical subtypes

in LRRK2-associated Parkinson's disease. *Eur J Neurol.* (2017) 24:427–e6. doi: 10.1111/ene.13223

17. Rusjan P, Mamo D, Ginovart N, Hussey D, Vitcu I, Yasuno F, et al. An automated method for the extraction of regional data from PET images. *Psychiatry Res.* (2006) 147:79–89. doi: 10.1016/j.pscychresns.2006.01.011

18. Armstrong RA. When to use the Bonferroni correction. *Ophthalmic Physiol Opt.* (2014) 34:502–8. doi: 10.1111/opo.12131

19. Qin XY, Zhang SP, Cao C, Loh YP, Cheng Y. aberrations in peripheral inflammatory cytokine levels in parkinson disease. *JAMA Neurol.* (2016) 73:1316–24. doi: 10.1001/jamaneurol.2016.2742

20. Menza M, Dobkin RD, Marin H, Mark MH, Gara M, Bienfait K, et al. The role of inflammatory cytokines in cognition and other non-motor symptoms of Parkinson's disease. *Psychosomatics* (2010) 51:474–9. doi: 10.1176/appi.psy.51.6.474

21. Scalzo P, Kümmer A, Bretas TL, Cardoso F, Teixeira AL. Serum levels of brain-derived neurotrophic factor correlate with motor impairment in Parkinson's disease. *J Neurol.* (2010) 257:540–5. doi: 10.1007/s00415-009-5357-2

22. Lindqvist D, Kaufman E, Brundin L, Hall S, Surova Y, Hansson O. Non-motor symptoms in patients with Parkinson's disease - correlations with inflammatory cytokines in serum. *PLoS ONE* (2012) 7:e47387. doi: 10.1371/journal.pone.0047387

23. Wang XM, Zhang YG, Li AL, Long ZH, Wang D, Li XX, et al. Relationship between levels of inflammatory cytokines in the peripheral blood and the severity of depression and anxiety in patients with Parkinson's disease. *Eur Rev Med Pharmacol Sci.* (2016) 20:3853–6.

24. Williams-Gray CH, Wijeyekoon R, Yarnall AJ, Lawson RA, Breen DP, Evans JR, et al. Serum immune markers and disease progression in an incident Parkinson's disease cohort (ICICLE-PD). *Mov Disord.* (2016) 31:995–1003. doi: 10.1002/mds.26563

25. Alcalay RN. Cytokines as potential biomarkers of parkinson disease. *JAMA Neurol.* (2016) 73:1282–4. doi: 10.1001/jamaneurol.2016.3335

26. Liu J, Marino MW, Wong G, Grail D, Dunn A, Bettadapura J, et al. TNF is a potent anti-inflammatory cytokine in autoimmune-mediated demyelination. *Nat Med.* (1998) 4:78–83. doi: 10.1038/nm0198-078

27. Scheller J, Chalaris A, Schmidt-Arras D, Rose-John S. The pro- and anti-inflammatory properties of the cytokine interleukin-6. *Biochim Biophys Acta* (2011) 1813:878–88. doi: 10.1016/j.bbamcr.2011.01.034

28. Wilke CM, Wei S, Wang L, Kryczek I, Kao J, Zou W. Dual biological effects of the cytokines interleukin-10 and interferon-γ. *Cancer Immunol Immunother.* (2011) 60:1529–41. doi: 10.1007/s00262-011-1104-5

29. Shachar I, Karin N. The dual roles of inflammatory cytokines and chemokines in the regulation of autoimmune diseases and their clinical implications. *J Leukoc Biol.* (2013) 93:51–61. doi: 10.1189/jlb.0612293

30. Cavaillon JM. Pro- versus anti-inflammatory cytokines: myth or reality. *Cell Mol Biol (Noisy-le-grand).* (2001) 47:695–702.

31. Johansson P, Almqvist EG, Wallin A, Johansson JO, Andreasson U, Blennow K, et al. Reduced cerebrospinal fluid concentration of interleukin-12/23 subunit p40 in patients with cognitive impairment. *PLoS ONE* (2017) 12:e0176760. doi: 10.1371/journal.pone.0176760

32. Rentzos M, Nikolaou C, Andreadou E, Paraskevas GP, Rombos A, Zoga M, et al. Circulating interleukin-10 and interleukin-12 in Parkinson's disease. *Acta Neurol Scand.* (2009) 119:332–7. doi: 10.1111/j.1600-0404.2008.01103.x

33. Ampatzoglou A, Williams CL, Atwal KK, Maidens CM, Ross AB, Thielecke F, et al. Effects of increased wholegrain consumption on immune and inflammatory markers in healthy low habitual wholegrain consumers. *Eur J Nutr.* (2016) 55:183–95. doi: 10.1007/s00394-015-0836-y

34. Khaodhiar L, Ling PR, Blackburn GL, Bistrian BR. Serum levels of interleukin-6 and C-reactive protein correlate with body mass index across the broad range of obesity. *J Parenter Enter Nutr.* (2004) 28:410–5. doi: 10.1177/0148607104028006410

35. Irwin MR, Wang M, Campomayor CO, Collado-Hidalgo A, Cole S. Sleep deprivation and activation of morning levels of cellular and genomic markers of inflammation. *Arch Intern Med.* (2006) 166:1756. doi: 10.1001/archinte.166.16.1756

36. Shiels MS, Katki HA, Freedman ND, Purdue MP, Wentzensen N, Trabert B, et al. Cigarette smoking and variations in systemic immune and inflammation markers. *JNCI J Natl Cancer Inst.* (2014) 106:dju294. doi: 10.1093/jnci/dju294

37. Fabris N, Mocchegiani E, Provinciali M. Pituitary-thyroid axis and immune system: a reciprocal neuroendocrine-immune interaction. *Horm Res.* (1995) 43:29–38. doi: 10.1159/000184234

38. Hopps E, Canino B, Caimi G. Effects of exercise on inflammation markers in type 2 diabetic subjects. *Acta Diabetol.* (2011) 48:183–9. doi: 10.1007/s00592-011-0278-9

39. Kasapis C, Thompson PD. The effects of physical activity on serum C-reactive protein and inflammatory markers: a systematic review. *J Am Coll Cardiol.* (2005) 45:1563–9. doi: 10.1016/j.jacc.2004.12.077

40. Zampelas A, Panagiotakos DB, Pitsavos C, Chrysohoou C, Stefanadis C. Associations between coffee consumption and inflammatory markers in healthy persons: the ATTICA study. *Am J Clin Nutr.* (2004) 80:862–7. doi: 10.1093/ajcn/80.4.862

41. Loftfield E, Shiels MS, Graubard BI, Katki HA, Chaturvedi AK, Trabert B, et al. Associations of coffee drinking with systemic immune and inflammatory markers. *Cancer Epidemiol Biomarkers Prev.* (2015) 24:1052–60. doi: 10.1158/1055-9965.EPI-15-0038-T

42. Velissaris D, Pantzaris N, Koniari I, Koutsogiannis N, Karamouzos V, Kotroni I, et al. C-reactive protein and frailty in the elderly: a literature review. *J Clin Med Res.* (2017) 9:461–5. doi: 10.14740/jocmr2959w

43. Dowlati Y, Herrmann N, Swardfager W, Liu H, Sham L, Reim EK, et al. A meta-analysis of cytokines in major depression. *Biol Psychiatry* (2010) 67:446–57. doi: 10.1016/j.biopsych.2009.09.033

44. Birur B, Amrock EM, Shelton RC, Li L. Sex differences in the peripheral immune system in patients with depression. *Front Psychiatry* (2017) 8:108. doi: 10.3389/fpsyt.2017.00108

45. Rentzos M, Nikolaou C, Andreadou E, Paraskevas GP, Rombos A, Zoga M, et al. Circulating interleukin-15 and RANTES chemokine in Parkinson's disease. *Acta Neurol Scand.* (2007) 116:374–9. doi: 10.1111/j.1600-0404.2007.00894.x

46. Gangemi S, Basile G, Merendino RA, Epifanio A, Di Pasquale G, Ferlazzo B, et al. Effect of levodopa on interleukin-15 and RANTES circulating levels in patients affected by Parkinson's disease. *Mediators Inflamm.* (2003) 12:251–3. doi: 10.1080/0962935031000159971

47. Dursun E, Gezen-Ak D, Hanagasi H, Bilgiç B, Lohmann E, Ertan S, et al. The interleukin 1 alpha, interleukin 1 beta, interleukin 6 and alpha-2-macroglobulin serum levels in patients with early or late onset Alzheimer's disease, mild cognitive impairment or Parkinson's disease. *J Neuroimmunol.* (2015) 283:50–7. doi: 10.1016/j.jneuroim.2015.04.014

48. Selikhova MV, Kushlinskii NE, Lyubimova NV, Gusev EI. Impaired production of plasma interleukin-6 in patients with Parkinson's disease. *Bull Exp Biol Med.* (2002) 133:81–3. doi: 10.1023/A:1015120930920

49. Brodacki B, Staszewski J, Toczyłowska B, Kozłowska E, Drela N, Chalimoniuk M, et al. Serum interleukin (IL-2, IL-10, IL-6, IL-4), TNFα, and INFγ concentrations are elevated in patients with atypical and idiopathic parkinsonism. *Neurosci Lett.* (2008) 441:158–62. doi: 10.1016/j.neulet.2008.06.040

50. Dobbs RJ, Charlett A, Purkiss AG, Dobbs SM, Weller C, Peterson DW. Association of circulating TNF-alpha and IL-6 with ageing and parkinsonism. *Acta Neurol Scand.* (1999) 100:34–41. doi: 10.1111/j.1600-0404.1999.tb00721.x

51. Rota E, Bellone G, Rocca P, Bergamasco B, Emanuelli G, Ferrero P. Increased intrathecal TGF-beta1, but not IL-12, IFN-gamma, and IL-10 levels in Alzheimer's disease patients. *Neurol Sci.* (2006) 27:33–9. doi: 10.1007/s10072-006-0562-6

52. Dufek M, Hamanová M, Lokaj J, Goldemund D, Rektorová I, Michálková Z, et al. Serum inflammatory biomarkers in Parkinson's disease. *Parkinsonism Relat Disord.* (2009) 15:318–20. doi: 10.1016/j.parkreldis.2008.05.014

53. Tang P, Chong L, Li X, Liu Y, Liu P, Hou C, et al. Correlation between Serum RANTES Levels and the Severity of Parkinson's Disease. *Oxid Med Cell Longev.* (2014) 2014:208408. doi: 10.1155/2014/208408

54. Scalzo P, Kümmer A, Cardoso F, Teixeira AL. Serum levels of interleukin-6 are elevated in patients with Parkinson's disease and correlate with physical performance. *Neurosci Lett.* (2010) 468:56–8. doi: 10.1016/j.neulet.2009.10.062

55. Brosseron F, Krauthausen M, Kummer M, Heneka MT. Body fluid cytokine levels in mild cognitive impairment and alzheimer's disease: a comparative overview. *Mol Neurobiol.* (2014) 50:534–44. doi: 10.1007/s12035-014-8657-1

56. Basu S, Dasgupta PS. Dopamine, a neurotransmitter, influences the immune system. *J Neuroimmunol.* (2000) 102:113–24. doi: 10.1016/S0165-5728(99)00176-9

57. Carr L, Tucker A, Fernandez-Botran R. The enhancement of T cell proliferation by L-dopa is mediated peripherally and does not involve interleukin-2. *J Neuroimmunol.* (2003) 142:166–9. doi: 10.1016/S0165-5728(03)00270-4

58. Sanchez-Guajardo V, Tentillier N, Romero-Ramos M. The relation between α-synuclein and microglia in Parkinson's disease: Recent developments. Neuroscience. (2015) 302:47–58.

59. Garcia-Esparcia P, Llorens F, Carmona M, Ferrer I. Complex deregulation and expression of cytokines and mediators of the immune response in parkinson's disease brain is region dependent. *Brain Pathol.* (2014) 24:584–98. doi: 10.1111/bpa.12137

60. Reynolds AD, Kadiu I, Garg SK, Glanzer JG, Nordgren T, Ciborowski P, et al. Nitrated alpha-synuclein and microglial neuroregulatory activities. *J Neuroimmune Pharmacol.* (2008) 3:59–74. doi: 10.1007/s11481-008-9100-z

18

Brainstem Raphe Alterations in TCS: A Biomarker for Depression and Apathy in Parkinson's Disease Patients

Daniel Richter[1], Dirk Woitalla[1,2], Siegfried Muhlack[1], Ralf Gold[1,3], Lars Tönges[1,3] and Christos Krogias[1]*

[1] Department of Neurology, St. Josef-Hospital, Ruhr University Bochum, Bochum, Germany, [2] Department of Neurology, Katholische Kliniken Ruhrhalbinsel, Essen, Germany, [3] Neurodegeneration Research, Protein Research Unit Ruhr (PURE), Ruhr University Bochum, Bochum, Germany

Correspondence:
Christos Krogias
christos.krogias@rub.de

Depression and apathy can both be present in patients with Parkinson's disease (PD) while e. g., essential tremor (ET) patients mostly only report depressive symptoms. In PD, depression has been linked with brainstem raphe (BR) signal alterations in transcranial sonography (TCS) but apathy has not been evaluated in such terms as a putative biomarker. Furthermore, the BR has only been investigated using a singular axial TCS examination plane, although coronal TCS examination allows a much more accurate evaluation of the craniocaudal formation of serotonergic raphe structures in the midbrain area. The objective of this study was to investigate the value of coronal TCS examination for the detection of BR signal alterations and clinically correlate it to apathy in patients with PD, ET and healthy controls (HC). We prospectively included PD patients ($n = 31$), ET patients ($n = 16$), and HC ($n = 16$). All were examined by TCS in the axial and coronal plane with focus on BR signal alterations. LARS and BDI-II scores were conducted to assess apathic and depressive symptoms in the study population. In a detailed analysis we found that the correlation of coronal and axial TCS alterations of BR was very high (rho = 0.950, $p < 0.001$). BR signal alterations were more frequent in PD patients than in ET patients and HC, while it was not different between ET patients and HC. In the PD patient group, BDI-II and LARS scores were negatively correlated to BR signal changes in TCS in a significant manner (BDI-II and axial BR: $p = 0.019$; BDI-II and coronal BR: $p = 0.011$; LARS and axial BR: $p = 0.017$; LARS and coronal BR: $p = 0.023$). Together in this brainstem ultrasound study we find a significant association of BR signal alterations with clinically evident apathy and depression in patients with PD. Therefore, TCS might enable the identification of a subgroup of PD patients which are at higher risk to suffer from or to develop depression or apathy.

Keywords: sonography, TCS, raphe, apathy, depression

INTRODUCTION

Transcranial sonography (TCS) is increasingly applied for the differential diagnosis of Parkinson's disease (PD) patients. Hyperechogenicity of substantia nigra (SN) has been identified as a biomarker and risk factor for PD patients and thus has been included as a diagnostic item in the new MDS research criteria for prodromal PD (1).

Depression and apathy frequently appear in PD patients and can represent early non-motor symptoms (2–4). Several studies have shown that many PD patients are affected by depression, even in the prodromal state of disease (5). Apathy has been described to appear independently from depression (6) and can severely impact quality of life (7). Brainstem raphe (BR) alterations in TCS have been associated with depressed PD patients (8, 9) but were not observed in patients with essential tremor (ET). So far, BR signal alterations have never been examined in relation to apathy and, furthermore, have only been evaluated using a singular axial TCS plane in spite of an additional coronal examination (10).

In this study, we investigated symptoms of apathy and depression by using the Lille apathy rating scale (LARS) and the Beck Depression Inventory II (BDI-II) in PD patients, ET patients and healthy controls. Recently, a new coronal examination plane has been introduced in the field of TCS by our group in order to study Substantia nigra echogogenicity (10). We applied this methodology of an additional coronal TCS examination now for BR alterations and evaluated this finding as a putative biomarker for depression and apathy in PD.

MATERIALS AND METHODS

Subjects

We prospectively included patients fulfilling the clinical diagnostic criteria of the UK Parkinson's Disease Society Brain Bank for idiopathic PD (11) or patients meeting the diagnostic criteria for ET (12). Participants with an insufficient transtemporal bone window were excluded. All patients received best medical treatment according to international guidelines for the treatment of advanced Parkinson's disease (13) or essential tremor (14). None of the participants of this study received anti-depressive therapy. Additionally, healthy controls (HC) were included to serve as an age-matched control group. The same clinical assessment and TCS imaging was performed for every subject in this study.

All subjects were included after detailed information about the study and gave written informed consent. In accordance to the Helsinki Declaration of 1975, the study was approved by the local university ethics committee of the Ruhr University Bochum, Germany (approval no. 4961-14).

Clinical Assessment

All PD and ET patients as well as the group of HC underwent clinical neurological assessment, done by a trained and experienced interviewer. Demographic and clinical data was assessed including disease duration and comorbidity (**Table 1**).

To evaluate motor symptoms of PD, part III of the Unified Parkinson's Disease Rating Scale (UPDRS) (15) was conducted in the entire study cohort. Definition of depression and apathy was based on established scores: using the Beck Depression Inventory II (16) to investigate severity of depression symptoms. A score of ≥19 points was defined as cut-off value for depression (17). Using the Lille Apathy Rating Scale (LARS) (18) to assess apathy, a cut-off-score of ≥-16 was chosen for apathy, since this cut-off-value has shown a high sensitivity of 87% and a high specificity of 93% in diagnosing apathy (18).

Transcranial Sonography

Transcranial sonographic (TCS) examination was performed on the same day as clinical assessment, and was performed by two experienced investigators (DR, CK) being blinded to clinical scores using a phased array ultrasound system equipped with a 2.5-MHz transducer (Aplio® XG Ultrasound System, Toshiba Medicals, Tochigi, Japan). A penetration depth of 150 mm and a dynamic range of 45–50 dB were chosen. Image brightness and time gain compensations were adapted as needed for each examination.

The examination protocol of the axial examination plane was based on previous published recommendations for TCS (19). Using the transtemporal approach, the midbrain and diencephalic examination planes were visualized in axial section. To evaluate SN hyperechogenicity, a planimetric measurement of SN was performed. According to previously published studies (20), we used the mean + 1 SD of SN echogenic area in the group of HC for each plane as upper normal value defining SN hyperechogenicty. In general, an enlarged echogenic area of the SN is a predictive biomarker with high sensitivity and specificity for the diagnosis of PD (10).

The echogenicity of brainstem raphe (BR) was classified semi-quantitatively on a three-point scale: 0 = raphe structure not visible, 1 = slight and interrupted echogenic raphe structure, 2 = normal echogenicity (echogenicity of raphe structure is not interrupted) (**Figure 1**). Different to the enlarged echogenic area of the SN in PD, a reduced echogenic signal of the BR is thought to visualize changes in the serotonergic system (9).

Similar to the axial examination plane protocol, the temporal bone window was used to assess also the coronal TCS plane: by rotating the transducer for 90°, the hypoechogenic midbrain is visualized in longitudinal view including SN and BR (**Figure 2**).

The sonographic findings were stored, so that the investigators could perform a second evaluation and classification of the results from the other investigator. In the case of discrepant ratings, a consensus was accomplished, subsequently.

Statistical Analysis

The descriptive statistics are given as median and interquartile range throughout the manuscript. As needed, the range is given additionally. Using appropriate nonparametric tests, the groups were statistically compared and correlation analysis were performed (Kruskal-Wallis H test, Mann-Whitney–U test,

TABLE 1 | Demographic, clinical and sonographic data.

	Parkinson's disease (n = 31)	Essential tremor (n = 16)	HC (n = 16)	p-value
Age (years)	69.0 (14.0)	63.5 (21.25)	58.0 (9.25)	0.079[H]
Female (%)/	10 (32.3)/	8 (50)/	10 (62.5)/	0.129[F]
Male (%)	21 (67.7)	8 (50)	6 (37.5)	
Time to first suspected disease	9.0 (6.0)	4.5 (9.75)	–	0.220[U]
Hoehn and Yahr	2.0 (0)	–	–	
MDR-UPDRS III	28.0 (14.0)	7.5 (5.0)	0.5 (2.0)	**<0.001**[H,b]
BDI-II	10.0 (14.0)	12.0 (12.5)	5.0 (8.25)	**0.050**[H,c]
LARS	−24.0 (15.0)	−30.0 (9.0)	−31.0 (4.75)	**<0.001**[H,b]
TCS				
Axial SN echogenicity in cm²	0.27 (0.10)	0.14 (0.04)	0.145 (1.0)	**<0.001**[H,a]
(Hyperechogen in %)	(90.3)	(12.5)	(18.8)	**<0.001**[F,a]
Reduced BR signal axial (%)	32.3	6.7	6.3	**0.044**[F,a]
Reduced BR signal coronal (%)	29.0	6.7	6.7	0.119[F]

Boldface p-values indicate statistical sgnificance. Values are given in median and (interquartile range). MDR-UPDRS, Part 3 of the Movement Disorder Society Unified Parkinson Disease Rating Scale, BDI-II, Becks Depression Inventory II; LARS, Lille Apathy Rating Scale; TCS, Transcranial sonography.
[a] Significant difference between the three groups but not between ET patients and HC; [b] Significant difference between the three groups and also between ET patients and HC; [c] Significant difference between the three groups but not between PD and ET patients; [H]Kruskal-Wallis H test; [U]Mann-Whitney-U test;
[F]Freeman-Halton extension of Fisher's exact test.

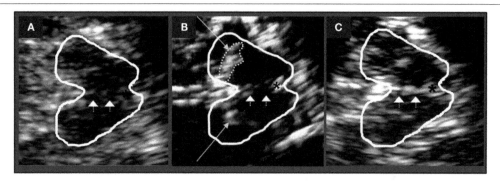

FIGURE 1 | Corresponding mesencephalic axial examination planes. The butterfly-shaped midbrain is outlined for better visualization. The asterisk indicates the aqueduct. Arrowheads indicate the brain stem raphe. **(A)** Raphe structure not visible, grade 0, pathologic finding. **(B)** Echogenic line of the raphe is interrupted, grade 1, pathologic finding. Long arrows indicating the hyperechogenic enlarged area of Substania nigra **(C)** Normal echogenicity, grade 2, normal finding.

Wilcoxon-Test, Fisher's exact test, Freeman-Halton extension of Fisher's exact test, Spearman rho analysis) with SPSS 23.0 for Mac.

RESULTS

Study Population and Clinical Features
We screened 36 patients with Parkinson's disease; four patients (11.1%) were excluded owing to an inadequate temporal bone window and one patient (2.7%) was excluded owing to severe dementia. Thus, 31 PD-patients (21 men, 10 women; age = 69.0 [14.0] years) were included into the study. Furthermore, one of the initially 17 patients with essential Tremor was excluded owing to an inadequate temporal bone window resulting in 16 ET patients (8 men, 8 women; age = 63.5 [21.25] years) being

included. As control group, 16 healthy subjects were recruited (6 men, 10 women; age = 58.0 [9.25] years). LARS could be performed in 44 participants of the patient population. Detailed information about the clinical characteristics of all participants is demonstrated in **Table 1**.

Symptoms of Depression and Apathy
Prevalence of depression based on BDI-II definition value differed significantly over the three groups. Owing to the definition, 10 (32.3%) PD patients, 3 (18.8%) ET patients and none of the HC were depressive in our investigation (Freeman-Halton extension of Fisher's exact test, $p = 0.024$). Additionally, there was a strong tendency for difference between PD-patients, ET-patients and HC regarding to the BDI-II Score (Kruskal-Wallis H test, $p = 0.05$). BDI-II scores of PD-patients and

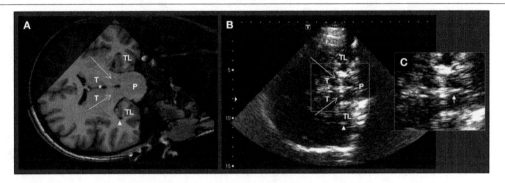

FIGURE 2 | Corresponding MRI and TCS images of coronal examination planes in a patient with idiopathic Parkinson's disease. Coronal MR scanning plane **(A)** and corresponding TCS examination plane **(B)** at brainstem level. **(C)** Zoom in of midbrain structures for planimetric assessment of the echogenic area of substantia nigra and evaluation of brainstem raphe. The large arrows in **(A)** and **(B)** indicate substantia nigra (note that in TCS the SN is displayed echogenic). White asterisks mark the third ventricle. Arrowheads in **(A)** and **(B)** indicate the inferior horn of lateral ventricle. Small arrow in **(C)** indicates the normal appearing brainstem raphe. TL, temporal lobe; P, Pons; T, thalamus.

ET-patients showed comparable results (Mann-Whitney–U test $p = 0.770$). The BDI-II score was significantly different between PD-patients and HC (Mann-Whitney–U test, $p = 0.02$) while the BDI-II scores of ET-patients and HC did not show a substantial difference as the postulated p-value level of statistical significance could not be reached (Mann-Whitney–U test, $p = 0.056$).

Analyzing the appearance of apathy, 12 (38.7%) PD patients, one (7.7%) ET patient and none of the HC were apathic indicating a significant difference in apathy prevalence over the groups (Freeman-Halton extension of Fisher's exact test, $p = 0.002$). Between ET patients and HC no difference in apathy prevalence was found (Fisher's exact test, $p = 1.000$). Regarding to LARS scores, there was also significant difference over the three groups (Kruskal-Wallis H test, $p < 0.001$). This difference in LARS scores appeared significant between PD and ET patients (Mann-Whitney–U test, $p = 0.023$) and significant between ET patients and HC (Mann-Whitney–U test, $p = 0.045$) and PD patients and HC (Mann-Whitney–U test, $p < 0.001$), respectively.

In respect to coexisting apathy and depression, 5 (41.6%) of the apathic PD patients had only apathy and 7 (58.3%) had apathy and depression. Concerning depressive PD patients, 3 (30.0%) had only depression and 7 (70.0%) had both depression and apathy. Interestingly, in these subgroups of PD patients with isolated either depressive (3 patients, 9.7%) or apathic (5 patients, 16.1%) symptoms, only one (3.2%) PD patient with isolated apathy showed an altered BR Signal in TCS.

Correlation of LARS and BDI-II

For each group of the study population BDI-II and LARS scores were correlated. Only for PD patients a significant positive correlation was found (PD: rho $= 0.657$, $p < 0.001$). In ET patients and in the group of HC, no significant correlation was determined (ET: rho $= 0.075$, $p = 0.808$; HC: rho $= 0.131$, $p = 0.630$).

Transcranial Sonography Findings

In one ET patient the BR could not sufficiently be evaluated. In one HC only the axial sonographic BR analyzes could be examined. In both cases there was a partially insufficient bone window. Evaluation of BR echogenicity revealed that 10 (32.3%) of the 31 patients with PD, but only one (6.7%) of the remaining 15 patients with ET and only one (6.3%) of the 16 healthy controls exhibited a reduced BR signal in the axial TCS plane indicating structural alterations in this area (Freeman-Halton extension of Fisher's exact test, $p = 0.044$). Using the coronal TCS plane, almost the same distribution of BR alterations in the groups was found (Freeman-Halton extension of Fisher's exact test, $p = 0.119$). Correlation of axial and coronal TCS results in BR region was very high (rho $= 0.950$, $p < 0.001$) (**Table 1**).

As BR signal alterations in TCS were very rare in ET patients und HC, correlation analysis of BDI-II, LARS and the sonographic BR results was only performed in the PD group determining a significant negative correlation between BDI-II and BR (rho $= -0.420$, $p = 0.019$) and LARS and BR (rho $= -0.427$, $p = 0.017$) using the axial TCS plane. Assessing BR through the coronal TCS plane in the PD population, the negative correlation values between BDI-II and BR (rho $= -0.434, p = 0.015$) and LARS and BR (rho $= -0.407$, $p = 0.023$) were comparable to the axial TCS assessment. The correlation analysis is also visualized as scatterplots in **Figure 3**.

Comparing BDI-II and LARS scores between PD patients with and without BR signal alterations in TCS, a significant difference was found. PD patients with BR alterations in axial TCS plane had higher scores in BDI-II (Mann-Whitney–U test, $p = 0.025$) and LARS (Mann-Whitney–U test, $p = 0.022$) compared to PD patients without BR signal changes. The same relation was found for coronal TCS plane by comparing the BDI-II and LARS scores in PD patients and without BR signal changes (BDI-II: Mann-Whitney–U test, $p = 0.029$; LARS: Mann-Whitney–U test, $p = 0.018$). Findings are summarized in **Table 2**.

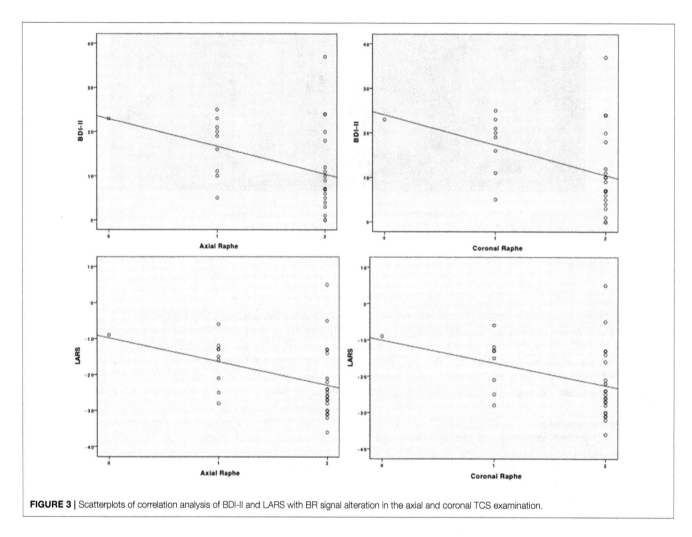

FIGURE 3 | Scatterplots of correlation analysis of BDI-II and LARS with BR signal alteration in the axial and coronal TCS examination.

No differences in BDI-II scores were found if depressive PD patients with and without BR signal alteration in TCS were compared irrespective of applying the axial (Kruskal Wallis H Test, $p = 0.469$) or coronal TCS plane (Mann-Whitney–U test, $p = 0.257$). Moreover, no differences in LARS scores were found, comparing apathic PD patients with and without BR signal alteration in TCS, neither for the axial (Kruskal Wallis H Test, $p = 0.683$) nor for the coronal TCS plane (Mann-Whitney–U test, $p = 0.792$).

Concerning SN hyperechogenicity, the mean $\pm$ 1 SD in the group of HC was calculated as 0.19 cm^2 for axial TCS plane resulting in a robust cut-off value for SN hyperechogenicity of unilateral echogenic SN area of at least 0.20 cm^2.

28 PD patients (90.3%), *three* HC (18.8%) and two ET patients (12.5%) showed SN hyperechogenicity (Freemann-Halton extension of Fisher's exact test, $p < 0.001$). Relating to the appearance of axial SN hyperechogenicity in the ET patients compared with the HC, no difference between these groups was found (Fisher's exact test, $p = 1.000$).

In the group of PD patients, the area of the SN in TCS was significantly larger than the SN area of the ET patients and HC (Kruskal-Wallis H test, $p < 0.001$), respectively. No

difference in SN areas was found between ET patients and HC (Mann-Whitney–U test, $p = 1.000$).

DISCUSSION

To our knowledge, this is the first study to correlate BR signal alterations with symptoms of apathy in PD patients. Furthermore, this is the first study which detects BR echogenicity additionally in the recently introduced coronal TCS examination plane. We could show, that BR signal alterations detected by axial TCS examination plane appear more frequently in PD patients compared to ET patients and HC. Similarly, concerning the coronal TCS examination plane, we could confirm a higher prevalence of BR signal alterations in PD patients compared to ET patients and HC. With regard to BR signal changes, the correlation of axial and coronal TCS examination planes was very high indicating no superiority of one TCS plane compared to the other. However, as sonographic raphe analysis is based on a three-point scale we did not expect a substantial difference between the results of both TCS planes a priori.

In other studies, there have been discrepancies in the prevalence of apathy and its status as an independent symptom

TABLE 2 | Relation of BR, LARS, and BDI-II.

PD patients (n = 31)

	BDI-II		LARS	
	Spearman rho	p-value	Spearman rho	p-value
Axial BR evaluation in TCS	−0.420	**0.019**	−0.427	**0.017**
Coronal BR evaluation in TCS	−0.434	**0.011**	−0.407	**0.023**

	Axial BR evaluation in TCS		Coronal BR evaluation in TCS		p-value	
	BR-	BR+	BR-	BR+	Axial	Coronal
BDI-II	19.5 (12.25)	7.0 (11.5)	20.0 (9.5)	7.0 (8.75)	**0.025**[U]	**0.029**[U]
LARS	−14 (10.75)	−26.0 (17.5)	−13.0 (12.5)	−25.5 (14.5)	**0.022**[U]	**0.018**[U]

Boldface p-values indicate statistical significance. Values are given in median and (interquartile range). BDI-II, Becks Depression Inventory II; LARS, Lille Apathy Rating Scale; TCS, Transcranial sonography; BR, Brainstem raphe; BR–, With brainstem raphe alterations; BR+, Without brainstem raphe alterations; [U]Mann-Whitney-U test.

of PD. Brok et al. found that about 40% of PD patients are suffering from apathy (21). In our study, we found comparable results by determining apathy in about 38.7% of our PD patient population. We could show that a higher grade of apathy was negatively correlated to BR signal alterations in TCS and that PD patients with BR signal changes in TCS had higher scores in LARS. BR alterations in TCS might appear as a structural correlate to apathic symptoms and thus could serve as a correlating biomarker for apathy in PD. Furthermore, TCS might allow to identify PD patients which are at high risk of developing apathy. To validate these findings, a prospective longitudinal study paradigm is needed.

One of the ET patients and none of the HC were apathic according to the definition. Apathy has been occasionally described to occur independently from depression in ET patients (22). In our study, ET patients had higher overall scores in LARS compared to HC indicating a difference in the magnitude of apathic symptoms between these two groups.

In our study, PD patients with BR signal alterations showed significantly higher scores in BDI-II compared to those without BR signal alterations. Independently of the applied TCS plane, the BR signal alteration in TCS was significantly negatively correlated to the BDI-II scores in the PD patients group. This suggests that a structural change in the BR could be associated with the occurrence of depression as well as the severity of depressive symptoms in PD patients and thus might also have a value as a biomarker for depression in PD. Therefore, BR evaluation by TCS might allow to identify a subpopulation of PD patients which are at higher risk to develop a depressive symptomatology and would benefit from a more frequent follow up or more intensive medical treatment. Additionally, we have found a correlation of BR signal changes and apathic symptoms indicating that BR alterations in PD could serve as a biomarker for both apathy and depression. In most of the PD patients apathy and depression were present simultaneously and BDI-II and LARS scores were significantly positively correlated

indicating a coexistence of apathic and depressive symptoms in PD.

A reduced BR signal, seen as absent or interrupted echogenic midline structure, is thought to reflect alterations in the serotonergic system and has been reported to be associated with depression in PD patients and with other extrapyramidal neuropsychiatric disorders like Huntington's disease (8, 9, 23). Anatomically, the echogenic midline in general represents various nuclei and fiber tracts of which the dorsal raphe nucleus is one of the main structures. The raphe nucleus is the major origin for serotonin release in the brain (24). A reduced echogenic signal of the BR could be due to alterations in the micro-architecture of this region (25, 26) and thus reflect a serotonin deficiency which is involved in depression pathophysiology.

The pathophysiological basis of apathy is still unknown. Concerning PD, this study found a correlation between sonographic BR alteration and apathy. As the echogenic raphe midline has much more fine anatomical structures than the raphe nuclei, it is also possible that microanatomical changes in other brain regions involved in the serotonin metabolism exist in addition. To our knowledge, sonographic BR signal alterations in PD have only been associated to mood disorders. Interestingly, a recent study has found a significant correlation between tremor severity in PD and raphe dysfunction measured by 123 ioflupane-fluoropropyl-carbomethoxy-3-beta-4-iodophenyltropane single photon emission computed tomography images (27). Further studies should check if sonographic BR signal changes are also linked to motor symptoms in PD.

Because the current BR evaluation in TCS is limited to a three-point scale, the discrimination of BR assessment might not be precise enough to detect differences in the severity of depression. We could not correlate the severity of depression in depressive PD patients to the extent of BR alterations in our study.

Interestingly, no difference with regard to BR signal alterations was found between ET patients and HC, although depression was present in some cases and BDI-II scores were higher in ET patients compared to HC as has been shown before (28, 29). This implies that depression in ET in contrast to PD does not seem to be associated with BR alterations in TCS.

In conclusion, BR signal alterations were found more frequently in PD patients compared to ET patients and HC independent of the applied axial or coronal TCS examination plane. BDI-II and LARS scores of PD patients could be correlated to BR signal alterations of both TCS planes. This indicates that a serotonergic signal disturbance might exist for both depression and apathy and that pharmacologic therapy should take these findings into account. In the case of depression, it has been already reported that a reduced BR signal might be associated with better treatment responses to serotonin-reuptake-inhibitors (SSRI) (30). Further prospective and longitudinal studies are urgently needed to validate these study results in PD

in order to substantiate this novel tool to more precisely identify PD and ET patients at risk to develop depression and apathy.

AUTHOR CONTRIBUTIONS

DR contributed to conceptualizing, organizing the project, analyzing, acquiring, and interpreting the data and writing of the first draft. DW contributed to conceptualizing and revising the manuscript. SM and RG contributed to conceptualizing, organizing the project and revising the manuscript. LT contributed to organizing the project, analyzing, acquiring and interpreting the data and revising the manuscript. CK contributed to conceptualizing, organizing the project, analyzing, acquiring and interpreting the data and revising the manuscript.

REFERENCES

1. Berg D, Postuma RB, Adler CH, Bloem BR, Chan P, Dubois B, et al. MDS research criteria for prodromal Parkinson's disease. *Mov Disord.* (2015) 12:1600–11. doi: 10.1002/mds.26431
2. Aarsland D, Marsh L, Schrag A. Neuropsychiatric symptoms in Parkinson's disease. *Mov Disord.* (2009) 24:2175–86. doi: 10.1002/mds.22589
3. Reijnders JS, Ehrt U, Weber WE, Aarsland D, Leentjens AF. A systematic review of prevalence studies of depression in Parkinson's disease. *Mov Disord.* (2008) 23:183–9. doi: 10.1002/mds.21803
4. Pedersen KF, Larsen JP, Alves G, Aarsland D. Prevalence and clinical correlates of apathy in Parkinson's disease: a community-based study. *Parkinsonism Relat Disord.* (2009) 15:295–9. doi: 10.1016/j.parkreldis.2008.07.006
5. Gaenslen A, Wurster I, Brockmann K, Huber H, Godau J, Faust B, et al. Prodromal features for Parkinson's disease–baseline data from the TREND study. *Eur J Neurol.* (2014) 21:766–72. doi: 10.1111/ene.12382
6. Oguru M, Tachibana H, Toda K, Okuda B, Oka N. Apathy and depression in Parkinson disease. *J Geriatr Psychiatry Neurol.* (2010) 23:35–41. doi: 10.1177/0891988709351834
7. Prakash KM, Nadkarni NV, Lye WK, Yong MH, Tan EK. The impact of non-motor symptoms on the quality of life of Parkinson's disease patients: a longitudinal study. *Eur J Neurol.* (2016) 23:854–60. doi: 10.1111/ene.12950
8. Walter U, Hoeppner J, Prudente-Morrissey L, Horowski S, Herpertz SC, Benecke R. Parkinson's disease-like midbrain sonography abnormalities are frequent in depressive disorders. *Brain* (2007) 130:1799–807.doi:10.1093/brain/awm017
9. Krogias C, Walter U. Transcranial sonography findings in depression in association with psychiatric and neurologic diseases: a review. *J Neuroimaging* (2016) 26:257–63. doi: 10.1111/jon.12328
10. Richter D, Woitalla D, Muhlack S, Gold R, Tönges L, Krogias C. Coronal transcranial sonography and m-mode tremor frequency determination in Parkinson's disease and essential tremor. *J Neuroimaging* (2017) 27:524–30. doi: 10.1111/jon.12441
11. Hughes AJ, Daniel SE, Kilford L, Lees AJ. Accuracy of clinical diag- nosis of idiopathic Parkinson's disease: a clinico-pathological study of 100 cases. *J Neurol Neurosurg Psychiatry* (1992) 55:181–4.
12. Deuschl G, Bain P, Brin M. Consensus statement of the movement disorder society on tremor. ad hoc scientific committee. *Mov Disord.* (1998) 13:2–23.
13. Horstink M, Tolosa E, Bonuccelli U, Deuschl G, Friedman A, Kanovsky P, et al. European federation of neurological societies; movement disorder society-european section. review of the therapeutic management of Parkinson's disease. report of a joint task force of the european federation of neurological

societies and the movement disorder society-european section. *Eur J Neurol.* (2006) 13:1186–202. doi: 10.1111/j.1468-1331.2006.01548.x
14. Zesiewicz TA, Elble RJ, Louis ED, Gronseth GS, Ondo WG, Dewey RB Jr, et al. Evidence-based guideline update: treatment of essential tremor: report of the quality standards subcommittee of the american academy of neurology. *Neurology* (2011) 77:1752–5. doi: 10.1212/WNL.0b013e318236f0fd
15. Movement Disorder Society Task Force on Rating Scales for Parkinson's Disease. The Unified Parkinson's Disease Rating Scale (UPDRS): status and recommendations. *Mov Disord.* (2003) 18:738–50. doi: 10.1002/mds.10473
16. Beck AT, Steer RA, Ball R, Ranieri W. Comparison of beck depression inventories–IA and –II in psychiatric outpatients. *J Personal Assess.* (1996) 67:588–97.
17. Arnau RC, Meagher MW, Norris MP, Bramson R. Psychometric evaluation of the beck depression inventory-II with primary care medical patients. *Health Psychol.* (2001) 20:112–9. doi: 10.1037//0278-6133.20.2.112
18. Sockeel P, Defebvre L, Denève C, Destèe A, Devos D, Dujardin K. The Lille apathy rating scale (LARS), a new instrument for detecting and quantifying apathy: validation in Parkinson's disease. *J Neurol Neurosurg Psychiatry* (2006) 77:579–84. doi: 10.1136/jnnp.2005.075929
19. Walter U, Skoloudik D. Transcranial sonography (TCS) of brain parenchyma in movement disorders: quality standards, diagnostic applications, and novel technologies. *Ultraschall Med.* (2014) 35:322–31. doi: 10.1055/s-0033-1356415
20. Doepp F, Plotkin M, Siegel L, Kivi A, Gruber D, Lobsien E, et al. Brain parenchyma sonography and ^{123}I-FP-CIT SPECT in Parkinson's disease and essential tremor. *Mov Disord.* (2008) 23:405–10. doi: 10.1002/mds.21861
21. den Brok MG, van Dalen JW, van Gool WA, Moll van Charante EP, de Bie RM, Richard E. Apathy in Parkinson's disease: a systematic review and meta-analysis. *Mov Disord.* (2015) 30:759–69. doi: 10.1002/mds.26208
22. Louis ED. Non-motor symptoms in essential tremor: a review of the current data and state of the field. *Parkinsonism Relat Disord.* (2016) 22(Suppl. 1):115–8. doi: 10.1016/j.parkreldis.2015.08.034
23. Krogias C, Strassburger K, Eyding J, Gold R, Norra C, Juckel G, et al. Depression in patients with Huntington disease correlates with alterations of the brain stem raphe depicted by transcranial sonography. *J Psychiatry Neurosci.* (2011) 36:187-94. doi: 10.1503/jpn.100067
24. Carpenter MB, Sutin J. *Human Neuroanatomy*. Baltimore: Williams and Wilkins (1983).
25. Berg D, Supprian T, Hofmann E, Zeiler B, Jäger A, Lange KW, et al. Depression in Parkinson's disease: brainstem midline alteration on transcranial sonography and magnetic resonance imaging. *J Neurol.* (1999) 246:1186–93.

26. Becker G, Berg D, Lesch KP, Becker T. Basal limbic system alteration in major depression: a hypothesis supported by transcranial sonography and MRI findings. *Int J Neuropsychopharmacol.* (2001) 4:21–31. doi: 10.1017/S1461145701002164

27. Pasquini J, Ceravolo R, Qamhawi Z, Lee JY, Deuschl G, Brooks DJ, et al. Progression of tremor in early stages of Parkinson's disease: a clinical and neuroimaging study. *Brain* (2018) doi: 10.1093/brain/awx376)

28. Sengul Y, Sengul HS, Yucekaya SK, Yucel S, Bakim B, Pazarci NK, et al. Cognitive functions, fatigue, depression, anxiety, and sleep disturbances: assessment of nonmotor features in young patients with essential tremor. *Acta Neurol Belg.* (2014) 115:281–7. doi: 10.1007/s13760-014-0396-6

29. Louis ED, Cosentino S, Huey ED. Depressive symptoms can amplify embarrassment in essential tremor. *J Clin Mov Disord.* (2016) 3:11. doi: 10.1186/s40734-016-0039-6

30. Walter U, Prudente-Morrissey L, Herpertz SC, Benecke R, Hoeppner J. Relationship of brainstem raphe echogenicity and clinical findings in depressive states. *Psychiatry Res.* (2007) 155:67–73. doi: 10.1016/j.pscychresns.2006.12.001

19

Biomarkers for Dementia, Fatigue and Depression in Parkinson's Disease

Tino Prell[1,2]*, Otto W. Witte[1,2] and Julian Grosskreutz[1,2]

[1] Department of Neurology, Jena University Hospital, Jena, Germany, [2] Center for Healthy Ageing, Jena University Hospital, Jena, Germany

*Correspondence:
Tino Prell
tino.prell@med.uni-jena.de

Parkinson's disease is a common multisystem neurodegenerative disorder characterized by typical motor and non-motor symptoms. There is an urgent need for biomarkers for assessment of disease severity, complications and prognosis. In addition, biomarkers reporting the underlying pathophysiology assist in understanding the disease and developing neuroprotective therapies. Ultimately, biomarkers could be used to develop a more efficient personalized approach for clinical trials and treatment strategies. With the goal to improve quality of life in Parkinson's disease it is essential to understand and objectively monitor non-motor symptoms. This narrative review provides an overview of recent developments of biomarkers (biofluid samples and imaging) for three common neuropsychological syndromes in Parkinson's disease: dementia, fatigue, and depression.

Keywords: Parkinson's disease, biomarker, non-motor syndromes, depression, fatigue, dementia

INTRODUCTION

Parkinson's disease (PD) is now considered as progressive and multisystem α-synucleinopathy. Therefore, PD is characterized not only by motor symptoms, but also a broad range of non-motor symptoms (NMS) (1). NMS can aggravate disease burden and significantly contribute to worsening of quality of life (2). Biomarkers which are associated with worse motor performance as well as development of NMS are of special importance in PD. A biomarker is "a characteristic that is objectively measured and evaluated as an indicator of normal biological processes, pathogenic processes, or pharmacologic responses to a therapeutic intervention" (3). The ideal PD biomarkers should have a reasonable effect size, are reproducible across different cohorts and are ideally verified in neuropathological proven PD cases. Biomarkers in PD can include (i) biomarker for prodromal stage to identify PD before motor symptoms occur, (ii) biomarkers of susceptibility to identify persons who are at risk for PD, (iii) biomarkers for motor and non-motor burden to assess disease severity and monitor the efficacy of therapies. The last one can help to identify patients who are at risk to develop complications and may lead to individual optimization and prevention in health care. This review provides an update on recent advances in the development of biomarkers (biofluid samples and neuroimaging) for three common neuropsychological syndromes: dementia, fatigue and depression.

COGNITIVE IMPAIRMENT

Cognitive deficits are common in PD and can present as mild dysfunction in the prodromal and early stages, or as dementia (PDD) in advanced stages (4). Approximately 20%

of patients with *de novo* PD have mild cognitive impairment (MCI) (5). The concept of PD-MCI was introduced 2012 (MDS Task Force) and characterizes a cognitive decline that is assessed during neuropsychological testing but does not impair activities of daily living (6). MCI is considered an intermediate state of cognitive dysfunction in PD that may progress to PDD. Up to 75% of patients will develop dementia over the longterm disease course (7). However, the rate to PDD, the cognitive profile and severity of cognitive dysfunction show high interindividual variation. Given its high medical and social impact and its health-related costs, the identification of biomarkers for PDD is of high priority (8). Biomarkers reflecting cognitive decline can facilitate early diagnosis and may indicate response to therapeutic interventions.

Clinical factors, such as higher age, male sex, low level of education, longer disease duration, higher Hoehn & Yahr stage, axial impairment, excessive daytime sleepiness, cardiovascular autonomic dysfunction, REM sleep behavior disorder, hallucinations and PD-MCI were found to strongly predict the development of PDD (9–13). Moreover, impairment of memory and language (posterior-cortical dysfunction) seems to be linked to a higher risk of PDD (14, 15).

Given the neuropathology of PDD several studies aimed to identify biomarkers which reflect proteinopathy, neuronal loss, abnormal neurotransmitters, and structural and functional brain changes. Lewy bodies and amyloid plaques in the neocortex and limbic system are typical neuropathological features of Alzheimer's disease and PDD (16, 17). Hence, the majority of studies investigated amyloid-ß 1–42 (Aß), tau protein, and α-synuclein in the cerebrospinal fluid (CSF) of PD patients (**Table 1**). In many studies the level of Aß was reduced in PDD. Low CSF levels of Aß were found to be related to deterioration in attention, executive function, semantic fluency and memory (21, 38, 40, 45). One-half of PDD patients had the CSF biomarker signature of Alzheimer's disease (46) suggestive of an overlap with Alzheimer's disease pathology (47). Low baseline CSF Aß was associated with more rapid cognitive decline later in disease. By contrast, the levels of total (t-tau) and phosphorylated tau (p-tau) were found to be increased or unchanged in PDD (**Table 1**). For clinicians it is highly relevant to know which biomarkers accurately predict the progression from MCI to PDD. Therefore, based on the data from cross-sectional and longitudinal studies one can assume that reduced Aß predicts cognitive decline in PD (40, 42, 48).

Several studies assessed the CSF levels of α-synuclein in PD. Meta-analyses demonstrated that total α-synuclein levels are lower in PD compared to controls (49, 50). However, in terms of α-synuclein and cognitive decline there are conflicting results with both low and high levels in the presence of cognitive impairment (29, 41, 48). In the DATATOP study with up to 8 years of follow-up, lower α-synuclein levels predicted better preservation of cognitive function (verbal learning and memory, visuospatial working memory) in early disease. Thus, α-synuclein may reflect changes in multiple cognitive domains and may predict cognitive decline in PD (29, 41, 48). On the other hand most studies of non-demented PD failed to find any association between α-synuclein levels and cognition

(51, 52). It seems that CSF α-synuclein levels may increase with disease stage. This could explain why cognitive deficits in connection with high levels of α- synuclein were found in more advanced disease stages (53). Isoforms of α-synuclein (e.g., phosphorylated, ubiquitinated, oligomeric) are potentially more sensitive to cognitive decline than the total α-synuclein level (24, 30). Another study examining plasma levels of α-synuclein found higher levels in PDD and a correlation with mini mental state examination scores (54). This finding, however, requires further investigations.

In another longitudinal study, high neurofilament light chain protein, low Aβ and high heart fatty acid–binding protein at baseline were related to future PDD with a relatively high diagnostic accuracy (19). Also several serum proteins, such as C-reactive protein, interleukins, interferon-γ, tumor necrosis factor α, uric acid, and cystatin C were found to be associated with cognition in PD (55). In particular, low uric acid concentrations, low levels of epidermal growth factor (EGF) and insulin-like growth factor (ILGF) seems to have predictive value for deterioration of cognitive function in PD (56–61). In combination with clinical markers, a study of 390 patients from the Progression Markers Initiative study with newly diagnosed PD, the occurrence of cognitive impairment at 2 years follow-up could be predicted with good accuracy using a model combining information on age, non-motor assessments, DAT imaging, and CSF biomarkers. Here, the Montreal Cognitive Assessment (MoCA) scores and low CSF Aβ to t-tau ratio and DAT imaging results were the best predictors of cognitive impairment (39). Using data from the Parkinson's Progression Markers Initiative, Fereshtehnejad et al., identified distinct subgroups via a cluster analysis of a comprehensive dataset consisting of clinical characteristics, neuroimaging, biospecimen and genetic information. Here, the CSF biomarkers differed between these PD subtypes. Patients with diffuse malignant disease course and fast cognitive decline, showed an Alzheimer's disease-like CSF profile (low Aβ, low Aβ/t-tau ratio) (62).

Applying computerized neuroimaging analyses several MRI studies have found gray matter atrophy and disruptions of white matter integrity in PDD, although findings in non-demented PD and PD-MCI remain inconsistent (63) (**Tables 2, 3**). A longitudinal study using voxel-based morphometry (VBM) found neocortical volume reduction (temporo-occipital region, hippocampal and parahippocampal) as the most relevant finding in patients who develop PDD (97). Another study has identified a validated Alzheimer's disease pattern of brain atrophy as an independent predictor of cognitive impairment in PD (64). More specifically cortical thinning in the right precentral, frontal, and in the anterior cingulate cortex as well as gray matter atrophy (prefrontal, insula, caudate nucleus, hippocampal) predicted cognitive decline in PD (23, 66, 70, 76, 98). Cognitive impairment was also found to be associated with lower gray matter volume and increased mean diffusivity in the nucleus basalis of Meynert, compared to non-demented patients. Moreover, these changes were predictive for developing cognitive impairment in cognitively intact patients with PD, independent of other clinical and non-clinical markers of the disease (99). The nucleus basalis of Meynert and the pedunculopontine nucleus

TABLE 1 | Cerebrospinal-fluid (CSF) biomarkers of cognitive impairment and dementia in Parkinson's disease.

Study	CSF biomarker						Participants	Methods	Result
	Aβ1-42	t-tau	p-tau	t-α-syn	o-α-syn	other			
Alves et al. (18)*	+	+	+				PDND 104	MDS Task Force	Low Aβ predicted early dementia
Bäckström et al. (19)*	+	+	+	+		+	PDND 104 C 30 PSP 13 MSA 11	NFL H-FABP	Low Aβ, NFL and H-FABP predicted PDD
Brockmann et al. (20)	+					+	PDND 353 PDD 103	Genetic variants known to be involved in Aβ clearance	Risk variants in *APOE* and cystatin C genes were associated with lower Aβ
Compta et al. (21)	+	+					PDND 20 PDD 20 C 30	MMSE DSM-IV-R MDS Task Force	PDD: ↑ t-tau PDND: ↓ Aβ positively correlated with phonemic fluency
Compta et al. (22)	+	+	+				PDND 19 PDD 29 C 9	MMSE MDS Task Force	PDD: ↓ Aβ ↑ t-tau and p-tau in a subgroup
Compta et al. (23)*	+	+	+				PDND 27	MMSE MDS Task Force	Low Aβ predicted PDD
Compta et al. (24)	+	+		+	+		PDND 21 PDD 20 C 13	MMSE/PDD by MDS Task Force	PDD: ↓ Aβ, ↑ t-tau, ↑ o-α-syn
Ffytche et al. (25)	+						PD 423 3-4 years of follow-up	Compare baseline structural imaging and CSF data in patients who go on to develop illusions or hallucinations in newly diagnosed PD	Patients with early onset PD psychosis: Aβ ↓
Gmitterová et al. (26)	+	+	+			+	PDND 22 PDD 31 DLB 51 C 32	Discriminatory potential of tau, p-tau, Aβ, NSE and S100B across the spectrum of LBD	PDD Aβ ↓, tau ↑ Rapid disease course not associated with decrease of Aβ
Halbgebauer et al. (27)						+	PDND 22 PDD 29 C 36	Modified serpinA1	PDD: acidic serpinA1 isoform ↑
Hall et al. (28)	+	+	+	+		◦	PDND 90 PDD 33 C 107	MMSE MDS Task Force	PDD: ↑ p-tau, Aβ or t-α-syn no differences
Hall et al. (29)*	+	+	+	+		+	PDND 42 C 69		Low Aβ predicted memory decline, high α-syn predicted reduced cognitive speed
Hansson et al. (30)				+	+		PDND 30 C 98	MMSE MDS Task Force	PDD: ↑ o-α-syn
Janssens et al. (31)	+	+	+			+	probable AD 52 FTD 59 DLB 39 PDD 14 C 88 young C 32	3-methoxy-4-hydroxyphenylglycol (MHPG)	Aβ young C > C > FTD > PDD, DLB > AD tau AD > FTD > PDD, DLB > C > young C p-tau AD > FTD = PDD,DLB = C> young C MHPG PDD, DLB > AD > C

(Continued)

TABLE 1 | Continued

Study	CSF biomarker						Participants	Methods	Result
	Aβ1-42	t- tau	p-tau	t-α-syn	o-α-syn	other			
Lindqvist et al. (32)						+	PDND 71 PDD 16 C 33	MMSE	PDD: C-reactive protein ↑ IL6 ↑ TNF-Alpha → Eotaxin→ MCP-1→ MIP-1beta→ IP-10→
Maetzler et al. (33)	+						PDND 14 PDD 12	MMSE	PDD: Aβ ↓
Maetzler et al. (34)	+	+					PDND 21 PDD 10 C 39	MMSE	No difference
Maetzler et al. (35)	+	+					PDND 77 PDD 26 C 72	MMSE MDS Task Force	No difference
Modreanu et al. (36)	+	+	+				PD 37 PDD 21 PDD at 18-months 35	Spatial disorientation, memory complaints over disease course	PDD: Aβ ↓ tau and p-tau no difference 'PDD -converters' had significantly lower Aβ at baseline
Parnetti et al. (37)		+	+				PDND 67 PDD 48 C 41	MMSE	No difference
Parnetti et al. (38)*	+	+	+	+	+		PDND 44 Disease C 25	MMSE MoCa	Low Aβ predicted more rapid decline
Schrag et al. (39)*	+	+					PDND 390 C 178	MoCa over 2 years	Low Aβ/t-tau ratio predicts cognitive decline
Siderowf et al. (40)*	+	+	+				PDND: 45	Dementia rating scale	Low Aβ predicted rapid decline in Dementia rating scale
Stewart et al. (41)*	+	+	+	+			PDND 350	Verbal memory, cognitive processing speed, and visuospatial working memory	Lower α-synuclein predicted better preservation of cognitive function
Terrelonge et al. (42)*	+	+	+	+			PDND 341	Memory, visuospatial, working memory–executive function, and attention processing speed	Low Aβ predicted cognitive impairment
Vranová et al. (43)	+	+					PDND 27 PDD 14 C 14	MMSE MDS Task Force	PDD: ↑ t-tau/ Aβ index Aβ or t-tau no differences
Wennström et al. (44)				+			PDND 38 PDD 22 C 52	MMSE MDS Task Force	No difference

PD, Patients with Parkinson's disease; PD-MCI, Parkinson's disease patients with mild cognitive impairment; PDD, Parkinson's disease patients with dementia; PDND, non-demented PD; MSA, multiple system atrophy; PSP, progressive supranuclear palsy; AD, Patients with Alzheimer's disease; DLB, Dementia with Lewy body; C, Controls; MoCA, Montreal Cognitive Assessment; MMSE, Mini Mental Status Examination; Aβ, Aβ1–42 amyloid; NFL, neurofilament light chain protein; H-FABP, heart fatty acid-binding protein; *longitudinal studies.

in the brainstem are important cholinergic projections in and post-mortem studies have shown that neuronal loss in in the nucleus basalis is an early phenomenon in PD (100, 101). Combining many modalities, Compta et al. (23) performed a longitudinal study in non-demented PD patients including CSF, neuropsychological and MRI studies at baseline and 18 months follow up. Here, a combination of lower CSF Aβ, reduced verbal learning, semantic fluency and visuoperceptual scores, as well

TABLE 2 | Cortical and subcortical structural changes related to cognitive impairment and dementia in Parkinson's disease.

Study	Participants	Methods	Result
Weintraub et al. (64)	PDND 60	VBM*	In PD-MCI hippocampal and temporal gray matter atrophy.
Melzer et al. (65)	PDND 57 PD-MCI 23 PDD 16 C 34	VBM	In PD-MCI gray matter atrophy in temporal, parietal, frontal cortex, amygdala, right putamen, and hippocampus. In PDD additional atrophy in medial temporal lobe, lingual gyrus, posterior cingulate gyrus, and bilateral caudate.
Lee et al. (66)	PD-MCI 51 C 25	VBM*	PD-MCI to PDD converters had lower GM density in the left prefrontal areas, left insular cortex and bilateral caudate nucleus compared with that in PD-MCI non-converters.
Borroni et al. (67)	PDND 11 PDD 10 LBD 13 C 10	VBM	In PDD bilateral frontal and subcortical (caudate nucleus) gray matter atrophy.
Duncan et al. (68)	PDND 125 C 50	VBM DTI	Frontal and parietal gray matter volume reductions were associated with reduced executive function. Increased mean diffusivity was associated with performance on the semantic fluency and Tower of London tasks in frontal and parietal white matter tracts.
Hattori et al. (69)	PDND 32 PD-MCI 28 PDD 25 DLB 29 C 40	VBM TBSS	In PDD more atrophy in the cerebellum, thalami, insula, parietal cortex and occipital cortex.
Kandiah et al. (70)	PDND 97	Hippocampal volume White matter hyperintensities*	Hippocampal volume predicts PD-MCI and PDD.
Rektorova et al. (71)	PDND 75 PD-MCI 29 PDD 22	Spatial Independent Component Analysis	In PDD gray matter volume reductions in the hippocampus and temporal lobes, fronto-parietal regions and increases in the midbrain/cerebellum correlated with visuospatial deficits and letter verbal fluency, respectively.
Biundo et al. (72)	PDND 15 PD-MCI 14 HC 21	Cortical thickness	In PD-MCI cortical thinning in right supramarginal, dorsolateral prefrontal cortex, hippocampus, orbito-frontal, fusiform, superior parietal, and cuneus.
Pereira et al. (73)	PDND 90 PD-MCI 33 H 56	Cortical thickness	In PD-MCI cortical thinning in left precuneus, inferior temporal precentral, superior parietal, and lingual regions.
Hanganu et al. (74)	PDND 15 PD-MCI 17 H 18	Cortical thickness *	In PD-MCI thinning in temporal and medial occipital lobe, nucleus accumbens and amygdala correlate with cognitive decline.
Ibarretxe-Bilbao et al. (75)	PDND 16 C 15	Cortical thickness*	In PD cortical thinning in bilateral fronto-temporal regions and reduced amygdala volume.
Mak et al. (76)	PDND 66 PD-MCI 39 H 37	Cortical thickness*	PD-MCI converters showed bilateral temporal cortex thinning at baseline.
Hwang et al. (77)	PDND 12 PDD 11 C 14	Cortical pattern matching Cortical thickness	PDD showed thinning bilateral sensorimotor, lateral parietal, right posterior cingulate, parieto-occipital, inferior temporal and lateral frontal relative to C and PDND.
Zarei et al. (78)	Early PD 24 moderate PD 18 PDD 15 C 39	Cortical thickness	MMSE correlated positively with cortical thickness in the anterior temporal, dorsolateral prefrontal, posterior cingulate, temporal fusiform and occipitotemporal cortex.
Pagonabarraga et al. (79)	PDND 26 PD-MCI 26 PDD 20 C 18	Cortical thickness	From PDND to PDD a linear and progressive cortical thinning was observed in areas functionally specialized in declarative memory (entorhinal cortex, anterior temporal pole), semantic knowledge (parahippocampus, fusiform gyrus), and visuoperceptive integration (banks of the superior temporal sulcus, lingual gyrus, cuneus and precuneus).
Carlesimo et al. (80)	PDND 25 C 25	DTI	Increased mean diffusivity in the PD hippocampi; high hippocampal mean diffusivity values obtained low memory scores.
Chen et al. (81)	PDND 19 PDD 11 C 21	DTI	In PDD lower fractional anisotropy in the left hippocampus, higher mean diffusivity in widespread white matter regions. In PD positive correlation between MoCA score and fractional anisotropy of left inferior longitudinal and hippocampus, and bilateral superior longitudinal fasciculus.

*PD, Patients with Parkinson's disease; PD-MCI, Parkinson's disease patients with mild cognitive impairment; PDD, Parkinson's disease patients with dementia; PDND, non-demented PD; DLB, Dementia with Lewy body; C, Controls; MoCA, Montreal Cognitive Assessment; MMSE, Mini Mental Status Examination; * **longitudinal studies.***

TABLE 3 | Changes of function and connectivity related to cognitive impairment and dementia in Parkinson's disease.

Study	Participants	Methods	Result
Gorges et al. (82)	PDND 14 PDD 17 C 22	Resting-state fMRI	In PDND hyperconnectivity (network expansions) in cortical, limbic, and basal ganglia-thalamic areas. In PDD decreased intrinsic functional connectivity compared with controls (predominantly between major nodes of the default mode network).
Baggio et al. (83)	PDND 32 PD-MCI 23 C 36	Resting-state fMRI	In PD-MCI reduced connectivity between dorsal attention network and right fronto-insular regions (worse performance in executive functions) and increased connectivity between default mode network and medial and lateral occipito-parietal regions (worse visuo-spatial performance).
Amboni et al. (84)	PDND 21 PD-MCI 21 C 20	Resting-state fMRI	In PD-MCI patients decreased functional connectivity in bilateral prefrontal cortex (fronto-parietal network).
Tessitore et al. (85)	PDNT 16 C 16	Resting-state fMRI	In PDND decreased default mode network connectivity correlated with cognitive parameters.
Rektorova et al. (86)	PDND 18 PDD 14 C 18	Resting-state fMRI	In PDD decreased connectivity in the right inferior frontal gyrus compared to PDND and C (using posterior cingulate cortex/precuneus as seed for analysis).
Borroni et al. (67)	PDND11 PDD 10 LBD 13 C 10	Resting-state fMRI	Reduced local coherence of frontal regions in PD and in PDD.
Olde et al. (87)	PDND 55 C 15	Resting-state fMRI	In PDND longitudinally decreases in functional connectivity most prominent for posterior brain regions correlated with disease progression and cognitive decline.
Seibert et al. (88)	C 19 PDND 19 PDD 18	Resting-state fMRI	In PDD corticostriatal functional correlations were decreased in bilateral prefrontal regions.
Lin et al. (89)	PDND 17 PDD 17 C 17	Arterial spin labeling (ASL) magnetic resonance imaging (ASL-MRI)	In PDND and PDD progressive widespread cortical hypoperfusion.
Le Heron et al. (90)	PDD 20 AD 17 C 37	Arterial spin labeling (ASL) magnetic resonance imaging (ASL-MRI)	In AD and PDD posterior hypoperfusion (including posterior cingulate gyrus, precuneus, occipital regions). Perfusion in medial temporal lobes (AD<PDD) and right frontal cortex (PDD<AD) differed between PDD and AD.
Vander Borght et al. (91)	PDD 9 AD 9 C 9	[18F]fluorodeoxyglucose-PET	In PDD and AD hypometabolism with similar regional accentuation (lateral parietal, lateral temporal and lateral frontal association cortices and posterior cingulate cortex). In contrast to AD PDD showed greater metabolic reduction in the visual cortex and relatively preserved metabolism in the medial temporal cortex.
Gonzalez-Redondo et al. (92)	PDND 14 PD-MCI 17 PDD 15 C 19	[18F]fluorodeoxyglucose-PET	In PD-MCI the hypometabolism exceeded atrophy in the angular gyrus, occipital, orbital and anterior frontal lobes. In PDD these areas were atrophic and surrounded by extensive hypometabolism.
Shinotoh et al. (93)	PDND 14 PDD 2 PSP 12 C 13	Acetylcholinesterase activity using N-methyl-4-[11C]piperidyl acetate PET	In PDD higher reduction of choline acetyltransferase and acetylcholinesterase than in PDND.
Bohnen et al. (94)	PDND 11 PDD 14 AD 12 C 10	Acetylcholinesterase activity using [11C]Methylpiperidin-4-ylpropionate PET	Mean cortical acetylcholinesterase activity was lowest in PDD.
Hiraoka et al. (95)	PDD 12 C 13	[5-(11)C-methoxy]donepezil-PET	In PDD density of acetylcholinesterase in the cerebral cortices correlated with improvements in visuoperceptual function after 3 months of donepezil therapy.
Kotagal et al. (96)	PDND 11 PDD 6 DLB 6 C 14	Acetylcholinesterase activity using [11C]Methylpiperidin-4-ylpropionate PET	Thalamic cholinergic denervation is present in PD, PDD, and DLB but not in AD.

PD, Patients with Parkinson's disease; PD-MCI, Parkinson's disease patients with mild cognitive impairment; PDD, Parkinson's disease patients with dementia; PDND, non-demented PD; DLB, Dementia with Lewy body; AD, Patients with Alzheimer's disease; C, Controls; MoCA, Montreal Cognitive Assessment; MMSE, Mini Mental Status Examination; PET, positron emission tomography.

as cortical thinning in superior-frontal/anterior cingulate and precentral regions were found to be predictive for PDD.

For the assessment of white matter pathology using DTI and imaging of metabolites (Proton magnetic resonance spectroscopy) there is currently not enough longitudinal data available and the value of these techniques to predict cognitive decline has to be further explored. The existing studies indicate that microstructural changes, such as increased mean diffusivity or reduced fractional anisotropy in the hippocampus, the frontal and parietal white matter tracts are associated with cognitive decline in PD (68, 80, 81, 102–104). In particular, an increased mean diffusivity may be predictive for cognitive decline before fractional anisotropy decreases. However, these findings need further validation in longitudinal studies.

FATIGUE

Fatigue is a common symptom that includes both mental and physical aspects. Up to 70% of individuals with PD experience fatigue every day (105). Fatigue dramatically impairs quality of life (106). It is a complex syndrome emerging from dysfunction in the nervous, endocrine and immune system (107). From a clinical point of view fatigue is frequently associated with other non-motor syndromes, like sleepiness, apathy, depression and autonomic dysfunction (105, 108). However, fatigue can also occur as an isolated syndrome; it is therefore important to understand that fatigue and sleepiness or depression is not the same condition (109, 110). Central fatigue is commonly measured through questionnaires, such as the Fatigue Severity Scale (111) which is recommended by the Movement Disorder Society (MDS) task force (112). Central fatigue can be described as a feeling of constant exhaustion and can occur in various chronic disorders. Peripheral fatigue is characterized by failure to sustain the force of muscle contraction and is more readily accessible to quantification (106, 113).

A key mechanism underlying fatigue is the activation of the inflammatory cytokine network (107, 114). Therefore, inflammatory markers serve as potential biomarkers of fatigue. In particular, higher serum levels of IL-6, IL1-Ra, sIL-2R, and VCAM-1 were associated with higher fatigue levels in patients with newly diagnosed, drug-naïve PD (115, 116). This neuroinflammatory processes may promote glutamate dysregulation and further influence neuronal activity and neuroplasticity, and impact neuronal circuits mediating distress and motivation in PD (117–119). Interestingly, higher serum uric acid levels were significantly associated with less fatigue (120).

In addition, dysfunction of the endocrine system, such as hypothalamic-pituitary-adrenal system which is connected to basal ganglia, amygdala, thalamus and frontal cortex, seems to contribute to the pathophysiology of fatigue (113). Although there are no neuropathological studies of PD-fatigue supporting this model so far, several neuroimaging studies showed that multiple brain areas are involved in fatigue in PD. These include frontal, temporal and parietal regions

indicative of emotion, motivation and cognitive functions (121–126). In SPECT imaging with technetium-99 hexamethyl-propylene-amine-oxime PD-fatigue was associated with reduced perfusion in the frontal lobe (125). Others used PET with dopaminergic and serotonergic markers in fatigued vs. non-fatigued PD patients. Less serotonergic marker binding was found in striatal and limbic regions (thalamus, anterior cingulate, amygdala, insula) in PD-fatigue. The striatal ^{18}F-dopa uptake was similar in fatigued and non-fatigued groups, but voxel-based analysis localized the reduced dopamine uptake to the caudate and insula in PD-fatigue (127). In addition the serotonin transporter (SERT) availability was significantly reduced in the striatum and thalamus of fatigued PD patients, suggesting that increasing the brain level of serotonin may improve PD-fatigue (127). The reduced serotonergic transmission suggests that a disturbed neurotransmitter balance within the basal ganglia and associated regions changes the integration of emotional and motor information in limbic regions, thus resulting in fatigue symptoms (128). With regard to striatal dopamine transporter uptake, results are conflicting. Two studies found no difference between fatigued and non-fatigued PD (127, 129). In the study by Chou et al., striatal dopamine transporter uptake was a significant predictor of fatigue in mild but not moderate-to-severe PD. They postulated that the lack of association between fatigue and nigrostriatal loss in advanced PD may reflect a denervation "floor" effect (130). Many of these studies have assessed advanced disease stages and patients on dopaminergic treatment. In contrast, Tessitore et al. studied fatigue in drug-naïve early PD using resting-state functional MRI (fMRI). Fatigue itself, and fatigue severity were associated with a decreased connectivity within the supplementary motor area and an increased connectivity within the default mode network (121). Importantly, these functional abnormalities occur independently from both dopamine-induced connectivity and structural changes. This study is in line with earlier neurophysiological studies suggesting that abnormal premotor and primary motor cortices connectivity correlate with fatigue (131, 132). Tessitore et al. hypothesized that the increased connectivity of the default mode network represents an initial cognitive compensatory response to the fatigue-related motor connectivity changes. In this sense fatigued PD-patients, when internally oriented, have to increase mental expenditure to maintain the same level of motor planning performance in order to switch more easily to externally oriented processing (121).

In summary, abnormalities in motivation of self-initiated tasks and motor function may play a significant role in the pathophysiology of fatigue (133). While non-dopaminergic basal ganglia pathways seem to be involved in PD-fatigue, the dopaminergic dysfunction may only play a role through extrastriatal projections.

DEPRESSION

PD patients are twice as likely to develop depression compared to healthy individuals (134). Depressive symptoms affect 40–50%

of PD patients and significantly impact quality of life in PD (2). In particular, patients with cognitive impairment, longer disease duration, motor fluctuations, female gender, and higher doses of levodopa are at risk to develop depression (9).

Like other NMS, depression seems to be linked to inflammatory signaling. Increased inflammatory responses have been described both in the brain and peripheral blood of PD patients (135). Depression correlated with a high serum level of IL-10 (136) and IL-6 (137). High levels of both sIL-2R and TNF-α in blood samples from PD patients were significantly associated with more severe depression and anxiety (119). As reflection of CNS involvement, high CRP levels in CSF of PD patients were associated with more severe symptoms of depression (32). However, these findings are not specific for PD. Chronic inflammation in physically ill patients is often associated with symptoms of depression and also occurs in normal aging (138–140). Moreover, PD in general is characterized by elevated levels of inflammatory cytokines, such as IL-6, tumor necrosis factor, IL-1β, IL-2, IL-10, C-reactive protein, and RANTES (141).

Depression in PD is associated with several structural and functional changes in the limbic system. In particular, changes in the amygdala, hippocampus and orbitofrontal cortex were frequently reported in PD depression (142–151). The involvement of the serotonergic system was demonstrated in post-mortem tissue and validated *in vivo* by several PET imaging studies (152–155). Compared to controls the serotonin transporter binding in non-depressed PD was lower in the striatal region, the orbitofrontal cortex, and the dorsolateral pre-frontal cortex which is an area known to be involved in major depression (155). Using dopaminergic and serotonergic presynaptic transporter radioligands a prominent role of serotonergic degeneration in limbic regions such as the anterior cingulate cortex was demonstrated (156, 157). Other PET studies observed a higher availability of the serotonin transporter in the raphe nuclei and limbic regions of depressed PD patients (152, 153). Likewise, decreased plasma levels of serotonin were found to be correlated with severity of depression (158). However, studies of the serotonin metabolite 5-hydroxyindoleacetic acid (5-HIAA) in CSF from depressed and non-depressed PD patients, have yielded contradictory results (159), and serotonergic dysfunction alone may only explain vulnerability to depression in PD. Yet, symptoms of depression are also linked to mesolimbic dopaminergic degeneration (160, 161) which is in line with the clinical observation of improvement of depression by dopaminergic treatment (162).

CONCLUSION

From this overview emerges a comprehensive picture of recent fluid and imaging biomarkers which have been studied in a number of clearly defined and sizable cohorts of PD patients with PD. Especially longitudinal studies are necessary to make the biomarkers potentially useful for therapeutic or even clinical trial evaluation. A number of recent studies have provided ample evidence for specific predictive biomarkers across multiple domains combining clinical, biochemical, and neuroimaging information. Yet, at this stage a lack of standardized and comparable methods preclude clinical everyday use of these biomarkers beyond their value as diagnostic or prognostic tools in cohorts of patients. Thus, more research needs to be undertaken into finding reliable combinations of predictors of NMS in PD on an individual level, and standardization and harmonization of protocols in particular in CSF handling and neuroimaging has to be taken further.

AUTHOR CONTRIBUTIONS

TP and JG: conception, collection of data, interpretation of data, drafting the work; OW: revising the work critically for important intellectual content.

ACKNOWLEDGMENTS

We thank Elena Huß for assistance of data collection.

REFERENCES

1. Schapira AHV, Chaudhuri KR, Jenner P. Non-motor features of Parkinson disease. *Nat Rev Neurosci.* (2017) 18:509. doi: 10.1038/nrn.2017.91
2. van Uem JM, Marinus J, Canning C, van Lummel R, Dodel R, Liepelt-Scarfone I, et al. Health-related quality of life in patients with parkinson's disease–a systematic review based on the ICF model. *Neurosci Biobehav Rev.* (2016) 61:26–34. doi: 10.1016/j.neubiorev.2015.11.014
3. Biomarkers Definitions Working Group. Biomarkers and surrogate endpoints: preferred definitions and conceptual framework. *Clin Pharmacol Ther.* (2001) 69:89–95. doi: 10.1067/mcp.2001.113989
4. Fengler S, Liepelt-Scarfone I, Brockmann K, Schäffer E, Berg D, Kalbe E. Cognitive changes in prodromal Parkinson's disease: a review. *Mov Disord.* (2017) 32:1655–66. doi: 10.1002/mds.27135
5. Aarsland D, Brønnick K, Larsen JP, Tysnes OB, Alves G, Norwegian ParkWest Study Group. Cognitive impairment in incident, untreated Parkinson disease: the Norwegian ParkWest study. *Neurology.* (2009) 72:1121–6. doi: 10.1212/01.wnl.0000338632.00552.cb

6. Litvan I, Goldman JG, Tröster AI, Schmand BA, Weintraub D, Petersen RC, et al. Diagnostic criteria for mild cognitive impairment in Parkinson's disease: movement disorder society task force guidelines. *Mov Disord.* (2012) 27:349–56. doi: 10.1002/mds.24893
7. Aarsland D, Andersen K, Larsen JP, Lolk A, Kragh-Sørensen P. Prevalence and characteristics of dementia in Parkinson disease: an 8-year prospective study. *Arch Neurol.* (2003) 60:387–92. doi: 10.1001/archneur.60.3.387
8. Svenningsson P, Westman E, Ballard C, Aarsland D. Cognitive impairment in patients with Parkinson's disease: diagnosis, biomarkers, and treatment. *Lancet Neurol.* (2012) 11:697–707. doi: 10.1016/S1474-4422(12)70152-7
9. Marinus J, Zhu K, Marras C, Aarsland D, van Hilten JJ. Risk factors for non-motor symptoms in Parkinson's disease. *Lancet Neurol.* (2018) 17:559–68. doi: 10.1016/S1474-4422(18)30127-3
10. Anang JB, Gagnon JF, Bertrand JA, Romenets SR, Latreille V, Panisset M, et al. Predictors of dementia in Parkinson disease: a prospective cohort study. *Neurology.* (2014) 83:1253–60. doi: 10.1212/WNL.0000000000000842
11. Zhu K, van Hilten JJ, Marinus J. Predictors of dementia in Parkinson's dise findings from a 5-year prospective study using

the SCOPA-COG. *Parkinsonism Relat Disord.* (2014) 20:980–5. doi: 10.1016/j.parkreldis.2014.06.006

12. Litvan I, Aarsland D, Adler CH, Goldman JG, Kulisevsky J, Mollenhauer B, et al. MDS Task Force on mild cognitive impairment in Parkinson's disease: critical review of PD-MCI. *Mov Disord.* (2011) 26:1814–24. doi: 10.1002/mds.23823

13. Pagano G, De Micco R, Yousaf T, Wilson H, Chandra A, Politis M. REM behavior disorder predicts motor progression and cognitive decline in Parkinson disease. *Neurology.* (2018) 91:e894–e905. doi: 10.1212/WNL.0000000000006134

14. Williams-Gray CH, Foltynie T, Brayne CE, Robbins TW, Barker RA. Evolution of cognitive dysfunction in an incident Parkinson's disease cohort. *Brain.* (2007) 130(Pt 7):1787–98. doi: 10.1093/brain/awm111

15. Kehagia AA, Barker RA, Robbins TW. Cognitive impairment in Parkinson's disease: the dual syndrome hypothesis. *Neurodegener Dis.* (2013) 11:79–92. doi: 10.1159/000341998

16. Braak H, Rüb U, Jansen Steur EN, Del Tredici K, de Vos RA. Cognitive status correlates with neuropathologic stage in Parkinson disease. *Neurology.* (2005) 64:1404–10. doi: 10.1212/01.WNL.0000158422.41380.82

17. Aarsland D, Perry R, Brown A, Larsen JP, Ballard C. Neuropathology of dementia in Parkinson's disease: a prospective, community-based study. *Ann Neurol.* (2005) 58:773–6. doi: 10.1002/ana.20635

18. Alves G, Lange J, Blennow K, Zetterberg H, Andreasson U, Førland MG, et al. CSF Aβ42 predicts early-onset dementia in Parkinson disease. *Neurology.* (2014) 82:1784–90. doi: 10.1212/WNL.0000000000000425

19. Bäckström DC, Eriksson Domellöf M, Linder J, Olsson B, Öhrfelt A, Trupp M, et al. Cerebrospinal fluid patterns and the risk of future dementia in early, incident Parkinson disease. *JAMA Neurol.* (2015) 72:1175–82. doi: 10.1001/jamaneurol.2015.1449

20. Brockmann K, Lerche S, Dilger SS, Stirnkorb JG, Apel A, Hauser AK, et al. SNPs in Aβ clearance proteins: lower CSF Aβ1–42 levels and earlier onset of dementia in PD. *Neurology.* (2017) 89:2335–40. doi: 10.1212/WNL.0000000000004705

21. Compta Y, Martí MJ, Ibarretxe-Bilbao N, Junqué C, Valldeoriola F, Mu-oz E, et al. Cerebrospinal tau, phospho-tau, and beta-amyloid and neuropsychological functions in Parkinson's disease. *Mov Disord.* (2009) 24:2203–10. doi: 10.1002/mds.22594

22. Compta Y, Ezquerra M, Mu-oz E, Tolosa E, Valldeoriola F, Rios J, et al. High cerebrospinal tau levels are associated with the rs57 tau gene variant and low cerebrospinal β-amyloid in Parkinson disease. *Neurosci Lett.* (2011) 487:169–73. doi: 10.1016/j.neulet.2010.10.015

23. Compta Y, Pereira JB, Ríos J, Ibarretxe-Bilbao N, Junqué C, Bargalló N, et al. Combined dementia-risk biomarkers in Parkinson's disease: a prospective longitudinal study. *Parkinsonism Relat Disord.* (2013) 19:717–24. doi: 10.1016/j.parkreldis.2013.03.009

24. Compta Y, Valente T, Saura J, Segura B, Iranzo Á, Serradell M, et al. Correlates of cerebrospinal fluid levels of oligomeric- and total-α-synuclein in premotor, motor and dementia stages of Parkinson's disease. *J Neurol.* (2015) 262:294–306. doi: 10.1007/s00415-014-7560-z

25. Ffytche DH, Pereira JB, Ballard C, Chaudhuri KR, Weintraub D, Aarsland D. Risk factors for early psychosis in PD: insights from the Parkinson's progression markers initiative. *J Neurol Neurosurg Psychiatry.* (2017) 88:325–31. doi: 10.1136/jnnp-2016-314832

26. Gmitterová K, Gawinecka J, Llorens F, Varges D, Valkovič P, Zerr I. Cerebrospinal fluid markers analysis in the differential diagnosis of dementia with Lewy bodies and Parkinson's disease dementia. *Eur Arch Psychiatry Clin Neurosci.* (2018). doi: 10.1007/s00406-018-0928-9

27. Halbgebauer S, Nagl M, Klafki H, Haußmann U, Steinacker P, Oeckl P, et al. Modified serpinA1 as risk marker for Parkinson's disease dementia: analysis of baseline data. *Sci Rep.* (2016) 6:26145. doi: 10.1038/srep26145

28. Hall S, Öhrfelt A, Constantinescu R, Andreasson U, Surova Y, Bostrom F, et al. Accuracy of a panel of 5 cerebrospinal fluid biomarkers in the differential diagnosis of patients with dementia and/or parkinsonian disorders. *Arch Neurol.* (2012) 69:1445–52. doi: 10.1001/archneurol.2012.1654

29. Hall S, Surova Y, Öhrfelt A, Zetterberg H, Lindqvist D, Hansson O. CSF biomarkers and clinical progression of Parkinson disease. *Neurology.* (2015) 84:57–63. doi: 10.1212/WNL.0000000000001098

30. Hansson O, Hall S, Ohrfelt A, Zetterberg H, Blennow K, Minthon L, et al. Levels of cerebrospinal fluid α-synuclein oligomers are increased in Parkinson's disease with dementia and dementia with Lewy bodies compared to Alzheimer's disease. *Alzheimers Res Ther.* (2014) 6:25. doi: 10.1186/alzrt255

31. Janssens J, Vermeiren Y, Fransen E, Aerts T, Van Dam D, Engelborghs S, et al. Cerebrospinal fluid and serum MHPG improve Alzheimer's disease versus dementia with Lewy bodies differential diagnosis. *Alzheimers Dement.* (2018) 10:172–81. doi: 10.1016/j.dadm.2018.01.002

32. Lindqvist D, Hall S, Surova Y, Nielsen HM, Janelidze S, Brundin L, et al. Cerebrospinal fluid inflammatory markers in Parkinson's disease: associations with depression, fatigue, and cognitive impairment. *Brain Behav Immun.* (2013) 33:183–9. doi: 10.1016/j.bbi.2013.07.007

33. Maetzler W, Liepelt I, Reimold M, Reischl G, Solbach C, Becker C, et al. Cortical PIB binding in Lewy body disease is associated with Alzheimer-like characteristics. *Neurobiol Dis.* (2009) 34:107–12. doi: 10.1016/j.nbd.2008.12.008

34. Maetzler W, Stapf AK, Schulte C, Hauser AK, Lerche S, Wurster I, et al. Serum and cerebrospinal fluid uric acid levels in lewy body disorders: associations with disease occurrence and amyloid-β pathway. *J Alzheimers Dis.* (2011) 27:119–26. doi: 10.3233/JAD-2011-110587

35. Maetzler W, Tian Y, Baur SM, Gauger T, Odoj B, Schmid B, et al. Serum and cerebrospinal fluid levels of transthyretin in Lewy body disorders with and without dementia. *PLoS ONE.* (2012) 7:e48042. doi: 10.1371/journal.pone.0048042

36. Modreanu R, Cerquera SC, Martí MJ, Ríos J, Sánchez-Gómez A, Cámara A, et al. Cross-sectional and longitudinal associations of motor fluctuations and non-motor predominance with cerebrospinal τ and Aβ as well as dementia-risk in Parkinson's disease. *J Neurol Sci.* (2017) 373:223–9. doi: 10.1016/j.jns.2016.12.064

37. Parnetti L, Tiraboschi P, Lanari A, Peducci M, Padiglioni C, D'Amore C, et al. Cerebrospinal fluid biomarkers in Parkinson's disease with dementia and dementia with Lewy bodies. *Biol Psychiatry.* (2008) 64:850–5. doi: 10.1016/j.biopsych.2008.02.016

38. Parnetti L, Farotti L, Eusebi P, Chiasserini D, De Carlo C, Giannandrea D, et al. Differential role of CSF alpha-synuclein species, tau, and Aβ42 in Parkinson's Disease. *Front Aging Neurosci.* (2014) 6:53. doi: 10.3389/fnagi.2014.00053

39. Schrag A, Siddiqui UF, Anastasiou Z, Weintraub D, Schott JM. Clinical variables and biomarkers in prediction of cognitive impairment in patients with newly diagnosed Parkinson's disease: a cohort study. *Lancet Neurol.* (2017) 16:66–75. doi: 10.1016/S1474-4422(16)30328-3

40. Siderowf A, Xie SX, Hurtig H, Weintraub D, Duda J, Chen-Plotkin A, et al. CSF amyloid β 1-42 predicts cognitive decline in Parkinson disease. *Neurology.* (2010) 75:1055–61. doi: 10.1212/WNL.0b013e3181f39a78

41. Stewart T, Liu C, Ginghina C, Cain KC, Auinger P, Cholerton B, et al. Parkinson Study Group DATATOP Investigators. Cerebrospinal fluid α-synuclein predicts cognitive decline in Parkinson disease progression in the DATATOP cohort. *Am J Pathol.* (2014) 184:966–75. doi: 10.1016/j.ajpath.2013.12.007

42. Terrelonge M Jr, Marder KS, Weintraub D, Alcalay RN. CSF β-amyloid 1-42 predicts progression to cognitive impairment in newly diagnosed parkinson disease. *J Mol Neurosci.* (2016) 58:88–92. doi: 10.1007/s12031-015-0647-x

43. Vranová HP, Hényková E, Kaiserová M, Menšíková K, Vaštík M, Mareš J, et al. Tau protein, beta-amyloid1–42 and clusterin CSF levels in the differential diagnosis of Parkinsonian syndrome with dementia. *J Neurol Sci.* (2014). 343:120–4. doi: 10.1016/j.jns.2014.05.052

44. Wennström M, Surova Y, Hall S, Nilsson C, Minthon L, Boström F, et al. Low CSF levels of both α-synuclein and the α-synuclein cleaving enzyme neurosin in patients with synucleinopathy. *PLoS ONE.* (2013) 8:e53250. doi: 10.1371/journal.pone.0053250

45. Liu C, Cholerton B, Shi M, Ginghina C, Cain KC, Auinger P, et al. CSF tau and tau/Aβ42 predict cognitive decline in Parkinson's disease. *Parkinson Relat Disord.* (2015). 21:271–6. doi: 10.1016/j.parkreldis.2014.12.027

46. Montine TJ, Shi M, Quinn JF, Peskind ER, Craft S, Ginghina C, et al. CSF Aβ42 and tau in Parkinson's disease with cognitive impairment. *Mov Disord.* (2010) 25:2682–5. doi: 10.1002/mds.23287

47. Palmqvist S, Zetterberg H, Blennow K, Vestberg S, Andreasson U, Brooks DJ, et al. Accuracy of brain amyloid detection in clinical practice using cerebrospinal fluid β-amyloid 42: a cross-validation study against amyloid positron emission tomography. *JAMA Neurol.* (2014) 71:1282–9. doi: 10.1001/jamaneurol.2014.1358

48. Skogseth RE, Bronnick K, Pereira JB, Mollenhauer B, Weintraub D, Fladby T, et al. Associations between cerebrospinal fluid biomarkers and cognition in early untreated Parkinson's disease. *J Parkinsons Dis.* (2015) 5:783–92. doi: 10.3233/JPD-150682

49. Zhou B, Wen M, Yu WF, Zhang CL, Jiao L. The diagnostic and differential diagnosis utility of cerebrospinal fluid α-synuclein levels in Parkinson's disease: a meta-analysis. *Parkinsons Dis.* (2015) 2015:567386 doi: 10.1155/2015/567386

50. Gao L, Tang H, Nie K, Wang L, Zhao J, Gan R, et al. Cerebrospinal fluid alpha-synuclein as a biomarker for Parkinson's disease diagnosis: a systematic review and meta-analysis. *Int J Neurosci.* (2015) 125:645–54. doi: 10.3109/00207454.2014.961454

51. Stav AL, Aarsland D, Johansen KK, Hessen E, Auning E, Fladby T. Amyloid-β and α-synuclein cerebrospinal fluid biomarkers and cognition in early Parkinson's disease. *Parkinsonism Relat Disord.* (2015) 21:758–64. doi: 10.1016/j.parkreldis.2015.04.027

52. Buddhala C, Campbell MC, Perlmutter JS, Kotzbauer PT. Correlation between decreased CSF α-synuclein and Aβ$_{1-42}$ in Parkinson disease*Neurobiol Aging.* (2015) 36:476–84. doi: 10.1016/j.neurobiolaging.2014.07.043

53. Hall S, Surova Y, Öhrfelt A, Swedish BioFINDER Study, Blennow K, Zetterberg H, et al. Longitudinal measurements of cerebrospinal fluid biomarkers in Parkinson's Disease. *Mov Disord.* (2016) 31:898–905. doi: 10.1002/mds.26578

54. Lin CH, Yang SY, Horng HE, Yang CC, Chieh JJ, Chen HH, et al. Plasma α-synuclein predicts cognitive decline in Parkinson's disease. *J Neurol Neurosurg Psychiatry.* (2017) 88:818–24. doi: 10.1136/jnnp-2016-314857

55. Delgado-Alvarado M, Gago B, Navalpotro-Gomez I, Jiménez-Urbieta H, Rodriguez-Oroz MC. Biomarkers for dementia and mild cognitive impairment in Parkinson's disease. *Mov Disord.* (2016) 31:861–81. doi: 10.1002/mds.26662

56. Annanmaki T, Pessala-Driver A, Hokkanen L, Murros K. Uric acid associates with cognition in Parkinson's disease. *Parkinsonism Relat Disord.* (2008) 14:576–8. doi: 10.1016/j.parkreldis.2007.11.001

57. Moccia M, Picillo M, Erro R, Vitale C, Longo K, Amboni M, et al. Is serum uric acid related to non-motor symptoms in de-novo Parkinson's disease patients? *Parkinsonism Relat Disord.* (2014) 20:772–5. doi: 10.1016/j.parkreldis.2014.03.016

58. Moccia M, Picillo M, Erro R, Vitale C, Longo K, Amboni M, et al. Presence and progression of non-motor symptoms in relation to uric acid in *de novo* Parkinson's disease. *Eur J Neurol.* (2015) 22:93–8. doi: 10.1111/ene.12533

59. Pellecchia MT, Santangelo G, Picillo M, Pivonello R, Longo K, Pivonello C, et al. Serum epidermal growth factor predicts cognitive functions in early, drug-naive Parkinson's disease patients. *J Neurol.* (2013) 260:438–44. doi: 10.1007/s00415-012-6648-6

60. Chen-Plotkin AS, Hu WT, Siderowf A, Weintraub D, Goldmann Gross R, Hurtig HI, et al. Plasma epidermal growth factor levels predict cognitive decline in Parkinson disease. *Ann Neurol.* (2011) 69:655–63. doi: 10.1002/ana.22271

61. Pellecchia MT, Santangelo G, Picillo M, Pivonello R, Longo K, Pivonello C, et al. Insulin-like growth factor-1 predicts cognitive functions at 2-year follow-up in early, drug-naïve Parkinson's disease. *Eur J Neurol.* (2014) 21:802–7. doi: 10.1111/ene.12137

62. Fereshtehnejad SM, Zeighami Y, Dagher A, Postuma RB. Clinical criteria for subtyping Parkinson's disease: biomarkers and longitudinal progression. *Brain.* (2017) 140:1959–76. doi: 10.1093/brain/awx118

63. Prell T. Structural and functional brain patterns of non-motor syndromes in Parkinson's Disease. *Front Neurol.* (2018) 9:138. doi: 10.3389/fneur.2018.00138

64. Weintraub D, Dietz N, Duda JE, Wolk DA, Doshi J, Xie SX, et al. Alzheimer's disease pattern of brain atrophy predicts cognitive decline in Parkinson's disease. *Brain.* (2012) 135(Pt 1):170–180. doi: 10.1093/brain/awr277

65. Melzer TR, Watts R, MacAskill MR, Pitcher TL, Livingston L, Keenan RJ, et al. Grey matter atrophy in cognitively impaired Parkinson's disease. *J Neurol Neurosurg Psychiatry.* (2012) 83:188–94. doi: 10.1136/jnnp-2011-300828

66. Lee JE, Cho KH, Song SK, Kim HJ, Lee HS, Sohn YH, et al. Exploratory analysis of neuropsychological and neuroanatomical correlates of progressive mild cognitive impairment in Parkinson's disease. *J Neurol Neurosurg Psychiatry.* (2014) 85:7–16. doi: 10.1136/jnnp-2013-305062

67. Borroni B, Premi E, Formenti A, Turrone R, Alberici A, Cottini E, et al. Structural and functional imaging study in dementia with Lewy bodies and Parkinson's disease dementia. *Parkinsonism Relat Disord.* (2015) 21:1049–55. doi: 10.1016/j.parkreldis.2015.06.013

68. Duncan GW, Firbank MJ, Yarnall AJ, Khoo TK, Brooks DJ, Barker RA, et al. Gray and white matter imaging: a biomarker for cognitive impairment in early Parkinson's disease? *Mov Disord.* (2016) 31:103–10. doi: 10.1002/mds.26312

69. Hattori T, Orimo S, Aoki S, Ito K, Abe O, Amano A, et al. Cognitive status correlates with white matter alteration in Parkinson's disease. *Hum Brain Mapp.* (2012) 33:727–39. doi: 10.1002/hbm.21245

70. Kandiah N, Zainal NH, Narasimhalu K, Chander RJ, Ng A, Mak E, et al. Hippocampal volume and white matter disease in the prediction of dementia in Parkinson's disease. *Parkinsonism Relat Disord.* (2014) 20:1203–8. doi: 10.1016/j.parkreldis.2014.08.024

71. Rektorova I, Biundo R, Marecek R, Weis L, Aarsland D, Antonini A. Grey matter changes in cognitively impaired Parkinson's disease patients. *PLoS ONE.* (2014) 9:e85595. doi: 10.1371/journal.pone.0085595

72. Biundo R, Calabrese M, Weis L, Facchini S, Ricchieri G, Gallo P, et al. Anatomical correlates of cognitive functions in early Parkinson's disease patients. *PLoS ONE.* (2013) 8:e64222. doi: 10.1371/journal.pone.0064222

73. Pereira JB, Svenningsson P, Weintraub D, Brønnick K, Lebedev A, Westman E, et al. Initial cognitive decline is associated with cortical thinning in early Parkinson disease. *Neurology.* (2014) 82:2017–25. doi: 10.1212/WNL.0000000000000483

74. Hanganu A, Bedetti C, Degroot C, Mejia-Constain B, Lafontaine AL, Soland V, et al. Mild cognitive impairment is linked with faster rate of cortical thinning in patients with Parkinson's disease longitudinally. *Brain.* (2014) 137(Pt 4):1120–9. doi: 10.1093/brain/awu036

75. Ibarretxe-Bilbao N, Junque C, Segura B, Baggio HC, Marti MJ, Valldeoriola F, et al. Progression of cortical thinning in early Parkinson's disease. *Mov Disord.* (2012) 27:1746–53. doi: 10.1002/mds.25240

76. Mak E, Su L, Williams GB, Firbank MJ, Lawson RA, Yarnall AJ, et al. Baseline and longitudinal grey matter changes in newly diagnosed Parkinson's disease: ICICLE-PD study. *Brain.* (2015) 138(Pt 10):2974–86. doi: 10.1093/brain/awv211

77. Hwang KS, Beyer MK, Green AE, Chung C, Thompson PM, Janvin C, et al. Mapping cortical atrophy in Parkinson's disease patients with dementia. *J Parkinsons Dis.* (2013) 3:69–76. doi: 10.3233/JPD-120151

78. Zarei M, Ibarretxe-Bilbao N, Compta Y, Hough M, Junque C, Bargallo N, et al. Cortical thinning is associated with disease stages and dementia in Parkinson's disease. *J Neurol Neurosurg Psychiatry.* (2013) 84:875–81. doi: 10.1136/jnnp-2012-304126

79. Pagonabarraga J, Corcuera-Solano I, Vives-Gilabert Y, Llebaria G, García-Sánchez C, Pascual-Sedano B, et al. Pattern of regional cortical thinning associated with cognitive deterioration in Parkinson's disease. *PLoS ONE.* (2013) 8:e54980. doi: 10.1371/journal.pone.0054980

80. Carlesimo GA, Piras F, Assogna F, Pontieri FE, Caltagirone C, Spalletta G. Hippocampal abnormalities and memory deficits in Parkinson disease: a multimodal imaging study. *Neurology.* (2012) 78:1939–45. doi: 10.1212/WNL.0b013e318259e1c5

81. Chen B, Fan GG, Liu H, Wang S. Changes in anatomical and functional connectivity of Parkinson's disease patients according to cognitive status. *Eur J Radiol.* (2015) 84:1318–24. doi: 10.1016/j.ejrad.2015.04.014

82. Gorges M, Müller HP, Lulé D; LANDSCAPE Consortium, Pinkhardt EH, Ludolph AC,et al. To rise and to fall: functional connectivity in cognitively normal and cognitively impaired patients with Parkinson's disease. *Neurobiol Aging.* (2015) 36:1727–35. doi: 10.1016/j.neurobiolaging.2014.12.026

83. Baggio HC, Segura B, Sala-Llonch R, Marti MJ, Valldeoriola F, Compta Y, et al. Cognitive impairment and resting-state network

connectivity in Parkinson's disease. *Hum Brain Mapp.* (2015) 36:199–212. doi: 10.1002/hbm.22622

84. Amboni M, Tessitore A, Esposito F, Santangelo G, Picillo M, Vitale C, et al. Resting-state functional connectivity associated with mild cognitive impairment in Parkinson's disease. *J Neurol.* (2015) 262:425–34. doi: 10.1007/s00415-014-7591-5

85. Tessitore A, Esposito F, Vitale C, Santangelo G, Amboni M, Russo A, et al. Default-mode network connectivity in cognitively unimpaired patients with Parkinson disease. *Neurology.* (2012) 79:2226–32. doi: 10.1212/WNL.0b013e31827689d6

86. Rektorova I, Krajcovicova L, Marecek R, Mikl M. Default mode network and extrastriate visual resting state network in patients with Parkinson's disease dementia. *Neurodegener Dis.* (2012) 10:232–7. doi: 10.1159/000334765

87. Olde Dubbelink KT, Schoonheim MM, Deijen JB, Twisk JW, Barkhof F, Berendse HW. Functional connectivity and cognitive decline over 3 years in Parkinson disease. *Neurology.* (2014) 83:2046–53. doi: 10.1212/WNL.0000000000001020

88. Seibert TM, Murphy EA, Kaestner EJ, Brewer JB. Interregional correlations in Parkinson disease and Parkinson-related dementia with resting functional MR imaging. *Radiology.* (2012) 263:226–34. doi: 10.1148/radiol. 12111280

89. Lin WC, Chen PC, Huang YC, Tsai NW, Chen HL, Wang HC, et al. Dopaminergic therapy modulates cortical perfusion in parkinson disease with and without dementia according to arterial spin labeled perfusion magnetic resonance imaging. *Medicine.* (2016) 95:e2206. doi: 10.1097/MD.0000000000002206

90. Le Heron CJ, Wright SL, Melzer TR, Myall DJ, MacAskill MR, Livingston L, et al. Comparing cerebral perfusion in Alzheimer's disease and Parkinson's disease dementia: an ASL-MRI study. *J Cereb Blood Flow Metab.* (2014) 34:964–70. doi: 10.1038/jcbfm.2014.40

91. Vander Borght T, Minoshima S, Giordani B, Foster NL, Frey KA, Berent S, et al. Cerebral metabolic differences in Parkinson's and Alzheimer's diseases matched for dementia severity. *J Nucl Med.* (1997) 38: 797–802.

92. González-Redondo R, García-García D, Clavero P, Gasca-Salas C, García-Eulate R, Zubieta JL, et al. Grey matter hypometabolism and atrophy in Parkinson's disease with cognitive impairment: a two-step process. *Brain.* (2014) 137(Pt 8):2356–67. doi: 10.1093/brain/awu159

93. Shinotoh H, Namba H, Yamaguchi M, Fukushi K, Nagatsuka S, Iyo M, et al. Positron emission tomographic measurement of acetylcholinesterase activity reveals differential loss of ascending cholinergic systems in Parkinson's disease and progressive supranuclear palsy. *Ann Neurol.* (1999) 46:62–9. doi: 10.1002/1531-8249(199907)46:1<62::AID-ANA10>3.0.CO;2-P

94. Bohnen NI, Kaufer DI, Ivanco LS, Lopresti B, Koeppe RA, Davis JG, et al. Cortical cholinergic function is more severely affected in parkinsonian dementia than in Alzheimer disease: an *in vivo* positron emission tomographic study. *Arch Neurol.* (2003) 60:1745–8. doi: 10.1001/archneur.60.12.1745

95. Hiraoka K, Okamura N, Funaki Y, Hayashi A, Tashiro M, Hisanaga K, et al. Cholinergic deficit and response to donepezil therapy in Parkinson's disease with dementia. *Eur Neurol.* (2012) 68:137–143. doi: 10.1159/000338774

96. Kotagal V, Müller ML, Kaufer DI, Koeppe RA, Bohnen NI. Thalamic cholinergic innervation is spared in Alzheimer disease compared to parkinsonian disorders. *Neurosci Lett.* (2012) 514:169–72. doi: 10.1016/j.neulet.2012.02.083

97. Ramírez-Ruiz B, Martí MJ, Tolosa E, Bartrés-Faz D, Summerfield C, Salgado-Pineda P, et al. Longitudinal evaluation of cerebral morphological changes in Parkinson's disease with and without dementia. *J Neurol.* (2005) 252:1345–52. doi: 10.1007/s00415-005-0864-2

98. Morales DA, Vives-Gilabert Y, Gómez-Ansón B, Bengoetxea E, Larra-aga P, Bielza C, et al. Predicting dementia development in Parkinson's disease using bayesian network classifiers. *Psychiatry Res.* (2013) 213:92–8. doi: 10.1016/j.pscychresns.2012.06.001

99. Schulz J, Pagano G, Fernández Bonfante JA, Wilson H, Politis M. Nucleus basalis of Meynert degeneration precedes and predicts cognitive impairment in Parkinson's disease. *Brain.* (2018) 141:1501–16. doi: 10.1093/brain/awy072

100. Arendt T, Bigl V, Arendt A, Tennstedt A. Loss of neurons in the nucleus basalis of Meynert in Alzheimer's disease, paralysis agitans and Korsakoff's Disease. *Acta Neuropathol.* (1983) 61:101–8. doi: 10.1007/BF006 97388

101. Candy JM, Perry RH, Perry EK, Irving D, Blessed G, Fairbairn AF, et al. Pathological changes in the nucleus of meynert in Alzheimer's and Parkinson's diseases. *J Neurol Sci.* (1983) 59:277–89. doi: 10.1016/0022-510X(83)90045-X

102. Agosta F, Canu E, Stefanova E, Sarro L, Tomić A, Špica V, et al. Mild cognitive impairment in Parkinson's disease is associated with a distributed pattern of brain white matter damage. *Hum Brain Mapp.* (2014) 35:1921–9. doi: 10.1002/hbm.22302

103. Theilmann RJ, Reed JD, Song DD, Huang MX, Lee RR, Litvan I, et al. White-matter changes correlate with cognitive functioning in Parkinson's disease. *Front Neurol.* (2013) 4:37. doi: 10.3389/fneur.2013.00037

104. Zheng Z, Shemmassian S, Wijekoon C, Kim W, Bookheimer SY, Pouratian N. DTI correlates of distinct cognitive impairments in Parkinson's disease. *Hum Brain Mapp.* (2014) 35:1325–33. doi: 10.1002/hbm. 22256

105. Friedman JH, Brown RG, Comella C, Garber CE, Krupp LB, Lou JS, et al. (2007). Working Group on Fatigue in Parkinson's Disease. Fatigue in Parkinson's disease: a review. *Mov Disord.* 22:297–308. doi: 10.1002/mds.21240

106. Friedman JH, Beck JC, Chou KL, Clark G, Fagundes CP, Goetz CG, et al. Fatigue in Parkinson's disease: report from a mutidisciplinary symposium. *NPJ Parkinsons Dis.* (2016) 2:15025. doi: 10.1038/npjparkd.2015.25

107. Klimas NG, Broderick G, Fletcher MA. Biomarkers for chronic fatigue. *Brain Behav Immun.* (2012) 26:1202–10. doi: 10.1016/j.bbi.2012.06.006

108. Chou KL, Gilman S, Bohnen NI. Association between autonomic dysfunction and fatigue in Parkinson disease. *J Neurol Sci.* (2017) 377:190–2. doi: 10.1016/j.jns.2017.04.023

109. Alves G, Wentzel-Larsen T, Larsen JP. Is fatigue an independent and persistent symptom in patients with Parkinson disease? *Neurology.* (2004) 63:1908–11. doi: 10.1212/01.WNL.0000144277.06917.CC

110. van Hilten JJ, Weggeman M, van der Velde EA, Kerkhof GA, van Dijk JG, Roos RA. Sleep, excessive daytime sleepiness and fatigue in Parkinson's disease. *J Neural Transm Park Dis Dement Sect.* (1993) 5:235–44. doi: 10.1007/BF02257678

111. Krupp LB, LaRocca NG, Muir-Nash J, Steinberg AD. The fatigue severity scale. Application to patients with multiple sclerosis and systemic lupus erythematosus. *Arch Neurol.* (1989) 46:1121–3. doi: 10.1001/archneur.1989.00520460115022

112. Kluger BM, Herlofson K, Chou KL, Lou JS, Goetz CG, Lang AE, et al. Parkinson's disease-related fatigue: A case definition and recommendations for clinical research. *Mov Disord.* (2016) 31:625–31. doi: 10.1002/mds.26511

113. Chaudhuri A, Behan PO. Fatigue in neurological disorders. *Lancet.* (2004) 363:978–88. doi: 10.1016/S0140-6736(04)15794-2

114. Bower JE. Cancer-related fatigue: links with inflammation in cancer patients and survivors. *Brain Behav Immun.* (2007) 21:863–71. doi: 10.1016/j.bbi.2007.03.013

115. Herlofson K, Heijnen CJ, Lange J, Alves G, Tysnes OB, Friedman JH, et al. Inflammation and fatigue in early, untreated Parkinson's disease. *Acta Neurol Scand.* (2018) 138:394–9. doi: 10.1111/ane.12977

116. Pereira JR, Santos LVD, Santos RMS, Campos ALF, Pimenta AL, de Oliveira MS, et al. IL-6 serum levels are elevated in Parkinson's disease patients with fatigue compared to patients without fatigue. *J Neurol Sci.* (2016) 370:153–6. doi: 10.1016/j.jns.2016.09.030

117. Eyre H, Baune BT. Neuroplastic changes in depression: a role for the immune system. *Psychoneuroendocrinology.* (2012) 37:1397–416. doi: 10.1016/j.psyneuen.2012.03.019

118. Miller AH, Haroon E, Raison CL, Felger JC. Cytokine targets in the brain: impact on neurotransmitters and neurocircuits. *Depress Anxiety.* (2013) 30:297–306. doi: 10.1002/da.22084

119. Lindqvist D, Kaufman E, Brundin L, Hall S, Surova Y, Hansson O. Non-motor symptoms in patients with Parkinson's disease - correlations with inflammatory cytokines in serum. *PLoS ONE.* (2012) 7:e47387. doi: 10.1371/journal.pone.0047387

120. Huang X, Ng SY, Chia NS, Acharyya S, Setiawan F, Lu ZH, et al. Serum uric acid level and its association with motor subtypes and non-motor symptoms in early Parkinson's disease: PALS study. *Parkinsonism Relat Disord.* (2018) 55:50–54. doi: 10.1016/j.parkreldis.2018.05.010

121. Tessitore A, Giordano A, De Micco R, Caiazzo G, Russo A, Cirillo M, et al. Functional connectivity underpinnings of fatigue in "Drug-Naïve" patients with Parkinson's disease. *Mov Disord.* (2016) 31:1497–505. doi: 10.1002/mds.26650

122. Zhang JJ, Ding J, Li JY, Wang M, Yuan YS, Zhang L, et al. Abnormal resting-state neural activity and connectivity of fatigue in Parkinson's disease. *CNS Neurosci Ther.* (2017) 23:241–7. doi: 10.1111/cns.12666

123. Li J, Yuan Y, Wang M, Zhang J, Zhang L, Jiang S, et al. Alterations in regional homogeneity of resting-state brain activity in fatigue of Parkinson's disease. *J Neural Transm.* (2017) 124:1187–95. doi: 10.1007/s00702-017-1748-1

124. Cho SS, Aminian K, Li C, Lang AE, Houle S, Strafella AP. Fatigue in Parkinson's disease: The contribution of cerebral metabolic changes. *Hum Brain Mapp.* (2017) 38:283–92. doi: 10.1002/hbm.23360

125. Abe K, Takanashi M, Yanagihara T. Fatigue in patients with Parkinson's disease. *Behav Neurol.* (2000) 12:103–6. doi: 10.1155/2000/580683

126. Zhang L, Li T, Yuan Y, Tong Q, Jiang S, Wang M, et al. Brain metabolic correlates of fatigue in Parkinson's disease: a PET study. *Int J Neurosci.* (2018) 128:330–6. doi: 10.1080/00207454.2017.1381093

127. Pavese N, Metta V, Bose SK, Chaudhuri KR, Brooks DJ. Fatigue in Parkinson's disease is linked to striatal and limbic serotonergic dysfunction. *Brain.* (2010) 133:3434–43. doi: 10.1093/brain/awq268

128. Politis M, Loane C. Serotonergic dysfunction in Parkinson's disease and its relevance to disability. *Scientific World Journal.* (2011) 11:1726–34. doi: 10.1100/2011/172893

129. Schifitto G, Friedman JH, Oakes D, Shulman L, Comella CL, Marek K, et al. Investigators. Fatigue in levodopa-naive subjects with Parkinson disease. *Neurology.* (2008) 71:481–5. doi: 10.1212/01.wnl.0000324862.29733.69

130. Chou KL, Kotagal V, Bohnen NI. Neuroimaging and clinical predictors of fatigue in Parkinson disease. *Parkinsonism Relat Disord.* (2016) 23:45–9. doi: 10.1016/j.parkreldis.2015.11.029

131. Lou JS, Benice T, Kearns G, Sexton G, Nutt J. Levodopa normalizes exercise related cortico-motoneuron excitability abnormalities in Parkinson's disease. *Clin Neurophysiol.* (2003) 114:930–7. doi: 10.1016/S1388-2457(03)00040-3

132. Berardelli A, Rothwell JC, Thompson PD, Hallett M. Pathophysiology of bradykinesia in Parkinson's disease. *Brain.* (2001) 124(Pt 11):2131–46. doi: 10.1093/brain/124.11.2131

133. Fabbrini G, Latorre A, Suppa A, Bloise M, Frontoni M, Berardelli A. Fatigue in Parkinson's disease: motor or non-motor symptom? *Parkinsonism Relat Disord.* (2013) 19:148–52. doi: 10.1016/j.parkreldis.2012.10.009

134. Becker C, Brobert GP, Johansson S, Jick SS, Meier CR. Risk of incident depression in patients with Parkinson disease in the UK. *Eur J Neurol.* (2011) 18:448–53. doi: 10.1111/j.1468-1331.2010.03176.x

135. Pessoa Rocha N, Reis HJ, Vanden Berghe P, Cirillo C. Depression and cognitive impairment in Parkinson's disease: a role for inflammation and immunomodulation? *Neuroimmunomodulation.* (2014) 21:88–94. doi: 10.1159/000356531

136. Karpenko MN, Vasilishina AA, Gromova EA, Muruzheva ZM, Bernadotte A. Interleukin-1β, interleukin-1 receptor antagonist, interleukin-6, interleukin-10, and tumor necrosis factor-α levels in CSF and serum in relation to the clinical diversity of Parkinson's disease. *Cell Immunol.* (2018) 327:77–82. doi: 10.1016/j.cellimm.2018.02.011

137. Veselý B, Dufek M, Thon V, Brozman M, Királová S, Halászová T, et al. Interleukin 6 and complement serum level study in Parkinson's disease. *J Neural Transm.* (2018). 125:875–81. doi: 10.1007/s00702-018-1857-5

138. Bruunsgaard H, Pedersen M, Pedersen BK. Aging and proinflammatory cytokines. *Curr Opin Hematol.* (2001) 8:131–6. doi: 10.1097/00062752-200105000-00001

139. Chen WW, Zhang X, Huang WJ. Role of neuroinflammation in neurodegenerative diseases (Review). *Mol Med Rep.* (2016) 13:3391–6. doi: 10.3892/mmr.2016.4948

140. Brites D, Fernandes A. Neuroinflammation and depression: microglia activation, extracellular microvesicles and microRNA dysregulation. *Front Cell Neurosci.* (2015) 9:476. doi: 10.3389/fncel.2015.00476

141. Qin XY, Zhang SP, Cao C, Loh YP, Cheng Y. Aberrations in peripheral inflammatory cytokine levels in Parkinson disease: a systematic review and meta-analysis. *JAMA Neurol.* (2016) 73:1316–24. doi: 10.1001/jamaneurol.2016.2742

142. Matsui H, Nishinaka K, Oda M, Niikawa H, Komatsu K, Kubori T, et al. Depression in Parkinson's disease. Diffusion tensor imaging study. *J Neurol.* (2007) 254:1170–3. doi: 10.1007/s00415-006-0236-6

143. Feldmann A, Illes Z, Kosztolanyi P, Illes E, Mike A, Kover F, et al. Morphometric changes of gray matter in Parkinson's disease with depression: a voxel-based morphometry study. *Mov Disord.* (2008) 23:42–6. doi: 10.1002/mds.21765

144. Kostić VS, Agosta F, Petrović I, Galantucci S, Spica V, Jecmenica-Lukic M, et al. Regional patterns of brain tissue loss associated with depression in Parkinson disease. *Neurology.* (2010) 75:857–63. doi: 10.1212/WNL.0b013e3181f11c1d

145. Surdhar I, Gee M, Bouchard T, Coupland N, Malykhin N, Camicioli R. Intact limbic-prefrontal connections and reduced amygdala volumes in Parkinson's disease with mild depressive symptoms. *Parkinsonism Relat Disord.* (2012) 18:809–13. doi: 10.1016/j.parkreldis.2012.03.008

146. van Mierlo TJ, Chung C, Foncke EM, Berendse HW, van den Heuvel OA. Depressive symptoms in Parkinson's disease are related to decreased hippocampus and amygdala volume. *Mov Disord.* (2015) 30:245–52. doi: 10.1002/mds.26112

147. Huang C, Ravdin LD, Nirenberg MJ, Piboolnurak P, Severt L, Maniscalco JS, et al. Neuroimaging markers of motor and nonmotor features of Parkinson's disease: an 18f fluorodeoxyglucose positron emission computed tomography study. *Dement Geriatr Cogn Disord.* (2013) 35:183–96. doi: 10.1159/000345987

148. O'Callaghan C, Shine JM, Lewis SJ, Hornberger M. Neuropsychiatric symptoms in Parkinson's disease: fronto-striatal atrophy contributions. *Parkinsonism Relat Disord.* (2014) 20:867–72. doi: 10.1016/j.parkreldis.2014.04.027

149. Huang P, Lou Y, Xuan M, Gu Q, Guan X, Xu X, et al. Cortical abnormalities in Parkinson's disease patients and relationship to depression: A surface-based morphometry study. *Psychiatry Res Neuroimag.* (2016) 250:24–8. doi: 10.1016/j.pscychresns.2016.03.002

150. Cardoso EF, Maia FM, Fregni F, Myczkowski ML, Melo LM, Sato JR, et al. Depression in Parkinson's disease: convergence from voxel-based morphometry and functional magnetic resonance imaging in the limbic thalamus. *Neuroimage.* (2009) 47:467–72. doi: 10.1016/j.neuroimage.2009.04.059

151. Lou Y, Huang P, Li D, Cen Z, Wang B, Gao J, et al. Altered brain network centrality in depressed Parkinson's disease patients. *Mov Disord.* (2015) 30:1777–84. doi: 10.1002/mds.26321

152. Boileau I, Warsh JJ, Guttman M, Saint-Cyr JA, McCluskey T, Rusjan P, et al. Elevated serotonin transporter binding in depressed patients with Parkinson's disease: a preliminary PET study with [11C]DASB. *Mov Disord.* (2008) 23:1776–80. doi: 10.1002/mds.22212

153. Politis M, Wu K, Loane C, Turkheimer FE, Molloy S, Brooks DJ, et al. Depressive symptoms in PD correlate with higher 5-HTT binding in raphe and limbic structures. *Neurology.* (2010) 75:1920–7. doi: 10.1212/WNL.0b013e3181feb2ab

154. Ballanger B, Klinger H, Eche J, Lerond J, Vallet AE, Le Bars D, et al. Role of serotonergic 1A receptor dysfunction in depression associated with Parkinson's disease. *Mov Disord.* (2012) 27:84–9. doi: 10.1002/mds.23895

155. Guttman M, Boileau I, Warsh J, Saint-Cyr JA, Ginovart N, McCluskey T, et al. Brain serotonin transporter binding in non-depressed patients with Parkinson's disease. *Eur J Neurol.* (2007) 14:523–8. doi: 10.1111/j.1468-1331.2007.01727.x

156. Maillet A, Krack P, Lhommée E, Météreau E, Klinger H, Favre E, et al. The prominent role of serotonergic degeneration in apathy, anxiety and depression in de novo Parkinson's disease. *Brain.* (2016) 139(Pt 9):2486–502. doi: 10.1093/brain/aww162

157. Skidmore FM, Yang M, Baxter L, von Deneen K, Collingwood J, He G, et al. Apathy, depression, and motor symptoms have distinct and separable resting activity patterns in idiopathic Parkinson disease. *Neuroimage.* (2013) 81:484–95. doi: 10.1016/j.neuroimage.2011.07.012

158. Tong Q, Zhang L, Yuan Y, Jiang S, Zhang R, Xu Q, et al. Reduced plasma serotonin and 5-hydroxyindoleacetic acid levels in Parkinson's disease are associated with nonmotor symptoms. *Parkinsonism Relat Disord*. (2015) 21:882–7. doi: 10.1016/j.parkreldis.2015.05.016

159. Svenningsson P, Pålhagen S, Mathé AA. Neuropeptide Y and calcitonin gene-related peptide in cerebrospinal fluid in parkinson's disease with comorbid depression versus patients with major depressive disorder. *Front Psychiatry*. (2017) 8:102. doi: 10.3389/fpsyt.2017.00102

160. Thobois S, Ardouin C, Lhommée E, Klinger H, Lagrange C, Xie J, et al. Non-motor dopamine withdrawal syndrome after surgery for Parkinson's disease: predictors and underlying mesolimbic denervation. *Brain*. (2010) 133(Pt 4):1111–27. doi: 10.1093/brain/awq032

161. Koerts J, Leenders KL, Koning M, Portman AT, van Beilen M. Striatal dopaminergic activity (FDOPA-PET) associated with cognitive items of a depression scale (MADRS) in Parkinson's disease. *Eur J Neurosci*. (2007) 25:3132–6. doi: 10.1111/j.1460-9568.2007.05580.x

162. Barone P, Poewe W, Albrecht S, Debieuvre C, Massey D, Rascol O, et al. Pramipexole for the treatment of depressive symptoms in patients with Parkinson's disease: a randomised, double-blind, placebo-controlled trial. *Lancet Neurol*. (2010) 9:573–80. doi: 10.1016/S1474-4422(10)70106-X

20

Potential of Sodium MRI as a Biomarker for Neurodegeneration and Neuroinflammation in Multiple Sclerosis

Konstantin Huhn[1]*, Tobias Engelhorn[2], Ralf A. Linker[3] and Armin M. Nagel[4,5]

[1] Department of Neurology, Friedrich-Alexander-University of Erlangen-Nuremberg, Erlangen, Germany, [2] Department of Neuroradiology, Friedrich-Alexander-University of Erlangen-Nuremberg, Erlangen, Germany, [3] Department of Neurology, University of Regensburg, Regensburg, Germany, [4] Department of Radiology, Friedrich-Alexander-University of Erlangen-Nuremberg, Erlangen, Germany, [5] Division of Medical Physics in Radiology, German Cancer Research Center (DKFZ), Heidelberg, Germany

*Correspondence:
Konstantin Huhn
konstantin.huhn@uk-erlangen.de

In multiple sclerosis (MS), experimental and *ex vivo* studies indicate that pathologic intra- and extracellular sodium accumulation may play a pivotal role in inflammatory as well as neurodegenerative processes. Yet, *in vivo* assessment of sodium in the microenvironment is hard to achieve. Here, sodium magnetic resonance imaging (^{23}NaMRI) with its non-invasive properties offers a unique opportunity to further elucidate the effects of sodium disequilibrium in MS pathology *in vivo* in addition to regular proton based MRI. However, unfavorable physical properties and low *in vivo* concentrations of sodium ions resulting in low signal-to-noise-ratio (SNR) as well as low spatial resolution resulting in partial volume effects limited the application of ^{23}NaMRI. With the recent advent of high-field MRI scanners and more sophisticated sodium MRI acquisition techniques enabling better resolution and higher SNR, ^{23}NaMRI revived. These studies revealed pathologic total sodium concentrations in MS brains now even allowing for the (partial) differentiation of intra- and extracellular sodium accumulation. Within this review we (1) demonstrate the physical basis and imaging techniques of ^{23}NaMRI and (2) analyze the present and future clinical application of ^{23}NaMRI focusing on the field of MS thus highlighting its potential as biomarker for neuroinflammation and -degeneration.

Keywords: multiple sclerosis, magnetic resonance imaging, sodium MRI, ^{23}Na MRI, neurodegeneration, biomarker

SODIUM AND THE PATHOPHYSIOLOGY OF MULTIPLE SCLEROSIS (MS)

As a widely accepted paradigm, the pathology of MS is hallmarked by inflammatory demyelination but also neuro-axonal damage. In fact, neurodegeneration occurs already at the early stages of the disease constituting a primary contributor to sustained or progressive disability in the longer disease course (1, 2). On a cellular level, the maintenance of a transmembrane ion gradient resulting in a negatively charged intracellular and positively charged extracellular space is crucial to enable vital electrochemical signal transduction in humans. This process strongly depends on sodium: the ion gradient is largely created and maintained by the energy consuming Na^+/K^+-ATPase, leading to cellular efflux of 3 Na^+ ions and influx of 2 K^+ ions. Independent of its origin, loss of ATPase function leads to breakdown of the resting transmembrane potential difference, intracellular sodium accumulation, deficiency of the ATP generating mitochondrial respiratory chain and finally to expiring signal transduction and cell death as well as increase of the extracellular volume fraction (3, 4).

In MS, chronically demyelinated axons are prone to degeneration and trophic failure as consequence of an increased energy demand. Maladaptive repair and neuro-axonal rearrangements as well as a decreased ATP supply may further contribute to this process. Finally, lack of energy may lead to breakdown of the Na^+/K^+-ATPase as a major energy consumer in the CNS (5). In fact, chronically demyelinated MS lesions display a substantially reduced axonal Na^+/K^+-ATPase expression (6).

Additionally, the pivotal role of pathologic sodium accumulation in MS was previously demonstrated in several *ex vivo* and *in vivo* studies (7). These studies point to a compensatory redistribution or over-expression of distinct voltage-gated Na^+ channels (e. g. Nav1.2, Nav1.6) on demyelinated axons in order to compensate for demyelination. This is an energy demanding process that is hardly sustained in already energy deprived axons. Thus, energy failure and toxic sodium accumulation may initiate a vicious cycle. Consecutively, increased intracellular sodium concentrations may provoke reverse action of the Na^+/Ca^{2+} exchanger and thus calcium accumulation, which leads to activation of neurodegenerative signaling cascades (8–11). Hence, application of therapeutic Na^+ channel blockers like amiloride, lamotrigine, phenytoin, or carbamazepine display some neuroprotective properties in experimental MS models (12–16). However, clinical trials with

---

Abbreviations: ADEM, acute disseminated encephalomyelitis; AnaWeTV, anatomically weighted second-order total variation; ATP, adenosine triphosphate; ATPase, adenosine triphosphatase; Ca^{2+}, calcium; CAG, trinucleotide of cytosine, adenine, guanine; cho, choline; ^{35}Cl, chlorine; CNS, central nervous system; CSF, cerebrospinal fluid; CVF, cell volume fraction; DA-3DPR, density-adapted 3D projection reconstruction; DTI, diffusion tensor imaging; EAE, experimental autoimmune encephalomyelitis; EDSS, expanded disability status scale; ESC, extracellular sodium concentration; ^{19}F, fluorine; FLAIR, fluid-attenuated inversion recovery; Glx, glutamate/glutamine; GM, gray matter; H^+, Proton hydrogen; H-EPSI, proton echo planar spectroscopic imaging; IR, inversion recovery; ISC, intracellular sodium concentration; ISVF, intracellular sodium volume fraction; ^{39}K, potassium; K^+, potassium; l, liter; m-Ins, myo-inositol; mM, millimolar; mm, millimeter; MQF, multiple quantum filtering; MRI, magnetic resonance imaging; MRS, magnetic resonance spectroscopy; MS, multiple sclerosis; ms, millisecond; MSFC, multiple sclerosis functional composite; MTR, magnetization transfer ratio; MWI, myelin water imaging; n, number; ^{23}Na, sodium; Na^+, sodium; NAA, N-acetyl aspartate; NaCl, sodium chloride, salt; NAGM, normal-appearing gray matter; Nav, voltage gated sodium channel; NAWM, normal-appearing white matter; NMO-SD, neuromyelitis optica spectrum diseases; ^{17}O, oxygen; OCT, optical coherence tomography; ^{31}P, phosphorous; PET, positron emission tomography; PPMS, primary progressive multiple sclerosis; r, correlation coefficient; RF, radiofrequency; ROI, region of interest; RRMS, relapsing remitting multiple sclerosis; SDWA, sampling density weighted apodization; SNR, signal-to-noise ratio; SPMS, secondary progressive multiple sclerosis; SQF, single quantum filtering; T, Tesla; T1, T1-weighted MRI sequence; T2, T2-weighted MRI sequence; tCr, total creatine; Th, T-helper cell; TSC, tissue sodium concentration; TPI, twisted projection imaging; TQF, triple quantum filtering; UTE, ultra-short echo time; WM, white matter.

Na^+ channel blockers in MS are few and report conflicting results on potential neuroprotective properties, yet (17–19).

In addition, the so-called fat- and salt- (NaCl) rich "western-diet" has recently been implicated in the etiology of MS (20, 21). In this context, sodium reappeared in the center of (experimental) MS studies as a mediator of pro-inflammatory effects (21, 22). In cell culture, an excess of NaCl up to 40 mM led to enhanced pro-inflammatory Th17 cell differentiation. In experimental autoimmune encephalomyelitis (EAE), an animal model for MS, a high salt diet was associated with increased disease severity mediated by enhanced levels of pro-inflammatory Th17 cells (23). However, transfer from experimental to clinical studies has been difficult and results of clinical studies on the influence of sodium to MS are conflicting: In a first study, high salt intake was partly associated with disease activity (24). Yet, a retrospective analysis of a large interferon-beta treated cohort with clinically isolated syndrome (BENEFIT study) showed no relevant association of further disease activity with blood or urine sodium levels (25). Similarly, a study investigating MS with early onset failed to demonstrate an association of relapse activity and the amount of dietary salt intake (26). However, the retrospective nature of sodium exposure analysis and the lack of standardized sodium load quantification limit the definite validity of these studies.

In consequence of these conflicting study results and with the advance of sodium magnetic resonance imaging ($^{23}NaMRI$) techniques, sodium MRI drew growing interest for the analysis of pathologic sodium accumulation and its consequences in MS. However, the history of sodium MRI application in the field of MS is short, only comprising about a decade to date. In addition to regular proton based MRI, $^{23}NaMRI$ with its ability to measure brain sodium *in vivo* along with additional advantages of modern imaging techniques may constitute a promising biomarker for the influence of sodium on neurodegeneration and -inflammation in MS and vice versa. In our review, we aim at (1) demonstrating the physical basis and imaging techniques of sodium MRI and at (2) analyzing previous and future clinical applications of sodium MRI in the field of MS.

PHYSICAL BASICS AND IMAGING TECHNIQUES OF SODIUM MRI

Conventional MRI is based on the signal of protons (hydrogen, H^+). Protons exhibit the best properties for *in vivo* MRI due to their large gyromagnetic ratio and their high abundance in human tissues, predominantly contained in water or fat (27, 28). Besides protons, MR imaging of other so called "X-nuclei" is feasible in principle if they inhere a non-zero nuclear magnetic spin moment, which requires an odd number of protons or neutrons (29). Almost all elements of the periodic table have at least one isotope that fulfills this requirement (30). However, the most limiting issue for X-nuclei MRI is the signal-to-noise ratio (SNR), which is proportional to the *in vivo* concentration, the physical MR sensitivity of the nucleus and the voxel volume. For most isotopes either the physical MR sensitivity or the *in vivo* concentration is too low to achieve sufficient SNR and reasonable voxel volumes. Thus, only a few X-nuclei, such as oxygen (^{17}O) (31), fluorine (^{19}F) (32), phosphorous (^{31}P) (33), chlorine (^{35}Cl) (34), potassium (^{39}K) (35, 36) and especially sodium (^{23}Na) (37–39) have been used for MR imaging so far.

Among these, Na$^+$ exhibits the best properties for *in vivo* MRI (40, 41).

Yet, ^{23}NaMRI is challenged by low tissue sodium concentrations and an approximately 4-fold lower gyromagnetic ratio of sodium as compared to protons. For brain white matter, these shortcomings result in a roughly 5.500 times lower *in vivo* SNR of ^{23}NaMRI vs. ^{1}HMRI, if the similar acquisition times and voxel sizes would be used (41). Furthermore, Na$^+$ highly interacts with surrounding macromolecules resulting in short biexponential T2 times (fast: 0.5–8 ms; slow: 15–40 ms; T1 time: 30–40 ms) (4, 42–45). To achieve sufficient SNR, only images with low spatial resolution can be acquired, which results in partial volume effects. In addition, longer acquisition times can be used to increase SNR. These effects limit the application of ^{23}NaMRI. Additionally, distinction of different sodium compartments, i.e., intra-/extracellular, is difficult (29, 46–48).

Hence, dedicated acquisition techniques and elaborated postprocessing may help to improve ^{23}NaMRI imaging technologies. Above all, application of ultra-short echo-time (UTE) sequences is the common basis of quantitative sodium MRI (29, 49).

Additionally, ^{23}NaMRI requires dedicated hardware, such as an appropriate radiofrequency (RF) amplifier and RF coils. Yet, both hardware components are not standard on routine clinical MRI scanners (50). Optimized scanner hardware may further improve the detection of the weak ^{23}NaMRI signal. In detail, special dual-tuned ^{23}Na/^{1}H head array coils with up to 32 multichannel receive arrays enable a synchronized registration of proton and sodium images with sufficient SNR (51–53).

As reviewed elsewhere, specialized ^{23}NaMRI acquisition techniques, image reconstruction and post-processing techniques further improve SNR and spatial resolution. At the same time they reduce partial volume effects as well as acquisition time. Such techniques comprise compressed sensing with iterative reconstruction, sampling density weighted apodization (SDWA), twisted projection imaging (TPI), density-adapted 3D projection reconstruction (DA-3DPR), multi-echo radial sequences or different trajectories, i.e., 3D cones (29, 54–62).

In principle, sodium MR imaging is feasible at any magnetic field strength. However, due to the physical properties of Na$^+$, application of at least 3 Tesla (T) field strength is warranted for a sufficient SNR and resolution. Modern 7 or 9.4 T ultra-high field MRI scanners further reduce the limitation of low signal strength, resulting in higher SNR (**Figure 1**) or improved spatial resolution (63). Nowadays, modern techniques enable sodium MRI of human brain at nominal spatial resolutions of $1 \times 1 \times 5$ mm^3 to $4 \times 4 \times 4$ mm^3 within 10–35 min acquisition time (48, 57, 64–67). Along with the development and advantages of high-field MRI scanners, research in the field of ^{23}NaMRI has been prospering within the last decade without signs of any harm to study participants (51, 66, 68, 69). Comparing ^{23}NaMRI signal intensities of brain tissue regions of interest (ROI) to control

tubes containing predefined liquid saline solutions (i.e., 0–150 mM) placed beside the patient's head enables quantification of sodium concentrations (66).

MRI total tissue sodium concentrations (TSC) are the volume-weighted average of respective intracellular (normal: 10–15 mmol/l) and extracellular (normal: 140–150 mmol/l) sodium compartments. Typical intracellular volume fractions are on the order of 80% and extracellular volume fractions are around 20% (70). This leads to a TSC of ∼40 mmol/l, which is close to results of studies directly analyzing the sodium concentration in brain white matter (3, 4, 47, 48, 71).

While classic ^{23}NaMRI sequences only allow for quantification of TSC, differentiation between sodium accumulation in extracellular and intracellular compartments is even more interesting. Yet, the single resonance spectrum of sodium ions limits such discrimination. Use of paramagnetic shift reagents, which cannot pass cell membranes like anionic complexes of dysprosium or thulium, principally enables discrimination of intra- and extracellular sodium. Thus, MRI may detect shift of resonance lines exclusively in the extracellular space. However, clinical application of these compounds is not readily feasible for CNS studies due to their inability to cross the blood brain barrier and possible toxic effects (29, 72–74).

Instead, the application of relaxation-weighted imaging may be better suited for human studies. Preclinical studies showed that intracellular sodium exhibits shorter relaxation times (75). Thus, inversion recovery imaging (IR) can be utilized to suppress signals originating from sodium with a distinct T1 relaxation time. This may enable a weighting of the signal toward the intracellular compartment (29). At the same time, suppression of the CSF sodium signal also reduces disturbing partial volume effects when analyzing brain regions close to the CSF (71, 76–78). Sodium MRI IR sequences with a specific suppression of Na$^+$ signals are comparable to the established fluid-attenuated-inversion-recovery (FLAIR) sequence of proton based MRI.

Sodium MRI IR sequences may be also the basis for the calculation of (pseudo) intracellular sodium concentrations and extracellular volume fractions (79). If additional anatomical masks from proton MRI are used, these techniques may even discriminate between intracellular sodium of white and gray matter (4). However, IR techniques only enable indirect calculation of compartmental sodium concentrations and are susceptible for confounders. In detail, the required intra- and extracellular relaxation times need to be estimated from preclinical studies and cannot be measured directly in humans, which might introduce a potential bias. In addition, relaxation times in pathologic structures are unknown and altered relaxation times may affect quantification. In consequence, some authors prefer the terms "pseudo-"intracellular sodium and "pseudo-"extracellular sodium for such analyses (79).

Alternatively, the use of two or more excitation pulses along with multiple quantum filtering (MQF; usually triple quantum filters = TQF) may also facilitate sodium compartment differentiation (80–82). In principle, the T2 relaxation based MQF allows for separation of different signals from sodium ions due to their variably restricted mobility within different compartments (81–86). However, MQF are

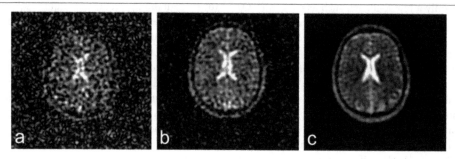

FIGURE 1 | ^{23}NaMRI at 1.5 **(A)**, 3 **(B)**, and 7 T **(C)**. Similar acquisition parameters and a nominal spatial resolution of (4 mm)^3 were applied. SNR increases approximately linearly with magnetic field strengths. Figure reproduced from (63) with permission of John Wiley and Sons, Journal of Magnetic Resonance Imaging.

prone to artifacts caused by field-inhomogeneity, low SNR or long acquisition times and its indirect calculation of sodium concentrations, similar to IR techniques (87). Recent quantitative multicompartment-multipulse techniques aim at exploiting differences in T1 and T2 relaxation times of different sodium compartments. This approach may enable separation of intracellular, extracellular and cerebrospinal fluid (CSF) signals, but is still hampered by low SNR (67).

SODIUM MRI IN NEUROLOGICAL DISORDERS OTHER THAN MS

First *in vivo* investigations using sodium MRI already stem from the 1980's: in an experimental model and in human investigations of stroke, Hilal and colleagues detected temporal changes of sodium levels over time. These studies already indicated the potential of sodium MRI as a biomarker for brain disorders (37, 46). However, technical restrictions limited brain sodium imaging to the investigation of widespread cerebral lesions or CSF (see above).

Yet, with the rapid development in scanner hardware and MRI software, several consecutive sodium MRI studies for stroke were conducted confirming highly elevated TSC in acute stroke due to estimated Na$^+$/K$^+$ ATPase breakdown, consecutive sodium accumulation, hypoxic cell death and perifocal edema (88). Furthermore, sodium MRI may represent a biomarker of viable, but hypoxic tissue-at-risk ("penumbra") in stroke (88–90).

In primary brain tumors like low- and high-grade glioma, exaggerated proliferation rates lead to cellular membrane depolarization preceding cell division. Here, ^{23}NaMRI may additionally be useful as a predictive biomarker for the discrimination of therapy responsive tissue (45, 77, 91–95).

Sodium MRI analysis of neurodegenerative diseases revealed whole-brain TSC increase in Huntington's disease independently of structural changes depicted by proton MRI. The caudate nucleus exhibited the highest TSC which correlated with gray matter atrophy and CAG repeat length (96). In addition, a small study in Alzheimer's disease ($n = 5$) reported a 7.5% brain TSC increase with an inverse correlation to hippocampal volume (97). Similarly, 9.4T sodium MRI of subjects with structural brain damage revealed loss of "cell volume fraction" (CVF) indicating

a reduced CNS cell density. In contrast, individuals with a constant CVF may represent aging patients without disease. Hence, sodium MRI may evolve as a predictive biomarker for neurodegenerative diseases which are often hallmarked by early regional neuronal loss before the onset of clinical symptoms (98).

SODIUM MRI IN MULTIPLE SCLEROSIS (MS)

Sodium MRI Alterations in Cerebral Lesions, NAWM, and NAGM in MS

In 2010, Inglese and colleagues published the first study applying ^{23}NaMRI in 17 relapsing-remitting MS (RRMS) patients and 13 healthy controls, using a 3D radial gradient-echo UTE sequence at 3T (64). In MS, lesional (**Figure 2**) and gray-matter (GM) TSC was increased as compared to normal appearing white matter (NAWM). Further studies confirmed these findings (65, 99–101). As compared to healthy controls, the NAWM of MS patients exhibited an elevated TSC (mean 19.4 vs. 26.9 mM). This increase was particularly predominant in the cerebellum and splenium, yet without statistical significance. The normal-appearing gray matter (NAGM) displayed even higher sodium levels, but without any regional predominance (64). In this study, MS lesion analysis was restricted to plaques with a diameter >5 mm due to potential partial volume effects. The mean lesion sodium concentration was 35.3 mM, clearly higher than TSC of NAWM.

Gadolinium-enhancing acute MS lesions showed the highest TSC. This finding may be the direct consequence of inflammatory processes in the cell (e.g., mitochondrial failure, ATP deprivation, sodium accumulation) and the extracellular space (e.g., tissue damage, edema, enlarged extracellular space, infiltrating immune cells). However, analyses only comprised a low number of acute MS lesions and did not discriminate between intra- and extracellular sodium compartments. Therefore, it was not possible to determine the exact source of lesional sodium accumulation.

A study of Eisele et al. further analyzed neuroinflammatory aspects and studied the evolution of lesional sodium accumulation by ^{23}Na MRI with a 3D radial sequence and SDWA at 3T. The authors analyzed acute and chronic lesions

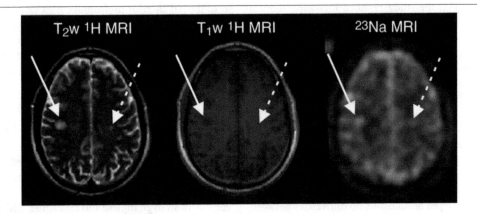

FIGURE 2 | MR images in a 33-years-old man with early RRMS. Examples of substantial sodium accumulation in two macroscopic T2 lesions with two different signal intensity patterns at T1-weighted imaging: one lesion was hypointense (solid arrows) and one was isointense (dashed arrows) to normal-appearing white matter on T1-weighted image. Figure reproduced from (99) with permission of the Radiological Society of North America (RSNA).

in 65 relapsing MS patients as compared to 10 controls (102). Mean TSC was quantified in all MS lesions with a diameter of >5 mm and in the NAWM as well as GM. First, TSC in NAWM and GM were higher in MS patients than in controls. Second, all types of MS lesions displayed a TSC increase. The most pronounced accumulation was seen in contrast-enhancing T1 lesions > T1 hypointense lesions > T1 isointense lesions. Interestingly, non-enhancing, hyperacute lesions with restricted diffusion on proton based diffusion-weighted MRI sequences showed a TSC comparable to the NAWM. Thus, TSC may not only serve as a biomarker for chronic tissue pathology and neurodegeneration, but also allow the detection and monitoring of inflammatory processes. Thus, this study further supported the use of TSC measured by sodium MRI as a potential biomarker for neuroinflammation. ^{23}Na MRI may enable visualization of blood-brain barrier disruption without need for application of contrast-enhancing agents.

Another study used ^{23}NaMRI in a case report on a large open-ring enhancing MS lesion. The authors reported intralesional sodium heterogeneity with declining TSC from the center of the active plaque (TSC: 50 mmol/l) across the enhanced periphery (33 mmol/l) toward the NAWM (26 mmol/l) (103). This gradual and centripetal TSC increase may result from the underlying degree of inflammation and mitochondrial dysfunction within acute MS lesions. Therefore, ^{23}NaMRI may constitute a future biomarker for the extent of neuroinflammation. It may even point to inflammatory "tissue at risk" before persistent neuro-axonal damage occurs.

Our group additionally studied ^{23}NaMRI in a case with an acute, enhancing tumefactive MS lesion over a follow-up of 5 weeks. Sodium accumulation outlasted contrast enhancement after steroid treatment as a potential sign of prolonged metabolic dysfunction and delayed recovery. At the same time, TSC in NAWM remained unaffected by steroid therapy (104).

However, comprehensive longitudinal studies reporting temporal evolution of sodium accumulation in acute MS lesions are still lacking. Upon repeated sodium MRI investigations in five healthy controls, WM and GM areas revealed a coefficient of

variation for TSC < 5% and an intra-class correlation coefficient of > 0.9. These data indicate sufficient reproducibility of ^{23}NaMRI as a basis for future longitudinal studies (64).

Zaaroui and colleagues used a DA-3DPR sequence for sodium MRI at 3T to analyze 26 RRMS patients. They compared patients with a disease duration <5 vs. >5 years to healthy controls (99). The authors investigated TSC in three different compartments: GM, NAWM, and T2 lesions. In T2 lesions of all MS patients, TSC was higher than in WM of controls. In contrast, only the RRMS cohort with advanced disease duration exhibited a significantly increased TSC of GM and NAWM. Both MS groups displayed a similar TSC in T2 lesions and NAWM. Yet, GM TSC was higher in the advanced duration RRMS cohort. Nevertheless, this study was able to detect brain sodium accumulation even at the early stages of RRMS. When analyzing for anatomic distribution of TSC, the same study found widespread brain regions with elevated TSC in both MS cohorts. In advanced RRMS, TSC increase was scattered in the splenial, thalamic, cingular, parietal, frontal, and prefrontal cortices. A recent 7T study further complemented these findings of a widespread distribution of increased TSC in various MS GM and WM regions (101).

Sodium MRI and MS Disease Course
Paling and colleagues conducted an investigation of 70 MS patients comprising three MS clinical subtypes (27 RRMS, 23 SPMS, 20 PPMS patients, and 27 controls). They applied a ramp sampled radial UTE sequence at 3 T with additional partial volume correction (65).

The authors analyzed TSC in cortical and deep GM, NAWM and in MS lesions, differentiated in T1 hypo- or isointense lesions. Independent of the disease course, MS patients exhibited an increased TSC of GM and NAWM as compared to controls. Additionally, deep GM and NAWM TSC were higher in the progressive MS subtypes. SPMS patients showed pronounced TSC in GM and NAWM as compared to RRMS. Further testing between MS subgroups was not significant. However, TSC of T1 hypointense lesions was higher in progressive MS subtypes than in RRMS. In conclusion, the study revealed increased sodium accumulation within MS lesions, NAWM and GM in all clinical MS courses. TSC accumulation was pronounced in SPMS and in patients with increased disability. This finding may serve as a hint for neuro-axonal damage, thus emphasizing the potential of ^{23}NaMRI to provide a biomarker for neurodegeneration.

An investigation of Maarouf and colleagues included 20 progressive MS patients (11 PPMS, 9 SPMS) and 15 controls. The authors applied a DA-3DPR sequence at 3 T analyzing TSC of GM, NAWM and T2 lesions (100). They also found that TSC of T2 lesions and GM were significantly elevated in progressive forms as compared to controls. However, NAWM TSC was not significantly elevated in both progressive forms vs. controls. Independent of the analyzed brain tissue, no differences between PPMS and SPMS were detected. In this study, TSC accumulated to a higher degree in distinct brain areas of SPMS patients than in PPMS: Above all, it involved primary or supplementary locomotor areas consistent with the pronounced disability of patients with a median expanded disability status scale (EDSS) score of 5.5.

Interestingly, early sodium MRI studies and a study performed at 9.4 T did not find relevant age-dependent changes in TSC (64, 65, 98–100). However, a 7 T study described a positive correlation of age with WM and GM TSC as well as with GM intracellular sodium accumulation in healthy controls. In contrast, a negative association of age with intracellular sodium concentration (ISC) but not with extracellular sodium concentration (ESC) or TSC was detected in MS patients. The same study also showed correlations between disease duration, WM TSC and ISC for both, GM and WM as well as between extracellular sodium accumulation in GM and EDSS (101).

Sodium MRI and MS Disability

In the first ever conducted MS sodium MRI study, Inglese and colleagues reported a low correlation of EDSS as a measure of disability with the mean TSC in T1-hypointense lesions ($r = 0.22$) as well as in NAWM and GM ($r = 0.20$). However, they did not find an association between disease duration, age or gender and TSC in lesions, GM or NAWM of RRMS patients (64).

Zaaroui et al. described no correlation of the TSC in T2 lesions or NAWM of RRMS patients with disability as measured by EDSS. However, GM TSC was significantly associated with EDSS as a potential biomarker for the degree of MS disability. In particular, the EDSS showed a positive correlation with the local TSC of the right primary motor area, middle frontal, and bilateral superior gyrus as well as the bilateral cerebellum (99).

In a study including progressive forms of MS, disability was correlated with TSC in deep GM and T1 isointense lesions. In addition, the authors showed independent associations of deep GM TSC with EDSS and features of the clinical assessment tool "Multiple Sclerosis Functional Composite" (MSFC). These data further support sodium MRI as a new method for monitoring disability and neurodegeneration (65).

In contrast, Maarouf et al. reported no significant correlation between TSC in T2 lesions or GM and EDSS or MSFC in their progressive MS study. Solely, the authors found an association between local TSC of the left premotor cortex and EDSS as well

as of the left anterior prefrontal cortex and MSFC (100). Further brain regions of the limbic and the frontal areas displayed an increased TSC only in SPMS. Thus, the authors concluded that in PPMS, sodium accumulation was restricted to the motor system. In SPMS, it was more widespread involving regions related to higher cognitive functions.

Sodium MRI and Correlation With Markers of Neurodegeneration

To date, brain atrophy is the "goldstandard" MRI marker. Yet, sodium MRI may provide additional information for imaging clinically relevant neurodegeneration (28, 105). Indeed, in the early 2010 study of Inglese and colleagues, RRMS patients already displayed a significantly lower normalized brain volume and GM volume. They also showed a trend toward lower WM volume as compared to controls.

TSC negatively associated with regional GM volume. However, there was no correlation of TSC with whole brain volume. TSC of NAWM did not correlate with any brain volume. In the respective control cohort, TSC in WM and GM showed an inverse correlation with normalized brain volume. Furthermore, TSC in RRMS associated with total T1 and T2 lesion volume (64).

An additional 3 T study showed an association of TSC in NAWM and GM with T2 lesion load. However, this study did not analyze brain atrophy (99). Application of 7 T ultra-highfield MRI showed no correlation of global and regional TSC, neither of intracellular or extracellular sodium concentrations to measures of brain volumes. In contrast, there was a trend for correlation of extracellular sodium accumulation and GM volume (101).

In 2017, Maarouf and colleagues investigated if brain TSC and GM atrophy were associated with cognitive dysfunction. They analyzed 58 RRMS patients in the early course and 31 controls using DA-3DPR at 3 T (106). The TSC increase in GM and NAWM was associated with cognitive dysfunction and predominantly located in neocortical regions. GM TSC even outmatched GM atrophy as a better predictor of cognitive dysfunction in MS patients. These data further emphasize the potential of sodium MRI for depiction of neurodegeneration, probably even at earlier stages than the "goldstandard" MRI brain atrophy. Hence, sodium MRI may show early neuronal dysfunction even before final neuronal damage occurs. Only the latter can be demonstrated by proton based MRI techniques (106).

To gain complementary information on microstructural pathologies, a recent analysis of 21 RRMS patients and 20 controls applied a DA-3DPR sodium MRI sequence at 3 T in combination with a proton based MR spectroscopy (proton echo planar spectroscopic imaging, 3D ^{1}H-EPSI). Spectroscopy studies included N-acetyl aspartate (NAA; marker for mitochondrial activity), glutamate/glutamine (Glx; marker for neuro-astrocytic metabolism), total creatine (tCr; marker for cellularity), choline (Cho; marker for inflammatory demyelination) and myo-inositol (m-Ins; marker for glial activation) (107). TSC was elevated in all types of brain tissue in MS patients. MR spectroscopy revealed decreased Cho and

Glx in GM, an increase of m-Ins but a decrease of NAA and Glx in NAWM and an increase in m-Ins but decrease in NAA in T2 lesions. In sum, TSC was negatively correlated with NAA as a marker for mitochondrial dysfunction and consecutive neuro-axonal damage. These data are consistent with findings from experimental studies pointing to mitochondrial damage as a consequence of toxic sodium accumulation (3, 108, 109). However, these studies did not correct for the influence of different sodium compartments.

Sodium MRI and Differentiation of Intra- vs. Extracellular Sodium

In the early MS sodium MRI studies, the distinction of different sodium compartments was not possible, mainly due to limited MRI techniques. However, such a differentiation was regarded as highly relevant for a better understanding of MS pathogenesis. Yet, it remained unclear if elevated TSC was the result of rising extracellular fluid sodium due to edema, neuro-axonal damage or demyelination on the one hand, or the result of intracellular sodium accumulation due to inflammatory toxicity on the other (64, 65, 99).

The first study enabling differentiation of cellular compartments in 19 RRMS patients and 17 controls applied a combined single (SQ) and triple quantum filtered (TQF) 3D gradient echo ^{23}NaMRI sequence at 7 T ultra-high field (101). The applied TQF technique used the different relaxation properties and signals of intracellular and extracellular distributed sodium ions. It thus enabled measurement of TSC, but also differentiation of the intracellular sodium concentration (ISC) and the intracellular sodium volume fraction (ISVF). ISVF is an indirect, inversely correlated measure of the extracellular sodium concentration (ESC): ISVF reduction is assumed to be a marker for a diminished intracellular volume and, accordingly, an increase of the extracellular space and ESC. As a limitation discussed by the authors, the applied model is based on the assumption, that the pathology itself does not change the ^{23}Na relaxation times and that the TQF sequence enables a precise and unbiased sodium compartment differentiation. However, the quantitative accuracy of ISC measurements in MS patients is still undefined, since there is no non-invasive "goldstandard" that the ISC measurement can be compared to *in vivo*.

In accordance with previous 3 T studies, TSC of GM and MS lesions was higher than in WM and higher in MS than in healthy controls. ISC did not differ between the respective GM and WM but was higher in MS patients than in controls in GM and WM. In contrast, ISVF was lower in MS patients than in controls and higher in WM than in GM of both groups. In conclusion, TSC accumulation was in part depending on the growth of the extracellular compartment as potential consequence of axonal loss in MS. Nevertheless, it also depended on a distinct intracellular sodium increase. These results support findings of *ex vivo* and experimental studies suggesting a concomitant toxic metabolic dysfunction due to sodium imbalance (101).

Another study aimed at elucidating (1) differences in sodium levels between acute (= contrast enhancing) and chronic MS lesions and (2) differences between intracellular (ISC) and total

sodium concentrations. Besides a regular DA-3DPR sequence, the authors also employed a fluid-attenuated sodium signal at 7 T in 29 MS patients (78). The applied fluid-attenuated sequence with a relaxation-weighted sodium signal preferentially depicts sodium ions with short relaxation times as found intracellularly. Thus, the setting enables a weighting toward the intracellular sodium compartment similar to previous approaches (4, 76, 77, 110). The study demonstrated that TSC and ISC were higher in acute as compared to chronic MS lesions. Hence, the fluid-attenuated sequence was useful to differentiate both types of lesions. TSC was positively correlated with T1 and T2 proton based lesion signals. In contrast, ISC only correlated with acute contrast enhancing T1 lesions. Interestingly, TSC and ISC levels were not associated. These data further support the additional biological significance of intracellular sodium accumulation measured by ^{23}NaMRI. Thus, ISC increase may occur independently of extracellular sodium increase due to inflammatory edema or cell loss. This observation renders ISC a useful biomarker of metabolic neuroinflammatory processes.

In addition, this study contributed rare longitudinal sodium MRI data. Three patients were analyzed before and after steroid treatment indicating decrease of both sodium signals after treatment. Besides intracellular sodium accumulation, a distinct inflammatory hyper-cellularity may lead to elevated ISC in acute lesions. A combination of proton (lesion detection) and sodium (lesion differentiation) MRI may yield a neurodegenerative and neuroinflammatory biomarker and potentially an alternative to contrast agent application in the future (78).

Additionally, in the above mentioned case report of an acute enhancing MS lesion with open ring sign, also ISC was analyzed. ISC was reduced in the center of the acute lesion as compared to the periphery and NAWM. The low central ISC may be explained by enhanced cellular necrosis as compared to a more viable periphery. Thus, sodium MRI may constitute a useful biomarker for the degree of acute neuroinflammatory damage in MS (103).

Sodium MRI and Further Fields of Applications in MS

Since low SNR and low spatial resolution is a major issue in sodium MRI, the incorporation of proton based anatomical MRI data in the reconstruction process enables improved image quality (111). A recent study described the application of an anatomically weighted second-order total variation (AnaWeTV) interative construction constraint in a MS patient including anatomical weighted MRI. AnaWeTV resulted in improved sodium MRI quality and less confounding partial volume effects, particularly in tissues or lesions that are visible in sodium and proton base MRI (60).

Another study was particularly engaged in the detection of potential errors of sodium MRI. Here, partial volume effects and spatially correlated noise artifacts impede quantification of sodium in small MS lesions (112). Besides a sodium-phantom analysis with given sodium concentration, sodium MRI signal variation in small lesions of five MS patients was compared to a computed predictive value using twisted projection imaging. Both, theoretical and *in vivo* sodium measurement pointed to a variation error of 20% in large, and even of 40–50% in small lesions as defined by the investigators. These data suggest underestimation of Na^+ signals especially in small lesions and emphasize the limitations of sodium MRI despite improved imaging techniques.

Regular proton based MRI often requires gadolinium containing contrast agents. At the same time, several previous studies detected distinct MRI signal alterations of the dentate nucleus as a potential consequence of multiple gadolinium applications. Consequently, a recent study aimed at investigation of the dentate nucleus by sodium MRI at 3 T (113): in 12 MS patients and 6 controls, there was no difference in TSC between both groups despite a signal-altered dentate nucleus. These results suggest sustained tissue integrity of dentate nuclei with gadolinium deposition.

Finally, a recent study was able to exclude relevant influences of a preceding gadolinium application to the subsequent sodium MRI measurement. Despite a distinct quantitative influence of gadolinium on sodium relaxation times, this study further emphasized the compatibility and potential of combined proton and sodium MRI (114).

CONCLUSIONS AND PERSPECTIVES

Within the last decade, there was increasing evidence for the value of sodium accumulation measured by $^{23}NaMRI$ as a biomarker for neurodegeneration and -inflammation in MS. Studies point to a widespread increase of TSC in MS as compared to healthy populations with a pronounced increase in the GM and in MS lesions as well as in progressive disease courses. Furthermore, sodium accumulation partly correlated with disability (as measured by EDSS) and brain atrophy as the proton based MRI "goldstandard" for monitoring neurodegeneration in MS. Moreover, the TSC increase occurs even in "unaffected" NAWM as defined by standard proton based MRI. Thus, TSC as measured by sodium MRI is discussed as an early biomarker of neurodegenerative changes in MS brains.

The value of $^{23}NaMRI$ as a potential tool for monitoring of neuroinflammation has mainly been restricted to lesional TSC measurements. These studies consistently showed highest TSC in acute contrast-enhancing lesions as compared to NAWM. To date, the investigation of intra- vs. extracellular sodium accumulation in inflammatory lesions is limited to case reports or studies including very few MS patients.

Moreover, the analysis of acute MS lesions still necessitates a large lesion size of roughly >5 mm to minimize partial volume effects. Furthermore, large longitudinal studies to examine the temporal evolution of the sodium content in MS lesions and the correlation to conventional markers of inflammation are still lacking. Meanwhile, novel imaging techniques allowing for discrimination of tissue compartments are in part capable to delineate increased extracellular sodium. These studies analyze the expanded extracellular space as consequence of neuro-axonal damage or inflammatory edema caused by increased intracellular sodium due to intraneuronal/-axonal sodium accumulation with its consecutive toxic intracellular signal cascades (4, 67, 78,

101). Preceding findings indicate that ISC in MS are elevated in different brain regions as compared to healthy controls. However, TSC accumulation in MS was shown to depend on both, ESC and ISC increase. These findings suggest an expanded extracellular compartment i.e., due to axonal loss in MS on the one hand, but also on a distinct intracellular accumulation on the other. However, the precise differentiation of intra- vs. extracellular sodium via $^{23}NaMRI$ is still limited. In particular, a mutual influence of intra- and extracellular spaces on each other cannot be definitely excluded. Progress in the development of respective imaging techniques will enable a more detailed insight in the diverse origin and effects of intra- vs. extracellular sodium accumulation.

Despite all progress, sodium MRI still has to overcome several limitations: initial studies displayed huge range of TSC quantification of more than 40 mM, mainly due to different scanner hardware, acquisition protocols or quantification models. Novel sodium imaging techniques improved the quantification range to roughly 10 mM but still may vary significantly (39). Thus, comparability of results from different study groups is complicated. Using the intraventricular CSF sodium signal as an intra-individual reference signal for quantification of sodium concentrations was recently discussed to specify sodium measurement. This approach is based in the observation that sodium levels in the CSF may be stable at the levels of extracellular fluid i.e., 140 mM (66, 115).

Yet, as a consequence of the physical properties of Na^+, application of ultra-high field ≥ 7 T scanners and/or long acquisition times is warranted for "state-of-the-art" sodium MRI. This is of particular relevance when aiming at the precise differentiation of sodium compartments.

In consequence, further development of sodium MRI techniques and hardware is crucial (1) to improve SNR and resolution, (2) to diminish partial volume effects and scanning times, and (3) to enable precise differentiation of sodium compartments.

The future technical improvement together with the demonstrated high potential of brain sodium as a biomarker in neurological disorders may pave the way for the implementation of sodium MRI in clinical routine. The implementation of this ambitious goal may be further supported by affordable sodium MRI head coils and software packages enabling widespread sodium measurement at commercial MRI systems (39).

Since $^{23}NaMRI$ requires no contrast agents, similar contraindications as for conventional proton MRI apply. Even at ultra-high field strengths, MRI is well-tolerated, thus further supporting an extended application of $^{23}NaMR$ investigations (29, 68, 116). However, none of the published studies so far comprised an MS collective with $n > 100$ thus in part limiting their significance. In consequence, multi-center studies with strictly defined MS patient cohorts and sodium MRI methods are warranted to improve the validity of future studies.

Furthermore, improved sodium MRI techniques may enable the future investigation of smaller regions of interest i.e., inflammatory brain lesions with a diameter <5 mm or spinal cord sodium concentrations. Analyzing the spinal cord would add useful information about disability-relevant MS pathology beyond previous *ex vivo* or proton based MRI analyses (117).

As another attractive location for sodium MRI, studies of hypertension, renal and rheumatological diseases displayed elevated sodium deposition in the skin and muscle (118–120). Together with experimental findings of proinflammatory properties of elevated sodium levels in the skin, analysis of dermal and muscular soft tissue sodium could also be interesting in the field of MS. Here, the inflammatory pathogenesis may likely be initiated in the periphery before immune cells enter the CNS (23). Hence, sodium MRI may help to elucidate sodium dependent effects of the yet scarcely characterized origin of inflammatory processes in the periphery of MS patients.

Finally, sodium MRI has not been applied in other acute or chronic inflammatory diseases of the CNS, such as acute disseminated encephalomyelitis (ADEM), vasculitis, granulomatous diseases, or aquaporine-4-antibody associated neuromyelitis optica spectrum diseases (NMO-SD). Here, the technique may add further valuable insights beyond conventional proton MRI which often cannot sufficiently differentiate between these entities (28). In addition, the effects of underlying disease-modifying therapies on MRI brain sodium levels have not been analyzed yet and remain to be demonstrated. Such studies warrant longitudinal investigations of MS patients under immunomodulatory treatment.

Combination of sodium MRI with additional imaging tools beyond standard proton MRI may gain novel information about pathological metabolic processes associated with sodium accumulation. Here, additional MRI techniques [i.e., myelin water imaging (MWI), magnetization transfer ratio (MTR), diffusion tensor imaging (DTI), magnetic resonance spectroscopy (MRS), optical coherence tomography (OCT) or metabolic imaging techniques, such as positron emission tomography (PET)] would be promising candidates (48).

In conclusion, modern sodium MRI has in part overcome its inherent physical limitations, but still is in need for further development. With its capability to give yet unknown insights in the pathology of MS, this imaging technique deserves further investigation aiming at implementation of sodium accumulation as a biomarker for neurodegeneration and -inflammation in the future.

AUTHOR CONTRIBUTIONS

KH drafted the work, contributed to the conception and interpretation of the work, and acquired the included data and references. TE contributed to the conception and interpretation of the work and revised it critically for important intellectual content. RL contributed to drafting the work, contributed to the conception and interpretation of the work, and revised it critically for important intellectual content. AN contributed to drafting the work, acquired the included data and references, contributed to the conception and interpretation of the work, and revised it critically for important intellectual content. All authors provide approval for publication of the content.

FUNDING

We acknowledge support by Deutsche Forschungsgemeinschaft and Friedrich-Alexander-Universität Erlangen-Nürnberg (FAU) within the funding programme Open Access Publishing for the publication fee.

REFERENCES

1. Trapp BD, Stys PK. Virtual hypoxia and chronic necrosis of demyelinated axons in multiple sclerosis. *Lancet Neurol.* (2009) 8:280–91. doi: 10.1016/S1474-4422(09)70043-2
2. Haider L, Zrzavy T, Hametner S, Hoftberger R, Bagnato F, Grabner G, et al. The topograpy of demyelination and neurodegeneration in the multiple sclerosis brain. *Brain* (2016) 139(Pt 3):807–15. doi: 10.1093/brain/awv398
3. Murphy E, Eisner DA. Regulation of intracellular and mitochondrial sodium in health and disease. *Circ Res.* (2009) 104:292–303. doi: 10.1161/CIRCRESAHA.108.189050
4. Madelin G, Kline R, Walvick R, Regatte RR. A method for estimating intracellular sodium concentration and extracellular volume fraction in brain *in vivo* using sodium magnetic resonance imaging. *Sci Rep.* (2014) 4:4763. doi: 10.1038/srep04763
5. Paling D, Golay X, Wheeler-Kingshott C, Kapoor R, Miller D. Energy failure in multiple sclerosis and its investigation using MR techniques. *J Neurol.* (2011) 258:2113–27. doi: 10.1007/s00415-011-6117-7
6. Young EA, Fowler CD, Kidd GJ, Chang A, Rudick R, Fisher E, et al. Imaging correlates of decreased axonal Na$^+$/K$^+$ ATPase in chronic multiple sclerosis lesions. *Ann Neurol.* (2008) 63:428–35. doi: 10.1002/ana.21381
7. Smith KJ. Sodium channels and multiple sclerosis: roles in symptom production, damage and therapy. *Brain Pathol.* (2007) 17:230–42. doi: 10.1111/j.1750-3639.2007.00066.x

8. Moll C, Mourre C, Lazdunski M, Ulrich J. Increase of sodium channels in demyelinated lesions of multiple sclerosis. *Brain Res.* (1991) 556:311–6.
9. Black JA, Dib-Hajj S, Baker D, Newcombe J, Cuzner ML, Waxman SG. Sensory neuron-specific sodium channel SNS is abnormally expressed in the brains of mice with experimental allergic encephalomyelitis and humans with multiple sclerosis. *Proc Natl Acad Sci USA.* (2000) 97:11598–602. doi: 10.1073/pnas.97.21.11598.
10. Craner MJ, Newcombe J, Black JA, Hartle C, Cuzner ML, Waxman SG. Molecular changes in neurons in multiple sclerosis: altered axonal expression of Nav1.2 and Nav1.6 sodium channels and Na$^+$/Ca^{2+} exchanger. *Proc Natl Acad Sci USA.* (2004) 101:8168–73. doi: 10.1073/pnas.0402765101
11. Waxman SG. Mechanisms of disease: sodium channels and neuroprotection in multiple sclerosis-current status. *Nat Clin Pract Neurol.* (2008) 4:159–69. doi: 10.1038/ncpneuro0735
12. Stys PK, Ransom BR, Waxman SG. Tertiary and quaternary local anesthetics protect CNS white matter from anoxic injury at concentrations that do not block excitability. *J Neurophysiol.* (1992) 67:236–40. doi: 10.1152/jn.1992.67.1.236
13. Fern R, Ransom BR, Stys PK, Waxman SG. Pharmacological protection of CNS white matter during anoxia: actions of phenytoin, carbamazepine and diazepam. *J Pharmacol Exp Ther.* (1993) 266:1549–55.
14. Bechtold DA, Kapoor R, Smith KJ. Axonal protection using flecainide in experimental autoimmune encephalomyelitis. *Ann Neurol.* (2004) 55:607–16. doi: 10.1002/ana.20045

15. Bechtold DA, Miller SJ, Dawson AC, Sun Y, Kapoor R, Berry D, et al. Axonal protection achieved in a model of multiple sclerosis using lamotrigine. *J Neurol.* (2006) 253:1542–51. doi: 10.1007/s00415-006-0204-1

16. Vergo S, Craner MJ, Etzensperger R, Attfield K, Friese MA, Newcombe J, et al. Acid-sensing ion channel 1 is involved in both axonal injury and demyelination in multiple sclerosis and its animal model. *Brain* (2011) 134(Pt 2):571–84. doi: 10.1093/brain/awq337

17. Kapoor R, Furby J, Hayton T, Smith KJ, Altmann DR, Brenner R, et al. Lamotrigine for neuroprotection in secondary progressive multiple sclerosis: a randomised, double-blind, placebo-controlled, parallel-group trial. *Lancet Neurol.* (2010) 9:681–8. doi: 10.1016/S1474-4422(10)70131-9

18. Arun T, Tomassini V, Sbardella E, de Ruiter MB, Matthews L, Leite MI, et al. Targeting ASIC1 in primary progressive multiple sclerosis: evidence of neuroprotection with amiloride. *Brain* (2013) 136(Pt 1):106–15. doi: 10.1093/brain/aws325

19. Yang C, Hao Z, Zhang L, Zeng L, Wen J. Sodium channel blockers for neuroprotection in multiple sclerosis. *Cochrane Database Syst Rev.* (2015) CD010422. doi: 10.1002/14651858.CD010422.pub2

20. Haghikia A, Jorg S, Duscha A, Berg J, Manzel A, Waschbisch A, et al. Dietary fatty acids directly impact central nervous system autoimmunity via the small intestine. *Immunity* (2015) 43:817–29. doi: 10.1016/j.immuni.2015.09.007

21. Jorg S, Grohme DA, Erzler M, Binsfeld M, Haghikia A, Muller DN, et al. Environmental factors in autoimmune diseases and their role in multiple sclerosis. *Cell Mol Life Sci.* (2016) 73:4611–22. doi: 10.1007/s00018-016-2311-1

22. Hammer A, Schliep A, Jorg S, Haghikia A, Gold R, Kleinewietfeld M, et al. Impact of combined sodium chloride and saturated long-chain fatty acid challenge on the differentiation of T helper cells in neuroinflammation. *J Neuroinflammation* (2017) 14:184. doi: 10.1186/s12974-017-0954-y

23. Kleinewietfeld M, Manzel A, Titze J, Kvakan H, Yosef N, Linker RA, et al. Sodium chloride drives autoimmune disease by the induction of pathogenic TH17 cells. *Nature* (2013) 496:518–22. doi: 10.1038/nature11868

24. Farez MF. Salt intake in multiple sclerosis: friend or foe? *J Neurol Neurosurg Psychiatry* (2016) 87:1276. doi: 10.1136/jnnp-2016-313768

25. Fitzgerald KC, Munger KL, Hartung HP, Freedman MS, Montalban X, Edan G, et al. Sodium intake and multiple sclerosis activity and progression in BENEFIT. *Ann Neurol.* (2017) 82:20–9. doi: 10.1002/ana.24965

26. Nourbakhsh B, Graves J, Casper TC, Lulu S, Waldman A, Belman A, et al. Dietary salt intake and time to relapse in paediatric multiple sclerosis. *J Neurol Neurosurg Psychiatry* (2016) 87:1350–3. doi: 10.1136/jnnp-2016-313410

27. Currie S, Hoggard N, Craven IJ, Hadjivassiliou M, Wilkinson ID. Understanding MRI: basic MR physics for physicians. *Postgrad Med J.* (2013) 89:209–23. doi: 10.1136/postgradmedj-2012-131342

28. Kaunzner UW, Gauthier SA. MRI in the assessment and monitoring of multiple sclerosis: an update on best practice. *Ther Adv Neurol Disord.* (2017) 10:247–61. doi: 10.1177/1756285617708911

29. Konstandin S, Nagel AM. Measurement techniques for magnetic resonance imaging of fast relaxing nuclei. *MAGMA* (2014) 27:5–19. doi: 10.1007/s10334-013-0394-3

30. Harris RK, Becker ED, Cabral de Menezes SM, Goodfellow R, Granger P. NMR nomenclature: nuclear spin properties and conventions for chemical shifts. IUPAC recommendations 2001. *Solid State Nucl Magn Reson.* (2002) 22:458–83. doi: 10.1006/snmr.2002.0063

31. Gordji-Nejad A, Mollenhoff K, Oros-Peusquens AM, Pillai DR, Shah NJ. Characterizing cerebral oxygen metabolism employing oxygen-17 MRI/MRS at high fields. *MAGMA* (2014) 27:81–93. doi: 10.1007/s10334-013-0413-4

32. Chen J, Lanza GM, Wickline SA. Quantitative magnetic resonance fluorine imaging: today and tomorrow. *Wiley Interdiscip Rev Nanomed Nanobiotechnol.* (2010) 2:431–40. doi: 10.1002/wnan.87

33. Lu A, Atkinson IC, Zhou XJ, Thulborn KR. PCr/ATP ratio mapping of the human head by simultaneously imaging of multiple spectral peaks with interleaved excitations and flexible twisted projection imaging readout trajectories at 9.4 T. *Magn Reson Med.* (2013) 69:538–44. doi: 10.1002/mrm.24281

34. Nagel AM, Lehmann-Horn F, Weber MA, Jurkat-Rott K, Wolf MB, Radbruch A, et al. *In vivo* 35Cl MR imaging in humans: a feasibility study. *Radiology* (2014) 271:585–95. doi: 10.1148/radiol.13131725

35. Umathum R, Rosler MB, Nagel AM. *In vivo* 39K MR imaging of human muscle and brain. *Radiology* (2013) 269:569–76. doi: 10.1148/radiol.13130757

36. Atkinson IC, Claiborne TC, Thulborn KR. Feasibility of 39-potassium MR imaging of a human brain at 9.4 Tesla. *Magn Reson Med.* (2014) 71:1819–25. doi: 10.1002/mrm.24821

37. Hilal SK, Maudsley AA, Ra JB, Simon HE, Roschmann P, Wittekoek S, et al. *In vivo* NMR imaging of sodium-23 in the human head. *J Comput Assist Tomogr.* (1985) 9:1–7.

38. Konstandin S, Schad LR. 30 Years of sodium/X-nuclei magnetic resonance imaging. *MAGMA* (2014) 27:1–4. doi: 10.1007/s10334-013-0426-z

39. Thulborn KR. Quantitative sodium MR imaging: a review of its evolving role in medicine. *Neuroimage* (2018) 168:250–68. doi: 10.1016/j.neuroimage.2016.11.056

40. Madelin G, Lee JS, Regatte RR, Jerschow A. Sodium MRI: methods and applications. *Prog Nucl Magn Reson Spectrosc.* (2014) 79:14–47. doi: 10.1016/j.pnmrs.2014.02.001

41. Ladd ME, Bachert P, Meyerspeer M, Moser E, Nagel AM, Norris DG, et al. Pros and cons of ultra-high-field MRI/MRS for human application. *Prog Nucl Magn Reson Spectrosc.* (2018) 109:1–50. doi: 10.1016/j.pnmrs.2018.06.001

42. Maudsley AA, Hilal SK. Biological aspects of sodium-23 imaging. *Br Med Bull.* (1984) 40:165–6.

43. Hirai H, Yamasaki K, Kidena H, Kono M. Quantitative analysis of sodium fast and slow component in *in vivo* human brain tissue using MR Na image. *Kaku Igaku* (1992) 29:1447–54.

44. Constantinides CD, Gillen JS, Boada FE, Pomper MG, Bottomley PA. Human skeletal muscle: sodium MR imaging and quantification-potential applications in exercise and disease. *Radiology* (2000) 216:559–68. doi: 10.1148/radiology.216.2.r00jl46559

45. Ouwerkerk R, Bleich KB, Gillen JS, Pomper MG, Bottomley PA. Tissue sodium concentration in human brain tumors as measured with 23Na MR imaging. *Radiology* (2003) 227:529–37. doi: 10.1148/radiol.2272020483

46. Hilal SK, Maudsley AA, Simon HE, Perman WH, Bonn J, Mawad ME, et al. *In vivo* NMR imaging of tissue sodium in the intact cat before and after acute cerebral stroke. *AJNR Am J Neuroradiol.* (1983) 4:245–9.

47. Petracca M, Fleysher L, Oesingmann N, Inglese M. Sodium MRI of multiple sclerosis. *NMR Biomed.* (2016) 29:153–61. doi: 10.1002/nbm.3289

48. Shah NJ, Worthoff WA, Langen KJ. Imaging of sodium in the brain: a brief review. *NMR Biomed.* (2016) 29:162–74. doi: 10.1002/nbm.3389

49. Boada FE, Christensen JD, Huang-Hellinger FR, Reese TG, Thulborn KR. Quantitative *in vivo* tissue sodium concentration maps: the effects of biexponential relaxation. *Magn Reson Med.* (1994) 32:219–23.

50. Wiggins GC, Brown R, Lakshmanan K. High-performance radiofrequency coils for (23)Na MRI: brain and musculoskeletal applications. *NMR Biomed.* (2016) 29:96–106. doi: 10.1002/nbm.3379

51. Qian Y, Zhao T, Wiggins GC, Wald LL, Zheng H, Weimer J, et al. Sodium imaging of human brain at 7 T with 15-channel array coil. *Magn Reson Med.* (2012) 68:1807–14. doi: 10.1002/mrm.24192

52. Benkhedah N, Hoffmann SH, Biller A, Nagel AM. Evaluation of adaptive combination of 30-channel head receive coil array data in 23Na MR imaging. *Magn Reson Med.* (2016) 75:527–36. doi: 10.1002/mrm.25572

53. Lommen JM, Resmer F, Behl NGR, Sauer M, Benkhedah N, Bitz AK, et al. Comparison of of a 30-channel head array with a birdcage for 23Na MRI at 7 Tesla. *Proc. Intl. Soc. Mag. Reson. Med.* (2016) 24:3974.

54. Irarrazabal P, Nishimura DG. Fast three dimensional magnetic resonance imaging. *Magn Reson Med.* (1995) 33:656–62.

55. Boada FE, Gillen JS, Shen GX, Chang SY, Thulborn KR. Fast three dimensional sodium imaging. *Magn Reson Med.* (1997) 37:706–15.

56. Stobbe R, Beaulieu C. Advantage of sampling density weighted apodization over postacquisition filtering apodization for sodium MRI of the human brain. *Magn Reson Med.* (2008) 60:981–6. doi: 10.1002/mrm.21738

57. Nagel AM, Laun FB, Weber MA, Matthies C, Semmler W, Schad LR. Sodium MRI using a density-adapted 3D radial acquisition technique. *Magn Reson Med.* (2009) 62:1565–73. doi: 10.1002/mrm.22157

58. Madelin G, Chang G, Otazo R, Jerschow A, Regatte RR. Compressed sensing sodium MRI of cartilage at 7T: preliminary study. *J Magn Reson.* (2012) 214:360–5. doi: 10.1016/j.jmr.2011.12.005

59. Gnahm C, Bock M, Bachert P, Semmler W, Behl NG, Nagel AM. Iterative 3D projection reconstruction of (23) Na data with an (1) H MRI constraint. *Magn Reson Med.* (2014) 71:1720–32. doi: 10.1002/mrm.24827

60. Gnahm C, Nagel AM. Anatomically weighted second-order total variation reconstruction of 23Na MRI using prior information from 1H MRI. *Neuroimage* (2015) 105:452–61. doi: 10.1016/j.neuroimage.2014.11.006

61. Behl NG, Gnahm C, Bachert P, Ladd ME, Nagel AM. Three-dimensional dictionary-learning reconstruction of (23)Na MRI data. *Magn Reson Med.* (2016) 75:1605–16. doi: 10.1002/mrm.25759

62. Ridley B, Nagel AM, Bydder M, Maarouf A, Stellmann JP, Gherib S, et al. Distribution of brain sodium long and short relaxation times and concentrations: a multi-echo ultra-high field (23)Na MRI study. *Sci Rep.* (2018) 8:4357. doi: 10.1038/s41598-018-22711-0

63. Kraff O, Fischer A, Nagel AM, Monninghoff C, Ladd ME. MRI at 7 Tesla and above: demonstrated and potential capabilities. *J Magn Reson Imaging* (2015) 41:13–33. doi: 10.1002/jmri.24573

64. Inglese M, Madelin G, Oesingmann N, Babb JS, Wu W, Stoeckel B, et al. Brain tissue sodium concentration in multiple sclerosis: a sodium imaging study at 3 tesla. *Brain* (2010) 133(Pt 3):847–57. doi: 10.1093/brain/awp334

65. Paling D, Solanky BS, Riemer F, Tozer DJ, Wheeler-Kingshott CA, Kapoor R, et al. Sodium accumulation is associated with disability and a progressive course in multiple sclerosis. *Brain* (2013) 136(Pt 7):2305–17. doi: 10.1093/brain/awt149

66. Mirkes CC, Hoffmann J, Shajan G, Pohmann R, Scheffler K. High-resolution quantitative sodium imaging at 9.4 Tesla. *Magn Reson Med.* (2015) 73:342–51. doi: 10.1002/mrm.25096

67. Gilles A, Nagel AM, Madelin G. Multipulse sodium magnetic resonance imaging for multicompartment quantification: proof-of-concept. *Sci Rep.* (2017) 7:17435. doi: 10.1038/s41598-017-17582-w

68. Atkinson IC, Renteria L, Burd H, Pliskin NH, Thulborn KR. Safety of human MRI at static fields above the FDA 8 T guideline: sodium imaging at 9.4 T does not affect vital signs or cognitive ability. *J Magn Reson Imaging* (2007) 26:1222–7. doi: 10.1002/jmri.21150

69. Shah NJ. Multimodal neuroimaging in humans at 9.4 T: a technological breakthrough towards an advanced metabolic imaging scanner. *Brain Struct Funct.* (2015) 220:1867–84. doi: 10.1007/s00429-014-0843-4

70. Madelin G, Regatte RR. Biomedical applications of sodium MRI *in vivo. J Magn Reson Imaging* (2013) 38:511–29. doi: 10.1002/jmri.24168

71. Niesporek SC, Hoffmann SH, Berger MC, Benkhedah N, Kujawa A, Bachert P, et al. Partial volume correction for *in vivo* (23)Na-MRI data of the human brain. *Neuroimage* (2015) 112:353–63. doi: 10.1016/j.neuroimage.2015.03.025

72. Naritomi H, Kanashiro M, Sasaki M, Kuribayashi Y, Sawada T. *In vivo* measurements of intra- and extracellular Na$^+$ and water in the brain and muscle by nuclear magnetic resonance spectroscopy with shift reagent. *Biophys J.* (1987) 52:611–6. doi: 10.1016/S0006-3495(87)83251-4

73. Bansal N, Germann MJ, Lazar I, Malloy CR, Sherry AD. *In vivo* Na-23 MR imaging and spectroscopy of rat brain during TmDOTP5-infusion. *J Magn Reson Imaging* (1992) 2:385–91.

74. Boada FE, LaVerde G, Jungreis C, Nemoto E, Tanase C, Hancu I. Loss of cell ion homeostasis and cell viability in the brain: what sodium MRI can tell us. *Curr Top Dev Biol.* (2005) 70:77–101. doi: 10.1016/S0070-2153(05)70004-1

75. Winter PM, Bansal N. TmDOTP^{5-} as a ^{23}Na shift reagent for the subcutaneously implanted 9L gliosarcoma in rats. *Magn Reson Med.* (2001) 45:436–42. doi: 10.1002/1522-2594(200103)45:3<436::AID-MRM1057>3.0.CO;2-6

76. Stobbe R, Beaulieu C. *In vivo* sodium magnetic resonance imaging of the human brain using soft inversion recovery fluid attenuation. *Magn Reson Med.* (2005) 54:1305–10. doi: 10.1002/mrm.20696

77. Nagel AM, Bock M, Hartmann C, Gerigk L, Neumann JO, Weber MA, et al. The potential of relaxation-weighted sodium magnetic resonance imaging as demonstrated on brain tumors. *Invest Radiol.* (2011) 46:539–47. doi: 10.1097/RLI.0b013e31821ae918

78. Biller A, Pflugmann I, Badde S, Diem R, Wildemann B, Nagel AM, et al. Sodium MRI in multiple sclerosis is compatible with intracellular sodium accumulation and inflammation-induced hyper-cellularity of acute brain lesions. *Sci Rep.* (2016) 6:31269. doi: 10.1038/srep31269

79. Madelin G, Babb J, Xia D, Regatte RR. Repeatability of quantitative sodium magnetic resonance imaging for estimating pseudo-intracellular sodium concentration and pseudo-extracellular volume fraction in brain at 3 T. *PLoS ONE* (2015) 10:e0118692. doi: 10.1371/journal.pone.0118692

80. Pike KJ, Malde RP, Ashbrook SE, McManus J, Wimperis S. Multiple-quantum MAS NMR of quadrupolar nuclei. Do five-, seven- and nine-quantum experiments yield higher resolution than the three-quantum experiment? *Solid State Nucl Magn Reson.* (2000) 16:203–15. doi: 10.1016/S0926-2040(00)00081-3

81. Fleysher L, Oesingmann N, Brown R, Sodickson DK, Wiggins GC, Inglese M. Noninvasive quantification of intracellular sodium in human brain using ultrahigh-field MRI. *NMR Biomed.* (2013) 26:9–19. doi: 10.1002/nbm.2813

82. Worthoff WA, Shymanskaya A, Shah NJ. Relaxometry and quantification in simultaneously acquired single and triple quantum filtered sodium MRI. *Magn Reson Med.* (2018) 81:303–15. doi: 10.1002/mrm.27387

83. Matthies C, Nagel AM, Schad LR, Bachert P. Reduction of B(0) inhomogeneity effects in triple-quantum-filtered sodium imaging. *J Magn Reson.* (2010) 202:239–44. doi: 10.1016/j.jmr.2009.11.004

84. Benkhedah N, Bachert P, Semmler W, Nagel AM. Three-dimensional biexponential weighted (23)Na imaging of the human brain with higher SNR and shorter acquisition time. *Magn Reson Med.* (2013) 70:754–65. doi: 10.1002/mrm.24516

85. Fiege DP, Romanzetti S, Mirkes CC, Brenner D, Shah NJ. Simultaneous single-quantum and triple-quantum-filtered MRI of 23Na (SISTINA). *Magn Reson Med.* (2013) 69:1691–6. doi: 10.1002/mrm.24417

86. Tsang A, Stobbe RW, Beaulieu C. Evaluation of B0-inhomogeneity correction for triple-quantum-filtered sodium MRI of the human brain at 4.7 T. *J Magn Reson.* (2013) 230:134–44. doi: 10.1016/j.jmr.2013.01.017

87. Gast LV, Gerhalter T, Hensel B, Uder M, Nagel AM. Double quantum filtered (23) Na MRI with magic angle excitation of human skeletal muscle in the presence of B0 and B1 inhomogeneities. *NMR Biomed.* (2018) 31:e4010. doi: 10.1002/nbm.4010

88. Thulborn KR, Gindin TS, Davis D, Erb P. Comprehensive MR imaging protocol for stroke management: tissue sodium concentration as a measure of tissue viability in nonhuman primate studies and in clinical studies. *Radiology* (1999) 213:156–66. doi: 10.1148/radiology.213.1.r99se15156

89. Hussain MS, Stobbe RW, Bhagat YA, Emery D, Butcher KS, Manawadu D, et al. Sodium imaging intensity increases with time after human ischemic stroke. *Ann Neurol.* (2009) 66:55–62. doi: 10.1002/ana.21648

90. Tsang A, Stobbe RW, Asdaghi N, Hussain MS, Bhagat YA, Beaulieu C, et al. Relationship between sodium intensity and perfusion deficits in acute ischemic stroke. *J Magn Reson Imaging* (2011) 33:41–7. doi: 10.1002/jmri.22299

91. Thulborn KR, Davis D, Adams H, Gindin T, Zhou J. Quantitative tissue sodium concentration mapping of the growth of focal cerebral tumors with sodium magnetic resonance imaging. *Magn Reson Med.* (1999) 41:351–9.

92. Kline RP, Wu EX, Petrylak DP, Szabolcs M, Alderson PO, Weisfeldt ML, et al. Rapid *in vivo* monitoring of chemotherapeutic response using weighted sodium magnetic resonance imaging. *Clin Cancer Res.* (2000) 6:2146–56.

93. Babsky AM, Zhang H, Hekmatyar SK, Hutchins GD, Bansal N. Monitoring chemotherapeutic response in RIF-1 tumors by single-quantum and triple-quantum-filtered (23)Na MRI, (1)H diffusion-weighted MRI and PET imaging. *Magn Reson Imaging* (2007) 25:1015–23. doi: 10.1016/j.mri.2006.11.004

94. Thulborn KR, Lu A, Atkinson IC, Damen F, Villano JL. Quantitative sodium MR imaging and sodium bioscales for the management of brain tumors. *Neuroimaging Clin N Am.* (2009) 19:615–24. doi: 10.1016/j.nic.2009.09.001

95. Nunes Neto LP, Madelin G, Sood TP, Wu CC, Kondziolka D, Placantonakis D, et al. Quantitative sodium imaging and gliomas: a feasibility study. *Neuroradiology* (2018) 60:795–802. doi: 10.1007/s00234-018-2041-1

96. Reetz K, Romanzetti S, Dogan I, Sass C, Werner CJ, Schiefer J, et al. Increased brain tissue sodium concentration in Huntington's disease–a sodium imaging study at 4 T. *Neuroimage* (2012) 63:517–24. doi: 10.1016/j.neuroimage.2012.07.009

97. Mellon EA, Pilkinton DT, Clark CM, Elliott MA, Witschey WR II, Borthakur A, et al. Sodium MR imaging detection of mild Alzheimer disease: preliminary study. *AJNR Am J Neuroradiol.* (2009) 30:978–84. doi: 10.3174/ajnr.A1495

98. Thulborn K, Lui E, Guntin J, Jamil S, Sun Z, Claiborne TC, et al. Quantitative sodium MRI of the human brain at 9.4 T provides assessment of tissue sodium concentration and cell volume fraction during normal aging. *NMR Biomed.* (2016) 29:137–43. doi: 10.1002/nbm.3312

99. Zaaraoui W, Konstandin S, Audoin B, Nagel AM, Rico A, Malikova I, et al. Distribution of brain sodium accumulation correlates with disability in multiple sclerosis: a cross-sectional 23Na MR imaging study. *Radiology* (2012) 264:859–67. doi: 10.1148/radiol.12112680

100. Maarouf A, Audoin B, Konstandin S, Rico A, Soulier E, Reuter F, et al. Topography of brain sodium accumulation in progressive multiple sclerosis. *MAGMA* (2014) 27:53–62. doi: 10.1007/s10334-013-0396-1

101. Petracca M, Vancea RO, Fleysher L, Jonkman LE, Oesingmann N, Inglese M. Brain intra- and extracellular sodium concentration in multiple sclerosis: a 7 T MRI study. *Brain* (2016) 139(Pt 3):795–806. doi: 10.1093/brain/awv386

102. Eisele P, Konstandin S, Griebe M, Szabo K, Wolf ME, Alonso A, et al. Heterogeneity of acute multiple sclerosis lesions on sodium (23Na) MRI. *Mult Scler.* (2016) 22:1040–7. doi: 10.1177/1352458515609430

103. Grist JT, Riemer F, McLean MA, Matys T, Zaccagna F, Hilborne SF, et al. Imaging intralesional heterogeneity of sodium concentration in multiple sclerosis: initial evidence from (23)Na-MRI. *J Neurol Sci.* (2018) 387:111–4. doi: 10.1016/j.jns.2018.01.027

104. Huhn K, Mennecke A, Linz P, Tschunko F, Kastle N, Nagel AM, et al. (23)Na MRI reveals persistent sodium accumulation in tumefactive MS lesions. *J Neurol Sci.* (2017) 379:163–6. doi: 10.1016/j.jns.2017.06.003

105. Filippi M, Rocca MA, De Stefano N, Enzinger C, Fisher E, Horsfield MA, et al. Magnetic resonance techniques in multiple sclerosis: the present and the future. *Arch Neurol.* (2011) 68:1514–20. doi: 10.1001/archneurol.2011.914

106. Maarouf A, Audoin B, Pariollaud F, Gherib S, Rico A, Soulier E, et al. Increased total sodium concentration in gray matter better explains cognition than atrophy in MS. *Neurology* (2017) 88:289–95. doi: 10.1212/WNL.0000000000003511

107. Donadieu M, Le Fur Y, Maarouf A, Gherib S, Ridley B, Pini L, et al. Metabolic counterparts of sodium accumulation in multiple sclerosis: a whole brain ^{23}Na-MRI and fast ^{1}H-MRSI study. *Mult Scler.* (2017) 25:39–47. doi: 10.1177/1352458517736146

108. Dutta R, McDonough J, Yin X, Peterson J, Chang A, Torres T, et al. Mitochondrial dysfunction as a cause of axonal degeneration in multiple sclerosis patients. *Ann Neurol.* (2006) 59:478–89. doi: 10.1002/ana.20736

109. Campbell GR, Ziabreva I, Reeve AK, Krishnan KJ, Reynolds R, Howell O, et al. Mitochondrial DNA deletions and neurodegeneration in multiple sclerosis. *Ann Neurol.* (2011) 69:481–92. doi: 10.1002/ana.22109

110. Nagel AM, Amarteifio E, Lehmann-Horn F, Jurkat-Rott K, Semmler W, Schad LR, et al. 3 Tesla sodium inversion recovery magnetic resonance imaging allows for improved visualization of intracellular sodium content changes in muscular channelopathies. *Invest Radiol.* (2011) 46:759–66. doi: 10.1097/RLI.0b013e31822836f6

111. Constantinides CD, Weiss RG, Lee R, Bolar D, Bottomley PA. Restoration of low resolution metabolic images with a priori anatomic information: ^{23}Na MRI in myocardial infarction. *Magn Reson Imaging* (2000) 18:461–71. doi: 10.1016/S0730-725X(99)00145-9

112. Stobbe RW, Beaulieu C. Calculating potential error in sodium MRI with respect to the analysis of small objects. *Magn Reson Med.* (2018) 79:2968–77. doi: 10.1002/mrm.26962

113. Eisele P, Konstandin S, Szabo K, Ong M, Zollner F, Schad LR, et al. Sodium MRI of T1 high signal intensity in the dentate nucleus due to gadolinium deposition in multiple sclerosis. *J Neuroimaging* (2017) 27:372–5. doi: 10.1111/jon.12448

114. Paschke NK, Neumann W, Uhrig T, Winkler M, Neumaier-Probst E, Fatar M, et al. Influence of gadolinium-based contrast agents on tissue sodium quantification in sodium magnetic resonance imaging. *Invest Radiol.* (2018) 53:555–62. doi: 10.1097/RLI.0000000000000487

115. Strange K. Regulation of solute and water balance and cell volume in the central nervous system. *J Am Soc Nephrol.* (1992) 3:12–27.

116. Rauschenberg J, Nagel AM, Ladd SC, Theysohn JM, Ladd ME, Moller HE, et al. Multicenter study of subjective acceptance during magnetic resonance imaging at 7 and 9.4 T. *Invest Radiol.* (2014) 49:249–59. doi: 10.1097/RLI.0000000000000035

117. Kearney H, Miller DH, Ciccarelli O. Spinal cord MRI in multiple sclerosis-diagnostic, prognostic and clinical value. *Nat Rev Neurol.* (2015) 11:327–38. doi: 10.1038/nrneurol.2015.80

118. Kopp C, Linz P, Dahlmann A, Hammon M, Jantsch J, Muller DN, et al. 23Na magnetic resonance imaging-determined tissue sodium in healthy subjects and hypertensive patients. *Hypertension* (2013) 61:635–40. doi: 10.1161/HYPERTENSIONAHA.111.00566

119. Titze J. Sodium balance is not just a renal affair. *Curr Opin Nephrol Hypertens.* (2014) 23:101–5. doi: 10.1097/01.mnh.0000441151.55320.c3

120. Wang P, Deger MS, Kang H, Ikizler TA, Titze J, Gore JC. Sex differences in sodium deposition in human muscle and skin. *Magn Reson Imaging* (2017) 36:93–7. doi: 10.1016/j.mri.2016.10.023

21

Dermal Phospho-Alpha-Synuclein Deposition in Patients with Parkinson's Disease and Mutation of the Glucocerebrosidase Gene

Kathrin Doppler[1][*][†], Kathrin Brockmann[2][†], Annahita Sedghi[1], Isabel Wurster[2], Jens Volkmann[1], Wolfgang H. Oertel[3] and Claudia Sommer[1]

[1] Department of Neurology, University Hospital Würzburg, Würzburg, Germany, [2] Department of Neurology, University Hospital Tübingen, Tubingen, Germany, [3] Department of Neurology, University Hospital Marburg, Marburg, Germany

*Correspondence:
Kathrin Doppler
Doppler_K@ukw.de

[†] These authors have contributed equally to this work

Heterozygous mutations in the glucocerebrosidase gene (GBA1) represent the most common genetic risk factor for Parkinson's disease (PD) and are histopathologically associated with a widespread load of alpha-synuclein in the brain. Therefore, PD patients with GBA1 mutations are a cohort of high interest for clinical trials on disease-modifying therapies targeting alpha-synuclein. There is evidence that detection of phospho-alpha-synuclein (p-syn) in dermal nerve fibers might be a biomarker for the histopathological identification of PD patients even at premotor or very early stages of disease. It is so far unknown whether dermal p-syn deposition can also be found in PD patients with GBA1 mutations and may serve as a biomarker for PD in these patients. Skin biopsies of 10 PD patients with different GBA1 mutations (six N370S, three E326K, one L444P) were analyzed by double-immunofluorescence labeling with anti-p-syn and anti-protein gene product 9.5 (PGP9.5, axonal marker) to detect intraaxonal p-syn deposition. Four biopsy sites (distal, proximal leg, paravertebral Th10, and C7) per patient were studied. P-syn was found in six patients (three N370S, three E326K). P-syn deposition was mainly detected in autonomic nerve fibers, but also in somatosensory fibers and was not restricted to a certain GBA1 mutation. In summary, dermal p-syn in PD patients with GBA1 mutations seems to offer a similar distribution and frequency as observed in patients without a known mutation. Skin biopsy may be suitable to study p-syn deposition in these patients or even to identify premotor patients with GBA1 mutations.

Keywords: Parkinson's disease, glucocerebrosidase mutation, alpha-synuclein, skin biopsy, biomarker

INTRODUCTION

Pre-mortal diagnosis of Parkinson's disease (PD) is based on its clinical presentation with tremor, rigor, akinesia, and postural instability. Alpha-synuclein aggregates in neurons of the substantia nigra represent the histopathological hallmark of the disease and are not only considered as post-mortem disease marker but also offer insights into the pathogenesis of the disease.

In the last few years, focus has been set on the onset of PD-associated neurodegeneration and it is known that the disease starts many years before the onset of motor symptoms (1). Non-motor symptoms such as obstipation, hyposmia, depression, or rapid eye movement sleep behavior disorder (RBD) may occur during the prodromal phase of PD when the patients do not show any motor symptoms but alpha-synuclein deposition and neuronal loss can already be found in the brain (2). Major efforts of drug development focus on the deposition of alpha-synuclein as a probable pathogenic key event. Clinical trials of drugs targeting alpha-synuclein deposition require reliable identification of patients with primarily alpha-synuclein-driven neurodegeneration who are in the prodromal stage of the disease and in whom pre-mortem non-invasive monitoring of alpha-synuclein deposition is possible. Within a high-risk cohort for PD, skin biopsy might be a potential tool to identify individuals at the earliest stages of the disease and to monitor progression of alpha-synuclein deposition. One of such a high-risk PD cohort are patients with RBD (3) and it has already been shown that p-syn deposition can be found in skin biopsies of RBD patients, rendering skin biopsy a potential biomarker for prodromal PD (4, 5). Another risk factor for the development of PD are glucocerebrosidase gene (GBA1) mutations that are supposed to be found in 4–10% of all PD patients (6–8) and increase the risk of developing PD 20-fold (8). PD patients carrying GBA1 mutations are of special interest as a first clinical trial with a substrate reduction inhibitor, GZ/SAR402671, has already started in in this subgroup of PD. However, alpha-synuclein deposition in skin biopsy has not yet been tested in PD patients with GBA1 mutations.

In the present study, we aimed to evaluate the use of skin biopsy for the detection of p- syn in PD patients with GBA1 mutations and to evaluate potential differences of dermal p-syn deposition in patients with GBA1 mutation associated PD compared to results from former studies on patients with idiopathic PD.

MATERIALS AND METHODS

Patients

Ten patients with a known GBA1 mutation were prospectively recruited at the University Hospital Tübingen (mean age 61.7 ($\pm$8.1) years. Initially, they had been recruited for the prospective observational MiGAP study (Markers in GBA1 associated Parkinson) funded by the DZNE (German Centre for Neurodegenerative Diseases, Site Tuebingen)[1] Out of 100 patients of the MIGAP study, we randomly selected and asked 10 PD patients to take part in the present sub-study. Diagnosis of PD was based on the UK brain bank criteria (9). Stage of disease was assessed using the Hoehn&Yahr scale (10), motor function was evaluated by Unified Parkinson's Disease Ranking Scale part III (UPDRS-III) (11). The bradykinesia score and annual UPDRSIII progression were calculated as previously described (12). Ten age and gender matched healthy controls who were recruited for former studies (5) and whose biopsy material was stored at our department were also investigated. All patients and controls gave oral and written informed consent to participate. The study was approved by the Ethic's committee of the University of Würzburg.

Abbreviations: GBA1, glucocerebrosidase gene; PD, Parkinson's disease; RBD, REM sleep behavior disorder; PGP9. 5, protein gene product 9.5; p-syn, phospho-alpha-synuclein.
[1]https://www.dzne.de/forschung/studien/klinische-studien/migap/

Demographic data of all patients and controls and the type of mutation are summarized in **Table 1**.

Skin Biopsy

Skin punch biopsies were taken from the distal and proximal leg, back (Th10), and neck (C7), fixed with paraformaldehyde and cryconserved until use as previously described (13). Twenty micrometer serial cryosections were cut. Double-immunofluorescence-labeling was performed using anti-PGP9.5 (axonal marker, Zytomed Systems, Berlin, Germany, 1:200) and anti-p-syn (Biolegend, San Diego, CA, United States, 1:500) and appropriate Cy3 and AlexaFluor488-conjugated secondary antibodies (Dianova, Hamburg, Germany, 1:100/1:400).

Microscopy

Double-immunofluorescence-labeling was assessed in a blinded manner using a fluorescence microscope with CARVII system (Ax10, Zeiss, Oberkochen, Germany/Visitron GmbH, Puchheim, Germany). All slides were scanned for p-syn-positive dermal nerve fibers. Nerve fibers were identified by staining with anti-PGP9.5 and only p-syn deposition within nerve fibers was considered "positive." A biopsy was assessed "positive" if at least one dermal nerve fiber was immunoreactive for p-syn. P-syn-positive nerve fibers were categorized as sudomotor, vasomotor, pilomotor, or somatosensory (subepidermal plexus or intraepidermal) according to their location. Nerve fibers that could not be assigned to a certain skin structure were assessed as dermal nerve bundles. P-syn deposition was quantified as the number of skin structures that contained at least one p-syn-positive nerve fiber.

Statistical Evaluation

Statistical analysis was calculated using SPSS Statistics 23 software (IBM, New York, United States). Two-sided Pearson's correlation test was used for correlation analysis. A significance level of 5% was applied.

RESULTS

P-syn deposition was found in 6/10 PD patients with GBA1 mutations, not in any healthy control (**Figure 1**). P-syn-positive nerve fibers were found in four biopsies of the distal leg, four of the proximal leg, two of the back, and two of the neck. Autonomic vasomotor fibers were affected in three cases, sudomotor fibers in one patient (**Figure 1C**), pilomotor in two (**Figure 1A**), and dermal nerve bundles in five cases. Somatosensory nerve fibers of the subepidermal plexus were found positive in two patients, in one of them, intraepidermal fibers were positive (**Figure 1B**). P-syn-positive fibers were not restricted to a certain mutation within GBA1 and were found in 3/6 patients with N370S mutation, 3/3 patients with E326K mutation, and 0/1 patient with L444P mutation. The number of p-syn positive dermal structures correlated with the duration of disease ($p = 0.02$, $r = 0.71$), but not with age at assessment. Correlation analysis between p-syn-positive structures and H&Y stage, bradykinesia score and annual UPDRSIII progression was not significant (H&Y: $p = 0.06$, $r = 0.61$, bradykinesia score: $p = 0.37$, $r = 0.32$, annual UPDRSIII progression: $p = 0.08$, $r = -0.58$).

TABLE 1 | Demographic data and p-syn deposition of patients with *GBA1* mutation.

Patient no.	Duration of disease (y)	H&Y stage	UPDRS part III	Annual UPDRS III progression	Bradykinesia score	Subtype	*GBA1* mut.	p-syn pos biopsy site	p-syn pos structures	No. of positive struct.
1	14	3	70	5	1.7	Equivalent	N370S	LL	ves, db, ep	3
2	6	2	48	8	1.5	Equivalent	N370S	–		0
3	17	2	34	2	0.6	Equivalent	N370S	LL, Th10	subepi, intraepi, ves, db	4
4	6	2.5	35	5.8	1.7	Equivalent	N370S	–		0
5	5	2	32	6.4	1.1	Equivalent	N370S	UL, Th10	db	2
6	1	2	10	10	0.5	Tremor dominant	L444P	–		0
7	8	3	49	6.1	2.5	Equivalent	E326K	UL, LL, C7	db, ves, ep	4
8	14	2	32	2.3	1.6	Equivalent	E326K	UL	subepi	1
9	14	3	53	3.8	2.6	Equivalent	E326K	UL, LL, C7	db, sg	4
10	2	2	36	18	1.8	Acinetic-rigid	N370S	–		0

No., number; y, years; H&Y, Hoehn&Yahr; GBA1, glucocerebrosidase gene; p-syn, phospho-alpha-synuclein; pos, positive; struct., structures; LL, lower leg; UL, upper leg; ves, vessel; db, dermal nerve bundle; ep, erector pilorum muscle; subepi, subepidermal; intraepi, intraepidermal; sg, sweat gland; UPDRS, Unified Parkinson Disease Rating Scale.

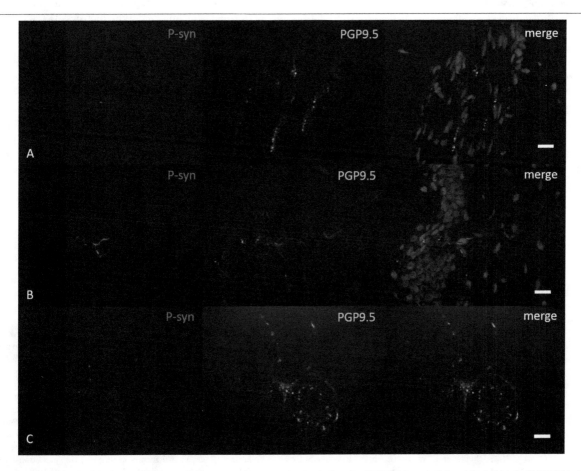

FIGURE 1 | Photomicrographs of a double-immunofluorescence staining with anti-p-syn (red) and anti-PGP9.5 (green). Cell nuclei are stained with DAPI (blue). P-syn deposition is detectable in pilomotor fibers **(A)**, intraepidermal fibers **(B)** and sudomotor fibers **(C)** of patients with *GBA1* mutation-associated PD. Scale Bar = 10 μm.

DISCUSSION

Here, we report p-syn deposition in dermal nerve fibers of PD patients carrying a mutation in *GBA1*.

The frequency of 60% in our study is comparable with former skin biopsy studies in idiopathic PD using similar protocols (5, 13, 14). Predominant autonomic involvement with vasomotor fibers as the mostly affected fibers is also in line with previous studies (13, 15). Our results indicate that dermal p-syn pathology of patients with *GBA1* mutations does not differ from idiopathic PD. This corresponds to findings from brain autopsy studies that also did not show a clear difference except for some studies describing more extensive diffuse cortical Lewy bodies (6, 16) that could not be confirmed by others (17, 18). Dermal p-syn deposition was not restricted to a certain mutation and was also found in patients with the E326K mutation which is considered a rather "mild" mutation (19). Our results indicate that clinical and neuropathological similarity between patients with *GBA1* mutations and without can be extended to the PNS, rendering skin biopsy a pre-mortem tool to investigate p-syn pathology in this patient group.

In recent studies no correlation between p-syn deposition and stage or duration of disease could be determined for PD (13, 15). Only in RBD, a potential prodromal stage of PD, a correlation between dermal p-syn and disease progression markers could be found, indicating a steady-state of dermal p-syn deposition during motor stages of disease. In the present study, p-syn positive structures correlated with duration of disease. This might indicate progressive p-syn deposition during the course of disease in patients with *GBA1* mutations. This is of special interest as this subgroup of PD patients was shown to present a more rapid disease progression (20). The frequency of p-syn deposition in early or even prodromal stages of *GBA1* associated PD needs to be investigated in future studies.

The exact underlying pathomechanism of p-syn deposition in patients with *GBA1* mutations is still unclear, but there is evidence that impaired lysosomal function and endoplasmatic reticulum stress play a role (21) and that accumulation of alpha synuclein is promoted by glucocerebrosidase deficiency (22).

Involvement of dermal nerve fibers in p-syn pathology in *GBA1* mutation associated PD provides the opportunity for the use of skin biopsy as a pre-mortem easily accessible tissue for the investigation of p-syn pathology in this subgroup of PD.

In summary, this pilot study gives evidence that dermal nerve fibers are affected by p-syn pathology in PD with *GBA1* mutations. A major limitation is the small sample size that does not allow a clear conclusion on the frequency and distribution of p-syn deposition in this subgroup compared to idiopathic PD. Detection of p-syn in skin biopsies of *GBA1*-associated PD is a basic prerequisite for future studies on prodromal *GBA1*-associated PD.

AUTHOR CONTRIBUTIONS

KD planned and designed the study, performed, and analyzed skin biopsies and wrote the first draft of the manuscript. KB planned and designed the study, recruited and characterized patients, performed skin biopsies, and revised the manuscript. AS performed and analyzed skin biopsies. IW recruited and characterized patients. JV and WO were involved in the study design. CS was involved in study design and revised the manuscript.

ACKNOWLEDGMENTS

We thank Barbara Dekant and Barbara Reuter for expert technical assistance. The study was funded by Parkinson Fonds Deutschland. WO is Hertie Senior Research Professor supported by the charitable Hertie Foundation, Frankfurt/Main, Germany.

REFERENCES

1. Berg D, Postuma RB, Adler CH, Bloem BR, Chan P, Dubois B, et al. MDS research criteria for prodromal Parkinson's disease. *Mov Disord.* (2015) 30:1600–11. doi: 10.1002/mds.26431

2. Braak H, Del Tredici K, Rub U, de Vos RA, Jansen Steur EN, Braak E. Staging of brain pathology related to sporadic Parkinson's disease. *Neurobiol Aging* (2003) 24:197–211. doi: 10.1016/S0197-4580(02)00065-9

3. Iranzo A, Tolosa E, Gelpi E, Molinuevo JL, Valldeoriola F, Serradell M, et al. Neurodegenerative disease status and post-mortem pathology in idiopathic rapid-eye-movement sleep behaviour disorder: an observational cohort study. *Lancet Neurol.* (2013) 12:443–53. doi: 10.1016/S1474-4422(13)70056-5

4. Antelmi E, Donadio V, Incensi A, Plazzi G, Liguori R. Skin nerve phosphorylated alpha-synuclein deposits in idiopathic REM sleep behavior disorder. *Neurology* (2017) 88:2128–31. doi: 10.1212/WNL.0000000000003989

5. Doppler K, Jentschke HM, Schulmeyer L, Vadasz D, Janzen A, Luster M, et al. Dermal phospho-alpha-synuclein deposits confirm REM sleep behaviour disorder as prodromal Parkinson's disease. *Acta Neuropathol.* (2017) 133:535–45. doi: 10.1007/s00401-017-1684-z

6. Neumann J, Bras J, Deas E, O'Sullivan SS, Parkkinen L, Lachmann RH, et al. Glucocerebrosidase mutations in clinical and pathologically proven Parkinson's disease. *Brain* (2009) 132:1783–94. doi: 10.1093/brain/awp044

7. Sidransky E, Nalls MA, Aasly JO, Aharon-Peretz J, Annesi G, Barbosa ER, et al. Multicenter analysis of glucocerebrosidase mutations in Parkinson's disease. *N Engl J Med.* (2009) 361:1651–61. doi: 10.1056/NEJMoa0901281

8. Schapira AH. Glucocerebrosidase and Parkinson disease: recent advances. *Mol Cell Neurosci.* (2015) 66:37–42. doi: 10.1016/j.mcn.2015.03.013

9. Hughes AJ, Daniel SE, Kilford L, Lees AJ. Accuracy of clinical diagnosis of idiopathic parkinson's disease: a clinico-pathological study of 100 cases. *J Neurol Neurosurg Psychiatr.* (1992) 55:181–4. doi: 10.1136/jnnp.55.3.181

10. Hoehn MM, Yahr MD. Parkinsonism: onset, progression and mortality. *Neurology* (1967) 17:427–42. doi: 10.1212/WNL.17.5.427

11. Goetz CG, Tilley BC, Shaftman SR, Stebbins GT, Fahn S, Martinez-Martin P, et al. Movement disorder society-sponsored revision of the unified parkinson's disease rating scale (MDS-UPDRS): scale presentation and clinimetric testing results. *Mov Disord.* (2008) 23:2129–70. doi: 10.1002/mds.22340

12. Szewczyk-Krolikowski K, Tomlinson P, Nithi K, Wade-Martins R, Talbot K, Ben-Shlomo Y, et al. The influence of age and gender on motor and non-motor features of early Parkinson's disease: initial findings from the Oxford Parkinson Disease Center (OPDC) discovery cohort. *Parkinsonism Relat Disord.* (2014) 20:99–105. doi: 10.1016/j.parkreldis.2013.09.025

13. Doppler K, Ebert S, Uceyler N, Trenkwalder C, Ebentheuer J, Volkmann J, et al. Cutaneous neuropathy in parkinson's disease: a window into brain pathology. *Acta Neuropathol.* (2014) 128:99–109. doi: 10.1007/s00401-014-1284-0

14. Doppler K, Weis J, Karl K, Ebert S, Ebentheuer J, Trenkwalder C, et al. Distinctive distribution of phospho-alpha-synuclein in dermal nerves in multiple system atrophy. *Mov Disord.* (2015) 30:1688–92. doi: 10.1002/mds.26293

15. Donadio V, Incensi A, Leta V, Giannoccaro MP, Scaglione C, Martinelli P, et al. Skin nerve alpha-synuclein deposits: a biomarker for idiopathic Parkinson disease. *Neurology* (2014) 82:1362–9. doi: 10.1212/WNL.0000000000000316

16. Clark LN, Kartsaklis LA, Wolf Gilbert R, Dorado B, Ross BM, Kisselev S, et al. Association of glucocerebrosidase mutations with dementia with lewy bodies. *Arch Neurol.* (2009) 66:578–83. doi: 10.1001/archneurol.2009.54

17. Parkkinen L, Neumann J, O'Sullivan SS, Holton JL, Revesz T, Hardy J, et al. Glucocerebrosidase mutations do not cause increased lewy body pathology in parkinson's disease. *Mol Genet Metab.* (2011) 103:410–2. doi: 10.1016/j.ymgme.2011.04.015

18. Adler CH, Beach TG, Shill HA, Caviness JN, Driver-Dunckley E, Sabbagh MN, et al. GBA mutations in Parkinson disease: earlier death but similar neuropathological features. *Eur J Neurol.* (2017) 24:1363–8. doi: 10.1111/ene.13395

19. Berge-Seidl V, Pihlstrom L, Maple-Grodem J, Forsgren L, Linder J, Larsen JP, et al. The GBA variant E326K is associated with Parkinson's disease and explains a genome-wide association signal. *Neurosci Lett.* (2017) 658:48–52. doi: 10.1016/j.neulet.2017.08.040

20. Brockmann K, Srulijes K, Pflederer S, Hauser AK, Schulte C, Maetzler W, et al. GBA-associated Parkinson's disease: reduced survival and more rapid progression in a prospective longitudinal study. *Mov Disord.* (2015) 30:407–11. doi: 10.1002/mds.26071

21. Beavan MS, Schapira AH. Glucocerebrosidase mutations and the pathogenesis of Parkinson disease. *Ann Med.* (2013) 45:511–21. doi: 10.3109/07853890.2013.849003

22. Bae EJ, Yang NY, Song M, Lee CS, Lee JS, Jung BC, et al. Glucocerebrosidase depletion enhances cell-to-cell transmission of alpha-synuclein. *Nat Commun.* (2014) 5:4755. doi: 10.1038/ncomms5755

α7 Nicotinic Acetylcholine Receptor Signaling Modulates Ovine Fetal Brain Astrocytes Transcriptome in Response to Endotoxin

Mingju Cao[1†], James W. MacDonald[2†], Hai L. Liu[1], Molly Weaver[3], Marina Cortes[4], Lucien D. Durosier[1], Patrick Burns[5], Gilles Fecteau[5], André Desrochers[5], Jay Schulkin[6], Marta C. Antonelli[7], Raphael A. Bernier[8], Michael Dorschner[3], Theo K. Bammler[2] and Martin G. Frasch[1,4,6,9]*

[1] Department of Obstetrics and Gynaecology and Department of Neurosciences, CHU Ste-Justine Research Centre, Faculty of Medicine, Université de Montréal, Montréal, QC, Canada, [2] Department of Environmental and Occupational Health Sciences, University of Washington, Seattle, WA, United States, [3] UW Medicine Center for Precision Diagnostics, University of Washington, Seattle, WA, United States, [4] Animal Reproduction Research Centre (CRRA), Faculty of Veterinary Medicine, Université de Montréal, Montréal, QC, Canada, [5] Department of Clinical Sciences, Faculty of Veterinary Medicine, Université de Montréal, Montréal, QC, Canada, [6] Department of Obstetrics and Gynecology, University of Washington, Seattle, WA, United States, [7] Instituto de Biología Celular y Neurociencia "Prof. Eduardo De Robertis", Facultad de Medicina, Universidad de Buenos Aires, Buenos Aires, Argentina, [8] Department of Psychiatry and Behavioral Sciences, University of Washington, Seattle, WA, United States, [9] Center on Human Development and Disability, University of Washington, Seattle, WA, United States

*Correspondence:
Martin G. Frasch
mfrasch@uw.edu

[†] These authors have contributed equally to this work

Neuroinflammation *in utero* may result in lifelong neurological disabilities. Astrocytes play a pivotal role in this process, but the mechanisms are poorly understood. No early postnatal treatment strategies exist to enhance neuroprotective potential of astrocytes. We hypothesized that agonism on α7 nicotinic acetylcholine receptor (α7nAChR) in fetal astrocytes will augment their neuroprotective transcriptome profile, while the inhibition of α7nAChR will achieve the opposite. Using an *in vivo–in vitro* model of developmental programming of neuroinflammation induced by lipopolysaccharide (LPS), we validated this hypothesis in primary fetal sheep astrocytes cultures re-exposed to LPS in the presence of a selective α7nAChR agonist or antagonist. Our RNAseq findings show that a pro-inflammatory astrocyte transcriptome phenotype acquired *in vitro* by LPS stimulation is reversed with α7nAChR agonistic stimulation. Conversely, α7nAChR inhibition potentiates the pro-inflammatory astrocytic transcriptome phenotype. Furthermore, we conducted a secondary transcriptome analysis against the identical α7nAChR experiments in fetal sheep primary microglia cultures. Similar to findings in fetal microglia, in fetal astrocytes we observed a memory effect of *in vivo* exposure to inflammation, expressed in a perturbation of the iron homeostasis signaling pathway (hemoxygenase 1, HMOX1), which persisted under pre-treatment with α7nAChR antagonist but was reversed with α7nAChR agonist. For both glia cell types, common pathways activated due to LPS included neuroinflammation signaling and NF-κB signaling in some, but not all comparisons. However, overall, the overlap on the level of signaling pathways was rather minimal. Astrocytes, not microglia—the primary immune cells of the brain, were characterized by unique inhibition patterns of STAT3 pathway due to agonistic stimulation of α7nAChR prior to LPS exposure. Lastly, we discuss the implications of our findings for fetal and postnatal brain development.

Keywords: neuroinflammation, LPS, CHRNA7, RNAseq, astrocyte, microglia, infection, fetal programming

INTRODUCTION

Glial cells (astrocytes and microglia) play a role in neuroinflammation and both cell types acquire a specific reactive phenotype when stimulated by lipopolysaccharide (LPS) (1). Activation of glial cells may lead to neuronal cell death. Activation of nicotinic α7 receptors (α7nAChR) suppresses the LPS-induced reactive phenotype of microglia and astrocytes and thus counteracts the deleterious effect regarding neuronal viability (2–8).

In the periphery the efferent fibers of the Vagus nerve activate α7nAChR on effector cells and inhibit inflammation (9). In the brain, fibers arising from the Nucleus tractus solitarii spread into both hemispheres and their activation may lead to a widespread central anti-inflammatory effect (5, 10, 11). It is currently insufficiently tested if this is also true for the fetal brain.

In a previous experiment we investigated the effect of α7nAChR stimulation on LPS-induced microglia-activation in a double hit model of sheep fetal microglia. In the current experiment, we extended this investigation to study the role of α7nAChR in fetal sheep astrocytes. These experiments may help to shed light on neurodevelopmental disorders such as autism spectrum disorder (ASD) or schizophrenia, that are thought to involve neuroinflammation during the fetal period (12, 13).

We hypothesized that (1) under exposure to LPS, α7nAChR agonist stimulation in fetal astrocytes augments their neuroprotective profile, while the inhibition reduces it; (2) a LPS double-hit (first *in vivo*, then *in vitro*) on astrocytes exacerbates these effects similar to microglia as demonstrated before. Using an *in vivo*—*in vitro* fetal sheep model (14), we validate these hypotheses via RNASeq analysis in primary fetal astrocyte cultures exposed to LPS in the presence of a selective α7nAChR agonist or antagonist. We compare these findings to the previously published results in identically conducted microglia experiments (3, 15).

METHODS

Study Approval

This study was carried out in strict accordance with the recommendations in the Guide for the Care and Use of Laboratory Animals of the National Institutes of Health. The respective *in vivo* and *in vitro* protocols were approved by the Committee on the Ethics of Animal Experiments of the Université de Montréal (Permit Number: 10-Rech-1560).

Anesthesia and Surgical Procedure

The detailed protocol has been presented elsewhere (3). Briefly, we instrumented pregnant time-dated ewes at 126 days of gestation (dGA, ~0.86 gestation) with arterial, venous and amniotic catheters and ECG electrodes. Ovine singleton fetuses of mixed breed were surgically instrumented with sterile technique under general anesthesia (both ewe and fetus). In case of twin pregnancy the larger fetus was chosen based on palpating and estimating the intertemporal diameter. The total duration of the procedure was approximately 2 h. Antibiotics were administered to the mother intravenously (trimethoprim sulfadoxine 5 mg/kg body weight) as well as to the fetus intravenously and into the amniotic cavity (ampicillin 250 mg). Amniotic fluid lost during surgery was replaced with warm saline. The catheters exteriorized through the maternal flank were secured to the back of the ewe in a plastic pouch. For the duration of the experiment the ewe was returned to a metabolic cage, where she could stand, lie and eat *ad libitum* while we monitored the non-anesthetized fetus without sedating the mother. During postoperative recovery antibiotic administration was continued for 3 days. Arterial blood was sampled for evaluation of maternal and fetal condition and catheters were flushed with heparinized saline to maintain patency.

In vivo Experimental Protocol

Postoperatively, all animals were allowed 3 days to recover before starting the experiments. On these 3 days, at 9.00 am 3 mL arterial plasma sample were taken for blood gasses and cytokine analysis. Each experiment commenced at 9.00 am with a 1 h baseline measurement followed by the respective intervention as outlined below. FHR and arterial blood pressure were monitored continuously (CED, Cambridge, UK, and NeuroLog, Digitimer, Hertfordshire, UK). Blood samples (3 mL) were taken for arterial blood gases, lactate, glucose, and base excess (ABL800Flex, Radiometer) and cytokines at the time points 0 (baseline), +1 (i.e., after LPS administration), +3, +6, +24, +48, and +54 h (i.e., before sacrifice at day 3). For the cytokine analysis, plasma was spun at 4°C (4 min, 4,000 g, Eppendorf 5804R, Mississauga, ON), decanted and stored at −80°C for subsequent ELISAs. After the +54 h (Day 3) sampling, the animals were sacrificed with an overdose of barbiturate (30 mg pentobarbital sodium, Fatal-Plus; Vortech Pharmaceuticals, Dearborn, MI) and a post mortem was carried out during which fetal gender and weight were determined. The fetal brain was then perfusion-fixed with 250 mL of cold saline followed by 250 mL of 4% paraformaldehyde and processed for histochemical analysis or dissected for cell culture (details see *in vitro* astrocytes culture paragraph). Fetal growth was assessed by body, brain, liver, and maternal weights.

Astrocytes Isolation and Purification

Briefly, fetal sheep brain tissues were obtained during sheep necropsy after completion of the *in vivo* experiment to conduct the *in vitro* study (**Figure 1**). In the *in vivo* experiments, three *in utero* instrumented fetal sheep were treated intravenously with LPS (400 ng/fetus/day) derived from *E. coli* (Sigma Cat. no L5293, *E. coli* O111:B4, ready-made stock solution at a concentration of 1 mg/ml) on experimental days 1 and 2 at 10:00 am to mimic high levels of endotoxin in fetal circulation (so-called first LPS exposure or first hit). Three *in utero* instrumented fetal sheep were used as control receiving sterile saline. The instrumented fetuses were referred to as primary fetuses. In case of twins, twin fetuses were not instrumented, and their brains directly used for subsequent cell culture. Fetuses not exposed to LPS, either primary or twins, were designated "naïve" (no LPS exposure *in vivo*). Instrumented animals that received LPS *in vivo* were used for second hit LPS exposure *in vitro*.

Astrocytes are the major adherent cell population in flask. Astrocytes were purified by passage into a new T75 flask for 4–5 times before any manipulations and treatments. After floating microglia collection, the adherent cells were detached by trypsinization (Trypsine 0.25% + EDTA 0.1%, Wisent Cat. No 325-043-EL) and re-plated into a new flask. Cells were cultured for another 7 days with 10% ready-to-use medium [DMEM plus 1% penicillin/streptomycin, 1% glutamine, in addition with 10% heat-inactivated fetal bovine serum (Gibco, Canada Origin)]. The cell passage procedure took 4–5 weeks until purified astrocytes could be used for the *in vitro* experiment. The cell culture conditions were 37°C, 5% CO_2.

Pure astrocytes were plated into a 24-well plate at 1×10^5 cells/mL with 10% DMEM for another 7 days, and then treated with LPS or saline for 6 h.

Cell-conditioned media were collected for cytokine analysis. To verify astrocytes purity, a portion of cells was plated into Lab-Tek 8 well chamber glass slide (Thermo Scientific) for immunocytochemistry (ICC) analysis. Glial fibrillary acidic protein (GFAP) was used as an astrocyte marker; cells were counterstained with Hoechst (15).

Astrocyte Cell Culture and Treatment

Prior to exposure to LPS (Sigma Cat. no L5024, *E. coli* O127:B8) at a concentration of 100 ng/ul, cells were pretreated for 1 h with either 10 nM AR-R17779 hydrochloride (Tocris Bioscience Cat# 3964), a selective α7nAChR agonist, or 100 nM α-Bungarotoxin (Tocris Bioscience Cat# 2133), a selective α7nAChR antagonist. Optimal dose of AR-R17779 (A) or α-Bungarotoxin (B) was chosen based on a dose-response experiment with LPS. We have tested 0, 10, 100, and 1,000 nM of α-Bungarotoxin and 0, 1, 10, and 100 nM of AR-R17779 in the absence or presence of 100 ng/ul LPS, and measured IL-1β concentrations in cultured media as the endpoint. The 100 nM α-Bungarotoxin and 10 nM AR-R17779 were chosen because the cells responded in a linear range as indicated by IL-1β production.

AR-R17779 was reconstituted in DMSO as stock solution, serial dilutions were made to prepare the working stock; to obtain 10 nM AR-R17779 in concentration per well, 5 ul working stock was added well by well containing 500 ul media; only DMSO was added in control well, therefore, the DMSO concentration per well was 1%. α-Bungarotoxin was reconstituted with culture media into a stock solution and underwent serial dilutions.

In a complete cell culture experiment, we had four experimental groups: Control (naïve control), LPS100 (naïve LPS), LPS100+B100 (naïve LPS+B) and LPS100+A10 (naïve LPS+A). Second hit cell cultures were designed with the same pattern and divided into four experimental groups: Control (SHC), LPS100, LPS100+B100 and LPS100+A10.

Measurement of the Cytokine IL-1β in Cell Culture Media

The approach is described elsewhere (14, 16). Briefly, IL-1β concentrations in cell culture media was determined by using an ovine-specific sandwich ELISA. Ninety-six-well plates were pre-coated with the mouse anti sheep monoclonal antibodies (IL-1β, MCA1658, Bio Rad AbD Serotec) at a concentration of 4 μg/ml on an ELISA plate at 4°C overnight. After 3 times wash with washing buffer (0.05% Tween 20 in PBS, PBST), plates were blocked for 1h with 1% BSA in PBST for plasma samples or 10% FBS for cell culture media. Recombinant sheep proteins (IL-1β, Protein Express Cat. no 968-405) were used as ELISA standard. All standards and samples were run in duplicate (50μl per well). Rabbit anti-sheep polyclonal antibodies (IL-1β, AHP423, Bio Rad AbD Serotec) at a concentration of 4 μg/ml were applied in wells and incubated for 30 min at room temperature. Plates were washed with washing buffer for 5–7 times between each step. Detection was accomplished by assessing the conjugated enzyme activity (goat anti-rabbit IgG-HRP, dilution 1:5000, Jackson ImmunoResearch, Cat. No 111-035-144) via incubation with TMB substrate solution (BD OptEIA TMB substrate Reagent Set, BD Biosciences Cat. No 555214); color development reaction was stopped with 2N sulphuric acid. Plates were read on an ELISA plate reader at 450 nm, with 570 nm wavelength correction (EnVision 2104 Multilabel Reader, Perkin Elmer). The sensitivity of IL-1β ELISA was 41.3 pg/ml. The intra-assay and inter-assay coefficients of variance were <5 and <10%, respectively.

RNAseq Approach

Nine replicates of astrocyte culture were studied, with one control and three treatment groups (Ctrl, LPS100, LPS+A10, LPS+B100) per replicate. Four replicates were used for RNAseq based on the RNA quality, of which 3 replicates of naive, one replicate of second-hit, with one treatment missing in this second-hit replicate (agonist treatment), fifteen samples in total were assessed with RNAseq in this study (**Table 1**).

RNA Extraction and Quantification

We used Qiagen RNeasy Mini Kit (Cat no 74104) for RNA extraction. RNA quantity and quality (RNA integrity number, RIN) was established by using a RNA Nano Chip (Agilent

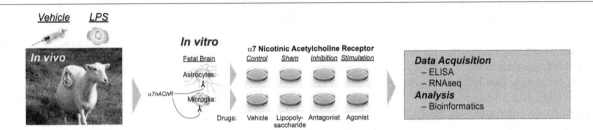

FIGURE 1 | Experimental design of modulating glial α7nAChR signaling in a double-hit fetal sheep model. *In vivo, in vitro*, and RNAseq experiments are illustrated. *In vivo* study includes Control (saline) or LPS-exposed sheep fetuses. LPS was administered intravenously to the instrumented fetus at 400 ng/fetus/day for two consecutive days 24 h apart, so-called first hit, inducing fetal inflammatory response with rising IL-6, but without cardiovascular component. For the *in vitro* study, cultured cells (microglia or astrocytes) were derived from an *in vivo* Control animal, named Naïve, or from an *in vivo* LPS-exposed animal, named second hit (SH). There were 8 experimental groups: naïve Control (NC, vehicle *in vivo*, vehicle *in vitro*), naïve LPS (NL, sham in reference to α7nAChR manipulation), naïve exposed to α-Bungarotoxin (NB, i.e., α7nAChR inhibition, preincubated followed by LPS exposure), naïve exposed to AR-R17779 (NA, i.e., α7nAChR stimulation, preincubated followed by LPS exposure), and each respective second-hit groups (SH, LPS *in vivo*). Reproduced with permission (16).

TABLE 1 | Sample inventory for RNAseq study in astrocytes samples.

Biological replicates	Serial#	Sample	Treatment	LPS hit number
Naïve R1	1	4414T1	Ctrl	0
	2	4414T1	LPS100	1
	3	4414T1	LPS100+B100	1
	4	4414T1	LPS100+A10	1
Naïve R2	5	4414T2	Ctrl	0
	6	4414T2	LPS100	1
	7	4414T2	LPS100+B100	1
	8	4414T2	LPS100+A10	1
Naïve R3	9	4502P	Ctrl	0
	10	4502P	LPS100	1
	11	4502P	LPS100+B100	1
	12	4502P	LPS100+A10	1
Second hit R1	13	711P	Ctrl	1
	14	711P	LPS100	2
	15	711P	LPS100+B100	2

Four replicates were used for RNAseq, with one control and three treatment groups (Ctrl, LPS100, LPS100+A10, LPS100+B100) per replicate. There were 3 replicates of naïve, one replicate of second-hit, with one treatment missing in this second-hit replicate (second-hit + Agonist). fifteen samples in total were assessed with RNAseq in this study. The instrumented fetuses were designated as primary fetus, identified as animal ID+P (stands for primary), whereas animal ID+T stands for non-instrumented twins.

RNA 6000 Nano Chips) with Agilent 2,100 BioAnalyzer. All samples had an acceptable RIN value ranging from 8.4 to 9.6. A total of 12 naïve astrocyte cultures from four sets of replicates was selected for RNA sequencing at high throughput, as well as three second hit astrocyte cultures (**Table 1**).

RNAseq libraries were prepared using the TruSeq stranded mRNA kit (Illumina cat #20020594) and quality control was performed on the Agilent TapeStation and using the KAPA SYBRFAST qPCR kit (Kapa Biosystems, Roche). Single read 100-bp sequencing was performed in rapid mode on a HiSeq 2,500 (Illumina Inc.) at the University of Washington Northwest Clinical Genomics Lab (Department of Pathology).

RNAseq Data Analyses

Astrocytes

The goal for this analysis was to compare the single hit LPS treated samples to Control, as well as making comparisons between the LPS treated samples (e.g., testing for changes due to the additional agonist or antagonist pre-treatment). The second hit samples had no replicates, so we could only make the directed comparisons between the single and second hit samples. For example, comparing the single and second hit LPS treated samples, as before (3).

We aligned the reads to the Oar_v3.1 transcriptome using the salmon aligner (17), which infers the most likely transcript for each read using a quasi-mapping algorithm. We then "collapsed" the transcript read counts to the gene level by summing up the reads for each gene's transcripts, using the Bioconductor tximport package (18). In the end, we had a set of read counts per gene, for each sample.

Four replicates were used for RNAseq, with one control and three treatment groups Ctrl, LPS, LPS+A10, LPS+B100) per replicate. There were 3 replicates of naïve, one replicate of second-hit, with one treatment missing in this second-hit replicate (second-hit + agonist, SHA), fifteen samples in total were assessed with RNAseq in this study (**Table 1**). The instrumented fetuses were designated as primary fetus, identified as animal ID+P (stands for primary), whereas animal ID+T stands for non-instrumented twins.

To compare astrocytes transcriptomes, we used the Bioconductor edgeR package (19), to fit a generalized linear model with a negative binomial link function, and made comparisons between groups using quasi-likelihood F-tests.

We fitted the model described above, including the treatment effect for each animal, and made the comparisons, incorporating a fold change criterion into the test. In other words, the conventional test for a difference is between the null hypothesis $H_0: \beta = 0$ vs. the alternative hypothesis $H_A: \beta \neq 0$, but this may include very small changes that are likely to be biologically meaningless. One alternative to exclude such genes is to use a *post hoc* fold change adjustment, where we select genes based on the observed fold change between groups. This is problematic because we ignore the imprecision in our estimate of fold change.

A better method is to incorporate the fold change into our inference, where we test $H_0 : \beta \leq |c|$ against the alternative $H_A : \beta \geq |c|$, for some constant fold change. By doing this, we are testing to see if we have evidence that the underlying population differences are larger than a given fold change, rather than simply testing that our sample data fulfill those criteria. We used a 1.5-fold change, and a false discovery rate (FDR) of 0.05 as criteria to define significantly differentially expressed genes, meaning that we expect that there are, at most, 5% false positives in our set of significant genes.

Microglia—Astrocytes Transcriptome Comparisons

We also made comparisons to the existing RNAseq data that our lab generated using primary cultures of fetal sheep microglia from the identical experimental design in three biological replicates. This data has been published and the data set is accessible online (14).

We downloaded the FASTQ data from SRA and processed using the same salmon/tximport pipeline we used for the astrocyte samples. The only difference was in the modeling step, where we converted the count data to log counts/million and estimated observation-level weights using the limma voom function. We also computed sample-specific weights that are intended to down-weight any samples that are not very similar to other samples of the same type. We then fit a conventional weighted linear model and made empirical Bayes adjusted contrasts between various groups. By incorporating sample-specific weights we were able to account for a single sample (LPS100 treated animal 4414T), which had significantly fewer reads, perhaps due to some technical problems.

Venn Diagrams

We sought to learn which genes are unique to a given comparison, and which are shared between two or more of those comparisons. Thus, we generated Venn diagrams for three sets of comparisons. We made a Venn diagram for the three comparisons of treated vs. control, a two-way Venn diagram of the agonist + LPS vs. either LPS alone or LPS plus antagonist (this shows that there is very little difference between LPS and LPS plus antagonist), and finally we made a Venn diagram of the one-hit vs. two-hit for all three treatments. The genes in any intersection between comparisons had to be significantly differentially expressed in both (or all three, depending on the intersection) of the comparisons. In addition, the direction of change had to be the same as well. For example, if a given gene was differentially expressed in LPS100 vs. control and LPS100+A10 vs. control, and it is either up or down-regulated in both comparisons as well, then it was listed in the intersection between those two comparisons. If it was significant in both comparisons, but was up-regulated in one comparison, but down-regulated in the other, then it was listed in the unique portion of the Venn diagram for each comparison.

Statistical Analyses and Data Repository

Generalized estimating equations (GEE) modeling approach was used to assess the effects of LPS and drug treatments on IL-1β. We used a linear scale response model with LPS/drug treatment

TABLE 2 | Astrocytes IL-1β secretion expressed as absolute values* in pg/ml (median and 25–75%).

LPS exposure	Ctrl	LPS	B100	A10
Single hit	1 (1,25)	429 (358,1034)	336 (285,928)	750 (439,1495)
Second hit	1 (1,1)	16 (15,16)	20 (17,22)	99 (95, 103)

*Values set to 1 where no signal was detected by the cytokine assay to compute fold-changes for **Figure 2**.

group (main term "treatment") and presence or absence of second hit exposure (main term "hit") as predicting factors to assess their interactions using maximum likelihood estimate and Type III analysis with Wald Chi-square statistic. SPSS Version 25 was used for these analyses (IBM SPSS Statistics, IBM Corporation, Armonk, NY). Significance was assumed for $p < 0.05$. Results are provided as median {25–75} percentiles. Not all measurements were obtained for each animal studied, as indicated.

Ingenuity Pathway Analysis (IPA, Qiagen, 2019) was used for identification of signaling pathways unique to each treatment.

The raw RNAseq data has been deposited under GEO accession number *GSE123713*. The analytical pipeline to allow reproduction of this analysis, in the form of a Rmarkdown document, will be made available upon request. Statistics from all comparisons (t-statistics, log fold changes, FDR values, dynamically linked Venn diagrams) can be found in supplemental document under the doi: 10.5281/zenodo.2609202.

RESULTS AND DISCUSSION
Cytokine Secretion Profile

The fetal *in vivo* exposure to LPS resulted in a rise of IL-6 as reported (14, 16).

The absolute values of IL-1β produced by naive (first hit) and second hit astrocytes at baseline, under LPS exposure and with preceding agonist or antagonist incubation are presented in **Table 2**. As reported, LPS treatment induced IL-1β increase in astrocytes (14). There was no difference in first and second hit astrocytes at baseline or when exposed to LPS alone. Our focus here was on the effect of α7nAChR modulation on LPS-triggered IL-1β production. Consequently, we expressed the data as fold-changes compared to sham treatment (LPS, **Figure 2**, LEFT). We present the response of primary microglia cultures side-by-side (**Figure 2**, RIGHT) in form of re-analysis of previously published data (3).

For astrocytes, the main terms "hit" and "treatment" as well as their interaction were significant (all p<0.001). Agonistic stimulation of the α7nAChR appeared, surprisingly, to result in a relative increase of IL-1β concentration, further potentiated in second hit astrocytes. This effect was absent in first hit astrocytes cultures treated with the α7nAChR antagonist and less pronounced but present in the second hit cultures.

For microglia, the main terms "hit" and "treatment" were not significant ($p = 0.716$ and $p = 0.666$, respectively), but their interaction was significant [$p = 0.026$, cf. Figure 1 in (3)].

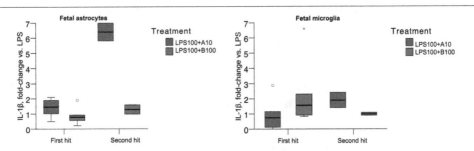

FIGURE 2 | (Left) IL-1β secretion in ovine primary astrocyte cultures in response to 6 h LPS exposure without or with pre-incubation with α7nAChR antagonist (B100) or agonist (A10) for 1 h. Single hit, *in vitro* only LPS exposure; second hit, *in vivo* systemic and subsequent *in vitro* LPS exposure 4 to 5 weeks later. Y axis shows fold changes in IL-1β in relation to the levels of sham treatment (LPS). Generalized estimating equations (GEE) modeling results are presented in text and no significance marks are provided in the figure. For both box plots, an asterisk represents an extreme outlier (a value more than 3 times the interquartile range from a quartile). A circle marks outlier with values between 1.5 and 3 box lengths from the upper or lower edge of the box. Briefly, we found significant main term effects ($p = 0.019$) "treatment" (LPS and α7nAChR drug) as well as main term "hit" ($p = 0.010$), i.e., the contribution of *in vivo* LPS exposure, the second hit effect on the IL-1β secretion profile. Results are provided as median {25–75} percentiles. **(Right)** Identical experimental results from microglia studies are presented for comparison. The main terms "hit" and "treatment" were not significant ($p = 0.716$ and $p = 0.666$, respectively), but their interaction was significant ($p = 0.026$, cf. Figure 1 in (3) where the original results have been published.

The overall pattern of IL-1β levels in response to LPS exposure with prior α7nAChR stimulation was inverted in astrocytes compared to microglia. In astrocytes, both first hit and second hit cell cultures responded under inhibition of α7nAChR with relative decrease of IL-1β production. In microglia, in contrast, first hit (naive) cultures behaved intuitively under the same conditions, showing a rise in IL-1β production. However, second hit microglia cultures, similar to second hit astrocytes, showed a drop in IL-1β production with α7nAChR inhibition. In contrast again, agonistic α7nAChR stimulation in both second hit glia cultures resulted in higher than first hit IL-1β production, albeit, the magnitude of this rise was ∼3.5-fold larger in astrocytes suggesting differences in sensitization of these glia cells to previous LPS exposure *in utero*. These counter-intuitive findings of α7nAChR stimulation in astrocytes on the individual IL-1β secretion stand in contrast to the transcriptome-level findings we discuss below. We attempt to tie together these results in the general discussion section.

Whole Transcriptome Analysis

Mapped reads aligned to any transcript from the Oar_v3.1 transcriptome at 66% which is good. Principal component analysis (PCA) showed large differences between the different treatment groups, and much smaller differences within each group, indicating that we have a good signal with likely many differentially expressed genes (DEG) to be found (**Figure 3**).

We present in **Table 3** the number of genes for each comparison as well as the top ten signaling pathways IPA identified. The results of the analysis on the entire data set are also accessible with search function via this repository.

PCA showed two transcriptome clusters (**Figure 3**):

1) Control, LPS single-hit and second-hit astrocytes pre-treated with α7nAChR agonist and

2) LPS single-hit and second-hit astrocytes pre-treated with α7nAChR antagonist.

That is, a pro-inflammatory transcriptome astrocyte phenotype acquired *in vivo* or *in vitro* by LPS stimulation is reversed

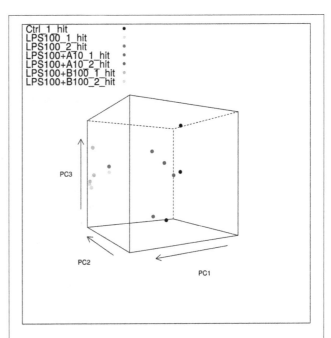

FIGURE 3 | Static 3D plot of the astrocyte RNAseq data with single and double-hit LPS treatment. The angle of the plot was chosen to give the best viewpoint to show differences between the sample types. Note that controls and α7nAChR agonistically pre-treated astrocytes cluster together and separately from those exposed to LPS w/o or with antagonistic α7nAChR pre-treatment. Note here that there are three of the LPS_100_1_hit samples in the plot shown in this figure; it just so happens that the third sample is obscured by the uppermost LPS+B100_1_hit sample.

with α7nAChR agonistic stimulation. Conversely, α7nAChR inhibition potentiates the pro-inflammatory astrocytic phenotype. The PCA level observations are substantiated further by the IPA analysis of key signaling pathways presented in **Table 3**. The visualization of the up or down regulation of the implicated pathways can be accessed on GitHub in its entirety. Here we focus on some key findings in top 10 signaling pathways.

TABLE 3 | Ingenuity Pathway Analysis of differentially expressed genes from the fetal sheep astrocytes whole transcriptome analysis: naïve and second hit astrocytes after modulation of α7nAChR signaling.

comparison	# genes	Top 10 signaling pathways	-log(p-value)
Single hit: LPS100 vs. Control	1835	NF-κB Signaling	15.8
		Role of Pattern Recognition Receptors in Recognition of Bacteria & Viruses	14
		Role of Macrophages, Fibroblasts and Endothelial Cells in Rheumatoid Arthritis	13.7
		Dendritic Cell Maturation	13
		Neuroinflammation Signaling Pathway	12.8
		Role of IL-17A in Arthritis	12.2
		Activation of IRF by Cytosolic Pattern Recognition Receptors	11.6
		Death Receptor Signaling	11.3
		Th1 and Th2 Activation Pathway	10.7
		TREM1 Signaling	10.5
Single hit: LPS100+A10 vs. Control	1725	**NF-κB Signaling**	14.7
		Role of Macrophages, Fibroblasts and Endothelial Cells in Rheumatoid Arthritis	13.7
		Role of Osteoblasts, Osteoclasts and Chondrocytes in Rheumatoid Arthritis	13.1
		Granulocyte Adhesion and Diapedesis	12.7
		Role of Pattern Recognition Receptors in Recognition of Bacteria and Viruses	12.5
		Hepatic Cholestasis	12.5
		Toll-like Receptor Signaling	11.7
		Axonal Guidance Signaling	11.5
		IL-10 Signaling	11.1
		Neuroinflammation Signaling Pathway	10.7
Single hit: LPS100+B100 vs. Control	1744	NF-κB Signaling	16.8
		Role of Macrophages, Fibroblasts and Endothelial Cells in Rheumatoid Arthritis	16
		Dendritic Cell Maturation	15.9
		Neuroinflammation Signaling Pathway	15
		Role of Pattern Recognition Receptors in Recognition of Bacteria & Viruses	14.8
		TREM1 Signaling	12.8
		Role of IL-17A in Arthritis	12.7
		T Cell Exhaustion Signaling Pathway	11.9
		Toll-like Receptor Signaling	11.8
		PI3K Signaling in B Lymphocytes	11.6
Single hit: LPS100+A10 vs. LPS100	273	Granulocyte Adhesion and Diapedesis	6.23
		Pathogenesis of Multiple Sclerosis	5.81
		Agranulocyte Adhesion and Diapedesis	5.12
		Th1 and Th2 Activation Pathway	4.45
		Th2 Pathway	4.4
		LPS/IL-1 Mediated Inhibition of RXR Function	3.81
		NF-κB Signaling	3.71
		Role of Osteoblasts, Osteoclasts and Chondrocytes in Rheumatoid Arthritis	3.63
		Inhibition of Angiogenesis by TSP1	3.33
		STAT3 Pathway	3.25
Single hit: LPS100+B100 vs. LPS100	0		
Single hit: LPS100+A10 vs. LPS100+B100	292	Granulocyte Adhesion and Diapedesis	5.25
		Agranulocyte Adhesion and Diapedesis	4.99
		LPS/IL-1 Mediated Inhibition of RXR Function	4.38
		Hepatic Fibrosis / Hepatic Stellate Cell Activation	4.35
		NF-κB Signaling	4.33
		Role of Osteoblasts, Osteoclasts and Chondrocytes in Rheumatoid Arthritis	4.18
		Pathogenesis of Multiple Sclerosis	3.97
		STAT3 Pathway	3.94
		p53 Signaling	3.57
		Sirtuin Signaling Pathway	3.36

(Continued)

TABLE 3 | Continued

comparison	# genes	Top 10 signaling pathways	-log(p-value)
LPS100: single hit vs. second hit	3761	Hepatic Fibrosis / Hepatic Stellate Cell Activation	10.7
		Fcγ Receptor-mediated Phagocytosis in Macrophages and Monocytes	7.69
		Leukocyte Extravasation Signaling	6.82
		Signaling by Rho Family GTPases	6.16
		Iron homeostasis signaling pathway	6.02
		LXR/RXR Activation	5.36
		Epithelial Adherens Junction Signaling	4.99
		Role of Osteoblasts, Osteoclasts and Chondrocytes in Rheumatoid Arthritis	4.96
		Axonal Guidance Signaling	4.91
		Tec Kinase Signaling	4.82
LPS100+A10: single hit vs. second hit	3307	Hepatic Fibrosis / Hepatic Stellate Cell Activation	13
		Leukocyte Extravasation Signaling	8.79
		Neuroinflammation Signaling Pathway	7.18
		Fcγ Receptor-mediated Phagocytosis in Macrophages and Monocytes	6.99
		Axonal Guidance Signaling	6.93
		Phagosome Formation	6.85
		Role of Pattern Recognition Receptors in Recognition of Bacteria and Viruses	6.67
		Agranulocyte Adhesion and Diapedesis	6.24
		GP6 Signaling Pathway	6.1
		Granulocyte Adhesion and Diapedesis	5.92
LPS100+B100: single hit vs. second hit	3860	Hepatic Fibrosis / Hepatic Stellate Cell Activation	8.89
		Fcγ Receptor-mediated Phagocytosis in Macrophages and Monocytes	8.03
		Leukocyte Extravasation Signaling	7.26
		Epithelial Adherens Junction Signaling	5.94
		Iron homeostasis signaling pathway	5.78
		Signaling by Rho Family GTPases	5.51
		Axonal Guidance Signaling	5.18
		Endothelin-1 Signaling	5.04
		Role of Macrophages, Fibroblasts and Endothelial Cells in Rheumatoid Arthritis	5.01
		Phagosome Formation	4.99

Differential analysis of count data was done with the Bioconductor limma package. Differentially expressed genes were selected, based on a 1.5-fold change and an FDR < 0.05. Up regulation and down regulation represent positive and negative log2 fold changes, respectively. For details on "raw gene" level, see our GitHub repository or directly here. Bold font highlights pathways common with microglia.
Orange: positive z-score; blue: negative z-score. For further details as raw data and visualized activity patterns see GitHub.
Significant genes in astrocytes cultures at an FDR < 0.05 and a 1.5-fold change sorted on log(p-value).

LPS treatment triggered activation of pro-inflammatory signaling pathways NF-κB and neuroinflammation. Compared to LPS exposure alone, pretreatment with α7nAChR agonist reversed both signaling pathways activation. Conversely, pretreatment with α7nAChR antagonist up regulated these pro-inflammatory pathways. Albeit the pattern overall was similar to the effect of LPS alone, activation of these signaling pathways under α7nAChR blockade stood out: Toll-like receptor signaling and PI3K signaling. Direct comparison of α7nAChR agonistic stimulation or inhibition yielded reduced activity of NF-κB and STAT3 pathways due to activation of α7nAChR, consistent with the expected intracellular anti-inflammatory effect of α7nAChR agonism. Another notable pathway activated in α7nAChR agonistically treated astrocytes was the Sirtuin signaling. Activation of this pathway in neurons and astrocytes has been implicated in AMPK-dependent neuroprotection from ischemic stroke (20, 21). Adenosine monophosphate kinase (AMPK) is a rapid key regulator of neuronal energy homeostasis implicated in fetal neuroinflammation (22).

The second half of **Table 3** documents some effects of astrocytes memory of LPS exposure *in vivo* when re-exposed *in vitro* (second hit effect). For comparison to microglial activity, see **Table 4**. Notably, we found a perturbation of the iron homeostasis signaling pathway in second hit LPS treated astrocytes which persisted under pre-treatment with α7nAChR antagonist but was reversed with α7nAChR agonist. Similar to our finding of second hit signature in microglia, here we observed hemoxygenase (HMOX)1 gene down regulation in second hit astrocytes compared to first hit cultures (3, 15). HMOX1 is a key gene of iron homeostasis. We observed a similar phenomenon in second hit fetal microglia compared to single hit microglia (15).

Together, observations on Sirtuin and iron homeostasis signaling reinforce the previously reported dual role of energy

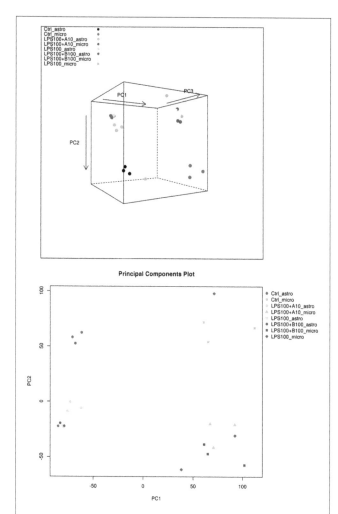

Principal Components Plot

FIGURE 4 | (Top) PCA plot of microglia and astrocyte samples. Here we can see that astrocytes and microglia separate on the first principal component, and the second principal component captures the LPS treatment differences. The third principal component captures some intra-treatment variability for the microglia samples, particularly for one of the LPS treated microglia samples. **(Bottom)** PCA plot of microglia and astrocyte samples, showing just the first two principal components. The largest differences appear to be between the cell types.

metabolism in determining inflammatory phenotype in glia cells (3, 15).

Based on the IPA analysis within the *Venn* diagrams, the top down-regulated signaling pathway unique to LPS treatment was Ephrin A signaling [log(*p*-value) 3.21, **Table 5**]. Analysis of genes unique to α7nAChR agonist treatment showed a reduction of this down-regulation [log(*p*-value)1.58, **Table 5**]. Analysis of genes unique to α7nAChR antagonist treatment had no significant effect on this signaling pathway (**Table 5**). Ephrin signaling has been implicated in neuroprotective astrocyte phenotype (23). Our findings suggest a neuroprotective effect of α7nAChR agonism on ephrin signaling pathway.

Consistent with the notion of cholinergic signaling involved in stress axis regulation (3), POMC was the second (by IPA ranking)

highest up-regulated gene under cholinergic agonist treatment, with a log ratio of 3.388 (Cf. GitHub repository).

Comparison to Fetal Sheep Microglial Transcriptome

PCA in **Figure 4** (top) shows that the main differences between astrocytes and microglia RNAseq data are captured on the first two principal components, so a 2D plot may be more useful (**Figure 4**, bottom). The intra-group variability is smaller for the astrocytes compared to the microglia. This may have to do with the total library sizes: there were several microglia samples with very few reads that aligned to any known transcript.

We compared the IPA-identified top signaling pathways in microglia and astrocytes under the LPS and α7nAChR signaling manipulation. **Table 4** presents the number of genes for each comparison and the corresponding findings of the IPA signaling pathway analysis. Overall, the response patterns to LPS and modulation of α7nAChR signaling were similar between the two glia cell types. The signaling pathways common to both astrocytes and microglia are bolded in **Tables 3**, **4**. Intuitively, common pathways activated due to LPS included neuroinflammation signaling and NF-κB signaling in some, but not all comparisons. However, overall, the overlap on the level of signaling pathway was rather minimal which may explain the strong separation by cell type on PCA. It is remarkable that astrocytes, not microglia— the primary immune cells of the brain, were characterized by unique inhibition patterns of STAT3 pathway due to agonistic stimulation of α7nAChR prior to LPS exposure.

The presented astrocytes—microglia comparison has limitations. The differences between the two cell types may be exaggerated by the inevitable technical differences (e.g., reagents). However, all these experiments were run from the same cohort, same animals (in some cases), at adjacent times and by the same people.

Do Fetal Neuroinflammation and Stress Mediate an Increased Risk for Autism Spectrum Disorder?

LPS effects on key genes involved in stress axis activity raised the question about the poorly understood role of astrocytes in the signaling pathways of neuroinflammation and prenatal stress (PS) (24).

Indeed, PS is accompanied by inflammation in the mother and offspring (24–29). Both, PS and fetal neuroinflammation have been implicated in the etiology of ASD (30, 31). PS increases expression of glutamate (Glu) transporter vGluT1 (SLC17A7) resulting in higher levels of GLT1 (32, 33).

Here, we sought to verify if the exposure of fetal astrocytes to LPS induces upregulation of Glu transporters in glia akin to PS (32, 33).

Given the known relationship between PS and VGLUT1 expression, we used IPA to annotate VGLUT1 gene network with our findings to test for evidence that the network is being perturbed by LPS treatment. Across all treatment comparisons, two DEGs were identified in astrocytes (common to all comparisons): JAK2 (2.732 (log ratio) upregulated, FDR

TABLE 4 | Ingenuity Pathway Analysis of differentially expressed genes from the fetal sheep microglia whole transcriptomes analysis.

Comparison	# genes	Top 10 signaling pathways	-log(p-value)
LPS100 vs. Control	1779	**Role of Macrophages, Fibroblasts and Endothelial Cells in Rheumatoid Arthritis**	16.7
		Dendritic Cell Maturation	12.9
		iNOS Signaling	12.6
		Role of IL-17A in Arthritis	12.5
		IL-10 Signaling	11.8
		Role of Tissue Factor in Cancer	11.6
		Production of Nitric Oxide and Reactive Oxygen Species in Macrophages	11.1
		Neuroinflammation Signaling Pathway	10.9
		Toll-like Receptor Signaling	10.7
		CD40 Signaling	10
LPS100+A10 vs. Control	4721	Molecular Mechanisms of Cancer	14.1
		Colorectal Cancer Metastasis Signaling	11.2
		Toll-like Receptor Signaling	11
		NF-κB Signaling	10.6
		Role of Macrophages, Fibroblasts and Endothelial Cells in Rheumatoid Arthritis	10.4
		PI3K Signaling in B Lymphocytes	10.4
		Role of Tissue Factor in Cancer	10.3
		B Cell Receptor Signaling	9.83
		TREM1 Signaling	7.83
		Protein Kinase A Signaling	7.81
LPS100+B100 vs. Control	4049	**Role of Macrophages, Fibroblasts and Endothelial Cells in Rheumatoid Arthritis**	13.6
		PI3K Signaling in B Lymphocytes	11.4
		Production of Nitric Oxide and Reactive Oxygen Species in Macrophages	10.2
		Molecular Mechanisms of Cancer	10.2
		Activation of IRF by Cytosolic Pattern Recognition Receptors	10.2
		IL-10 Signaling	9.63
		B Cell Receptor Signaling	9.55
		iNOS Signaling	9.21
		Role of Tissue Factor in Cancer	9.06
		Toll-like Receptor Signaling	8.93
LPS100+A10 vs. LPS100	8		
LPS100+B100 vs. LPS100	0		
LPS100+A10 vs. LPS100+B100	1132	T Cell Exhaustion Signaling Pathway	5.46
		Dendritic Cell Maturation	5.43
		Role of Macrophages, Fibroblasts and Endothelial Cells in Rheumatoid Arthritis	5.42
		Altered T Cell and B Cell Signaling in Rheumatoid Arthritis	5.22
		Th17 Activation Pathway	5.16
		Leukocyte Extravasation Signaling	4.81
		Superpathway of Cholesterol Biosynthesis	4.8
		IL-10 Signaling	4.49
		Role of Tissue Factor in Cancer	4.31
		Th1 and Th2 Activation Pathway	4.26

Differential analysis of count data was done with the Bioconductor limma package. Differentially expressed genes were selected, based on a 1.5-fold change and an FDR < 0.05. Up regulation and down regulation represent positive and negative log2 fold changes, respectively. For details on "raw gene" level, see our GitHub repository or directly here. Bold font highlights signaling pathways common with astrocytes. Orange: positive z-score; blue: negative z-score. For further details as raw data and visualized activity patterns see GitHub. Significant genes in microglia cultures at an FDR < 0.05 and a 1.5-fold change sorted on log(p-value).

3.91E-05) and SLC1A2 (2.350 upregulated, FDR 1.80E-04). JAK1 signaling is involved in glucocorticoid receptor signaling (34) and JAK1/2 signaling is involved in iron homeostasis signaling pathways(35), whereas JAK/Stat is involved in IL-6 signaling pathways. SLC1A2 is also known as GLT-1 or glial high affinity glutamate transporter; it is implicated in glutamate receptor signaling and neuroinflammation signaling pathways (36). Upregulation of glial GLT-1 in the hippocampus has been reported after chronic stress due to its control by glucocorticoids (37–39).

TABLE 5 | Genes unique to LPS, agonistic stimulation or inhibition of α7nAChR in single hit astrocytes cultures.

	Top 10 signaling pathways	-log(*p*-value)
Genes unique to LPS100	Ephrin A Signaling	3.21
	P2Y Purigenic Receptor Signaling Pathway	2.72
	Role of p14/p19ARF in Tumor Suppression	2.55
	Thiamin Salvage III	2.2
	Melanoma Signaling	2.14
	Lymphotoxin β Receptor Signaling	2.03
	CCR3 Signaling in Eosinophils	1.96
	CD40 Signaling	1.84
Genes unique to A10	Germ Cell-Sertoli Cell Junction Signaling	9.13
	Integrin Signaling	7.4
	Actin Cytoskeleton Signaling	5.84
	Leukocyte Extravasation Signaling	5.81
	Sertoli Cell-Sertoli Cell Junction Signaling	5.58
	GDP-glucose Biosynthesis	5.49
	Glucose and Glucose-1-phosphate Degradation	5.24
	Phagosome Formation	4.84
	Signaling by Rho Family GTPases	4.71
	HGF Signaling	4.6
Genes unique to B100	Apelin Cardiomyocyte Signaling Pathway	5.54
	Adrenomedullin signaling pathway	4.09
	Dendritic Cell Maturation	3.23
	Endothelin-1 Signaling	3.2
	UVA-Induced MAPK Signaling	3.2
	Renin-Angiotensin Signaling	2.97
	Role of NFAT in Cardiac Hypertrophy	2.95
	Phagosome Formation	2.95
	GP6 Signaling Pathway	2.91
	Wnt/Ca+ pathway	2.89

Again assessing the present findings together with the previously published RNAseq data from the identical experiment in ovine fetal microglia (3), we found GLT-1 to be upregulated in microglia and astrocytes regardless cholinergic manipulation (for details see GitHub repository). Albeit both pure primary cultures were exposed to LPS, we found the up regulation of JAK2 to be unique to astrocytes. This finding is conceptually in line with studies reporting brain cell-specific signaling pathways behavior in response to IL-1β (40). Much remains to be learned about the differences between second messenger signaling cascades involved in astrocytes, microglia and neurons in the developing fetal brain exposed to inflammatory stimuli. Furthermore, there is still a paucity of data about differences across the species for these signaling pathways.

General Discussion

Fetal sheep is the classic model of fetal physiology and neuroscience (41). It has been used successfully for both integrative physiological as well as genomic studies. In the present study, we expand the recently published series of experiments in the same animal model using primary microglia cultures to now include primary astrocytes cultures (3, 14–16).

Acetylcholine is synthesized by cultured microglia and astrocyte in mouse and rat (42, 43), however, there is no information from other species. It is plausible that the fetal sheep brain astrocytes in culture produce acetylcholine, because they appear to respond to α7nAChR stimulation. However, we do not know how much acetylcholine is produced, and whether or not the speculated endogenous acetylcholine can activate the α7nAChR. This remains worthwhile to investigate in future studies.

The antagonist drug for α7nAChR we used, α-bungarotoxin, is a selective inhibitor for α7 receptors acting by preventing the opening of nicotinic receptor-associated ion channels (Tocris α-bungarotoxin datasheet). By using optimized dose, we treated our astrocyte cells with α-bungarotoxin 1 h prior to LPS exposure, which would block LPS-induced cytokine production in the cells.

LPS exposure had the anticipated effect of increasing IL-1β production in astrocytes and we observed this consistently on the transcriptome level. However, our findings on protein level following pre-incubation with α7nAChR antagonist or agonist do not align with those on the transcriptome level: present results on protein level do not show a clear hypothesized effect of α7nAChR agonism or antagonism on LPS secretion in ovine fetal astrocytes. Such discordant behavior on protein and transcriptome levels has been reported and studied systematically to represent the rule rather than an exception to cellular biology in general (44).

Future studies will need to explore the protein responses in more depth and in different species to further delineate astrocytic behavior under α7nAChR stimulation, especially the peculiarly opposite effect of endotoxin memory in astrocytes and microglia on IL-1β secretion.

Microglia—astrocyte ensemble interactions need to be studied to bridge the methodological gap between *in vitro* experimental design and the *in situ* physiology. This can be done in co-cultures, feasible in ovine species, for example (14). Recent study in mice highlighted the importance of microglia—astrocyte interactions for understanding the polarization dynamics of astrocytes (45).

In an adult rodent model, cholinergic signaling reduced stress responsiveness via cortisol releasing hormone (CRH) receptor 1 with positive behavioral changes (46). We identified POMC as up regulated under α7nAChR stimulation. Considering that CRH is an upstream regulator of POMC, another question for future studies is whether we can implicate a direct interaction with the CRH receptor 1 in the developing brain.

We found that within its interaction network, GLT-1 was upregulated in microglia and astrocytes regardless of cholinergic manipulation, while the up-regulation of JAK1/2 was unique to astrocytes. This is in line with studies showing brain region specific overexpression of vGluT-1 (SLC17A7) both due to endotoxin stress and due to PS and puts the LPS exposure in the context of a more general brain stress exposure paradigm presenting with shared response patterns of neuroinflammation and metabolic adaptations in astrocytes (13, 47, 48). PS has long lasting consequences on α7nACh-ergic signaling in frontal cortex and hippocampus reducing the expression of α7nAChR protein expression in the brain of adult rats (47).

It is plausible to conclude that low grade neuroinflammation results in changes similar to those induced by PS with regard to reprogramming astrocytes to a higher glutamate uptake. As shown elsewhere (49), PS and exposure to endotoxin may act synergistically to exacerbate the impairment of neuron-glial glutamatergic interaction. For endotoxin exposure, this process is not subject to cholinergic modulation. Whether or not PS effects alone on astrocytes glutamate uptake can be ameliorated or reversed by α7nAChR agonism remains to be investigated.

The phylogenetically conserved interaction between neuroinflammation and chronic stress has been the subject of multiple studies (24), yet we are only beginning to unravel the complex web of interactions, across developmental stages, organs, cell types and species-specific differences, which connect these two phenomena. While the role of microglia in this context has been appreciated, the response of astrocytes we report here and their behavior on protein level under second hit scenario are novel observations warranting further studies in different species.

In summary, we show that genes involved in stress memory of the offspring are also impacted by LPS stress, this impact is further altered by a second hit (memory) and that such memory of LPS stress is amenable to cholinergic treatment via α7nAChR. It remains to be validated in future studies whether, when and which stimulation of the α7nAChR is favorable.

AUTHOR CONTRIBUTIONS

MCa, PB, GF, AD, and MF are responsible for conception and design. MCa, HL, MW, LD, PB, GF, AD, and MF acquired data. MCa, HL, MW, JM, MCo, MD, TB, JS, and MF did the analysis and interpretation of data. MCa, JM, MCo, TB, and MF drafted the manuscript. MCa, JM, MW, MCo, JS, MA, TB, and MF are responsible for revising it for intellectual content. MCa, JM, HL, MW, MCo, LD, PB, GF, AD, JS, MA, RB, MD, TB, and MF gave final approval of the completed manuscript.

FUNDING

Supported by grants from the Canadian Institute of Health Research (CIHR) (MF); Fonds de la recherche en santé du Québec (FRSQ) (MF) and Molly Towell Perinatal Research Foundation (MF); QTNPR (by CIHR) (LD). Supported in part by Illumina Inc.

ACKNOWLEDGMENTS

The authors thank Dr. Jack Antel lab, especially Manon Blain, and Dr. Craig Moore for invaluable assistance with the cell culture protocol, St-Hyacinthe CHUV team for technical assistance and Jan Hamanishi for graphical design. We also thank MD lab for skilful assistance with RNA samples pipeline on the Illumina platform and Lu Wang for assistance in RNAseq bioinformatics pipeline.

REFERENCES

1. Jassam YN, Izzy S, Whalen M, McGavern DB, El Khoury J. Neuroimmunology of traumatic brain injury: time for a paradigm shift. *Neuron.* (2017) 95:1246–65. doi: 10.1016/j.neuron.2017.07.010
2. Kalkman HO, Feuerbach D. Modulatory effects of α7 nAChRs on the immune system and its relevance for CNS disorders. *Cell Mol Life Sci.* (2016) 73:2511–30. doi: 10.1007/s00018-016-2175-4
3. Cortes M, Cao M, Liu HL, Moore CS, Durosier LD, Burns P, Fecteau G, et al. α7 nicotinic acetylcholine receptor signaling modulates the inflammatory phenotype of fetal brain microglia: first evidence of interference by iron homeostasis. *Sci Rep.* (2017) 7:10645. doi: 10.1038/s41598-017-09439-z
4. Kiguchi N, Kobayashi D, Saika F, Matsuzaki S, Kishioka S. Inhibition of peripheral macrophages by nicotinic acetylcholine receptor agonists suppresses spinal microglial activation and neuropathic pain in mice with peripheral nerve injury. *J Neuroinflamm.* (2018) 15:96. doi: 10.1186/s12974-018-1133-5
5. Frasch MG, Szynkaruk M, Prout AP, Nygard K, Cao M, Veldhuizen R, et al. Decreased neuroinflammation correlates to higher vagus nerve activity fluctuations in near-term ovine fetuses: a case for the afferent cholinergic anti-inflammatory pathway? *J Neuroinflamm.* (2016) 13:103. doi: 10.1186/s12974-016-0567-x
6. Han Z, Li L, Wang L, Degos V, Maze M, Su H. Alpha-7 nicotinic acetylcholine receptor agonist treatment reduces neuroinflammation, oxidative stress, and brain injury in mice with ischemic stroke and bone fracture. *J Neurochem.* (2014) 131:498–508. doi: 10.1111/jnc.12817

7. de Jonge WJ, Ulloa L. The alpha7 nicotinic acetylcholine receptor as a pharmacological target for inflammation. *Br J Pharmacol.* (2007) 151:915–29. doi: 10.1038/sj.bjp.0707264
8. Shytle RD, Mori T, Townsend K, Vendrame M, Sun N, Zeng J, Ehrhart J,et al. Cholinergic modulation of microglial activation by alpha 7 nicotinic receptors. *J Neurochem.* (2004) 89:337–43. doi: 10.1046/j.1471-4159.2004.02347.x
9. Rosas-Ballina M, Olofsson PS, Ochani M, Valdes-Ferrer SI, Levine YA, Reardon C, et al. Acetylcholine-synthesizing T cells relay neural signals in a vagus nerve circuit. *Science.* (2011) 334:98–101. doi: 10.1126/science.1209985
10. Cheyuo C, Jacob A, Wu R, Zhou M, Coppa GF, Wang P. The parasympathetic nervous system in the quest for stroke therapeutics. *J Cereb Blood Flow Metab.* (2011) 31:1187–95. doi: 10.1038/jcbfm.2011.24
11. Cao J, Lu K-H, Powley TL, Liu Z. Vagal nerve stimulation triggers widespread responses and alters large-scale functional connectivity in the rat brain. *PLoS ONE.* (2017) 12:e0189518. doi: 10.1371/journal.pone.0189518
12. al-Haddad BJS, Jacobsson B, Chabra S, Modzelewska D, Olson EM, Bernier R, et al. Long-term risk of neuropsychiatric disease after exposure to infection in utero. *JAMA Psychiatry.* (2019) doi: 10.1001/jamapsychiatry.2019.0029. [Epub ahead of print].
13. Elovitz MA, Brown AG, Breen K, Anton L, Maubert M, Burd I. Intrauterine inflammation, insufficient to induce parturition, still evokes fetal and neonatal brain injury. *Int J Dev Neurosci.* (2011) 29:663–71. doi: 10.1016/j.ijdevneu.2011.02.011
14. Cortes M, Cao M, Liu HL, Burns P, Moore C, Fecteau G, et al. RNAseq profiling of primary microglia and astrocyte cultures in near-term ovine fetus: a glial *in vivo-in vitro* multi-hit paradigm in large mammalian brain. *J Neurosci Methods.* (2017) 276:23–32. doi: 10.1016/j.jneumeth.2016.11.008

15. Cao M, Cortes M, Moore CS, Leong SY, Durosier LD, Burns P, et al. Fetal microglial phenotype in vitro carries memory of prior in vivo exposure to inflammation. *Front Cell Neurosci.* (2015) 9:294. doi: 10.3389/fncel.2015.00294

16. Frasch MG, Burns P, Benito J, Cortes M, Cao M, Fecteau G, et al. Sculpting the sculptors: methods for studying the fetal cholinergic signaling on systems and cellular scales. *Methods Mol Biol.* (2018) 1781:341–52. doi: 10.1007/978-1-4939-7828-1_18

17. Patro R, Duggal G, Kingsford C. Salmon: accurate, versatile and ultrafast quantification from rna-seq data using lightweight-alignment. *bioRxiv.* (2015) 021592. doi: 10.1101/021592

18. Soneson C, Love MI, Robinson MD. Differential analyses for RNA-seq: transcript-level estimates improve gene-level inferences. *F1000Res.* (2015) 4:1521. doi: 10.12688/f1000research.7563.2

19. Smyth GK. Linear models and empirical bayes methods for assessing differential expression in microarray experiments. *Stat Appl Genet Mol Biol.* (2004) 3:Article3. doi: 10.2202/1544-6115.1027

20. Wang P, Xu T-Y, Guan Y-F, Tian W-W, Viollet B, Rui Y-C, et al. Nicotinamide phosphoribosyltransferase protects against ischemic stroke through SIRT1-dependent adenosine monophosphate-activated kinase pathway. *Ann Neurol.* (2011) 69:360–74. doi: 10.1002/ana.22236

21. Li D, Liu N, Zhao H-H, Zhang X, Kawano H, Liu L, et al. Interactions between Sirt1 and MAPKs regulate astrocyte activation induced by brain injury *in vitro* and *in vivo*. *J Neuroinflamm.* (2017) 14:67. doi: 10.1186/s12974-017-0841-6

22. Frasch MG. Putative role of AMPK in fetal adaptive brain shut-down: linking metabolism and inflammation in the brain. *Front Neurol.* (2014) 5:150. doi: 10.3389/fneur.2014.00150

23. Tyzack GE, Hall CE, Sibley CR, Cymes T, Forostyak S, Carlino G, et al. A neuroprotective astrocyte state is induced by neuronal signal EphB1 but fails in ALS models. *Nat Commun.* (2017) 8:1164. doi: 10.1038/s41467-017-01283-z

24. Deak T, Kudinova A, Lovelock DF, Gibb BE, Hennessy MB. A multispecies approach for understanding neuroimmune mechanisms of stress. *Dialogues Clin Neurosci.* (2017) 19:37–53. Available online at: https://www.dialogues-cns.org/contents-19-1/dialoguesclinneurosci-19-37/

25. Diz-Chaves Y, Astiz M, Bellini MJ, Garcia-Segura LM. Prenatal stress increases the expression of proinflammatory cytokines and exacerbates the inflammatory response to LPS in the hippocampal formation of adult male mice. *Brain Behav Immun.* (2013) 28:196–206. doi: 10.1016/j.bbi.2012.11.013

26. Bronson SL, Bale TL. Prenatal stress-induced increases in placental inflammation and offspring hyperactivity are male-specific and ameliorated by maternal antiinflammatory treatment. *Endocrinology.* (2014) 155:2635–46. doi: 10.1210/en.2014-1040

27. Wu S, Gennings C, Wright RJ, Wilson A, Burris HH, Just AC, et al. Prenatal stress, methylation in inflammation-related genes, and adiposity measures in early childhood: the programming research in obesity, growth environment and social stress cohort study. *Psychosom Med.* (2018) 80:34–41. doi: 10.1097/PSY.0000000000000517

28. Shapiro GD, Fraser WD, Frasch MG, Séguin JR. Psychosocial stress in pregnancy and preterm birth: associations and mechanisms. *J Perinat Med.* (2013) 41:631–645. doi: 10.1515/jpm-2012-0295

29. Christian LM, Franco A, Glaser R, Iams JD. Depressive symptoms are associated with elevated serum proinflammatory cytokines among pregnant women. *Brain Behav Immun.* (2009) 23:750–4. doi: 10.1016/j.bbi.2009.02.012

30. El-Ansary A, Al-Ayadhi L. Neuroinflammation in autism spectrum disorders. *J Neuroinflamm.* (2012) 9:265. doi: 10.1186/1742-2094-9-265

31. Kinney DK, Munir KM, Crowley DJ, Miller AM. Prenatal stress and risk for autism. *Neurosci Biobehav Rev.* (2008) 32:1519–32. doi: 10.1016/j.neubiorev.2008.06.004

32. Barros VG, Duhalde-Vega M, Caltana L, Brusco A, Antonelli MC. Astrocyte-neuron vulnerability to prenatal stress in the adult rat brain. *J Neurosci Res.* (2006) 83:787–800. doi: 10.1002/jnr.20758

33. Barros VG, Berger MA, Martijena ID, Sarchi MI, Perez AA, Molina VA, et al. Early adoption modifies the effects of prenatal stress on dopamine and glutamate receptors in adult rat brain. *J Neurosci Res.* (2004) 76:488–96. doi: 10.1002/jnr.20119

34. Pace TWW, Miller AH. Cytokines and glucocorticoid receptor signaling. Relevance to major depression. *Ann N Y Acad Sci.* (2009) 1179:86–105. doi: 10.1111/j.1749-6632.2009.04984.x

35. Schmidt PJ. Regulation of iron metabolism by hepcidin under conditions of inflammation. *J Biol Chem.* (2015) 290:18975–83. doi: 10.1074/jbc.R115.650150

36. Jauregui-Huerta F, Ruvalcaba-Delgadillo Y, Gonzalez-Castañeda R, Garcia-Estrada J, Gonzalez-Perez O, Luquin S. Responses of glial cells to stress and glucocorticoids. *Curr Immunol Rev.* (2010) 6:195–204. doi: 10.2174/157339510791823790

37. Autry AE, Grillo CA, Piroli GG, Rothstein JD, McEwen BS, Reagan LP. Glucocorticoid regulation of GLT-1 glutamate transporter isoform expression in the rat hippocampus. *Neuroendocrinology.* (2006) 83:371–9. doi: 10.1159/000096092

38. Reagan LP, Rosell DR, Wood GE, Spedding M, Muñoz C, Rothstein J, et al. Chronic restraint stress up-regulates GLT-1 mRNA and protein expression in the rat hippocampus: reversal by tianeptine. *Proc Natl Acad Sci USA.* (2004) 101:2179–2184. doi: 10.1073/pnas.0307294101

39. Zschocke J, Bayatti N, Clement AM, Witan H, Figiel M, Engele J, Behl C. Differential promotion of glutamate transporter expression and function by glucocorticoids in astrocytes from various brain regions. *J Biol Chem.* (2005) 280:34924–32. doi: 10.1074/jbc.M502581200

40. Srinivasan D, Yen J-H, Joseph DJ, Friedman W. Cell Type-Specific Interleukin-1β Signaling in the CNS. *J Neurosci.* (2004) 24:6482–8. doi: 10.1523/JNEUROSCI.5712-03.2004

41. Morrison JL, Berry MJ, Botting KJ, Darby JRT, Frasch MG, Gatford KL, et al. Improving pregnancy outcomes in humans through studies in sheep. *Am J Physiol Regul Integr Comp Physiol.* (2018) 315:R1123–53. doi: 10.1152/ajpregu.00391.2017

42. Wessler I, Kirkpatrick CJ, Racké K. The cholinergic "pitfall": acetylcholine, a universal cell molecule in biological systems, including humans. *Clin Exp Pharmacol Physiol.* (1999) 26:198–205.

43. Wessler I, Reinheimer T, Klapproth H, Schneider FJ, Racké K, Hammer R. Mammalian glial cells in culture synthesize acetylcholine. *Naunyn Schmiedebergs Arch Pharmacol.* (1997) 356:694–7.

44. Ghazalpour A, Bennett B, Petyuk VA, Orozco L, Hagopian R, Mungrue IN, et al. Comparative analysis of proteome and transcriptome variation in mouse. *PLoS Genet.* (2011) 7:e1001393. doi: 10.1371/journal.pgen.1001393

45. Rothhammer V, Borucki DM, Tjon EC, Takenaka MC, Chao C-C, Ardura-Fabregat A, et al. Microglial control of astrocytes in response to microbial metabolites. *Nature.* (2018) 557:724–8. doi: 10.1038/s41586-018-0119-x

46. Farrokhi CB, Tovote P, Blanchard RJ, Blanchard DC, Litvin Y, Spiess J. Cortagine: behavioral and autonomic function of the selective CRF receptor subtype 1 agonist. *CNS Drug Rev.* (2007) 13:423–43. doi: 10.1111/j.1527-3458.2007.00027.x

47. Baier CJ, Pallares ME, Adrover E, Monteleone MC, Brocco MA, Barrantes FJ, et al. Prenatal restraint stress decreases the expression of alpha-7 nicotinic receptor in the brain of adult rat offspring. *Stress.* (2015) 18:435–45. doi: 10.3109/10253890.2015.1022148

48. Adrover E, Pallarés ME, Baier CJ, Monteleone MC, Giuliani FA, Waagepetersen HS, et al. Glutamate neurotransmission is affected in prenatally stressed offspring. *Neurochem Int.* (2015) 88:73–87. doi: 10.1016/j.neuint.2015.05.005

49. Cumberland AL, Palliser HK, Rani P, Walker DW, Hirst JJ. Effects of combined IUGR and prenatal stress on the development of the hippocampus in a fetal guinea pig model. *J Dev Orig Health Dis.* (2017) 8:584–96. doi: 10.1017/s2040174417000307

Real World Lab Data: Patterns of Lymphocyte Counts in Fingolimod Treated Patients

Maxi Kaufmann, Rocco Haase, Undine Proschmann, Tjalf Ziemssen*† and Katja Akgün†

MS Center, Center of Clinical Neuroscience, University Hospital Carl Gustav Carus, University of Technology Dresden, Dresden, Germany

*Correspondence:
Tjalf Ziemssen
tjalf.ziemssen@uniklinikum-dresden.de

†These authors share senior authorship

Objective: Fingolimod is approved for the treatment of highly active relapsing remitting multiple sclerosis (MS) patients and acts by its unique mechanism of action via sphingosine-1-phosphate receptor-modulation. Although fingolimod-associated lymphopenia is a well-known phenomenon, the exact cause for the intra- and inter-individual differences of the fluctuation of lymphocyte count and its subtypes is still subject of debate. In this analysis, we aim to estimate the significance of the individual variation of distinct lymphocyte subsets for differences in absolute lymphocyte decrease in fingolimod treated patients and discuss how different lymphocyte subset patterns are related to clinical presentation in a long-term real life setting.

Methods/Design: One hundred and thirteen patients with MS were characterized by complete blood cell count and immune cell phentopying of peripheral lymphocyte subsets before, at month 1 and every 3 months up to 36 months of fingolimod treatment. In addition, patients were monitored regarding clinical parameters (relapses, disability, MRI).

Results: There was no significant association of baseline lymphocyte count and lymphocyte subtypes with lymphocyte decrease after fingolimod start. The initial drop of the absolute lymphocyte count could not predict the level of lymphocyte count during steady state on fingolimod. Variable CD8+ T cell and NK cell counts account for the remarkable intra- and inter-individual differences regarding initial drop and steady state level of lymphocyte count during fingolimod treatment, whereas CD4+ T cells and B cells mostly present a quite uniform decrease in all treated patients. Selected patients with lymphocyte count >1.0 GPT/l differed by higher CD8+ T cells and NK cell counts compared to lymphopenic patients but presented comparable clinical effectiveness during treatment.

Conclusion: Monitoring of the absolute lymphocyte count at steady state seems to be a rough estimate of fingolimod induced lymphocyte redistribution. Our results suggest, that evaluation of distinct lymphocyte subsets as CD4+ T cells allow a more detailed evaluation to weigh and interpret degree of lymphopenia and treatment response in fingolimod treated patients.

Keywords: fingolimod, lymphopenia, lymphocyte subsets, real world lab data, monitoring

INTRODUCTION

Multiple sclerosis (MS) is a chronic inflammatory disease of the central nervous system (CNS) initiated and perpetuated by an imbalance in the immune-regulatory network. Different MS specific treatment regimens are available and aim to govern autoimmunity and CNS inflammation (1). For some years cellular anti-migratory strategies have been used to control cell migration and accumulation in the CNS (2). Fingolimod acts as sphingosine-1-phosphate (S1P) receptor modulator that inhibits S1P-mediated lymphocyte egress from lymph nodes impairing peripheral lymphocyte recirculation (3–5). This unique mechanism of action results in reduction of absolute lymphocyte counts including specific subsets as naïve T cells, central memory T and B cells but also pro-inflammatory Th1 and Th17 cell subsets in the peripheral and central compartment (3, 6–9). Natalizumab is a further effective therapy for MS patients also known by its anti-migratory mechanism of action. Compared to fingolimod, natalizumab is effective by the block of the α4-subunit of the very late antigen-4 that impairs transmigration of immune cells across the blood-brain barrier into the CNS. Although immune cell subsets are rapidly decreased in the CNS compartment as well, natalizumab lead to significant lymphocyte increase and distinct changes in CD4/CD8 ratio in peripheral blood of treated patients (10, 11). In contrast to other MS treatment regimens e.g., dimethylfumarate therapy even low levels of absolute lymphocyte count up to 0.2 GPT/l can be tolerated during fingolimod treatment (12–16). Other disease managing regimens e.g., in cancer treatment use scoring systems as the National Cancer Institute Common Terminology Criteria for Adverse Events (NCI-CTAE) for grading degree and severity of adverse events including lymphopenia to define risk of infectious complications (17). Interestingly, even though there is a potential increased risk for severe and opportunistic infections due to persistent decrease of CD4+ T cells, only herpes reactivation and infection is relevantly increased in fingolimod treatment (18). Although the peripheral decreased lymphocyte count is a well-known phenomenon for clinicians who are experienced with fingolimod, the exact details of the intra- and inter-individual differences regarding drop and fluctuation of lymphocyte count as well of its subtypes is still a subject of debate (19–22). Up to now, it is not clear which factors can lead to higher vs. lower lymphocyte counts during fingolimod treatment and whether distinct lymphocyte count patterns can assist to select patients that are at higher risk for infections or non-responsiveness to fingolimod treatment (20, 21, 23).

Real-world evidence (RWE) and observational studies are becoming increasingly popular because they provide longitudinal information on usefulness of drugs in real life and have the ability to discover uncommon or rare adverse drug reactions inclusive lab abnormalities (24, 25). Following this approach of real world lab data, here we aim to estimate the significance of the individual variation of distinct lymphocyte subsets for differences in absolute lymphocyte count decrease in fingolimod treated patients and discuss how different lymphocyte subset patterns are related to clinical presentation.

METHODS
Patients

In our observational real world cohort, we included 113 RRMS patients that were treated in our MS center in Dresden (65 females/48 males) with highly active disease course (**Supplementary Table 1**). After critical review of all relevant clinical and imaging parameters and available treatment options, fingolimod treatment was initiated at a dose of 0.5 mg fingolimod daily. Before fingolimod start, 80.5% of patients were pre-treated with different DMTs (**Supplementary Table 1**). During a standardized treatment switch procedure, injectables were stopped 2 weeks before fingolimod start, natalizumab was stopped 12 weeks before fingolimod start and other DMTs at least 6 months before fingolimod start. Blood samples were collected before (baseline), at month 1 and every 3 months up to 36 months of fingolimod treatment. Additionally patients were monitored regarding clinical parameters including infections, relapse activity, confirmed disability progression measured by EDSS (≥1.0 point increase if EDSS baseline score was <4.0; ≥0.5 point increase if EDSS baseline score was ≥4.0) and BMI three-monthly and MRI progression every year assessed by an examined neuro-radiologist. MRI progression was defined in case of appearance of new gadolinium enhancing lesions or new T2 lesions in cerebral MRI scan. No serious adverse events appeared in our cohort. Data have been collected from the MSDS3D database. The study was approved by the institutional review board of the University Hospital of Dresden. Patients gave their written informed consent.

Routine Blood Analysis

Standardized blood testing was performed for routine blood parameters at the Institute of Clinical Chemistry and Laboratory Medicine, University Hospital in Dresden, Germany. The institute complies with standards required by DIN-EN-ISO-15189:2014 for medical laboratories. Whole blood samples were collected in ethylene diamine tetra acetic acid (EDTA). Routine blood testing included complete blood cell count.

Immune Cell Phenotyping by Fluorescence-Activated Cell Sorting (FACS)

Whole blood samples were collected in EDTA. After collection blood samples were incubated with fluorescence labeled monoclonal antibodies including anti-CD3, anti-CD4, anti-CD8, anti-CD16, anti-CD19, anti-CD56 (BD Biosciences, Heidelberg, Germany) to define T cell, B cell, and natural killer (NK) cell subpopulations. Afterwards, red blood cells were lysed using BD FACS Lysing Solution (BD Bioscience). After washing with FACS

Abbreviations: BMI, Body Mass Index; CNS, central nervous system; CRP, C-reactive protein; DMT, disease modifying drug; gamma-GT, EDSS, Expanded Disability Status Scale; EDTA, ethylene diamine tetra acetic acid; GLMM, Generalized Linear Mixed Model; MRI, magnet resonance imaging; MS, multiples sclerosis; NCI-CTAE, National Cancer Institute Common Terminology Criteria for Adverse Events; NK cells, natural killer cells; RR, relapsing remitting; RWD, real-world data; RWE, real-world evidence; S1P, sphingosine-1-phosphate.

buffer (phosphate buffered saline, 0.2% fetal bovine serum, 0.02% sodium azide, all Biochrom) cells were evaluated on FACSCanto II flow cytometer.

Evaluations and Definition of the Groups

Different approaches were chosen to discuss our study objectives: (1) the whole cohort was examined to evaluate mean changes in peripheral immune cell subsets on group level. Ten patients out of our cohort presented lymphocyte count >1.0 GPT/L after fingolimod start. In addition, matched groups of patients with lymphocyte count 0.5–1.0 GPT/l and ≤0.5 GPT/l were defined and used for further considerations. Additionally intra-individual variability of lymphocytes and its subsets was evaluated in these subgroups. Intra-individual variability was calculated as the standard deviation of absolute cell counts measured every 3 months between month 1 to month 36 of fingolimod therapy in each patient (2). The impact of initial absolute lymphocyte drop was assessed. Median-split was done for the initial absolute drop of lymphocyte count at 1.40 GPT/l and the whole cohort was divided into a high vs. low lymphocyte drop group (3). For the third approach the relevance of high vs. low steady state lymphopenia during fingolimod treatment was assessed. Median-split for lymphocyte count was calculated for the steady state period

after month 6 at 0.48GPT/l and a lower steady state group vs. a higher steady state group was selected out of the whole cohort.

Scoring and grading of the level of lymphopenia was performed using the system of the National Cancer Institute Common Terminology Criteria for Adverse Events (NCI-CTAE). Characterization of levels of lymphopenia using NCI-CTAE grading was defined by lymphopenia grade 1: > 0.8 GPt/L, lymphopenia grade 2: 0.5-0.8 GPt/L, lymphopenia grade 3: 0.2-0.5 GPt/L, and lymphopenia grade 4: < 0.2 GPt/L.

Statistical Analysis

Data were analyzed applying Generalized Linear Mixed Models (GLMM) with Gamma distribution and log link function for evaluations with immune cell populations with skewed distribution. Absolute lymphocyte counts and lymphocyte steady state were skewed distributed and though groups of interest were defined using medians-split to define groups of same and comparable sample size. Although lymphocyte count drop was normal distributed medians-split was applied as well to use comparable methodology. Differences in patient characteristics were defined using Analysis of Variances (ANOVA), Kruskal-Wallis H test, Person's chi-square test or Fischer exact test, and an alpha error level of 5%. Correlation was calculated using

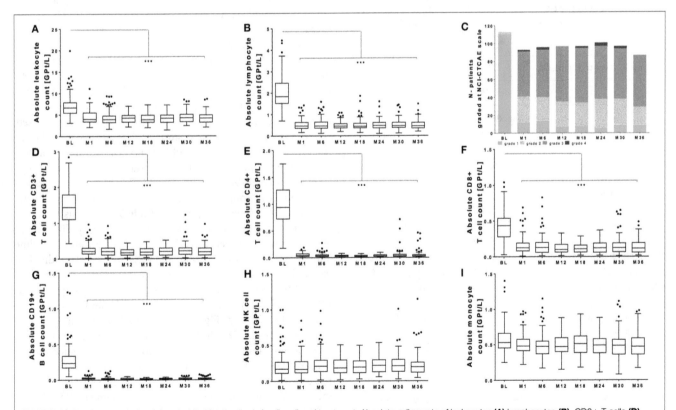

FIGURE 1 | Absolute count of peripheral white blood cells during fingolimod treatment. Absolute cell counts of leukocytes **(A)** lymphocytes **(B)**, CD3+ T cells **(D)**, CD4+ T cells **(E)**, CD8+ T cells **(F)**, CD19+ B cells **(G)** and NK cells **(H)**, and monocytes **(I)** are depicted. Data for the whole cohort are shown as Boxplot Tukey before fingolimod start (baseline, BL), month 1 and every 6 months follow up. **(C)** Distribution of different ranges of lymphocyte count are shown graded with NCI-CTCAE: lymphopenia grade 1 >0.8 GPt/L (green), lymphopenia grade 2 0.5-0.8 GPt/L (yellow), lymphopenia grade 3 0.2-0.5 GPt/L (orange) and lymphopenia grade 4 < 0.2 GPt/L (red). Asterisks indicate level of significance of pairwise comparison (***p < 0.001).

Spearman's correlation. In order to control for the familywise error rate of the multiple GLMM analyses, comparable alpha error rates were adjusted via Bonferroni correction as α/k were k is the number of analyses per parameter. Therefore, values of $p < 0.0125$ (0.05/4) were considered significant.

RESULTS

Lymphocyte Decrease and Its Relevance in Lymphocyte Variation During Fingolimod Treatment

All patients of our observational cohort demonstrated the well-known drop of absolute lymphocyte count after fingolimod initiation. There was a significant drop of leukocyte count and lymphocyte count (**Figures 1A,B**). Evaluating grading by NCI-CTAE demonstrated that most of the patients presented lymphopenia grade 2 or 3 after fingolimod start (**Figure 1C**). NCI-CTAE grade 4 was reached only at single time points in selected patients. None of the patients stopped fingolimod treatment due to lymphopenia during the observation period as retest revealed grade 3 lymphopenia. Monocytes and NK cells changed only mildly (**Figures 1H,I**), whereas the most intense decrease was seen on T and B cell subtypes (**Figures 1D–G**).

Within our cohort, 10 of 113 patients presented with lymphocyte counts ≥ 1.0 GPT/L. This specific high lymphocyte group (HL) was compared with a matched (sex, age) fingolimod

TABLE 1 | Patient characteristics.

	HL	ML	LL
Age (yr ± SD)	36.6 (9.9)	39.2 (8.6)	39.0 (8.1)
Duration since MS diagnosis (yr ± SD)	4.8 (2.1)	3.6 (4.0)	5.0 (3.6)
Sex (f/m)	3/7	3/7	3/7
Previous DMT use before fingolimod start [no. (%)]	10 (100)	7 (70)	7 (70)
Interferon beta	–	4 (40)	3 (26)
Glatirameracetat	8 (80)	3 (26)	3 (26)
Natalizumab	1 (10)	–	1 (10)
Others	1 (10)	–	–
None previous DMT use [no. (%)]	–	3 (26)	3 (26)
BMI at BL (± SD)	23.8 (2.5)	27.1 (4.0)	25.9 (4.8)
EDSS at BL (± SD)	2.4 (1.0)	2.0 (0.6)	3.6 (1.6)
Relapses during fingolimod (no.)	0	0	0
Confirmed EDSS progression during fingolimod (no.)	0	0	1
MRI progression during fingolimod (no.)	4	2	3
Adverse events—infections (no.)	23	14	15

Baseline characteristics of evaluated patients are depicted. HL (high lymphocyte group) includes patients with lymphocyte count ≥ 1.0 GPT/L after fingolimod start. ML (median lymphocyte group) with lymphocyte count of 0.5–1.0 GPT/l and LL (low lymphocyte group) with lymphocyte count ≤ 0.5 GPT/l. DMT, disease modifying treatment. Other previous treatments included: Laquinimod. Number of relapses, confirmed EDSS progression, MRI progression and infectious events during fingolimod treatment period are presented. Yr, year; SD, standard deviation; f, female; m, male; BL, baseline; no, number.

treated patient group with lymphocyte counts of 0.5-1.0 GPT/l (median lymphocyte group, ML) respective ≤ 0.5 GPT/l (low lymphocyte group, LL) (**Table 1**). Although characterized by varying levels in lymphocyte decrease, the patients did not differ regard clinical parameters including relapse activity, confirmed EDSS progression and MRI progression or occurrence of reported infectious events between all three groups (**Table 1**). Distribution of previous DMT use was different in all three groups with a higher proportion of interferon-beta use (30–40%) in the ML and LL group whereas glatiramer acetate was used more frequent in the HL group before fingolimod start (**Table 1**). At baseline, there was a trend to a higher absolute count of leukocytes and lymphocytes in HL group compared to ML and LL group. Nevertheless, this trend was not statistical significant (**Figures 2A,B**). After fingolimod start, all lymphocyte counts significantly decreased (**Table 2**). The HL group presented with the highest lymphocyte count at month 1. Thereafter, lymphocyte count decreased further on but was still higher and different compared to lymphocyte counts of ML and LL group (**Figure 2B, Table 2**). Additionally, intra-individual variability was evaluated in all three groups: there was a wide intra-individual variation in lymphocyte count in HL group after month 1 (**Figure 2G**). After the initial drop, ML group and LL group presented with quiet stable levels of lymphocyte count over the whole observation period (**Figure 2B**). Intra-individual variation of lymphocyte count presented at a smaller range compared to HL group (**Figure 2G**).

Lymphocyte subpopulations have been analyzed in all three groups: there were no significant differences at baseline between the three groups for CD4+ T cells and CD19+ B cells (**Figures 3C,E**). In contrast, highest CD8+ T cell and NK cell count was seen in HL group before fingolimod start (**Figures 2D,F**). After fingolimod start, T and B cell subsets significantly dropped in all groups (**Figures 2C–E, Table 2**). Interestingly, CD4+ T cells and CD19 B cells dropped similarly and did not differ even at steady state in all three groups (**Figures 2C,E, Table 2**), while CD8+ T cells were constantly higher in HL group compared to ML and LL group during fingolimod treatment (**Figure 2D, Table 2**). NK cells were not affected by fingolimod treatment but significantly different in absolute count between the HL, ML, and LL group at baseline and follow up (**Figure 2F, Table 2**). Evaluation of intra-individual variability of lymphocyte subtypes demonstrated high variability in CD8+ T cells and NK cells especially in HL group whereas ML and LL group presented comparable and lower intra-individual variability (**Figure 2G**). CD4+ T cells and CD19+ B cells were characterized by low variability reflecting constant and stable levels within observation period in all investigated groups (**Figure 2G**). Additional correlation analyses demonstrated that there was a comparable CD4+ T cell decrease irrespective of the lymphocyte count ($r = 0.2849$, n.s.; **Figure 2H**) whereas CD8+ T cell decrease was strongly correlated with lymphocyte decrease in our patients ($r = 0.5998$, $p < 0.001$; **Figure 2I**). These data indicate that variability and occasionally high levels of absolute lymphocyte count are primarily caused by the wide individual variation in CD8+ T cell count, while CD4+ T

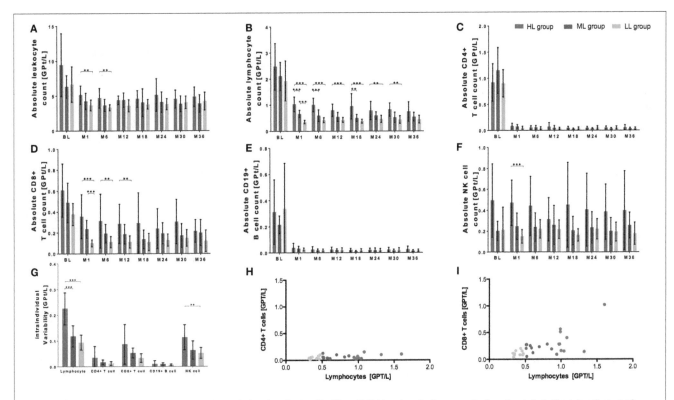

FIGURE 2 | Cell count of selective immune cell subpopulations in cohorts with different initial lymphocyte decrease after fingolimod start. Absolute cell count of leukocytes **(A)**, lymphocytes **(B)**, CD4+ T cells **(C)**, CD8+ T cells **(D)**, CD19+ B cells **(E)**, and NK cells **(F)** are depicted. Three groups of patients during fingolimod treatments are compared: HL group (high lymphocyte count 1 ≥ 1.0 GPt/L, red) ML group (medium lymphocyte count 0.5–1.0 GPt/L, blue) and LL group (low lymphocyte count ≤ 0.5 GPt/L, green). BL, month 1 and 6 months interval of evaluation up to 36 months of fingolimod therapy are depicted. **(G)** Intra-individual variability of lymphocytes, CD4+ T cells and CD8+ T cells, CD19+ B cells and NK cells compared between HL group, ML group and LL group are presented. Intra-individual variability was declared as the standard deviation of absolute cell counts between month 1 to month 36 of fingolimod therapy. Mean ± SD are depicted. Asterisks indicate level of significance of pairwise comparison. (**p < 0.01 and ***p < 0.001) **(H,I)** Correlation of decrease of CD4+ T cells resp. CD8+ T cells and lymphocytes are presented. Mean of absolute lymphocyte count, CD4+ T cell count and CD8+ T cell count between month 1, month 3, and month 6 after fingolimod start were calculated and depicted. Level of statistical significance was evaluated using Spearman's correlation. **(H)** r = 0.2849, n.s. **(I)** r = 0.5998, p < 0.001.

cells are more robust and less variable to evaluate fingolimod treatment effects.

Initial Drop of Lymphocyte Count Does Not Predict Long-Term Level of Lymphocyte Count

Lymphocyte decrease dependent on individual lymphocyte drop during fingolimod treatment is frequently discussed. Initial drop of lymphocyte count was individually calculated using lymphocyte count at baseline vs. steady state after 6 months for each patient. Median-split was performed for the initial absolute drop of lymphocyte count resulting at 1.40 GPT/l. A lower absolute drop group (LAD group; < 1.40 GPT/l) and a higher absolute drop group (HAD group; ≥ 1.40 GPT/l) were defined. Both groups were not significantly different in age, sex, disease duration, BMI, or EDSS at baseline (**Table 2**). In the HAD there was a significant higher number of patients that were pretreated with natalizumab (21.1% in the HAD vs. 3.6% in the LAD group, p < 0.01).

At baseline, absolute lymphocyte count was significantly higher in the HAD group (**Figure 3A**, **Table 2**). Highest

baseline lymphocyte counts were seen in previously natalizumab treated patients (treatment stopped 12 weeks before fingolimod initiation), whereas lymphocyte counts in patients with other DMT use or none previous treatments were at comparable range. By definition, the HAD group demonstrated significant higher absolute as well as relative lymphocyte drop compared to LAD group (**Table 3**, p < 0.001). Highest drop was found in patients with previous natalizumab treatment (mean absolute drop 2.52 GPT/l ± SD 1.00 GPT/l). During long-term observation, lymphocyte counts were significantly reduced to comparable levels in the LAD group vs. HAD group (**Figure 3A**, **Table 3**). There was no significant correlation between absolute lymphocyte drop and absolute lymphocyte count at steady state (r = −0.041, p = 0.668). Additional characterization of levels of lymphopenia using NCI-CTAE grading demonstrated that there was a similar distribution of grades of lymphopenia between the LAD group and HAD group threw the whole observation period (**Figures 3H,I**). There was no association between type of previous DMT use and grade of lymphopenia during fingolimod therapy. Independent of degree of lymphocyte drop, disease activity parameters including relapse activity, disability progression and MRI progression were comparable in both groups (**Table 3**).

TABLE 2 | Level of significance for comparing the groups—global effects.

HL/ML/LL group	Group-effect	Time-effect	Time-by-group interaction	HAD/LAD group	Group-effect	Time-effect	Time-by-group interaction	HSS/LSS group	Group-effect	Time-effect	Time-by-group interaction
Leukocyte	$p < 0.001$	$p < 0.001$	$p = 0.747$	Leukocyte	$p < 0.001$	$p < 0.001$	$p = 0.566$	Leukocyte	$p < 0.001$	$p < 0.001$	$p = 0.845$
Lymphocyte	$p < 0.001$	$p < 0.001$	$p = 0.008$	Lymphocyte	$p = 0.120$	$p < 0.001$	$p < 0.001$	Lymphocyte	$p < 0.001$	$p < 0.001$	$p < 0.001$
CD3+ T cell	$p < 0.001$	$p < 0.001$	$p = 0.040$	CD3+ T cell	$p = 0.236$	$p < 0.001$	$p < 0.001$	CD3+ T cell	$p < 0.001$	$p < 0.001$	$p < 0.001$
CD4+ T cell	$p = 0.048$	$p < 0.001$	$p = 0.264$	CD4+ T cell	$p = 0.381$	$p < 0.001$	$p < 0.001$	CD4+ T cell	$p < 0.001$	$p < 0.001$	$p = 0.013$
CD8+ T cell	$p < 0.001$	$p < 0.001$	$p = 0.450$	CD8+ T cell	$p = 0.383$	$p < 0.001$	$p < 0.001$	CD8+ T cell	$p < 0.001$	$p < 0.001$	$p = 0.073$
CD19+ B cell	$p = 0.017$	$p < 0.001$	$p = 0.957$	CD19+ B cell	$p < 0.001$	$p < 0.001$	$p = 0.004$	CD19+ B cell	$p = 0.043$	$p < 0.001$	$p = 0.877$
Monocyte	$p < 0.001$	$p = 0.558$	$p = 0.926$	Monocyte	$p = 0.002$	$p = 0.005$	$p = 0.592$	Monocyte	$p < 0.001$	$p = 0.003$	$p = 0.869$
NK cell	$p < 0.001$	$p = 0.981$	$p = 0.855$	NK cell	$p = 0.220$	$p = 0.955$	$p = 0.165$	NK cell	$p < 0.001$	$p = 0.811$	$p = 0.995$

Values of $p < 0.0125$ were considered significant.

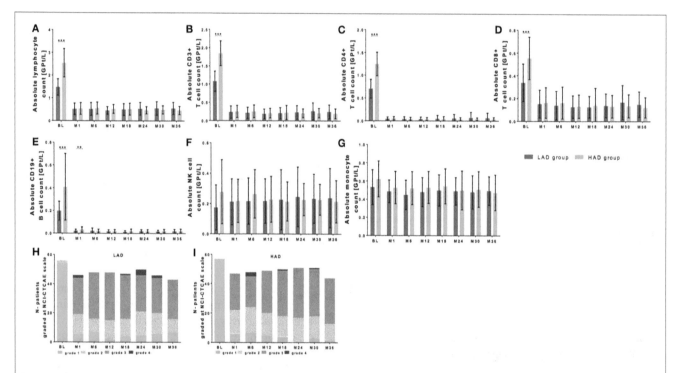

FIGURE 3 | Cell count of selective immune cell subpopulations in patients with high (HAD) vs. low absolute lymphocyte (HAD) drop. Absolute cell counts of lymphocytes **(A)**, CD3+ T cells **(B)**, CD4+ T cells **(C)**, CD8+ T cells **(D)**, CD19+ B cells **(E)**, NK-cells **(F)** and monocytes **(G)** are depicted. Comparison between two groups is presented: LAD group is defined as lower absolute lymphocyte drop group (< 1.40 GPT/l, red) and HAD group defined as higher lymphocyte drop group (≥ 1.40 GPT/l, green) after median-split. Data are shown before fingolimod start (baseline, BL), month 1 and every 6 months follow up. Mean ± SD are depicted. **(H,I)** Distribution of different ranges of lymphocyte count are shown graded with NCI-CTCAE: lymphopenia grade 1 >0.8 GPt/L (green), lymphopenia grade 2 0.5-0.8 GPt/L (yellow), lymphopenia grade 3 0.2-0.5 GPt/L (orange) and lymphopenia grade 4 < 0.2 GPt/L (red). Results are presented for LAD group **(H)** and HAD group **(I)** threw an observation period of 36 months. Asterisks indicate level of significance of pairwise comparison (**p < 0.01 and ***p < 0.001).

Furthermore, no significant differences in BMI or occurrence of acute infections in the LAD vs. HAD group could be confirmed.

Evaluation of lymphocyte subtypes demonstrated that T and B cells presented with significantly higher absolute cell counts at baseline in the HAD group (**Figures 3B–E, Table 3**). After significant drop, T and B cells were at comparable levels in both groups during fingolimod treatment (**Figures 3B–E, Table 3**). There were no differences in absolute NK cell at baseline and after

treatment initiation between HAD and LAD group (**Figure 3F, Table 3**). In monocytes only mild changes were found during fingolimod treatment in both groups (**Figure 3G, Table 3**).

Lymphocyte Subtypes Differ in Patients With High-Level vs. Low-Level Steady State Lymphopenia

It is known that lymphocyte count and changes of its subpopulations reach at latest their steady state 6 months after fingolimod start. Median-split was calculated for the steady state period after month 6 (lymphocyte count of 0.48GPT/l). A lower steady state group (LSS group; < 0.48 GPT/l) and a higher steady state group (HSS group; ≥ 0.48 GPT/l) was defined. There were no significant differences in age, disease duration, previous DMT use, EDSS or BMI at baseline (**Table 3**). In the LSS group a significant higher number of women (LSS group 70.3% vs. HSS group 45.7%) could be identified ($p < 0.05$).

Baseline lymphocyte levels demonstrated only a trend to higher baseline lymphocyte counts in the HSS group that were significantly decreased to different levels of lymphocyte steady state in both groups (**Figure 4A**, **Table 2**). As well after fingolimod start, the absolute lymphocyte drop was not different between LSS group and HSS group in reference to baseline levels; a higher significant relative lymphocyte drop ($p < 0.001$) could be shown for LSS group (**Table 4**). Grading with NCI-CTAE scale demonstrated that LSS group included single patients that presented with lymphocyte counts at grade 2 already before fingolimod start (**Figure 4H**). All of these patients were pretreated with interferon-beta treatment that was stopped two weeks before fingolimod start. During follow up, almost all patients in the LSS group presented with lymphocyte counts lower than grade 2 and up to grade 4 (**Figure 4H**). None of these patients stopped fingolimod treatment due to lymphopenia during the observation period as retest revealed grade 3 lymphopenia. HSS group included only patients with lymphocyte levels in the reference range before fingolimod start and none of the patients presented lymphocyte levels lower than grade 3 during follow up (**Figure 4I**). There was no association between type of previous DMT use and grade of lymphopenia during fingolimod therapy. Patients that presented lymphocyte counts at lower NCI-CTAE grade were not at risk for increased occurrence of infections compared to patients with higher lymphocyte count grade (**Table 4**). We could not find any differences in BMI between the LSS group and HSS group. There were no significant differences in clinical progression or MRI activity over the 36 months observation period in LSS vs. HSS patients (**Table 4**).

There were no significant differences regarding baseline levels of all analyzed T and B cell subpopulations between LSS group and HSS group (**Figures 4B–E**). After fingolimod start, CD4+ T cells and CD19+ B cells significantly decreased to comparable levels, whereas CD8+ T cells were significantly higher in the HSS group vs. LSS group (**Figures 4C–E, Table 2**). In addition, NK cells presented with higher counts at baseline and during treatment period in HSS patients (**Figure 4F, Table 2**). Interestingly, monocytes were higher at baseline and follow up in the HSS compared to the LSS group (**Figure 4G, Table 2**).

DISCUSSION

Lymphopenia is an integral part of fingolimod therapy based on its unique mechanism of action (8). Already initial clinical trials reported a decrease of lymphocyte count about 70% and

TABLE 3 | Patient characteristics.

	LAD group	HAD group
N patients	56	57
Age (yr ± SD)	39.9 (9.6)	39.0 (10.1)
Duration since MS diagnosis (yr ± SD)	6.4 (5.6)	7.1 (6.1)
Sex (f/m)	28/28	37/20
Previous DMT use before fingolimod start [no. (%)]	43 (76.8)	48 (84.2)
Interferon beta	23 (41.1)	22 (38.6)
Glatirameracetat	14 (25.0)	13 (22.8)
Natalizumab	2 (3.6)	12 (21.1)
Others	4 (7.1)	1 (1.8)
None previous DMT use [no. (%)]	13 (23.2)	9 (15.8)
BMI—BL (± SD)	24.1 (4.0)	25.6 (5.1)
EDSS—BL (± SD)	3.0 (1.6)	2.7 (1.3)
Lymphocyte absolute drop [GPT/L] Mean (95% CI)	0.95 (0.87; 1.03)	2.04 (1.88; 2.20)
Lymphocyte relative drop [%] Mean (95% CI)	64.01 (60.80; 67.21)	79.65 (78.03; 81.26)
Lymphocyte steady state [GPT/L] Mean (95% CI)	0.52 (0.46; 0.57)	0.50 (0.46; 0.55)
Relapse during fingolimod (no.)	13	12
Confirmed EDSS progression during fingolimod (no.)	9	11
MR progression during fingolimod (no.)	18	17
Adverse events—infections (no.)	38	40

Patient characteristics of evaluated patients are depicted. LAD group (lower absolute drop group) includes patients with an absolute lymphocyte drop < 1.40 GPT/l. HAD includes patients with an absolute lymphocyte drop ≥ 1.40 GPT/l. DMT, disease modifying treatment. Other previous treatments included: Azathioprin (2), Laquinimod (3). Number of relapses, confirmed EDSS progression, MRI progression and infectious events during fingolimod treatment period are presented. Yr, year; SD, standard deviation; f, female; m, male; BL, baseline; no, number.

discussed wide inter-individual differences in lymphocyte drop and fluctuation of total lymphocyte count in treated patients (27–29) There are different hypotheses which try to interpret the variation in levels of lymphopenia in fingolimod treated patients (19, 23, 30). Previous reports already discussed no relevant relation between degree of lymphopenia and clinical efficacy as well as occurrence of side effects (21, 28). Up to date it is unclear whether and why patients appear with less or marked decrease in lymphocyte count after fingolimod start.

Real-world data provide longitudinal information on different outcomes including effects on lab parameters (24). Implementing lab data into a comprehensive real world data approach can complete the fundamental quest of real world evidence for individually improved treatment decisions and balanced therapeutic risk assessment. In our observation, we evaluated individual variation of lymphocytes and its subsets in a long-term real life setting. There was a wide range of baseline lymphocyte levels in our cohort. Differences in baseline lymphocyte count dependent on previous DMT use cannot be excluded based on restricted washout periods. In our evaluation, moderate lymphopenia at baseline was more frequent in interferon-beta treated patients whereas natalizumab pretreatment lead

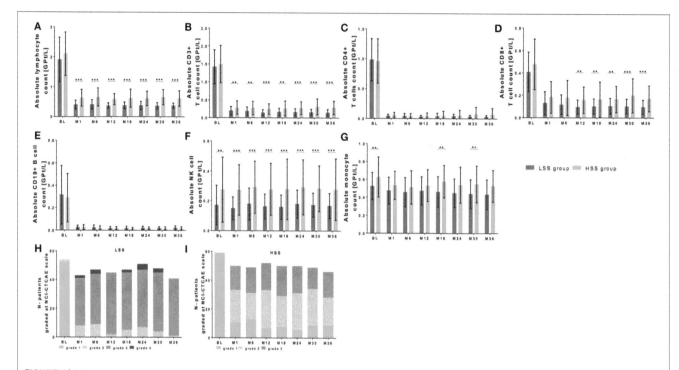

FIGURE 4 | Cell count of selective immune cell subpopulations in patients with high-level vs. low-level steady-state lymphopenia. Absolute cell counts of lymphocytes **(A)**, CD3+ T cells **(B)**, CD4+ T cells **(C)**, CD8+ T cells **(D)**, CD19+ B cells **(E)**, NK cells **(F)**, and monocytes **(G)** are depicted. Comparison between two groups is presented: LSS group defined as lower steady state group (< 0.48 GPT/l; red) and HSS group defined as higher steady state group (≥ 0.48 GPT/l; green) after median split. Data are shown before fingolimod start (baseline, BL), month 1 and every 6 month follow up. Mean ± SD are depicted. **(H,I)** Distribution of different ranges of lymphocyte count are shown graded with NCI-CTCAE: lymphopenia grade 1 >0,8 GPt/L (green), lymphopenia grade 2 0,5-0,8 GPt/L (yellow), lymphopenia grade 3 0,2-0,5 GPt/L (orange) and lymphopenia grade 4 < 0,2 GPt/L (red). Results are presented for LSS group **(H)** and HSS group **(I)** threw an observation period of 36 months. Asterisks indicate level of significance of pairwise comparison (**$p < 0.01$ and ***$p < 0.001$).

to higher levels at fingolimod start. Other reports discussed that higher baseline lymphocyte levels were associated with higher lymphocyte count threw follow up (20, 22). Furthermore, increased risk of fingolinod-associated lymphopenia in patients with interferon-beta pretreatment was suggested (20). In our cohort, we could not statistically prove that higher baseline levels or different pretreatment conditions were associated with the level of lymphocyte count or decrease at steady state during fingolimod therapy. Previous reports discussed an increased risk of lymphopenia in patients with BMI <18.5 kg/m^2 (20). Others presented data that could not confirm correlation between BMI and lymphopenia levels (22). In our observation, we could not define a significant relation between BMI and lymphocyte count, probably because only four patients presented persistent BMI levels <18.5 kg/m^2. Nevertheless, its lymphocyte count was reduced about 0.39–1.13 GPT/l at comparable range in contrast to other treated patients.

Interestingly, the absolute and relative lymphocyte drop after fingolimod start could not predict the level of lymphopenia in our cohort. Although marked differences in lymphocyte drop were present between patients, lymphocyte levels reached comparable levels independent of degree of lymphocyte drop. Most of the recent reports evaluating lymphopenia and its variation in fingolimod treated patients did not

analyze specific lymphocyte subtypes. Although absolute lymphocyte count differed in our patients, additional analysis of lymphocyte subtypes confirmed that CD4+ T cells and CD19+ B cells were decreased at a comparable level with narrow intra- and inter-individual variation in all fingolimod treated patients irrespective of the degree of lymphopenia.

In line with previous data, absolute NK cells count was not altered by fingolimod treatment in our cohort (26). NK cell recirculation is mediated by S1PR1 and S1PR5. It is suggested that S1PR5 is less susceptible to fingolimod than S1PR1, which is used by the other lymphocyte subtypes (31). These circulating NK cells maintain their functional capacity and contribute to the immunosurveillance by the innate immune system in fingolimod treated patients (32). In our study, patients with lower lymphocyte count during fingolimod treatment were associated with significant lower NK cell number. Intra-individual fluctuation of NK cell count was highest in patients with higher level of lymphocyte count compared to patients with lower level of lymphocyte count and did significantly differ compared to CD4+ T cells and CD19+ B cells. Main differences in absolute lymphocyte count were induced by variation in NK cell count.

Although initially supposed, degree of lymphopenia could not confirm a correlation with clinical treatment response (21).

TABLE 4 | Patient characteristics.

	LSS group	HSS group
N patients	54	59
Age (yr ± SD)	40.4 (10.0)	38.6 (9.6)
Duration since MS diagnosis (yr ± SD)	7.7 (6.0)	5.7 (5.6)
Sex (f/m)	38/16	27/32
Previous DMT use before fingolimod start [no. (%)]	45 (83.3)	46 (78.0)
Interferon beta	25 (46.3)	20 (33.9)
Glatirameracetat	10 (18.5)	17 (28.8)
Natalizumab	6 (11.1)	8 (13.6)
Others	4 (7.4)	1 (1.7)
None previous DMT use [no. (%)]	9 (16.7)	13 (22.0)
BMI—Baseline (± SD)	24.5 (4.6)	25.3 (4.7)
EDSS—Baseline (± SD)	3.0 (1.5)	2.7 (1.3)
Lymphocyte absolute drop [GPT/L] Mean (95% CI)	1.52 (1.32;1.73)	1.48 (1.29;1.66)
Lymphocyte relative drop [%] Mean (95% CI)	76.86 (74.05;79.68)	67.35 (64.16;70.54)
Lymphocyte steady state [GPT/L] Mean (95% CI)	0.38 (0.37;0.40)	0.63 (0.58;0.68)
Relapse during fingolimod (no.)	15	10
Confirmed EDSS progression during fingolimod (no.)	13	7
MR progression during fingolimod (no.)	15	20
Adverse events—infections (no.)	39	39

Patient characteristics of evaluated patients are depicted. LSS group (lower steady state group) includes patients with a lymphocyte count at steady state < 0.48 GPT/l. HSS group (higher steady state group) includes patients with a lymphocyte count at steady state ≥ 0.48 GPT/l. Number of relapses, confirmed EDSS progression, MRI progression and infectious events during fingolimod treatment period are presented. Yr, year; SD, standard deviation; f, female; m, male; BL, baseline; no, number.

Others discussed increased CD3+ and CD8+ T cell counts and decreased number of NK cells in first 6 months of fingolimod therapy as predictive marker for relapse activity (23). In our cohort, some patients presented with lymphocyte counts above 1.0 GPT/l. In these patients we could not confirm differences of clinical MS disease activity compared to patients with < 1.0 GPT/l or even < 0.5 GPT/l lymphopenia. Differences in lymphocyte count were caused by higher levels and of CD8+ T cell and NK cell count in higher lymphocyte cohort whereas CD4+ T cells and CD19+ B cells were markedly and comparable decreased in all three groups. Though, we suppose that decrease in CD4+ T cell count is associated with fingolimod efficacy and response rather than complete lymphocyte count.

During fingolimod treatment, the degree of lymphopenia and its clinical relevance defined by increased risk of infectious events is critically discussed (18, 30). Grading the level of lymphopenia using the NCI-CTAE is done especially for oncological diseases and treatment to define patients at higher risk for infections (17). Level of lymphopenia displayed in our cohort presented a wide range of distribution from grade 1 to grade 4 of the

NCT-CTAE scale. Nevertheless, we could not prove an increased incidence of infectious adverse events in the lower vs. higher-level lymphopenia group. These data are in line with several studies presenting primarily mild to moderate infections during fingolimod (8, 18, 28) The most relevant infectious complication in fingolimod treated patients is defined by varicella-zoster virus (VZV) and herpes simplex virus (HSV) infection or reactivation (8, 18, 33). However, individual variation of VZV specific T cell responses are assumed to be more relevant for upcoming VZV activation rather than absolute lymphocyte counts (34, 35). Up to date, we are not able to confirm that monitoring of absolute lymphocyte count or its subtypes can assist to predict higher infectious risk at lymphocyte counts of 0.2 GPT/l. Instead, cases of severe upcoming disease activity after fingolimod cessation because of lymphopenia (<0.2 GPT/l) are known (35, 36). Though, fingolimod interruption on the basis of lymphopenia of < 0.2 GPT/l has to be critically discussed in the individual context.

In summary, we demonstrate that CD4+ T cells and CD19+ B cells are comparably decreased in all fingolimod treated patients whereas grade of lymphopenia is primarily defined by individual variation of CD8+ T cell and NK cells. Monitoring of absolute lymphocyte drop and absolute lymphocyte count at steady state is only partially helpful as they do not cover distinct changes in the specific immune cell distribution. Our results suggest that monitoring of cellular target populations as CD4+ T cells seems to be more straight forward and probably clinically relevant to weigh and interpret the degree of immunological effects in fingolimod treated patients.

AUTHOR CONTRIBUTIONS

KA and TZ: Study concept and design; MK: Acquisition of data; MK, KA, RH, and UP: Analysis and interpretation of data; MK, KA, and TZ: Drafting of the manuscript; UP and RH: Critical revision of the manuscript for important intellectual content; MK, and RH: Statistical analysis.

ACKNOWLEDGEMENTS

We are grateful to Prof. Dr. T. Chavakis from the Institute of clinical chemistry and laboratory medicine, University clinic Dresden for performing the analysis and providing the data. We acknowledge support by the Open Access Publication Funds of the SLUB/TU Dresden.

REFERENCES

1. Ziemssen T, De Stefano N, Pia Sormani M, Van Wijmeersch B, Wiendl H, Kieseier BC. Optimizing therapy early in multiple sclerosis: an evidence-based view. *Mult Scler Relat Disord.* (2015) 4:460–9. doi: 10.1016/j.msard.2015.07.007

2. Wiendl H, Kieseier B. Multiple sclerosis: reprogramming the immune repertoire with alemtuzumab in MS. *Nat Rev Neurol.* (2013) 9:125–6. doi: 10.1038/nrneurol.2013.2

3. Brinkmann V, Davis MD, Heise CE, Albert R, Cottens S, Hof R, et al. The immune modulator FTY720 targets sphingosine 1-phosphate receptors. *J Biol Chem.* (2002) 277:21453–7. doi: 10.1074/jbc.C200176200

4. Brinkmann V, Cyster JG, Hla T. FTY720: sphingosine 1-phosphate receptor-1 in the control of lymphocyte egress and endothelial barrier function. *Am J Transplant* (2004) 4:1019–25. doi: 10.1111/j.1600-6143.2004.00476.x

5. Chun J, Hartung HP. Mechanism of action of oral fingolimod (FTY720) in multiple sclerosis. *Clin Neuropharmacol.* (2010) 33:91–101. doi: 10.1097/WNF.0b013e3181cbf825

6. Grutzke B, Hucke S, Gross CC, Herold MV, Posevitz-Fejfar A, Wildemann BT, et al. Fingolimod treatment promotes regulatory phenotype and function of B cells. *Ann Clin Transl Neurol.* (2015) 2:119–30. doi: 10.1002/acn3.155

7. Rudnicka J, Czerwiec M, Grywalska E, Siwicka-Gieroba D, Walankiewicz M, Grafka A, et al. Influence of fingolimod on basic lymphocyte subsets frequencies in the peripheral blood of multiple sclerosis patients - preliminary study. *Cent Eur J Immunol.* (2015) 40:354–9. doi: 10.5114/ceji.2015.54599

8. Thomas K, Proschmann U, Ziemssen T. Fingolimod hydrochloride for the treatment of relapsing remitting multiple sclerosis. *Expert Opin Pharmacother.* (2017) 18:1649–60. doi: 10.1080/14656566.2017.1373093

9. Thomas K, Sehr T, Proschmann U, Rodriguez-Leal FA, Haase R, Ziemssen T. Fingolimod additionally acts as immunomodulator focused on the innate immune system beyond its prominent effects on lymphocyte recirculation. *J Neuroinflammation* (2017) 14:41. doi: 10.1186/s12974-017-0817-6

10. Signoriello E, Lanzillo R, Brescia Morra V, Di Iorio G, Fratta M, Carotenuto A, et al. Lymphocytosis as a response biomarker of natalizumab therapeutic efficacy in multiple sclerosis. *Mult Scler.* (2016) 22:921–5. doi: 10.1177/1352458515604381

11. Carotenuto A, Scalia G, Ausiello F, Moccia M, Russo CV, Sacca F, et al. CD4/CD8 ratio during natalizumab treatment in multiple sclerosis patients. *J Neuroimmunol.* (2017) 309:47–50. doi: 10.1016/j.jneuroim.2017.05.006

12. Fox RJ, Miller DH, Phillips JT, Hutchinson M, Havrdova E, Kita M, et al. Placebo-controlled phase 3 study of oral BG-12 or glatiramer in multiple sclerosis. *N Engl J Med.* (2012) 367:1087–97. doi: 10.1056/NEJMoa1206328

13. Gold R, Kappos L, Arnold DL, Bar-Or A, Giovannoni G, Selmaj K, et al. Placebo-controlled phase 3 study of oral BG-12 for relapsing multiple sclerosis. *N Engl J Med.* (2012) 367:1098–107. doi: 10.1056/NEJMoa1114287

14. Thomas K, Ziemssen T. Management of fingolimod in clinical practice. *Clin Neurol Neurosurg.* (2013) 115(Suppl 1):S60–64. doi: 10.1016/j.clineuro.2013.09.023

15. Giovannoni G, De Jong B, Derfuss T, Izquierdo G, Mazibrada G, Molyneux P, et al. A pragmatic approach to dealing with fingolimod-related lymphopaenia in Europe. *Mult Scler Relat Disord.* (2015) 4:83–4. doi: 10.1016/j.msard.2014.09.215

16. Nakhaei-Nejad M, Barilla D, Lee CH, Blevins G, Giuliani F. Characterization of lymphopenia in patients with MS treated with dimethyl fumarate and fingolimod. *Neurol Neuroimmunol Neuroinflamm.* (2018) 5:e432. doi: 10.1212/NXI.0000000000000432

17. Trotti A, Colevas AD, Setser A, Rusch V, Jaques D, Budach V, et al. CTCAE v3.0: development of a comprehensive grading system for the adverse effects of cancer treatment. *Semin Radiat Oncol* (2003) 13:176–81. doi: 10.1016/S1053-4296(03)00031-6

18. Redelman-Sidi G, Michielin O, Cervera C, Ribi C, Aguado JM, Fernandez-Ruiz M, et al. ESCMID study group for infections in compromised hosts (ESGICH) consensus document on the safety of targeted and biological therapies: an infectious diseases perspective (Immune checkpoint inhibitors, cell adhesion inhibitors, sphingosine-1-phosphate receptor modulators and proteasome inhibitors). *Clin Microbiol Infect.* (2018) 24(Suppl 2):S95–107. doi: 10.1016/j.cmi.2018.01.030

19. Henault D, Galleguillos L, Moore C, Johnson T, Bar-Or A, Antel J. Basis for fluctuations in lymphocyte counts in fingolimod-treated patients with multiple sclerosis. *Neurology* (2013) 81:1768–72. doi: 10.1212/01.wnl.0000435564.92609.2c

20. Warnke C, Dehmel T, Ramanujam R, Holmen C, Nordin N, Wolfram K, et al. Initial lymphocyte count and low BMI may affect fingolimod-induced lymphopenia. *Neurology* (2014) 83:2153–7. doi: 10.1212/WNL.0000000000001049

21. Fragoso YD, Spelman T, Boz C, Alroughani R, Lugaresi A, Vucic S, et al. Lymphocyte count in peripheral blood is not associated with the level of clinical response to treatment with fingolimod. *Mult Scler Relat Disord.* (2018) 19:105–8. doi: 10.1016/j.msard.2017.11.018

22. Ohtani R, Mori M, Uchida T, Uzawa A, Masuda H, Liu J, et al. Risk factors for fingolimod-induced lymphopenia in multiple sclerosis. *Mult Scler J Exp Transl Clin.* (2018) 4:2055217318759692. doi: 10.1177/2055217318759692

23. Paolicelli D, Manni A, D'onghia M, Direnzo V, Iaffaldano P, Zoccolella S, et al. Lymphocyte subsets as biomarkers of therapeutic response in Fingolimod treated relapsing multiple sclerosis patients. *J Neuroimmunol.* (2017) 303:75–80. doi: 10.1016/j.jneuroim.2016.12.012

24. Ziemssen T, Hillert J, Butzkueven H. The importance of collecting structured clinical information on multiple sclerosis. *BMC Med.* (2016) 14:18. doi: 10.1186/s12916-016-0627-1

25. Haase R, Wunderlich M, Dillenseger A, Kern R, Akgun K, Ziemssen T. Improving multiple sclerosis management and collecting safety information in the real world: the MSDS3D software approach. *Expert Opinion on Drug Safety* (2018) 17:369–78. doi: 10.1080/14740338.2018.1437144

26. Vaessen LM, Van Besouw NM, Mol WM, Ijzermans JN, Weimar W. FTY720 treatment of kidney transplant patients: a differential effect on B cells, naive T cells, memory T cells and NK cells. *Transpl Immunol.* (2006) 15:281–8. doi: 10.1016/j.trim.2006.02.002

27. Kappos L, Radue EW, O'connor P, Polman C, Hohlfeld R, Calabresi P, et al. A placebo-controlled trial of oral fingolimod in relapsing multiple sclerosis. *N Engl J Med.* (2010) 362:387–401. doi: 10.1056/NEJMoa0909494

28. Kappos L, Cohen J, Collins W, De Vera A, Zhang-Auberson L, Ritter S, et al. Fingolimod in relapsing multiple sclerosis: An integrated analysis of safety findings. *Mult Scler Relat Disord.* (2014) 3:494–504. doi: 10.1016/j.msard.2014.03.002

29. Teniente-Serra A, Hervas JV, Quirant-Sanchez B, Mansilla MJ, Grau-Lopez L, Ramo-Tello C, et al. Baseline differences in minor lymphocyte subpopulations may predict response to fingolimod in relapsing-remitting multiple sclerosis patients. *CNS Neurosci Ther.* (2016) 22:584–92. doi: 10.1111/cns.12548

30. Francis G, Kappos L, O'connor P, Collins W, Tang D, Mercier F, et al. Temporal profile of lymphocyte counts and relationship with infections with fingolimod therapy. *Mult Scler.* (2014) 20:471–80. doi: 10.1177/1352458513500551

31. Gross CC, Schulte-Mecklenbeck A, Wiendl H, Marcenaro E, Kerlero De Rosbo N, Uccelli A, et al. Regulatory functions of natural killer cells in multiple sclerosis. *Front Immunol.* (2016) 7:606. doi: 10.3389/fimmu.2016.00606

32. Johnson TA, Evans BL, Durafourt BA, Blain M, Lapierre Y, Bar-Or A, et al. Reduction of the peripheral blood CD56(bright) NK lymphocyte subset in FTY720-treated multiple sclerosis patients. *J Immunol.* (2011) 187:570–9. doi: 10.4049/jimmunol.1003823

33. Quirant-Sanchez B, Hervas-Garcia JV, Teniente-Serra A, Brieva L, Moral-Torres E, Cano A, et al. Predicting therapeutic response to fingolimod treatment in multiple sclerosis patients. *CNS Neurosci Ther.* (2018) 24:1175–84. doi: 10.1111/cns.12851

34. Asanuma H, Sharp M, Maecker HT, Maino VC, Arvin AM. Frequencies of memory T cells specific for varicella-zoster virus, herpes simplex virus, and cytomegalovirus by intracellular detection of cytokine expression. *J Infect Dis.* (2000) 181:859–66. doi: 10.1086/315347

35. Avasarala J, Jain S, Urrea-Mendoza E. Approach to Fingolimod-induced lymphopenia in multiple sclerosis patients: do we have a roadmap? *J Clin Pharmacol.* (2017) 57:1415–8. doi: 10.1002/jcph.945

36. Hatcher SE, Waubant E, Nourbakhsh B, Crabtree-Hartman E, Graves JS. Rebound syndrome in patients with multiple sclerosis after cessation of fingolimod treatment. *JAMA Neurol.* (2016) 73:790–4. doi: 10.1001/jamaneurol.2016.0826

Permissions

List of Contributors

Gerard E. Dwyer, Alexander R. Craven, Marco Hirnstein and Kristiina Kompus
Department of Biological and Medical Psychology, University of Bergen, Bergen, Norway
NORMENT Centre of Excellence, Haukeland University Hospital, Bergen, Norway

Jörg Assmus
Centre for Clinical Research, Haukeland University Hospital, Bergen, Norway

Lars Ersland
Department of Biological and Medical Psychology, University of Bergen, Bergen, Norway
NORMENT Centre of Excellence, Haukeland University Hospital, Bergen, Norway
Department of Clinical Engineering, Haukeland University Hospital, Bergen, Norway

Kenneth Hugdahl
Department of Biological and Medical Psychology, University of Bergen, Bergen, Norway
NORMENT Centre of Excellence, Haukeland University Hospital, Bergen, Norway
Division of Psychiatry, Department of Clinical Medicine, Haukeland University Hospital, Bergen, Norway
Department of Radiology, Haukeland University Hospital, Bergen, Norway

Renate Grüner
Department of Radiology, Haukeland University Hospital, Bergen, Norway
Department of Physics and Technology, University of Bergen, Bergen, Norway

Maxi Kaufmann, Rocco Haase, Undine Proschmann, Tjalf Ziemssen and Katja Akgün
MS Center, Center of Clinical Neuroscience, University Hospital Carl Gustav Carus, University of Technology Dresden, Dresden, Germany

Florian Hatz, Antonia Meyer, Anne Roesch, Ute Gschwandtner and Peter Fuhr
Department of Neurology, Hospitals of University of Basel, Basel, Switzerland

Ethan Taub
Department of Neurosurgery, Hospitals of University of Basel, Basel, Switzerland

Daniela Parisi, Olimpia Musumeci, Rosaria Oteri, Annamaria Ciranni, Carmelo Rodolico, Giuseppe Vita and Antonio Toscano
Department of Clinical and Experimental Medicine, University of Messina, Messina, Italy

Stefania Mondello and Alba Migliorato
Department of Biomedical and Dental Sciences and Morphofunctional Imaging, University of Messina, Messina, Italy

Teresa Brizzi
Department of Clinical and Experimental Medicine, University of Messina, Messina, Italy
DIBIMIS University of Palermo, Palermo, Italy

Tiziana E. Mongini
Department of Neurosciences Rita Levi Montalcini, University of Turin, Turin, Italy

Benjamin Hotter, Sarah Hoffmann, Jochen B. Fiebach and Andreas Meisel
Charité – Universitätsmedizin Berlin, Corporate Member of Freie Universität Berlin, Berlin Institute of Health, Humboldt-Universität zu Berlin, Berlin, Germany
Center for Stroke Research Berlin, NeuroCure Clinical Research Center and Department of Neurology, Charité University Hospital Berlin, Berlin, Germany

Lena Ulm
Centre for Clinical Research, University of Queensland, Herston, QLD, Australia

Christian Meisel
Department of Medical Immunology, Charité University Medicine & Labor Berlin - Charité Vivantes, Berlin, Germany

Marc Pawlitzki
Department of Neurology, Otto-von-Guericke University, Magdeburg, Germany
Department of Neurology with Institute of Translational Neurology, University Hospital of Muenster, Münster, Germany

Catherine M. Sweeney-Reed, Daniel Bittner, Stefan Vielhaber, Stefanie Schreiber and Jens Neumann
Department of Neurology, Otto-von-Guericke University, Magdeburg, Germany

Anke Lux
Department for Biometrics and Medical Informatics, Otto-von-Guericke-University, Magdeburg, Germany

Friedemann Paul
Charité – Universitätsmedizin Berlin, Corporate Member of Freie Universität Berlin, Humboldt-Universität zu Berlin, and Berlin Institute of Health, NeuroCure Clinical Research Center, Berlin, Germany
Charité – Universitätsmedizin Berlin, Corporate Member of Freie Universität Berlin, Humboldt-Universität zu Berlin, and Berlin Institute of Health, Department of Neurology, Berlin, Germany
Experimental and Clinical Research Center, Max Delbrueck Center for Molecular Medicine and Charité – Universitätsmedizin Berlin, Corporate Member of Freie Universität Berlin, Humboldt-Universität zu Berlin, and Berlin Institute of Health, Berlin, Germany

Takao Yamasaki
Department of Clinical Neurophysiology, Neurological Institute, Graduate School of Medical Sciences, Kyushu University, Fukuoka, Japan
Department of Neurology, Minkodo Minohara Hospital, Fukuoka, Japan

Shozo Tobimatsu
Department of Clinical Neurophysiology, Neurological Institute, Graduate School of Medical Sciences, Kyushu University, Fukuoka, Japan

Julian Varghese, Iñaki Soto-Rey and Martin Dugas
Institute of Medical Informatics, University of Münster, Münster, Germany

Stephan Niewöhner
Department of Information Systems, University of Münster, Münster, Germany

Stephanie Schipmann-Miletić and Nils Warneke
Department of Neurosurgery, University Hospital Münster, Münster, Germany

Tobias Warnecke
Department of Neurology, University Hospital Münster, Münster, Germany

Fang Yao
Shenzhen Key Laboratory of Marine Biotechnology and Ecology, College of Life Science and Oceanography, Shenzhen University, Shenzhen, China
Key Laboratory of Optoelectronic Devices and Systems of Ministry of Education and Guangdong Province, College of Optoelectronic Engineering, Shenzhen University, Shenzhen, China

Kaoyuan Zhang, Yan Zhang, Shifeng Xiao, Qiong Liu, Liming Shen and Jiazuan Ni
Shenzhen Key Laboratory of Marine Biotechnology and Ecology, College of Life Science and Oceanography, Shenzhen University, Shenzhen, China

Yi Guo
Department of Neurology, Shenzhen People's Hospital, Shenzhen, China

Aidong Li
Department of Rehabilitation, The Eighth Affiliated Hospital of Sun Yat-sen University, Shenzhen, China

Peter Körtvelyessy
Department of Neurology, University Hospital Magdeburg, Magdeburg, Germany
German Center for Neurodegenerative Diseases Magdeburg, Magdeburg, Germany
Department of Neurology, Charité-Universitätsmedizin Berlin, Berlin, Germany
German Center for Neurodegenerative Diseases Berlin, Berlin, Germany

Harald Prüss
Department of Neurology, Charité-Universitätsmedizin Berlin, Berlin, Germany
German Center for Neurodegenerative Diseases Berlin, Berlin, Germany

Lorenz Thurner
José Carreras Center for Immuno- and Gene Therapy and Internal Medicine I, Saarland University Medical School, Homburg, Germany

Walter Maetzler
Department of Neurodegeneration, Hertie Institute for Clinical Brain Research (HIH), University of Tübingen, Tübingen, Germany
Department of Neurology, University Hospital Schleswig-Holstein, Christian-Albrechts-University, Kiel, Germany
German Center for Neurodegenerative Diseases Tübingen, Tübingen, Germany

Deborah Vittore-Welliong
Department of Neurology and Epileptology, Universitätsklinikum Tübingen, Universität Tübingen, Tübingen, Germany

Jörg Schultze-Amberger
Department of Neurology, Median Clinic Kladow, Kladow, Germany

Hans-Jochen Heinze
Department of Neurology, University Hospital Magdeburg, Magdeburg, Germany
German Center for Neurodegenerative Diseases Magdeburg, Magdeburg, Germany
Department of Behavioral Neurology, Leibniz Institute for Neurobiology, Magdeburg, Germany

Dirk Reinhold
Department of Immunohistopathology, Institute of Molecular and Clinical Immunology, Magdeburg, Germany

Frank Leypoldt
Department of Neurology, University Hospital Schleswig-Holstein, Kiel, Germany

Stephan Schreiber
Asklepios Department of Neurology, Brandenburg a.d. Havel, Germany

Daniel Bittner
Department of Neurology, University Hospital Magdeburg, Magdeburg, Germany
German Center for Neurodegenerative Diseases Magdeburg, Magdeburg, Germany

Christian Schlenstedt, Steffen Paschen, Jana Seuthe, Jan Raethjen and Günther Deuschl
Department of Neurology, University Hospital Schleswig-Holstein, Christian-Albrechts-University, Kiel, Germany

Yam Nath Paudel, Mohd. Farooq Shaikh, Yatinesh Kumari and Iekhsan Othman
Neuropharmacology Research Laboratory, Jeffrey Cheah School of Medicine and Health Sciences, Monash University Malaysia, Bandar Sunway, Malaysia

Ayanabha Chakraborti
Department of Surgery, University of Alabama at Birmingham, Birmingham, AL, United States

Ángel Aledo-Serrano
Department of Neurology, Epilepsy Program, Hospital Ruber Internacional, Madrid, Spain

Katina Aleksovska
Medical Faculty, Department of Neurology, "Saints Cyril and Methodius" University, Skopje, Macedonia

Marina Koutsodontis Machado Alvim
Department of Neurology, Neuroimaging Laboratory, State University of Campinas, Campinas, Brazil

Elsie Amedonu
Myocellular Electrophysiology and Molecular Biology, Institute for Genetics of Heart Diseases, University of Muenster, Muenster, Germany
Department of Neurology, University of Muenster, Muenster, Germany

Julian A. Schreiber, Sebastian Becker, Stefan Peischard, Nathalie Strutz-Seebohm and Guiscard Seebohm
Myocellular Electrophysiology and Molecular Biology, Institute for Genetics of Heart Diseases, University of Muenster, Muenster, Germany

Christine Strippel, Andre Dik, Heinz Wiendl, Sven G. Meuth and Nico Melzer
Department of Neurology, University of Muenster, Muenster, Germany

Christoph Brenker and Timo Strünker
Centre of Reproductive Medicine and Andrology, University of Muenster, Muenster, Germany

Sumanta Barman, Hans-Peter Hartung and Norbert Goebels
Department of Neurology, Universitätsklinikum and Center for Neurology and Neuropsychiatry LVR Klinikum, Heinrich Heine University Duesseldorf, Duesseldorf, Germany

Thomas Budde
Institute for Physiology I, University of Muenster, Muenster, Germany

Bernhard Wünsch
Institute for Pharmaceutical and Medical Chemistry, University of Muenster, Muenster, Germany

Boel De Paepe, Tea Šokčević and Jan L. De Bleecker
Department of Neurology and Neuromuscular Reference Center, Ghent University Hospital, Ghent, Belgium

Jana Zschüntzsch and Jens Schmidt
Department of Neurology, University Medical Center Göttingen, Göttingen, Germany

Joachim Weis
Institute for Neuropathology, Reinisch-Westfälische Technische Hochschule Aachen University Hospital, Aachen, Germany

Antoinette Depoorter and Peter Weber
Department of Neuropediatrics and Developmental Medicine, University Children's Hospital Basel, University of Basel, Basel, Switzerland

Roland P. Neumann and Sven Wellmann
Department of Neonatology, University Children's Hospital Basel, University of Basel, Basel, Switzerland

Christian Barro, Urs Fisch and Jens Kuhle
Neurologic Clinic and Policlinic, Departments of Medicine, Biomedicine and Clinical Research, University Hospital Basel, University of Basel, Basel, Switzerland

Katja Vohl, Alexander Duscha, Barbara Gisevius, Johannes Kaisler, Ralf Gold and Aiden Haghikia
Department of Neurology, Ruhr-University Bochum, St. Josef-Hospital, Bochum, Germany

Rezzak Yilmaz, Johanna Geritz, Clint Hansen and Sebastian Heinzel
Department of Neurology, Christian-Albrechts-University of Kiel, Kiel, Germany

Antonio P. Strafella
Institute of Medical Science, University of Toronto, Toronto, ON, Canada
Edmond J Safra Program in Parkinson's Disease and the Morton and Gloria Shulman Movement Disorders Clinic, University of Toronto, Toronto, ON, Canada
Division of Neurology, Department of Medicine, University of Toronto, Toronto, ON, Canada
Research Imaging Centre, Centre for Addiction and Mental Health, Toronto, ON, Canada
Division of Brain, Imaging and Behaviour-Systems Neuroscience, Toronto Western Research Institute, University Hospital Network, University of Toronto, Toronto, ON, Canada
Krembil Brain Institute, University Health Network, Toronto, ON, Canada

Alice Bernard
Department of Neurodegeneration, Hertie Institute for Clinical Brain Research, University of Tübingen, Tübingen, Germany

Claudia Schulte, Anja Apel and Thomas Gasser
Department of Neurodegeneration, Hertie Institute for Clinical Brain Research, University of Tübingen, Tübingen, Germany
German Center for Neurodegenerative Diseases (DZNE), Tübingen, Germany

Lieneke van den Heuvel and Connie Marras
Edmond J Safra Program in Parkinson's Disease and the Morton and Gloria Shulman Movement Disorders Clinic, University of Toronto, Toronto, ON, Canada
Division of Neurology, Department of Medicine, University of Toronto, Toronto, ON, Canada

Nicole Schneiderhan-Marra, Thomas Knorpp and Thomas O. Joos
Natural and Medical Sciences Institute (NMI) at the University of Tübingen, Reutlingen, Germany

Frank Leypoldt
Department of Neurology, Christian-Albrechts-University of Kiel, Kiel, Germany
Neuroimmunology, Institute of Clinical Chemistry, University Hospital Schleswig-Holstein, Kiel, Germany

Anthony E. Lang
Institute of Medical Science, University of Toronto, Toronto, ON, Canada
Edmond J Safra Program in Parkinson's Disease and the Morton and Gloria Shulman Movement Disorders Clinic, University of Toronto, Toronto, ON, Canada
Division of Neurology, Department of Medicine, University of Toronto, Toronto, ON, Canada
Krembil Brain Institute, University Health Network, Toronto, ON, Canada
Tanz Centre for Research in Neurodegenerative Diseases, University of Toronto, Toronto, ON, Canada

Daniela Berg
Department of Neurology, Christian-Albrechts-University of Kiel, Kiel, Germany
Department of Neurodegeneration, Hertie Institute for Clinical Brain Research, University of Tübingen, Tübingen, Germany
German Center for Neurodegenerative Diseases (DZNE), Tübingen, Germany

Daniel Richter, Siegfried Muhlack and Christos Krogias
Department of Neurology, St. Josef-Hospital, Ruhr University Bochum, Bochum, Germany

Dirk Woitalla
Department of Neurology, St. Josef-Hospital, Ruhr University Bochum, Bochum, Germany
Department of Neurology, Katholische Kliniken Ruhrhalbinsel, Essen, Germany

Ralf Gold and Lars Tönges
Department of Neurology, St. Josef-Hospital, Ruhr University Bochum, Bochum, Germany
Neurodegeneration Research, Protein Research Unit Ruhr (PURE), Ruhr University Bochum, Bochum, Germany

Tino Prell, Otto W. Witte and Julian Grosskreutz
Department of Neurology, Jena University Hospital, Jena, Germany
Center for Healthy Ageing, Jena University Hospital, Jena, Germany

Konstantin Huhn
Department of Neurology, Friedrich-Alexander-University of Erlangen-Nuremberg, Erlangen, Germany

Tobias Engelhorn
Department of Neuroradiology, Friedrich-Alexander-University of Erlangen-Nuremberg, Erlangen, Germany

Ralf A. Linker
Department of Neurology, University of Regensburg, Regensburg, Germany

Armin M. Nagel
Department of Radiology, Friedrich-Alexander-University of Erlangen-Nuremberg, Erlangen, Germany
Division of Medical Physics in Radiology, German Cancer Research Center (DKFZ), Heidelberg, Germany

Kathrin Doppler, Annahita Sedghi, Jens Volkmann and Claudia Sommer
Department of Neurology, University Hospital Würzburg, Würzburg, Germany

Kathrin Brockmann and Isabel Wurster
Department of Neurology, University Hospital Tübingen, Tubingen, Germany

Wolfgang H. Oertel
Department of Neurology, University Hospital Marburg, Marburg, Germany

Mingju Cao, Hai L. Liu and Lucien D. Durosier
Department of Obstetrics and Gynaecology and Department of Neurosciences, CHU Ste-Justine Research Centre, Faculty of Medicine, Université de Montréal, Montréal, QC, Canada

James W. MacDonald and Theo K. Bammler
Department of Environmental and Occupational Health Sciences, University of Washington, Seattle, WA, United States

Molly Weaver and Michael Dorschner
UW Medicine Center for Precision Diagnostics, University of Washington, Seattle, WA, United States

Marina Cortes
Animal Reproduction Research Centre (CRRA), Faculty of Veterinary Medicine, Université de Montréal, Montréal, QC, Canada

Patrick Burns, Gilles Fecteau and André Desrochers
Department of Clinical Sciences, Faculty of Veterinary Medicine, Université de Montréal, Montréal, QC, Canada

Jay Schulkin
Department of Obstetrics and Gynecology, University of Washington, Seattle, WA, United States

Marta C. Antonelli
Instituto de Biología Celular y Neurociencia "Prof. Eduardo De Robertis", Facultad de Medicina, Universidad de Buenos Aires, Buenos Aires, Argentina

Raphael A. Bernier
Department of Psychiatry and Behavioral Sciences, University of Washington, Seattle, WA, United States

Martin G. Frasch
Department of Obstetrics and Gynaecology and Department of Neurosciences, CHU Ste-Justine Research Centre, Faculty of Medicine, Université de Montréal, Montréal, QC, Canada
Animal Reproduction Research Centre (CRRA), Faculty of Veterinary Medicine, Université de Montréal, Montréal, QC, Canada
Department of Obstetrics and Gynecology, University of Washington, Seattle, WA, United States
Center on Human Development and Disability, University of Washington, Seattle, WA, United States

Tobias Ruck and Sven G. Meuth
Department of Neurology, University of Muenster, Muenster, Germany

Index